Genetic Disorders: Clinical Aspects

Genetic Disorders: Clinical Aspects

Edited by Luke Stanton

hayle medical

New York

Hayle Medical,
750 Third Avenue, 9th Floor,
New York, NY 10017, USA

Visit us on the World Wide Web at:
www.haylemedical.com

ISBN: 978-1-63241-498-4

The publisher's policy is to use permanent paper from mills that operate a sustainable forestry policy. Furthermore, the publisher ensures that the text paper and cover boards used have met acceptable environmental accreditation standards.

Printed in China.

Cataloging-in-Publication Data

Genetic disorders : clinical aspects / edited by Luke Stanton.
p. cm.
Includes bibliographical references and index.
ISBN 978-1-63241-498-4
1. Genetic disorders. 2. Medical genetics. I. Stanton, Luke.
RB155.5 .G46 2018
616.042--dc23

Table of Contents

Preface

The main aim of this book is to educate learners and enhance their research focus by presenting diverse topics covering this vast field. This is an advanced book which compiles significant studies by distinguished experts in the area of analysis. This book addresses successive solutions to the challenges arising in the area of application, along with it; the book provides scope for future developments.

The disorder caused by any abnormality found in an individual's genes is known as a genetic disorder. They are mostly hereditary or can also be caused by new mutations. Genetic disorders can be grouped into three types, single gene disorders, chromosome disorders and multifactorial disorders. With advanced research and technology, new approaches are being developed in treating genetic disorders. This book presents the complex subject of genetic disorders in the most comprehensible and easy to understand language.

It was a great honour to edit this book, though there were challenges, as it involved a lot of communication and networking between me and the editorial team. However, the end result was this all-inclusive book covering diverse themes in the field.

Finally, it is important to acknowledge the efforts of the contributors for their excellent chapters, through which a wide variety of issues have been addressed. I would also like to thank my colleagues for their valuable feedback during the making of this book.

Editor

Tumor Suppressor DYRK1A Effects on Proliferation and Chemoresistance of AML Cells by Downregulating c-Myc

Qiang Liu[1], Na Liu[2], Shaolei Zang[2], Heng Liu[1], Pin Wang[1], Chunyan Ji[2]*, Xiulian Sun[1]*

1 Key Lab of Otolaryngology, Qilu Hospital of Shandong University, Jinan, China, **2** Department of Hematology, Qilu Hospital of Shandong University, Jinan, China

Abstract

Acute myeloid leukemia (AML), caused by abnormal proliferation and accumulation of hematopoietic progenitor cells, is one of the most common malignancies in adults. We reported here DYRK1A expression level was reduced in the bone marrow of adult AML patients, comparing to normal controls. Overexpression of DYRK1A inhibited the proliferation of AML cell lines by increasing the proportion of cells undergoing G0/G1 phase. We reasoned that the proliferative inhibition was due to downregulation of c-Myc by DYRK1A, through mediating its degradation. Moreover, overexpression of c-Myc markedly reversed AML cell growth inhibition induced by DYRK1A. DYRK1A also had significantly lower expression in relapsed/refractory AML patients, comparing to newly-diagnosed AML patients, which indicated the role of DYRK1A in chemoresistance of AML. Our study provided functional evidences for DYRK1A as a potential tumor suppressor in AML.

Editor: Arun Rishi, Wayne State University, United States of America

Funding: This work was supported by National Natural Science Foundation of China Grant 81171030 (X. Sun), 81370662 (C. Ji), and 81000223 (S. Zang). The funders had no role in study design, data collection and analysis, decision to publish, or preparation of the manuscript.

Competing Interests: The authors have declared that no competing interests exist.

* E-mail: xiulians@gmail.com (XS); jichunyan@sdu.edu.cn (CJ)

Introduction

Acute myeloid leukemia (AML), caused by abnormal proliferation and accumulation of hematopoietic progenitor cells, is one of the most common malignancies in adults. The median age of AML patients at diagnosis is 69 [1]. Although improvement of AML treatment has been achieved during the last decades, but the five-year overall survival is still poor, especially in aged AML patients [1,2]. The pathogenesis of AML involves variety of molecular abnormalities, mainly including activation of oncogenes and dysfunction of tumor suppressor genes [3]. Exploring new molecular mechanisms of AML is necessary to develop revolutionary therapy strategies for AML patients.

Dual specificity tyrosine-phosphorylation-regulated kinase (DYRK), which is characterized by catalyzing autophosphorylation on tyrosine residue and phosphorylation of substrates strictly on serine/threonine residues, is an evolutionarily conserved kinase family belonging to CMGC family [4]. The DYRK family, including DYRK1A, DYRK1B, DYRK1C, DYRK2, DYRK3, DYRK4A, and DYRK4B, is involved in regulating neurogenesis and cellular processes such as differentiation, proliferation, and survival [5,6]. Recently, emerging studies have revealed their importance in development and progression of several malignancies. Taira et al. reported that DYRK2 directly phosphorylated p53 at Ser46 in osteosarcoma cells, resulting in apoptotic cell death in response to DNA damage [7]. Findings have shown that DYRK1A and DYRK2 inactivated NFATc by phosphorylation [8,9], which increased invasive ability of breast cancer cells and drug resistance of leukemia cells [10,11]. However, until recently, the functional role of DYRK1A in cancer is largely obscure. Interestingly, DYRK1A is localized within the Down Syndrome critical region (DSCR) on chromosome 21, and is considered to be a strong candidate gene for this genetic disorder [12,13]. Adult with Down syndrome (DS) have a markedly decreased risk of developing cancers compared with that without DS [14,15]. Although children with DS have a markedly increased risk of B cell precursor ALL, but T-ALL and non-megakaryoblastic myeloid leukemia are extremely rare in individuals without DS [15,16]. We recently reported that dysregulation of DYRK1A reduced RE1 silencing factor (REST) protein stability and transcriptional activity through ubiquitination and subsequent degradation of REST protein [17]. This strongly suggests that the DYRK1A has anti-tumor effects in adult.

We report here the identification of significant lower expression of DYRK1A in adult AML patients compared to their normal controls. Overexpression of DYRK1A, by increasing the proportion of cells in the G0/G1 phase, inhibited the proliferation of AML cells. We also found that DYRK1A phosphorylated c-Myc on Ser62, priming phosphorylation on Thr58 by GSK3β and subsequent degradation. c-Myc is a critical inducer of cellular proliferation, and its abnormal expression and activation are frequently observed in most human cancers [18,19]. Moreover, reduced AML cell growth induced by overexpression of DYRK1A was markedly reversed by c-Myc. DYRK1A also showed lower expression in relapsed/refractory patients compared to newly-diagnosed AML patents, which indicated the role of DYRK1A in drug sensitivity of AML cells. What's more, DYRK1A sensitized HL-60/ADM cell to doxorubicine. Our study contributes to reveal the molecular function of DYRK1A in pathological mechanism of AML.

Methods

Cell cultures and Reagents

Human myeloid leukemia cell line HEL, HL-60, NB4 and human embryonic kidney cell line HEK293 and HEK293T were purchased from the Cell Bank of the Chinese Academy of Medical Science (Shanghai, China). Human myeloid leukemia cell line HL-60/ADM were purchased from Chinese Academy of Medical Science and Peking Union Medical College(Tianjin, China). Human AML cell line HL-60, NB4, HEL, HL-60/ADM were grown in RPMI-1640 medium (Hyclone, South Logan, UT) supplemented with 10% FBS(Gibco, Gaithersburg, MD). HEK293 and HEK293T cells were cultured in high glucose Dulbecco's modified Eagle's medium (Hyclone, South Logan, UT) supplemented with 10% FBS. All cell lines were maintained at 37°C, 5% CO_2. Primary antibodies for DYRK1A, cyclin D1, $p21^{Waf1/Cip1}$ were purchased from CST (Beverly, MA), those for flag and β-actin were from Sigma-Aldrich (St Louis, MO), those for c-Myc was from Santa Cruz (Santa Cruz, CA), those for c-Myc pThr58 and pSer62 were from Immunoway (Newark, DE). All secondary antibodies were obtained from Jackson Immuno Research (West Grove, PA).

Clinical samples

Bone marrow samples of 55 initially diagnosed and 16 relapsed/refractory adult AML patients and 24 healthy donors were obtained after informed consent at the Qilu Hospital, Shandong University from May 2011 to December 2012. Mononuclear cells were prepared using Ficoll-Hypaque (Sigma–Aldrich, St Louis, MO), according to the manufacturer's protocol. All the study protocols involved with patients and healthy donors were approved by the Medical Ethics Committee of Qilu Hospital of Shandong University, Jinan, China, and written informed consents were obtained from all patients and healthy donors. The detailed clinical information of the 71 patients is presented in Table 1.

Plasmid construction and lentivirus packaging

Human *DYRK1A* cDNA was generated as described previously [17]. Human *c-Myc* CDS was amplified from NB4 cells by RT-PCR using the primer pair: 5′- GAAGATCTCTGGA TTTTTTTCGGGTAGTGG -3′ and 5′- CGGAATTCTTACG-CACAAGAGTTCCGTAG -3′. PCR products were cloned into eukaryotic expression vector pEGFP-C1. *DYRK1A* and *c-Myc* were subcloned into lentiviral vectors pWPXL. GV248-si-*c-Myc* lentiviral vectors were purchased from Genechem(Shanghai, China). 4×10^6 HEK293T cells were plated 1 day before transfection in 10 cm dish and 20 μg DNA were transfected per dish using the calcium phosphate precipitate method. The supernatant containing viral particles were collected at 48 and 72 hr after transfection, filtered through a 0.45 μm filter, concentrated by 100KD centrifugal filter(Millipore, Billerica, MA) and then stored at −80°C.

MTT assay

Cells (3×10^3) were seeded into 96-well culture plates. When measuring, cells were incubated with 10 μL MTT (5 mg/mL) at 37°C for 4 hrs, and then 100 μL 10% SDS(PH 4.0) was added to each well and incubated over night. The absorbance was measured at 570 nm. Each experiment was repeated at least three times.

Cell cycle analysis

Cells were harvested and washed twice in PBS, then fixed in 75% alcohol over night at 4°C. After washed in cold PBS thrice, cells were resuspended in 1 mL PBS with 40 μg PI and 100 μg RNase A (Sigma-Aldrich, St Louis, MO) and incubated for 30 min at 37°C. Samples were then analyzed by FACS(Beckman, CA).

Table 1. Characteristics of the 71 AML patients.

	No. of patients	
	Newly-diagnosed	**Relapsed/refractory**
No. of patients	55	16
Sex		
male	31	9
female	24	7
Age: median (range)	48 (16–77)	42.5 (17–61)
FAB Classification		
M0	2	0
M1	2	0
M2	6	5
M3	13	5
M4	15	4
M5	14	1
M6	3	1
Hemoglobin (g/l): median (range)	75 (33–136)	70.1 (48–135)
WBC (x109/l): median (range)	6.65 (1.18–169.5)	9.01 (0.88–146.1)
Neutrophils (%): median (range)	3.86 (0.09–129.9)	5.88 (0.16–122.71)

Abbreviations: FAB, French-American-British classification; WBC, white blood cells; PLT, platelets.

Apoptosis assay

The apoptosis assay was performed using the Annexin V-PE/7-AAD apoptosis detection kit(Ebioscience, San Diego, CA), according to the manufacturer's instructions. Fluorescence of at least 10,000 cells was collected by FACS(Beckman, CA). to determine the percentage of apoptotic cells.

Quantitative real-time RT-PCR

TRIzol reagent (Invitrogen, Carlsbad, CA) was applied to extract total RNA from cells or patient samples. Reverse transcription was performed using M-MLV reverse transcriptase cDNA Synthesis Kit(Takara, Japan). Real-time RT-PCR was carried out on ABI 7900HT Fast Real-Time PCR System(Foster City, CA) with SYBR-Green PCR Master Mix (Toyobo, Japan) as described previously[20]. Melting curves analysis and agarose gel electrophoresis were applied to guarantee the specificity of amplification. A comparative CT method ($2^{-\Delta\Delta CT}$) was used to analyze the gene expression level. *β-actin* or *GAPDH* were used as the internal control. The primers for real time quantitative were as follows: *DYRK1A*-F 5'-GCAATTTCCTGCTCCTCTTG-3'; *DYRK1A*-R 5'-TTACCCAAGGCTTGTTGTCC-3'; *c-Myc*-F 5'-TCAAGAGGTGCCACGTCTCC-3'; *c-Myc*-R, 5'-TCTTGG-CAGCAGGATAGTCCTT-3'; *cyclin D1*-F5'-GCTGCGAAG-TGGAAACCATC-3'; *cyclin D1*-R 5'-CCTCCTTCTGCACA-CATTTGAA-3'; $p21^{Waf1/Cip1}$-F 5'-TGTCCGTCAGAACCCAT-GC-3'; $p21^{Waf1/Cip1}$-R 5'-AAAGTCGAAGTTCCATCGCTC-3'; *CDK2*-F 5'-CCAGGAGTTACTTCTATGCCTGA-3'; *CDK2*-R 5'-TTCATCCAGGGGAGGTACAAC-3'; *β-actin*-F 5'-CACTG-TGTTGGCGTACAGGT-3'; *β-actin*-R 5'-TCATCACCATTG-GCAATGAG-3'; *GAPDH*-F 5'- TGTGGGCATCAATGGATT-TGG-3'; *GAPDH*-R 5'-ACACCATGTATTCCGGGTCAAT-3'.

Western Blot

For western blot analysis, cells were harvested and washed by ice-cold PBS and lysed by sonication in RIPA buffer (150 mM NaCl, 50 mM Tris-HCl, 1% Triton X-100, 2% SDS, and 1% sodium deoxycholate) containing protease inhibitor cocktail (Roche, Indianapolis, IN). Bio-Rad Dc protein assay kit (Bio-Rad, Richmond, CA) was used to measure the concentration of protein samples. Samples were denatured at 95°C with 4× SDS sample buffer for 5 min in metal bath and separated on 10% glycine SDS-PAGE gel. Membranes were blocked in 3% non-fat milk for 1 hous and incubated in primary antibodies with 1:1000 dilution (TBS with 0.1% Tween-20, 1% goat serum) overnight. After secondary antibody incubation, signals were detected and analyzed by the Li-Cor Odyssey imaging system.

CHX chase assay

c-Myc and DYRK1A or control vectors were co-transfected into HEK293 cells. 36 hrs after transfection, cells were treated with 50 μg/mL cycloheximide (Sigma-Aldrich, St Louis, MO) for 0, 1 and 2 hrs. Cells were then harvested and analyzed by western blot.

Co-immunoprecipitation

For co-immunoprecipitation, the cells were lysed in 1 mL 1% NP-40 lysis buffer(1% NP-40, 50 mM Tris-base, 150 mM NaCl). Cell lysates were gently shaken with 100 μL CL-4B (Sigma-Aldrich, St Louis, MO) at 4°C for 1 hr, then centrifuged at 15000 r/min 4°C for 15 min. The immunoprecipitation antibody recruited with 20 μL protein A/G (Santa Cruz Biotechnology, Santa Cruz, CA) were mixed with the supernatant and shaken at 4°C overnight. The protein-agarose beads mixture was washed once by 1% NP-40 lysis buffer and twice by ice-cold PBS, boiled with 4×SDS sample buffer, then analyzed on 10% glycine SDS-PAGE gel.

Data Analysis

All the experiments were repeated at least three times. For immunoblotting, one representative picture was shown, while quantifications were calculated from at least three independent experiments. The values represented means ± S.E. The data were evaluated for statistical significance by analysis of variance or Student's t test analysis. For patient samples, *DYRK1A* mRNA level was presented quantitatively as median. The differences in the newlydiagnosed, relapsed/refractory patients and normal controls were performed using a one-way ANOVA test. All statistical analysis were processed by SPSS 17.0 software.

Results

Aberrant expression profile of DYRK1A in adult AML patients

Relative *DYRK1A* mRNA levels of the newly diagnosed adult AML patients and healthy controls were measured by real-time RT-PCR. In spite of the wide range of individual values, median level of *DYRK1A* was significantly reduced in the AML patients compared with the normal controls (P = 0.004) (Figure 1). The attenuated level of *DYRK1A* was also observed in relapsed/refractory AML patients compared with untreated AML patients (p = 0.000) (Figure 1).

DYRK1A suppresses proliferation of AML cells by extending the G0/G1 phase

To observe the effects of DYRK1A on the growth of HEL, HL-60 and NB4 cells, cell proliferation assays were performed after infection with DYRK1A lentiviral particles or negative control for 72 hrs. RT-PCR and western blot assay showed that DYRK1A lentiviral particles could efficiently increase *DYRK1A* mRNA and protein levels in AML cells (Figure 2 A and B). As shown in Figure 2C, overexpression of DYRK1A led to consistently reduced

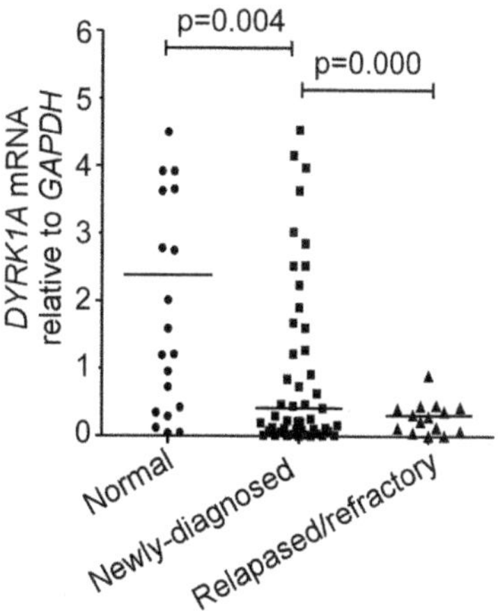

Figure 1. Real-time RT-PCR of *DYRK1A* mRNA level of in 55 newly diagnosed adult AML patients, 16 relapsed/refractory adult AML patients and 24 normal controls. *GAPDH* was used as internal control. Solid points indicate individual values and horizontal lines represent medians. The differences in copy number of each gene in the newly diagnosed, relapsed/refractory patients and normal controls were performed using a one-way ANOVA test.

cell growth compared with negative control in HEL, HL-60 and NB4 cells. We next questioned whether inhibited proliferation was induced through the arrest of cell cycle. As shown in Figure 2D, overexpression of DYRK1A significantly increased the ratio of cells in G0/G1 phase while concomitantly reduced the ratio of cells undergoing S phase, To exclude the influence of cell apoptosis, cells were stained with annexin V-PE/7-AAD and analyzed by flow cytometry. We did not find significant change of cell apoptosis between DYRK1A overexpression and control cells (data not shown). To further identified the genes that were responsible for the cell cycle arrest after DYRK1A overexpression, representative cell cycle regulators were studied. p21 was increased, while cyclin D1 and CDK2 were down-regulated by DYRK1A overexpression in AML cells (Figure 2E and F). These results provided evidences that DRYK1A suppressed proliferation of AML cells by extending the G0/G1 phase.

c-Myc expression is down-regulated by DYRK1A

c-Myc is a critical inducer of cellular proliferation, and its dysregulation is frequently observed in most human cancers. To determine whether DYRK1A can regulate c-Myc, we measured c-Myc protein and mRNA level in DYRK1A overexpressed AML cells. We found that c-Myc protein was downregulated by DYRK1A overexpression in HEL, HL-60 and NB4 cells (Figure 3A). Western blot quantification showed that c-Myc protein levels were markedly reduced by DYRK1A overexpression by 40.90±2.43%, 39.46±0.98% and 73.29±3.37% of controls in HEL, HL-60 and NB4 cells, respectively (P<0.01)(Figure 3B), while DYRK1A could not significantly change *c-Myc* mRNA level(Figure 3C), indicating that the reduction of c-Myc was due to post-translational regulation. To further investigate whether c-Myc reduction is due to decreased protein stability, HEK293 cells were co-transfected with c-Myc and DYRK1A or control and cycloheximide chase assay was performed to evaluate the degradation rate of c-Myc. Western blot clearly showed that the degradation of c-Myc protein was accelerated in the presence of DYRK1A overexpression (Figure 3D and E). Phosphorylation on Thr58 residue is necessary for binding between E3 ligase SCF^{Fbw7} and c-Myc, and subsequent ubiquitination and proteolysis [21]. Phosphorylation on c-Myc Thr58 is mainly catalyzed by GSK3β [21], which targets the first Serine or Threonine of the conserved sequence S/T PxxSP, primed by the phosphorylation of the second Serine. DYRK1A has been reported several times to act as a phosphorylation partner of GSK3β [9,22,23,24], which are aligned in Figure 3F. From Figure 3F we can see that c-Myc resembles a similar sequence from Thr58 to Ser62 with other GSK3β substrates. We speculate that DYRK1A phosphorylates on c-Myc Ser62, priming the phosphorylation of Thr58 by GSK3β and its degradation by ubiquitin-proteasome system. Three days after infection with lentiviral particles, HEL, HL-60 and NB4 cells were lysed for Western Blot. Our results showed overexpression of DYRK1A downregulated c-Myc protein level, consistent with our previous studies. Phosphorylation status of c-Myc Ser62 and Thr58 was significantly increased by DYRK1A overexpression (Figure 3G). To further assess whether there is a direct interaction between DYRK1A and c-Myc in mammalian cells, HEK293 cells were co-transfected with pCMV6-*DYRK1A* and pEGFP-c1 or pEGFP-C1-*c-Myc*. c-Myc was detected by anti-GFP antibody in co-immunoprecipitation assay pulling down with anti-flag antibody, indicating an direct interaction between DYRK1A and c-Myc (Figure 3H). These results strongly demonstrated that DYRK1A reduced c-Myc level via promoting its degradation.

DYRK1A suppresses proliferation of AML cells through downregulating c-Myc

To determine whether c-Myc affects proliferation of AML cells, we first silenced c-Myc (Figure 4A and B) and found significant reduction of *cyclin D1* mRNA level by 49.53±2.43% (p = 0.006), and marked elevation of *p21* mRNA level by 105.36±42.94% (p = 0.015), to negative controls, respectively (Figure 4C). Next, we confirmed whether cell growth inhibition induced by DYRK1A overexpression was reversed by upregulating c-Myc expression. We found reduced AML cells growth by overexpression of DYRK1A was markedly attenuated by expression of c-Myc (Figure 4D). This was further supported by changes of cell cycle markers. We found that overexpressing of c-Myc reversed the downregulation of cyclin D1 and upregulation of p21 caused by DYRK1A overexpression (Figure 4E and F). Our studies revealed DYRK1A suppressed AML cells proliferation through downregulation of c-Myc.

Upregulation of DYRK1A increases drug sensitivity of HL-60/ADM

As shown in Figure 1, the reduced level of *DYRK1A* was observed in relapsed/refractory AML patients compared with untreated AML patients, suggesting that DYRK1A could play an important role in chemoresistance of AML patients. We then investigated the effect of DYRK1A on drug sensitivity of HL-60/ADM, a multidrug resistant leukemia cell line. As shown in Figure 5A, DYRK1A sensitized HL-60/ADM cell to doxorubicine. IC50 values(drug concentration leads to 50% decrease of cell viability), is an intelligible indicator of drug sensitivity. IC50 value of HL-60/ADM cells transfected with DYRK1A was significantly lower than that of control group. The IC50 values of HL-60/ADM-DYRK1A and HL60/ADM control were 0.9389±0.063,2.3144±0.58299, respectively (P<0.01). Transfected or control HL-60/ADM cells were treated with 0.5 mg/L doxorubicin for 48 h. After labeled with Annexin V-PE/7-AAD, cells were analyzed by flow cytometry. HL-60/ADM cells overexpressing DYRK1A showed a higher percentage of apoptosis than control (Figure 5B). These results demonstrated that upregulation of DYRK1A promoted apoptosis induced by doxorubicin in HL-60/ADM.

Discussion

In this study, we found that DYRK1A mRNA level was reduced in newly-diagnosed adult AML patients comparing to normal controls and overexpression of DYRK1A markedly inhibited proliferation of in AML cell lines. What's more, DYRK1A has been recently reported to mediate inactivity of several oncogenic proteins including NFATc [8,9], cyclin D1 [25], and NOTCH [26]. These findings suggest the important role of DYRK1A as a tumor suppressor in adult AML.

Down syndrome (DS) associated neurogenesis defects are characterized by slowed proliferation of neural precursor cells. DYRK1A, as an important triggering protein in the pathogenesis of DS, was reported to impair G0/G1-S phase transition and alter neural precursor cell proliferation [27]. Litovchick et al. found DYRK1A inhibited various cells proliferation, including T98G brain glioblastoma cells, U-2 OS osteosarcoma cells and SW 1990 pancreatic adenocarcinoma cells [28]. Chen et al. reported DYRK1A increased G1 duration in BJ-5ta foreskin fibroblast cell line [25]. In our study, we found overexpression of DYRK1A inhibited the proliferation of AML cell lines by cell cycle arrest. Our results confirmed the previous study about the proliferation regulating functions of DYRK1A.

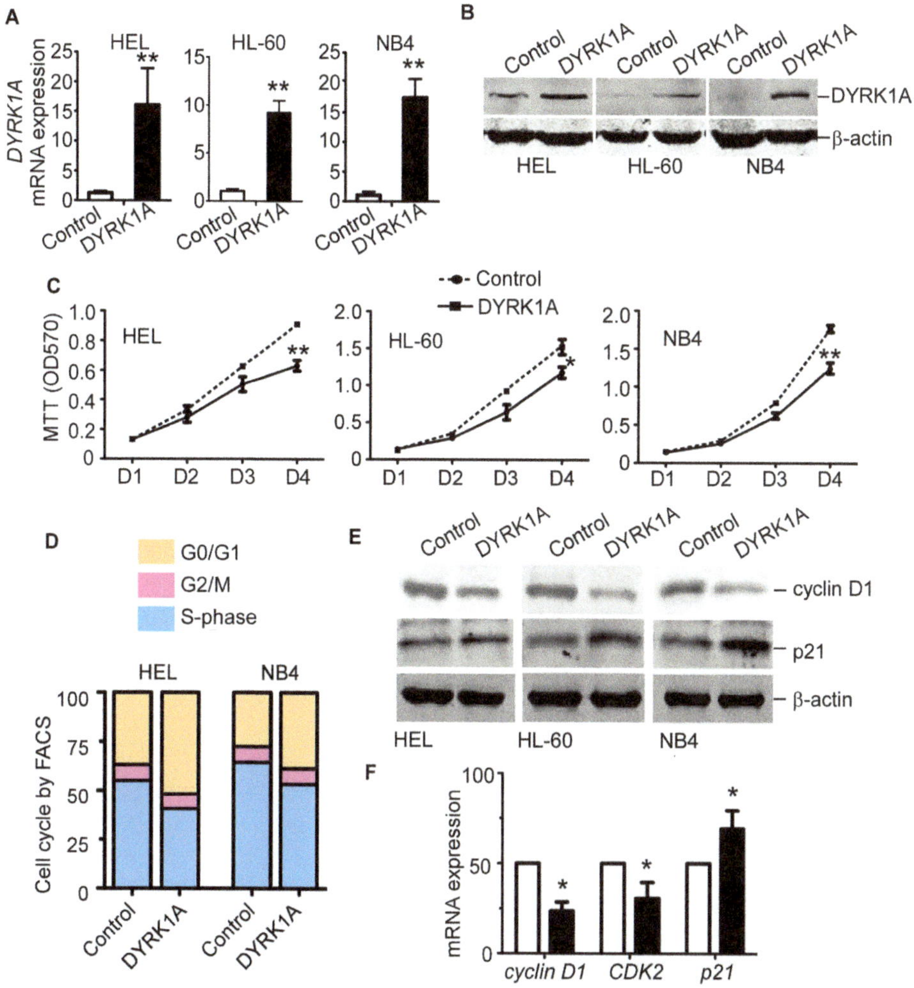

Figure 2. DYRK1A suppressed proliferation of AML cells by extending the G0/G1 phase. HEL, HL-60 and NB4 cells were infected with DYRK1A lentiviral particles(DYRK1A) or negative control (Control) for 72 hrs. (A) Real-time RT-PCR was performed to assess the increment of *DYRK1A* mRNA level. *DYRK1A* mRNA levels were normalized to *β-actin*. The results present the fold-increase relative to control. Data represents mean ± S.E. from three independent experiments. $^{**}P<0.01$, (B) Western Blot was used to detect the DYRK1A protein level increment. β-actin was used as loading control. Experiments were repeated three times, and one representative figure was shown, (C) After being infected with DYRK1A lentiviral particles for 72 hrs, HEL, HL-60 and NB4 cell proliferation were measured by MTT assay. The values represent the means ± S.E. (n = 3). $^{*}P<0.05$, $^{**}P<0.01$, (D) After being infected with DYRK1A lentiviral particles for 72 hrs, HEL and NB4 cells were stained with PI and analyzed for their DNA content using FACS Calibur. Results shown are representative of at least three independent experiments. (E) Western blot of cell cycle regulators cyclin D1, CDK2 and p21 in HEL, HL-60 and NB4 cells. β-actin was used as loading control. Results shown are representative of at least three independent experiments. (F) Real-time RT-PCR detected *cyclin D1*, *CDK2* and *p21* mRNA levels in HEL cells after being infected with DYRK1A lentiviral particles for 72 hrs. *β-actin* was used as control. The values represent the means ± S.E. (n = 3). $^{*}P<0.05$.

However, the mechanism of how DYRK1A regulates cell proliferation is still unclear. Litovchick et al. reported that DYRK1A specifically phosphorylated LIN52 on Ser28, which was required for DREAM complex assembly, repressing the expression of cell cycle-dependent genes during quiescence [28]. Chen et al. reported DYRK1A increased G1 duration via phosphorylation and subsequent degradation of cyclin D1 as well as stabilization of p21 [25]. In our study, we found that DYRK1A regulated cell cycle related genes, cyclin D1 and p21, at mRNA level, which prompted a new molecular mechanism.

The oncogene c-Myc plays an important role in tumorgenesis, e.g. lymphoma [29] and leukemia [30]. Over the past decades, however, a large body of research showed c-Myc activity were essential for cell cycle progression. Mateyak et al. reported c-Myc null cells ceased to proliferate and exited the cell cycle [31]. c-Myc played a central role in promoting G1 to S phase cell cycle transition. The possible mechanism was through regulating cyclins and CKIs [32]. Other studies reported similar results. Daksis et al. found the activation of c-Myc was sufficient to induce cyclin D1 mRNA as well as protein expression [33]. Seoane et al. reported c-Myc attenuated p21 expression by directly binding its promoter [34]. All these studies have proved that c-Myc acts as an upregulator of cyclin D1 and a repressor of p21 at transcription level, promoting G0/G1 to S phase transition. Here we found overexpression of DYRK1A downregulated c-Myc protein other than mRNA, indicating DYRK1A regulates c-Myc at post-transcription level. Moreover, DYRK1A had been reported to impact protein stability through phosphorylation, e.g. REST [17], RCAN1 [22] and CRY2 [24]. Here we confirmed when co-

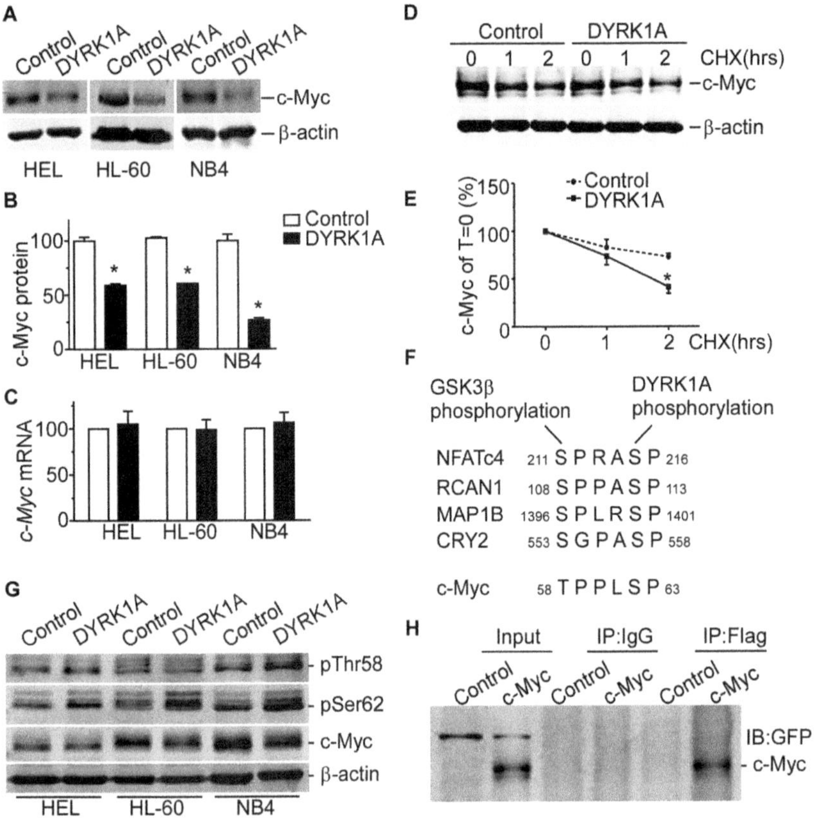

Figure 3. c-Myc expression is down-regulated by DYRK1A. (A and B) HEL, HL-60 and NB4 cells were infected with DYRK1A lentiviral particles or negative control for 72 hrs. Western blot showed that c-Myc were downregulated in AML cell lines, compared with negative control, respectively. β-actin was used as loading control. Results shown are representative of at least three independent experiments. The values represent the means ± S.E. (n = 3). *$P<0.05$. (C)HEL, HL-60 and NB4 cells were infected with DYRK1A lentiviral particles or negative control for 72 hrs. Real time RT-PCR showed the *c-Myc* mRNA levels in AML cell lines. The values represent the means ± S.E. (n = 3). *$P<0.05$. (D and E) HEK293 cells co-transfected with pEGFP-*c-Myc* vector and pCMV6 or pCMV6-*DYRK1A* were chased with 50 μg/mL cycloheximide(CHX) for 1 and 2 hrs. c-Myc expression was detected by anti-GFP antibody. β-actin was used as loading control. The values represent the means ± S.E.(n = 3). *$P<0.05$. (F) Sequence alignments around phosphorylation residues of GSK3β and DYRK1A substrates, as well as c-Myc. (G) HEL, HL-60 and NB4 cells were infected with DYRK1A lentiviral particles or negative control for 72 hrs. Cells were lysed for western blot. Anti-c-Myc, anti-c-Myc(pThr58), anti-c-Myc(pSer62) antibodies were applied for analysis.β-actin was used as loading control. (H) HEK293 cells co-transfected with pCMV6-*DYRK1A* and pEGFP-c1 or pEGFP-C1-*c-Myc* were lysed and immunoprecipitated with anti-flag antibody, anti-GFP antibody was used in immunoblotting.

expressed with DYRK1A in AML cells, c-Myc was accelerated for degradation when chased with cycloheximide. These studies suggest DYRK1A regulates cell cycle by influencing c-Myc degradation and subsequently cyclin D1 and p21.

We also observed downregulated *CDK2* mRNA induced by overexpression of DYRK1A, however, CDK2 is not a downstream target of c-Myc, indicating other mechanisms were involved in regulating *CDK2* mRNA level. *CDK2* mRNA expression is induced by MITF [35] and repressed by p53 and IRF1 [36]. MITF drives most of the melanocytic markers, and interestingly, *DYRK1A* mRNA is downregulated in melanoma cell lines [37]. DYRK1A phosphorylates p53 at Ser 15 and increases its transcriptional activity in H19-7 cells [27]. In Figure 2, we showed when DYRK1A was overexpressed in HEL cell, *CDK2* mRNA level was downregulated, which was consistent with these studies.

In Down Syndrome, DYRK1A overexpression is due to the extra copy of chromosome 21(or part of chromosome 21), which is known as gene dosage effect. But in most cases, *DYRK1A* gene dosage effect does not exist in pathological and physiological processes, whereas *DYRK1A* mRNA abundance differs strikingly in various tissues and time points of differentiation and proliferation. DYRK1A was found to be downregulated in melanoma [37], and overexpressed in the activation of T-cells [38]. In neural progenitor cells, *DYRK1A* expression was restricted to M-G1 phase [39]. These studies indicate that DYRK1A is tightly controlled at transcriptional level, however, the mechanisms are not clear. AP4 was reported to be strongly expressed in colorectal carcinomas [40] and repress the transcription of *DYRK1A* in coordinate with geminin [41]. E2F1 was shown to bind to the promoter of *DYRK1A* and activate its transcription [42], though E2F1 was reported to promote myeloid cell cycle progression and block granulocyte differentiation [43]. Youngkyun Lee et al. reported NFAFc1 regulated *DYRK1A* in a feedback loop [44]. Our study showed REST could directly bound to *DYRK1A* promoter, initiating the transcription [17], and previous research proved REST was an tumor suppressor in breast cancer cells [45,46]. Despite these studies, the mechanism in AML of downregulation of *DYRK1A* mRNA level is still unclear. More studies about the functions of these factors are necessary and researchers should take effort to discover new factors regulating *DYRK1A* transcription in AML.

In summary, we found that DYRK1A level was decreased in adult AML patients and overexpression of DYRK1A caused cell

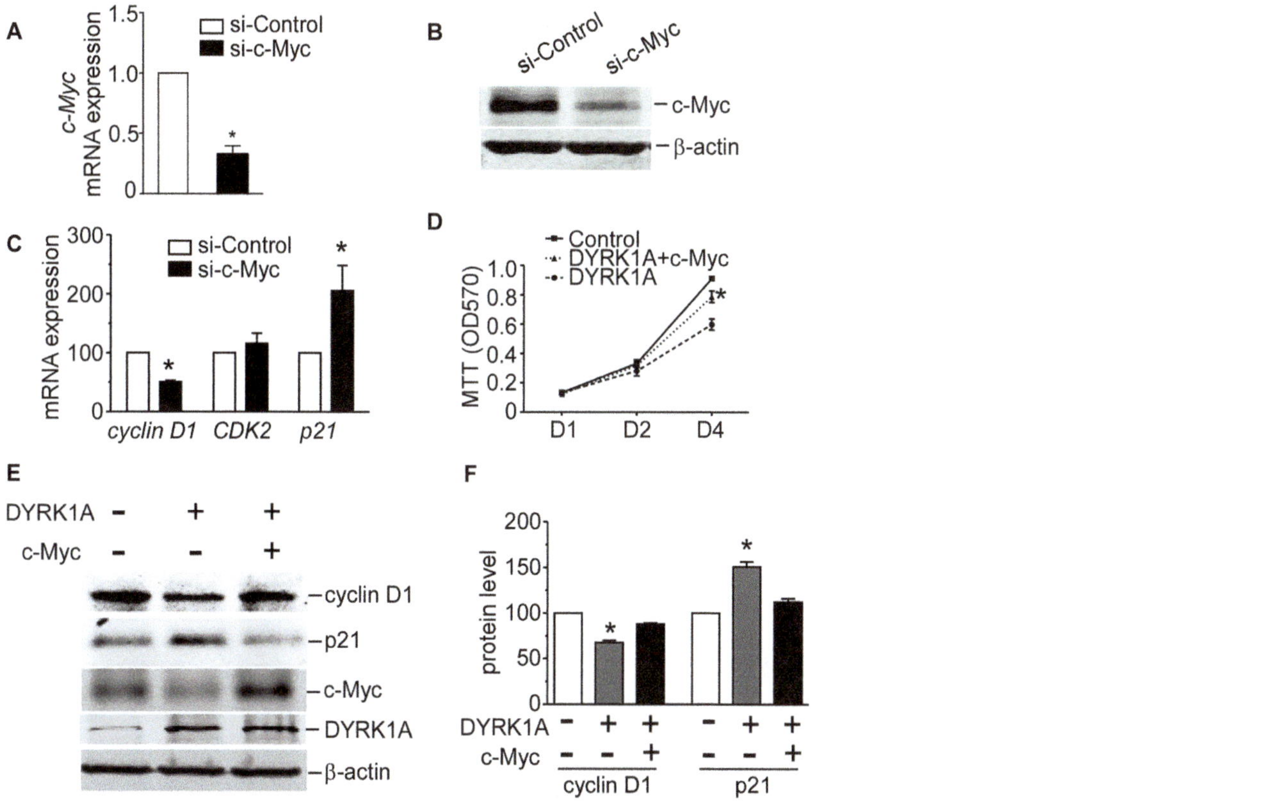

Figure 4. DYRK1A suppresses proliferation of AML cells through downregulating c-Myc. (A and B) HEL cells were infected with pSV248-sic-Myc lentiviral particles(si-c-Myc) or negative control(si-Control) for 72 hrs. Real-time RT-PCR and western blot was used to validate the siRNA effect on c-Myc expression. For real-time PCR, data were calculated from 3 experiments. Values represent the means ± S.E. (n = 3). *$P<0.05$. For western blot, one representative figure from three experiments was shown. (C) HEL cells were infected with pSV248-sic-*Myc* lentiviral particles(si-*c-Myc*) or negative control(si-Control) for 72 hrs. Real-time RT-PCR detected *cyclin D1*, *CDK2* and *p21* mRNA levels in HEL cells. *β-actin* was used as internal control. The values represent the means ± S.E. (n = 3). *$P<0.05$. (D)HEL cells were infected with DYRK1A lentiviral particles(DYRK1A) or negative control(Control) and c-Myc lentiviral particles(c-Myc) for 72 hrs. After infection, cells were subjected to the MTT assay. The values represent the means ± S.E.(n = 3). *$P<0.05$(DYRK1A+c-Myc vs DYRK1A) (E and F) HEL cells were infected with DYRK1A lentiviral particles(DYRK1A) or negative control(Control) and c-Myc lentiviral particles(c-Myc) for 72 hrs. Cell cycle regulators cyclin D1 and p21 were detected by western blot. Results shown are representative of at least three independent experiments. The values represent the means ± S.E. (n = 3). *$P<0.05$.

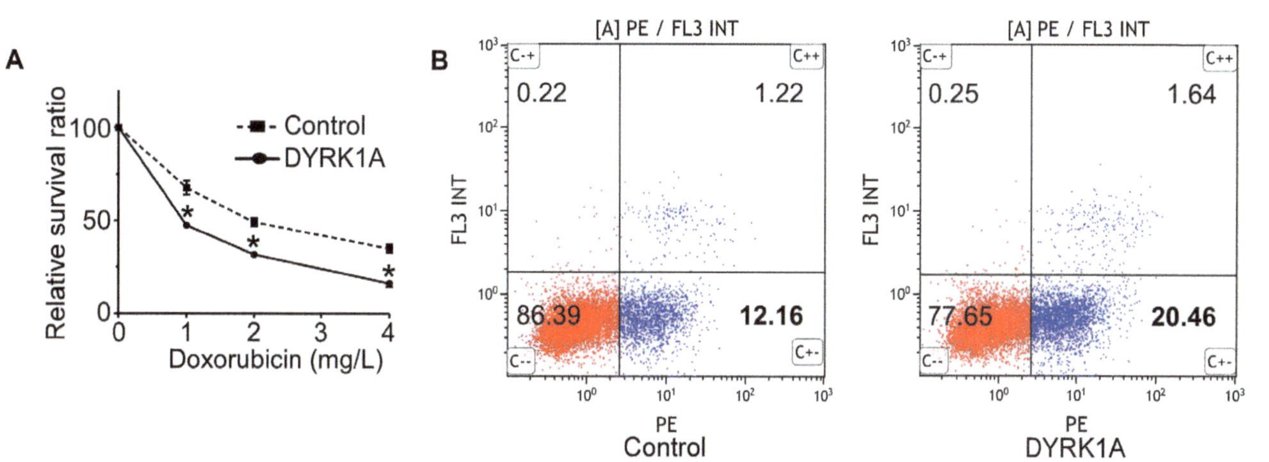

Figure 5. Upregulation of DYRK1A increases drug sensitivity of HL-60/ADM. (A) HL-60/ADM cells infected with DYRK1A lentiviral particles(DYRK1A) or negative control(Control) were treated with gradient dilutions of doxorubicin for 72 hrs (0, 1, 2, 4 mg/L). Cell viability was measured by MTT assays. Results represent the mean ± S.E. from three independent experiments. *$P<0.05$. (B) HL-60/ADM cells infected with DYRK1A lentiviral particles(DYRK1A) or negative control(Control) were cultured in 0.5 mg/L doxorubicin for 48 hrs. Apoptosis was quantified by flow cytometry with dual staining of Annexin V-PE and 7-AAD. Dot plots of representative experiments showing apoptotic cell detection after 48 hrs of treatment with doxorubicin. Percentages of early (AV+7-AAD-) and late (AV+7-AAD+) apoptotic cells were calculated.

cycle arrest and proliferation inhibition in AML cells. We reasoned that the proliferation inhibition could be due to the role of DYRK1A in downregulation of c-Myc by mediating its degradation. Our results clearly show DYRK1A acts as a potential tumor suppressor in AML. Our findings may also present new opportunities for exploitation in novel treatment strategies in AML.

Acknowledgments

We would like to thank Dr. William Tse for constructive suggestions.

Author Contributions

Conceived and designed the experiments: XS CJ. Performed the experiments: QL NL. Analyzed the data: SZ. Contributed reagents/materials/analysis tools: PW HL. Wrote the paper: QL NL XS.

References

1. Oran B, Weisdorf DJ (2012) Survival for older patients with acute myeloid leukemia: a population-based study. Haematologica 97: 1916–1924.
2. Pulte D, Redaniel MT, Jansen L, Brenner H, Jeffreys M (2013) Recent trends in survival of adult patients with acute leukemia: overall improvements, but persistent and partly increasing disparity in survival of patients from minority groups. Haematologica 98: 222–229.
3. Licht JD, Sternberg DW (2005) The molecular pathology of acute myeloid leukemia. Hematology Am Soc Hematol Educ Program: 137–142.
4. Becker W, Weber Y, Wetzel K, Eirmbter K, Tejedor FJ, et al. (1998) Sequence characteristics, subcellular localization, and substrate specificity of DYRK-related kinases, a novel family of dual specificity protein kinases. J Biol Chem 273: 25893–25902.
5. Yoshida K (2008) Role for DYRK family kinases on regulation of apoptosis. Biochem Pharmacol 76: 1389–1394.
6. Aranda S, Laguna A, de la Luna S (2011) DYRK family of protein kinases: evolutionary relationships, biochemical properties, and functional roles. FASEB J 25: 449–462.
7. Taira N, Nihira K, Yamaguchi T, Miki Y, Yoshida K (2007) DYRK2 is targeted to the nucleus and controls p53 via Ser46 phosphorylation in the apoptotic response to DNA damage. Mol Cell 25: 725–738.
8. Gwack Y, Sharma S, Nardone J, Tanasa B, Iuga A, et al. (2006) A genome-wide Drosophila RNAi screen identifies DYRK-family kinases as regulators of NFAT. Nature 441: 646–650.
9. Arron JR, Winslow MM, Polleri A, Chang CP, Wu H, et al. (2006) NFAT dysregulation by increased dosage of DSCR1 and DYRK1A on chromosome 21. Nature 441: 595–600.
10. Yiu GK, Toker A (2006) NFAT induces breast cancer cell invasion by promoting the induction of cyclooxygenase-2. J Biol Chem 281: 12210–12217.
11. Gregory MA, Phang TL, Neviani P, Alvarez-Calderon F, Eide CA, et al. (2010) Wnt/Ca2+/NFAT signaling maintains survival of Ph+ leukemia cells upon inhibition of Bcr-Abl. Cancer Cell 18: 74–87.
12. Altafaj X, Dierssen M, Baamonde C, Marti E, Visa J, et al. (2001) Neurodevelopmental delay, motor abnormalities and cognitive deficits in transgenic mice overexpressing Dyrk1A (minibrain), a murine model of Down's syndrome. Hum Mol Genet 10: 1915–1923.
13. Park J, Song WJ, Chung KC (2009) Function and regulation of Dyrk1A: towards understanding Down syndrome. Cell Mol Life Sci 66: 3235–3240.
14. Satge D, Sasco AJ, Carlsen NL, Stiller CA, Rubie H, et al. (1998) A lack of neuroblastoma in Down syndrome: a study from 11 European countries. Cancer Res 58: 448–452.
15. Malinge S, Izraeli S, Crispino JD (2009) Insights into the manifestations, outcomes, and mechanisms of leukemogenesis in Down syndrome. Blood 113: 2619–2628.
16. Birger Y, Izraeli S (2012) DYRK1A in Down syndrome: an oncogene or tumor suppressor? J Clin Invest 122: 807–810.
17. Lu M, Zheng L, Han B, Wang L, Wang P, et al. (2011) REST regulates DYRK1A transcription in a negative feedback loop. J Biol Chem 286: 10755–10763.
18. Adams JM, Harris AW, Pinkert CA, Corcoran LM, Alexander WS, et al. (1985) The c-myc oncogene driven by immunoglobulin enhancers induces lymphoid malignancy in transgenic mice. Nature 318: 533–538.
19. Nesbit CE, Tersak JM, Prochownik EV (1999) MYC oncogenes and human neoplastic disease. Oncogene 18: 3004–3016.
20. Zhang J, Ma D, Ye J, Zang S, Lu F, et al. (2012) Prognostic impact of delta-like ligand 4 and Notch1 in acute myeloid leukemia. Oncol Rep 28: 1503–1511.
21. Welcker M, Orian A, Jin J, Grim JE, Harper JW, et al. (2004) The Fbw7 tumor suppressor regulates glycogen synthase kinase 3 phosphorylation-dependent c-Myc protein degradation. Proc Natl Acad Sci U S A 101: 9085–9090.
22. Jung MS, Park JH, Ryu YS, Choi SH, Yoon SH, et al. (2011) Regulation of RCAN1 protein activity by Dyrk1A protein-mediated phosphorylation. J Biol Chem 286: 40401–40412.
23. Scales TM, Lin S, Kraus M, Goold RG, Gordon-Weeks PR (2009) Nonprimed and DYRK1A-primed GSK3 beta-phosphorylation sites on MAP1B regulate microtubule dynamics in growing axons. J Cell Sci 122: 2424–2435.
24. Kurabayashi N, Hirota T, Sakai M, Sanada K, Fukada Y (2010) DYRK1A and glycogen synthase kinase 3beta, a dual-kinase mechanism directing proteasomal degradation of CRY2 for circadian timekeeping. Mol Cell Biol 30: 1757–1768.
25. Chen JY, Lin JR, Tsai FC, Meyer T (2013) Dosage of Dyrk1a shifts cells within a p21-cyclin D1 signaling map to control the decision to enter the cell cycle. Mol Cell 52: 87–100.
26. Hammerle B, Ulin E, Guimera J, Becker W, Guillemot F, et al. (2011) Transient expression of Mnb/Dyrk1a couples cell cycle exit and differentiation of neuronal precursors by inducing p27KIP1 expression and suppressing NOTCH signaling. Development 138: 2543–2554.
27. Park J, Oh Y, Yoo L, Jung MS, Song WJ, et al. (2010) Dyrk1A phosphorylates p53 and inhibits proliferation of embryonic neuronal cells. J Biol Chem 285: 31895–31906.
28. Litovchick L, Florens LA, Swanson SK, Washburn MP, DeCaprio JA (2011) DYRK1A protein kinase promotes quiescence and senescence through DREAM complex assembly. Genes Dev 25: 801–813.
29. Ruggero D, Montanaro L, Ma L, Xu W, Londei P, et al. (2004) The translation factor eIF-4E promotes tumor formation and cooperates with c-Myc in lymphomagenesis. Nat Med 10: 484–486.
30. Reavie L, Buckley SM, Loizou E, Takeishi S, Aranda-Orgilles B, et al. (2013) Regulation of c-Myc ubiquitination controls chronic myelogenous leukemia initiation and progression. Cancer Cell 23: 362–375.
31. Mateyak MK, Obaya AJ, Adachi S, Sedivy JM (1997) Phenotypes of c-Myc-deficient rat fibroblasts isolated by targeted homologous recombination. Cell Growth Differ 8: 1039–1048.
32. Adhikary S, Eilers M (2005) Transcriptional regulation and transformation by Myc proteins. Nat Rev Mol Cell Biol 6: 635–645.
33. Daksis JI, Lu RY, Facchini LM, Marhin WW, Penn LJ (1994) Myc induces cyclin D1 expression in the absence of de novo protein synthesis and links mitogen-stimulated signal transduction to the cell cycle. Oncogene 9: 3635–3645.
34. Seoane J, Le HV, Massague J (2002) Myc suppression of the p21(Cip1) Cdk inhibitor influences the outcome of the p53 response to DNA damage. Nature 419: 729–734.
35. Du J, Widlund HR, Horstmann MA, Ramaswamy S, Ross K, et al. (2004) Critical role of CDK2 for melanoma growth linked to its melanocyte-specific transcriptional regulation by MITF. Cancer Cell 6: 565–576.
36. Xie RL, Gupta S, Miele A, Shiffman D, Stein JL, et al. (2003) The tumor suppressor interferon regulatory factor 1 interferes with SP1 activation to repress the human CDK2 promoter. J Biol Chem 278: 26589–26596.
37. de Wit NJ, Burtscher HJ, Weidle UH, Ruiter DJ, van Muijen GN (2002) Differentially expressed genes identified in human melanoma cell lines with different metastatic behaviour using high density oligonucleotide arrays. Melanoma Res 12: 57–69.
38. Teague TK, Hildeman D, Kedl RM, Mitchell T, Rees W, et al. (1999) Activation changes the spectrum but not the diversity of genes expressed by T cells. Proc Natl Acad Sci U S A 96: 12691–12696.
39. Hammerle B, Vera-Samper E, Speicher S, Arencibia R, Martinez S, et al. (2002) Mnb/Dyrk1A is transiently expressed and asymmetrically segregated in neural progenitor cells at the transition to neurogenic divisions. Dev Biol 246: 259–273.
40. Jung P, Menssen A, Mayr D, Hermeking H (2008) AP4 encodes a c-MYC-inducible repressor of p21. Proc Natl Acad Sci U S A 105: 15046–15051.
41. Kim MY, Jeong BC, Lee JH, Kee HJ, Kook H, et al. (2006) A repressor complex, AP4 transcription factor and geminin, negatively regulates expression of target genes in nonneuronal cells. Proc Natl Acad Sci U S A 103: 13074–13079.
42. Maenz B, Hekerman P, Vela EM, Galceran J, Becker W (2008) Characterization of the human DYRK1A promoter and its regulation by the transcription factor E2F1. BMC Mol Biol 9: 30.
43. Strom DK, Cleveland JL, Chellappan S, Nip J, Hiebert SW (1998) E2F-1 and E2F-3 are functionally distinct in their ability to promote myeloid cell cycle progression and block granulocyte differentiation. Cell Growth Differ 9: 59–69.
44. Lee Y, Ha J, Kim HJ, Kim YS, Chang EJ, et al. (2009) Negative feedback Inhibition of NFATc1 by DYRK1A regulates bone homeostasis. J Biol Chem 284: 33343–33351.
45. Reddy BY, Greco SJ, Patel PS, Trzaska KA, Rameshwar P (2009) RE-1-silencing transcription factor shows tumor-suppressor functions and negatively regulates the oncogenic TAC1 in breast cancer cells. Proc Natl Acad Sci U S A 106: 4408–4413.
46. Wagoner MP, Gunsalus KT, Schoenike B, Richardson AL, Friedl A, et al. (2010) The transcription factor REST is lost in aggressive breast cancer. PLoS Genet 6: e1000979.

2

Behavioral Characterization of a Mouse Model Overexpressing *DSCR1/ RCAN1*

Mara Dierssen[1]*, Gloria Arqué[1], Jerome McDonald[1], Nuria Andreu[1], Carmen Martínez-Cué[2], Jesús Flórez[2,3], Cristina Fillat[1]

1 Genes and Disease Program, Centre for Genomic Regulation (CRG), Barcelona Biomedical Research Park (PRBB), and CIBER de Enfermedades Raras (CIBERER), Barcelona, Catalonia, Spain, **2** Department of Physiology and Pharmacology, Faculty of Medicine, University of Cantabria, Santander, Spain, **3** Fundación Síndrome de Down de Cantabria, Fundación Iberoamericana Down21, Santander, Spain

Abstract

DSCR1/ RCAN1 is a chromosome 21 gene found to be overexpressed in the brains of Down syndrome (DS) and postulated as a good candidate to contribute to mental disability. However, even though *Rcan1* knockout mice have pronounced spatial learning and memory deficits, the possible deleterious effects of its overexpression in DS are not well understood. We have generated a transgenic mouse model overexpressing DSCR1/RCAN1 in the brain and analyzed the effect of RCAN1 overexpression on cognitive function. Tg*RCAN1* mice present a marked disruption of the learning process in a visuo-spatial learning task. However, no significant differences were observed in the performance of the memory phase of the test (removal session) nor in a step-down passive avoidance task, thus suggesting that once learning has been established, the animals are able to consolidate the information in the longer term.

Editor: Georges Chapouthier, Université Pierre et Marie Curie, France

Funding: The laboratories of MD and CF are supported by DURSI (Grups consolidats 09 2009SGR1313, SGR091527). This work was supported by FCT-08-0782, SAF2007-60827, SAF2010-16427, SAF2007-31093-E, FIS (PI 082038, PI041559), Marató TV3, Jerome Lejeune, Reina Sofia and Areces Foundations and EU (LSHG-CT-2006-037627; CureFXS E-Rare: EU/FIS PS09102673). The CIBER of Enfermedades Raras is an initiative of the ISCIII. The funders had no role in study design, data collection and analysis, decision to publish, or preparation of the manuscript.

Competing Interests: The authors have declared that no competing interests exist.

* E-mail: mara.dierssen@crg.es

Introduction

Mental disability in individuals with Down syndrome (DS) is produced by the increased expression of some of the 231 supernumerary genes on the extra copy of chromosome 21. One such gene is Down's syndrome candidate region-1 (*DSCR1*, also known as *RCAN1*) [1,2], which encodes a protein that is a functional inhibitor of calcineurin, a ubiquitous and multifunctional calcium-activated protein phosphatase. It is located in the Down syndrome critical region and its expression is consistently increased 1.8-fold in Down's syndrome human fetal tissues and in Ts65Dn mice [3].

RCAN1 physically and functionally interacts with calcineurin A, effectively inhibiting its phosphatase activity [4]. Calcineurin is the most abundant protein in brain where it regulates, among other neuronal functions, neurotransmitter release, neurite outgrowth and neuronal cell death. The only calcineurin inhibitor which expression is regulated by calcium-calcineurin signaling is RCAN1, indicating that this protein can function in a feedback inhibition loop to suppress sustained calcineurin activity. RCAN1 is widely expressed in brain, both during development and in the adult and it has been postulated as a good candidate to contribute to mental disability in DS [5,6,7]. Mouse models of RCAN1 overexpression have shown a role of RCAN1 regulating exocytosis in chromaffin cells and in mutant huntingtin phosphorilation, suggesting a role of RCAN1 in the Alzheimer's disease neuropathology associated to DS and in Huntington's disease [8,9,10]. Moreover, it has been identified as a gene involved in cognitive symptoms of schizophrenia patients by measuring differences in DNA copy number variants [11]. Evidences of an RCAN1 role in cognition also exist from studies in experimental models. *Drosophila* mutants with both loss-of-function or overexpression of nebula exhibit severe learning defects that are attributed by biochemical perturbations rather than maldevelopment of the brain [12] and the *Rcan1* knockout mice present pronounced spatial learning and memory deficits in the Morris water maze task and impaired long-term potentiation (LTP) [13]. However, the *in vivo* relevance of Rcan1 overexpression and its possible contribution to DS cognitive phenotypes has not yet been explored.

In the current study we have analyzed the effect of RCAN1 overexpression on the cognitive function using transgenic mice. We have focused on the potential role of this regulator in processes related to learning and memory in DS by characterizing the neurological and cognitive alterations in these mice. Our work confirms a role of RCAN1 overexpression in the visuo-spatial learning and memory tasks, with alterations similar to those present in DS persons.

Materials and Methods

Generation of TgRCAN1 transgenic mice

The transgenic cassette was generated by cloning a 1.3 Kb fragment of the human *PDGFβ* chain promoter in the 5′ region of a plasmid containing the second intron of the β-globin gene, flanked by part of exons 2 and 3, and the polyadenilation signal of the SV-40 virus. The 0.6 Kb *RCAN1* cDNA was introduced in the *EcoRI* site of the β-globin exon 3. The complete cassette was sequenced with specific primers in an automated sequencer (Applied Biosystems 373A) to ensure the integrity of the transgene. The *PDGFβ-RCAN1* construct was isolated from the plasmid sequences by digestion with *Xba*I and *Xho*I, gel purified using the GenClean spin kit (Q-Biogene) and microinjected (2–5 μg/ml) into B6/SJL zygotes, which were transferred to the oviducts of 0.5 dpc pseudopregnant CD1 females. Genotyping of founder mice was performed by Southern blotting. Genomic DNA was obtained from mice tail biopsy. Ten μg of DNA were digested with *EcoR*I, electrophoresed in 1% agarose and transferred to nitrocellulose membranes (Hybond-N+; Amersham Pharmacia Biotech). Hybridization of the filters was done according to manufacturer procedures (Amersham Pharmacia Biotech), using the human *RCAN1* cDNAs as a probe. Three transgenic lines were obtained and maintained in hemizygosity by crossing with B6/SJL mice. Transgene copy number was also determined by Southern blot analysis. Autoradiographies were analyzed using Phoretix 1D software (Nonlinear Dynamics Ltd, Newcastle Upon Tyne, UK). Genotyping of the progeny was performed by multiplex PCR analysis using the human specific primer pairs: *RCAN1*-F primer, 5′- AGGACGTATGACAAGGACAT -3′ and *RCAN1*-R primer, 5′-ATCAGAAACTGCTTGTCTGGA-3′; GdX-F primer, 5′-GGCAGCTGATCTCCAAAGTCCTGG-3′ and GdX-R primer, 5′- AACGTTCGATGTCATCCAGTGTTA -3′. PCR conditions were denaturation at 94°C for 15 sec, annealing at 56°C for 15 sec, and extension at 72°C for 30 sec, for 32 cycles.

RT-PCR analysis

Total RNA was prepared from different brain regions (hippocampus, cerebral cortex and cerebellum) of Tg*RCAN1* and control mice using TriPure reagent (Roche). To avoid genomic contamination RNA samples were treated with DNAse (DNAfree, Ambion), as described by manufacturer's protocol. One μg of total RNA from each sample was reverse transcribed with a Retroscript RT kit (Ambion). Two μl of cDNA was PCR amplified with the same conditions described above for genotyping with the human specific primers (*RCAN1*-F and *RCAN1*-R). Absence of genomic DNA contamination was determined by the amplification of a 126 bp PCR fragment from cDNA samples with primers for GdX transcript (GdX-F and GdX-R).

Western blot analysis

Western blot analysis from adult brain samples was performed as described by Porta et al. with minor modifications [5]. Briefly, individual samples were mechanically homogenized in a glass potter, with a lysis buffer, containing: 50 mM Tris-HCl pH 7.4, 10 mM EDTA, 320 mM sucrose, 1 mM phenylmethylsulfonyl fluoride and a protease inhibitor cocktail (Complete Mini, Roche Diagnostics, Mannheim, Germany). Extracts were centrifuged for 10 min at 800×g for 10 min at 4°C, and the protein concentration determined from the cleared lysate (BCA assay; Pierce, Rockford, IL). Proteins were separated by 12% SDS-PAGE gel and transferred onto nitrocellulose membranes (HybondTM-C, Amersham Biosciences, Freiburg, Germany). The membranes were blocked in 10% non-fat dried milk dissolved in TBS-T (10 mM Tris-HCl pH 7.5, 100 mM NaCl, 0,1% Tween 20) for 1 h at room temperature and then incubated overnight at 4°C with the primary antibody, a rabbit polyclonal anti-RCAN1 [5], diluted 1:1000 in 5% powdered milk in TBS-T. Protein loading was monitored using a mouse antibody against α-tubulin (1:5000, Sigma). Incubation with anti-rabbit or anti-mouse IgG/HRP (horseradish peroxidase) antibodies (1:2000; Dako, Glostrup, Denmark) was performed at room temperature for 1 h. Membranes were rinsed in PBS-T and the immunocomplexes were detected by enhanced chemiluminiscence with ECL™ Western blotting detection reagent (Amersham Bioscience). Chemiluminiscence was determined with a LAS-3000 image analyzer (Fuji PhotoFilm Co., Carrollton, TX, USA).

General histology

Mice were anaesthetized and then perfused transcardially with 0.1 M PBS, followed by chilled 4% paraformaldehyde in PBS. At least five animals were used per genotype and age. Brains were removed from the skull and postfixed in the same fixative for 24 h at 4°C overnight. After rinsing in PBS, brains of adult mice were cryoprotected in 30% sucrose and kept frozen at −80°C. Coronal sections 50 μm thick were cut with a cryostat and maintained in cryoprotective solution at −20°C until use. Sections were mounted in slices, air-dried, dehydrated in increasing concentrations of ethanol followed by xilene and coverslipped with DPX mounting medium. Cresyl violet staining was performed to determine the total cell population.

Behavioral analysis

Animals. Transgenic mice were obtained in heterozygosity in B6/SJL-F1J genetic background. Hybrid founders were crossed using B6/SJL-F1J females and all experiments were performed using mice from the F1–F5 generation to attenuate littermate's genetic differences. We have used male mice in order to avoid female estrous cycle variations. The non-transgenic (WT) littermates obtained from crosses of males Tg*RCAN1* mice and B6/SJL-F1J females served as controls. Mice were housed in groups of 3–5 animals per cage in standard macrolon cages (40 cm long×25 cm wide×20 cm high) under a 12 h light/dark schedule (lights on 08:00 to 20:00) in controlled environmental conditions of humidity (50%–70%) and temperature (22±2°C) with food and water supplied *ad libitum*. All experimental procedures were approved by the local ethical committee (CEEA-IMIM and CEEA-PRBB), and met the guidelines of the local (Catalan law 5/1995 and Decrees 214/97, 32/2007) and European regulations (EU directives 86/609 and 2001-486) and the Standards for Use of Laboratory Animals n° A5388-01 (NIH).

Neurological assessment (SHIRPA protocol). A comprehensive testing protocol was used to identify and characterize phenotype impairments as previously described [14,15]. Assessment of each animal began with observation of undisturbed behavior in a cylindrical clear Perspex viewing jar (15 cm height×11 cm diameter) for wild running or stereotypy. The mice were then transferred to an arena (56×34 cm) for observation of motor behavior and sensorial function. Animals underwent screening exams for visual acuity, vibrissae, corneal and pinna responses to an approaching cotton swab, auditory function (Preyer reflex), vestibular function (contact righting reflex and negative geotaxis), and grip strength and body tone. In the last part of the test, changes in excitability, aggression, general fear, vocalization and salivation and piloerection (for analysis of autonomic function) were recorded.

Coat-hanger test. Motor coordination was initially measured using the coat-hanger test, placing the mice in the middle of the wire in an upside-down position. First, the prehensile reflex was evaluated and was rated as (0) if the mouse fell off the hanger and as (1) if it remained hanging during a 5 sec period. During this period traction capacity was rated as (0) if mice did not lifted-up their hind limbs, (1) if they lifted one of the hind limbs, (2) if they lifted both, and (3) if they reached one of the ends of the hanger. After this initial evaluation, the latency to fall, time to reach one of the ends of the hanger, as well as the activity performed on the wire was measured in a single trial lasting 60 sec.

Balance beam test. The ability of the mice to maintain balance was evaluated on a wooden bar (9 cm diameter×50 cm long×12 mm thick) during a period of 40 sec. Mice were placed with their forelimbs on the bar and two trials were performed. The score was rated as follows: (0) if the mouse fell before the 40 sec period; (1) if the mouse remained in the center of the bar; (2) if it moved out of the center, but it did not reach the ends; (3) if it reached one of the ends.

Open field. The open field was a white Plexiglas apparatus (70 cm wide×70 cm long×25 cm high) divided into 25 equal squares, it were delimited with black lines on the white floor of the box and under high intensity light levels (300 luxes). Two zones, the centre and periphery, were delineated being the centre more anxiogenic. At the beginning of the test session, mice were left in the middle of the apparatus and the latency to cross from the centre to the periphery, the distance traveled, velocity and time spent in each zone and rearing activity, defecation (number of fecal boluses) and grooming behavior were scored during 5 min.

Rotating rod test. To test motor coordination and balance, the ability of each mouse to maintain balance was assessed on a rotating rod (5 cm diameter×10 cm long) with a plastic dowel surface (Rotarod LE8500, Panlab SA, Barcelona, Spain). The equipment consisted of a rotating spindle that is able to maintain a fixed rotational speed (revolutions per min, rpm) and to undergo an acceleration cycle, starting at 4 rpm and accelerating at a constant rate to 40 rpm over a 1 min period. The apparatus is provided with magnetic plates to detect when a mouse has fallen off the rod. Mice were placed on the middle of the rotating rod, its body axis being perpendicular to the rotation axis, and its head against the direction of rotation. All animals were tested for acquisition and maintenance of rotating performance. The experimental design consisted of two training sessions (day 1 and 2) in which the number of trials required to learn to remain on the rod during 180 sec at the minimum speed (4 rpm) was recorded. After the mice reached the criterion, a third session (day 3) was carried out in which two different tasks were performed: motor coordination and balance were assessed (a) by measuring the latency to fall off the rod in consecutive trials with increasing fixed rotational speeds (7, 10, 14, 19, 24, and 34 rpm), and the animals were allowed to stay on the rod for a maximum period of 240 sec per trial and a resting period of 15 min was left between trials; and (b) for the accelerating rod test, the rotation speed was increased during a single session of 60 sec from 4 to 40 rpm. For each trial, the elapsed time until the mouse fell off the rod was recorded.

Visuo-spatial learning and memory in the water maze test. To test hippocampal-dependent spatial cognition, Tg*RCAN1* mice were trained in the standard Morris water maze (MWM) with a hidden platform as previously described [16]. The mice were tested over 6 days (4 trials/session, 10 min inter-trial intervals). The water maze consisted of a circular pool (diameter, 1.20 m; height, 0.5 m). It was filled with tepid water (24°C) opacified by the addition of powdered milk (0.9 kg). A white escape platform (15 cm diameter, height 24 cm) was located 1 cm below the water surface in a fixed position (NE quadrant, 22 cm away from the wall). In each trial, mice were placed at one of the starting locations in random order [north, south, east, west (N, S, E, W), including permutations of the four starting points per session] and were allowed to swim until they located the platform. Mice failing to find the platform within 60 sec were placed on it for 20 sec (the same period of time as the successful animals). At the end of every trial the mice were allowed to dry for 15 min in a heated enclosure and were returned to their home cage. The cue session was performed to test the swimming speed and visual ability using the visible platform, elevated 1 cm above the water and its position was clearly indicated by a visible cue (black flag). White curtains with affixed black patterns to provide an arrangement of spatial cues surrounded the maze. It was performed 24 hours after the fourth training sessions and 5 days after completion of the hidden platform training protocol. To test whether the mice remembered the location of the platform, probe trials were performed. In the probe session the platform was removed and mice were allowed to swim for 60 sec. The time spent in the trained and non-trained quadrants as well as the number of platform annulus crossings during 60 sec were recorded. On the next day (5 days after the last acquisition session), mice performed the reversal learning session. In this test, the platform position was changed to the opposite quadrant (SW).

All the trials were recorded and traced with an image tracking system (SMART, Panlab, Spain) connected to a video camera placed above the pool. Escape latencies, length of the swimming paths and swimming speed for each animal and trial were monitored and computed. The more in detail analysis of the performance of the mice, was performed using a custom-designed analysis program the jTracks software [17].

Passive Avoidance. We used a step-down passive avoidance test, which consisted of a transparent Plexiglas circular cage (40 cm in height, 30 cm in diameter) with a grid floor and a circular platform (4 cm diameter) in the center. During the training session, animals were placed on the platform and their latency to step down with all four paws was measured. Immediately after stepping down on the grid, animals received an electric shock (0.6 mA, 2 sec). Retention test sessions were carried out 24 h (short-term) and 7 days after training (long-term). Step-down latency was used as a measure of memory retention. A cut-off time of 300 sec was set.

Data analysis

Simple comparisons between Tg*RCAN1* and control mice in various tasks were performed using the two-tailed unpaired Student *t* test with Mann-Withney's correction to account for the different variances in the populations being studied. Performances on the Rotarod were compared using repeated measures ANOVA. To assess significant differences in the behavior of both transgenic lines a one-way ANOVA with Bonferroni test for post hoc analyses was performed. In the Morris Water Maze a repeated measures ANOVA test was used. The passive avoidance test was analyzed using Mann-Withney U non-parametric test. Data were summarized as mean ± standard error of mean (S.E.M.). In all tests, a difference was considered to be significant if the obtained probability value was $P<0.05$. The statistical analysis was performed using the SPSS 12.0 software.

Results

Tg*RCAN1* mice are viable and show no gross abnormal phenotype

To generate the transgenic mice Tg*RCAN1*, the human isoform splice variant 1 was placed under the control of the PDGFβ promoter to drive transgene expression to brain areas [18,19] **(Fig. 1A)**. Three transgenic lines were generated **(Fig. 1B)** that expressed the human RCAN1 isoform in the brain regions analyzed, being more abundant in the hippocampus and cerebral cortex as shown by RT-PCR **(Fig. 1C)**. No expression of hRCAN1 was detected in WT mice. Western blot analysis confirmed RCAN1 overexpression that was estimated in 1.3-fold and 1.5-fold in the hippocampus and cerebral cortex respectively

(**Fig. 1D**). No differences among transgenic lines and between genotypes were observed in terms of viability. Neurological assesment using the comprehensive SHIRPA protocol did not reveal any differences between Tg*RCAN1* and the control littermates, suggesting no gross impairment in general neural function. The observational assessment of behaviour in basal conditions showed no changes in excitability, fear, or aggressive behaviour (**Table 1**). General histological staining did not reveal gross abnormalities in Tg*RCAN1* brains.

Sensorimotor evaluation

Tg*RCAN1* mice did not show differences in the performance of a battery of sensorimotor tasks. No significant differences were attained in traction capacity (χ^2 Pearson = 3.364, P = 0.762, data not shown), or when measuring the prehensile reflex, as shown by the similar latencies to fall in the 5 sec trial ($F_{(1,\ 54)} = 0.866$, P = 0.356, ANOVA). Similarly, in the balance beam test, the latencies to fall during 40 sec did not differ between genotypes ($F_{(1,\ 54)} = 0.006$, P = 0.938, ANOVA) thus suggesting that neither balance nor muscular strength were affected by RCAN1 overexpression. Also, no genotype-dependent differences were observed in the execution of the rotarod task (**Fig. 2**), neither during the training sessions (T1, T2), nor in the constant rotational speed sessions at low rpm ($F_{(1,\ 10)} = 2.296$, P = 0.161, MANOVA). However, at higher speed Tg*RCAN1* performed significantly worse than wild types (latency to fall from the rod at 24 rpm

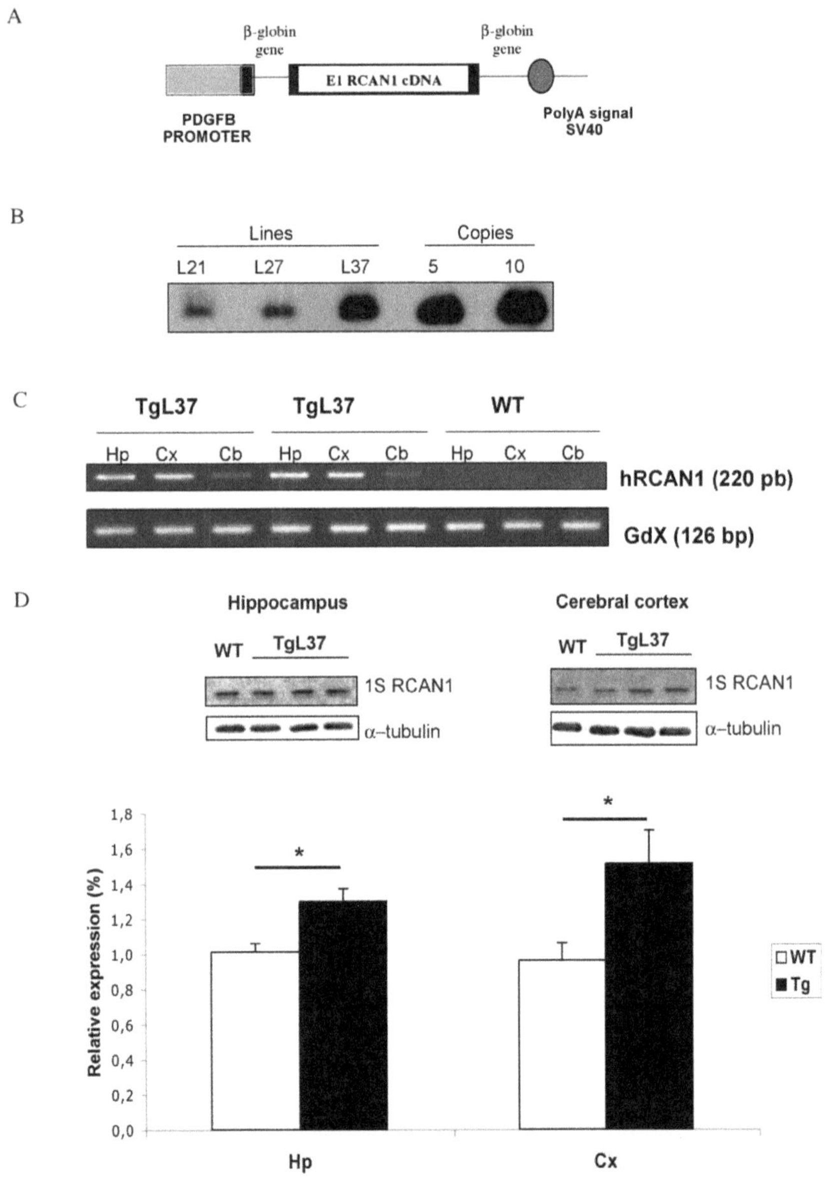

Figure 1. Genotyping and expression analysis of Tg*RCAN1* mice. A) Schematic representation of the *PDGFβ/RCAN1* chimeric gene. **B**) Southern blot analysis of three independent transgenic lines (L21, L27 and L37). **C**) Expression of the transgene by RT-PCR analysis in hippocampus (Hp), cerebral cortex (Cx) and cerebellum (Cb) of Tg*RCAN1* and control mice. **D**) Western blot analysis and relative quantification of RCAN1 protein levels from adult wild type (WT n = 6) and transgenic mice (TgL37 n = 8), in cerebral cortex and hippocampus. α-Tubulin was used as an internal loading control. Bars show densitometric analysis of Rcan1 normalized against the α-tubulin band (Hp: hippocampus, Cx: cerebral cortex). Data are represented as mean ± S.E.M. *P<0.05, Student's t test.

Table 1. SHIRPA primary behavioral screen.

	WT	TgRCAN1	P
Piloerection			
Absent	60%	75%	NS
Present	40%	25%	NS
Tail Elevation			
Horizontally extended	80%	100%	NS
Elevated /Straub tail	20%	0%	NS
Negative Geotaxis			
Turns and climbs the grid	100%	100%	NS
Touch escape			
Escape response to a firm stroke	20%	25%	NS
Escape response to a light stroke	80%	75%	NS
Trunk curling			
Absent	100%	100%	NS
Visual Placing			
Extension of forelimbs before contact	100%	100%	NS
Preyer Reflex			
Absent	20%	12,5%	NS
Flick of pinnae	60%	87,5%	NS
Startle	20%	0%	NS
Pinna Reflex			
Absent	40%	37,5%	NS
Active retraction	40%	62,5%	NS
Hyperactive, repetitive flicking	20%	0%	NS
Corneal Reflex			
Absent	10%	10%	NS
Active blink	90%	90%	NS
Provoked biting (absent)	100%	100%	NS
Righting Reflex (present)	100%	100%	NS
Toe Pinch			
Moderate withdrawal	80%	100%	NS
Brisk, rapid withdrawal	20%	0%	NS

Data are given as percentage of animals showing a specific phenotype. NS: non significant.

$F_{(1,\ 10)} = 5.111$, $P = 0.0473$, ANOVA). However, this may not be dependent on motor coordination since the more demanding acceleration trials showed no differences between genotypes ($F_{(1,\ 11)} = 0.915$, $P = 0.359$, ANOVA).

Open Field

In the open field, Tg*RCAN1* mice showed a tendency to hyperactivity with increased distance travelled in the periphery ($F_{(1,\ 11)} = 3.550$, $P = 0.086$, ANOVA, data not shown), along with an increase in the mean speed found in Tg*RCAN1* mice ($F_{(1,\ 11)} = 2.544$, $P = 0.139$, ANOVA) This phenotype probably reflects a higher anxiety level since the mice showed no increase in the distance traveled in the center.

Morris Water Maze

We used the standard paradigm of the Morris water maze to analyze the visuo-spatial learning and memory profile in Tg*RCAN1* mice (**Fig. 3**). No genotype-related differences were observed in the training session, as demonstrated by the similar escape latency (ANOVA, $F_{(1,25)} = 2.96$; $P = 0.87$) and distance travelled (data not shown), although a tendency to perform worse the procedural learning task was detected in transgenic mice. Along the acquisition sessions, all groups of animals were efficient in learning the location of the platform as indicated by the progressive decrease in escape latency (repeated measures ANOVA, wild type, $F_{(1,23)} = 100.7$, $P = 0.0001$; Tg*RCAN1*, $F_{(1,16)} = 110.5$, $P = 0.0001$) and distance travelled (repeated measures ANOVA, $P<0.001$). However, an important learning impairment was detected in Tg*RCAN1* (repeated measures ANOVA, "session×genotype", $F_{(1,28)} = 14.11$, $P<0.001$) mice as shown by the increased latencies (**Fig. 3**, left panel) to reach the platform and distances (repeated measures ANOVA, "session× genotype", $F_{(1,28)} = 16.14$, $P<0.001$) **Fig. 3**, right panel) travelled across acquisition sessions. This was specifically related to learning problems since swimming speed was not affected and in the cued session, where the goal was to find a visible platform (black stripped flag), no differences were detected in the latency to reach the platform when it was made visible (ANOVA, $F_{(1,40)} = 1.08$; $P = 0.31$) suggesting that RCAN1 overexpression did not produce significant motor or motivational problems. During the probe trial that is a measure of the visuo-spatial memory, the latency to cross the annulus of the hidden escape platform and the number of crosses was similar between genotypes thus suggesting that once learned the information is retained in transgenic mice. Moreover, in both groups we observed a significantly higher preference for the trained quadrant (northwest), as shown by the percentage of time spent in the trained quadrant (ANOVA, wild-type, $F_{(1,23)} = 58.6$, $P = 0.001$ and Tg*RCAN1*, $F_{(1,16)} = 56.7$, $P = 0.001$). These observations support the conclusion that Tg*RCAN1* mice indeed remember the location of the platform. Finally, in the reversal session the efficiency to unlearn the old platform position and learn a new one was not altered in Tg*RCAN1*.

Passive avoidance test

To further explore the learning and memory phenotypes, we used a step down passive avoidance paradigm. Retention memory was not altered either 24 hours or one week after training in transgenic mice, both genotypes showing increased retention latencies. This indicates that memory consolidation had taken place (data not shown).

Discussion

Efforts to identify genes on human chromosome 21 with the potential to cause the brain anomalies observed in Down syndrome (DS), led to the discovery of a gene, Down syndrome candidate region-1 (*DSCR1*) now renamed *RCAN1* (Regulator of Calcineurin-1). RCAN1 is a modulator of calcineurin, a protein phosphatase known to function in a variety of cellular processes, among which learning and memory are relevant for the mental impairment seen in DS. Specifically, Hoeffer et al [13] reported that *Rcan1* knockout mice have pronounced spatial learning and memory deficits in the Morris water maze task, along with significant deficits in long-term potentiation (LTP) in the hippocampal area CA1, similar to what was found in mice with inducible, hippocampal-restricted overexpression of constitutively active calcineurin [20]. In animals in which calcineurin was inhibited by either transgenic expression of a calcineurin inhibitory domain or application of antisense oligonucleotides [21,22] the opposite phenotypes were detected, thus suggesting that RCAN1 provides a constraint on calcineurin activity during learning and memory.

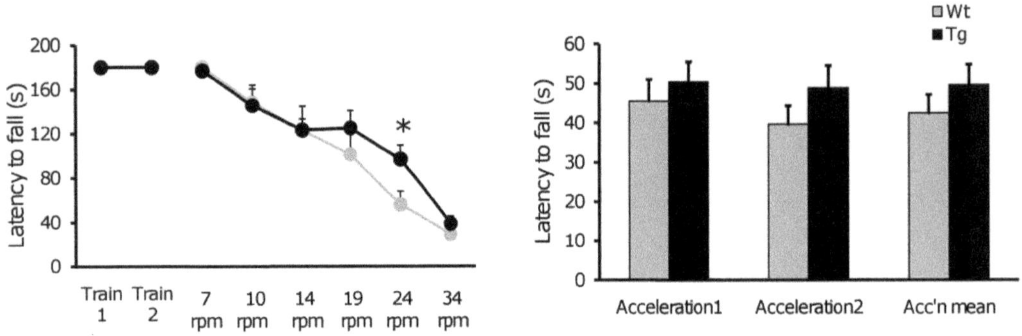

Figure 2. Motor learning and coordination in the Rotarod test. Left panel: Motor learning curve of Tg*RCAN1* and wild type mice. Tg*RCAN1* did not show impairment in motor learning but when submitted to consecutive trials at increasing rotational speeds (7, 10, 14, 24 and 34 rpm) performance in the more demanding trials was slightly improved in transgenic vs. wild type mice. **Right panel**: Acceleration trials. No differences were detected between genotypes. Each data point represents the mean ± S.E.M. $^*P \leq 0.05$. Abbreviations: NS: non significant; rpm: revolutions per min.

However, the threshold for hippocampal-dependent synaptic plasticity and memory storage seems to be determined by the balance between protein phosphorylation and dephosphorylation mediated by the kinase PKA and the phosphatase calcineurin. To establish whether an excessive inhibitory constraint on endogenous calcineurin in this balance may have a deleterious impact on learning and memory in DS, we examined the effect of genetically overexperessing *RCAN1*, and we have applied well-established mouse behavioral tests addressing hippocampal function. Moreover, we also explored other learning and memory processes, such as the recent memory, as tested in the passive avoidance paradigm.

Our data revealed neither motor nor sensory impairment in Tg*RCAN1* or changes in any of the neurological parameters tested. However, transgenic mice showed higher levels of activity in the open field similar to what was has been described in other DS models, such as Ts65Dn [16,23] and in DS persons. This hyperactivity was not related to changes in emotionality, as it did not affect the activity in the central part of the field.

However, a marked phenotype was attained in the visuo-spatial learning paradigm. Although procedural learning was not affected in the pre-training session, the acquisition of the allocentric learning was markedly impaired in transgenic mice, thus suggesting that RCAN1 overexpression is specifically affecting hippocampal function. Those learning defects are specific since no differences were observed in swimming speed or in the motivational/motor aspects in the cued session. Moreover, the Gallagher index was markedly altered indicating the use of non-spatial learning strategies, and thus reinforcing the concept that RCAN1 overexpression leads to a specific and marked learning deficit in mice. However, in our experiments, Tg*RCAN1* mice did not show any impairment in the removal session, thus indicating that once consolidation has taken place, memory is well established. The poorer execution of transgenic mice during the acquisition phase was correlated with the searching trajectory of the mice, that was significantly different, so that wild type mice develop a clear spatial preference, whereas transgenic mice distribute their activity similarly across all quadrants, indicating impaired spatial learning.

Since the training procedure we have used involves an extensive acquisition phase, we also tested recent memory in a one-trial passive avoidance test to specifically targeting memory [24]. Again Tg*RCAN1* mice did not show any impairment reinforcing the concept that RCAN1 overexpression leads to specific alterations in the acquisition process but does not influence memory.

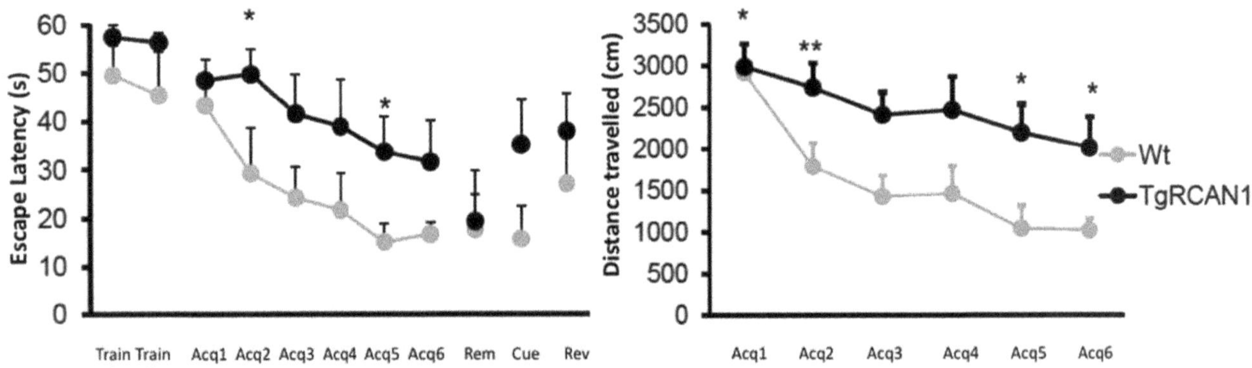

Figure 3. Visuo-spatial learning in the Morris water maze. Morris water maze performance of Tg*RCAN1* and wild type animals during the learning sessions expressed as (**left panel**) latency (s) to reach the platform along the acquisition phase, cue and reversal sessions. A clear deficit was observed in Tg*RCAN1* in all learning phases; (**Right panel**) Cumulative search-error on training trials and a learning index (Gallagher's proximity index) computed from the trials over the course of training. This measure relies on a computation of distance from the platform during the trial [17] and clearly indicated the use of poorer learning strategies in transgenic mice. White squares represent wild types and black squares represent Tg*RCAN1*. Data are represented as mean ± S.E.M. $^*P<0.05$, $^{**}P<0.01$.

In conclusion, our results suggest that RCAN1 may contribute to specific learning phenotypes in DS patients. We also propose that excess of inhibition of endogenous calcineurin, which in turn acts as an inhibitory constraint in the hippocampal phosphorilation/dephosphorilation balance, has a significant impact on learning but not on memory.

Acknowledgments

We thank Dr. Mariona Arbones for kindly providing RCAN1 antibodies.

Author Contributions

Supervised experiments: MD CF. Created the transgenic and performed molecular biology experiments: NA. In charge of colony expansion and maintenance and the genotyping: NA GA JM. Conceived and designed the experiments: MD CF JF. Performed the experiments: GA JM CM-C. Analyzed the data: GA JM CM-C. Wrote the paper: MD CF.

References

1. Casas C, Martinez S, Pritchard MA, Fuentes JJ, Nadal M, et al. (2001) Dscr1, a novel endogenous inhibitor of calcineurin signaling, is expressed in the primitive ventricle of the heart and during neurogenesis. Mech Dev 101: 289–292.
2. Guimera J, Pucharcos C, Domenech A, Casas C, Solans A, et al. (1997) Cosmid contig and transcriptional map of three regions of human chromosome 21q22: identification of 37 novel transcripts by direct selection. Genomics 45: 59–67.
3. Baek KH, Zaslavsky A, Lynch RC, Britt C, Okada Y, et al. (2009) Down's syndrome suppression of tumour growth and the role of the calcineurin inhibitor DSCR1. Nature 459: 1126–1130.
4. Fuentes JJ, Genesca L, Kingsbury TJ, Cunningham KW, Perez-Riba M, et al. (2000) DSCR1, overexpressed in Down syndrome, is an inhibitor of calcineurin-mediated signaling pathways. Hum Mol Genet 9: 1681–1690.
5. Porta S, Marti E, de la Luna S, Arbones ML (2007) Differential expression of members of the RCAN family of calcineurin regulators suggests selective functions for these proteins in the brain. Eur J Neurosci 26: 1213–1226.
6. Park J, Oh Y, Chung KC (2009) Two key genes closely implicated with the neuropathological characteristics in Down syndrome: DYRK1A and RCAN1. BMB Rep 42: 6–15.
7. Mitchell AN, Jayakumar L, Koleilat I, Qian J, Sheehan C, et al. (2007) Brain expression of the calcineurin inhibitor RCAN1 (Adapt78). Arch Biochem Biophys 467: 185–192.
8. Keating DJ, Dubach D, Zanin MP, Yu Y, Martin K, et al. (2008) DSCR1/RCAN1 regulates vesicle exocytosis and fusion pore kinetics: implications for Down syndrome and Alzheimer's disease. Hum Mol Genet 17: 1020–1030.
9. Ermak G, Hench KJ, Chang KT, Sachdev S, Davies KJ (2009) Regulator of calcineurin (RCAN1-1L) is deficient in Huntington disease and protective against mutant huntingtin toxicity in vitro. J Biol Chem 284: 11845–11853.
10. Sun X, Wu Y, Chen B, Zhang Z, Zhou W, et al. Regulator of calcineurin 1 (RCAN1) facilitates neuronal apoptosis through caspase 3 activation. J Biol Chem.
11. Tam GW, van de Lagemaat LN, Redon R, Strathdee KE, Croning MD, et al. (2010) Confirmed rare copy number variants implicate novel genes in schizophrenia. Biochem Soc Trans 38: 445–451.
12. Chang KT, Shi YJ, Min KT (2003) The Drosophila homolog of Down's syndrome critical region 1 gene regulates learning: implications for mental retardation. Proc Natl Acad Sci U S A 100: 15794–15799.
13. Hoeffer CA, Dey A, Sachan N, Wong H, Patterson RJ, et al. (2007) The Down syndrome critical region protein RCAN1 regulates long-term potentiation and memory via inhibition of phosphatase signaling. J Neurosci 27: 13161–13172.
14. Dierssen M, Fotaki V, Martinez de Lagran M, Gratacos M, Arbones M, et al. (2002) Neurobehavioral development of two mouse lines commonly used in transgenic studies. Pharmacol Biochem Behav 73: 19–25.
15. Martinez de Lagran M, Altafaj X, Gallego X, Marti E, Estivill X, et al. (2004) Motor phenotypic alterations in TgDyrk1a transgenic mice implicate DYRK1A in Down syndrome motor dysfunction. Neurobiol Dis 15: 132–142.
16. Escorihuela RM, Fernandez-Teruel A, Vallina IF, Baamonde C, Lumbreras MA, et al. (1995) A behavioral assessment of Ts65Dn mice: a putative Down syndrome model. Neurosci Lett 199: 143–146.
17. Arque G, Fotaki V, Fernandez D, Martinez de Lagran M, Arbones ML, et al. (2008) Impaired spatial learning strategies and novel object recognition in mice haploinsufficient for the dual specificity tyrosine-regulated kinase-1A (Dyrk1A). PLoS One 3: e2575.
18. Sasahara M, Fries JW, Raines EW, Gown AM, Westrum LE, et al. (1991) PDGF B-chain in neurons of the central nervous system, posterior pituitary, and in a transgenic model. Cell 64: 217–227.
19. Resnick N, Collins T, Atkinson W, Bonthron DT, Dewey Jr. CF, et al. (1993) Platelet-derived growth factor B chain promoter contains a cis-acting fluid shear-stress-responsive element. Proc Natl Acad Sci U S A 90: 4591–4595.
20. Mansuy IM, Mayford M, Jacob B, Kandel ER, Bach ME (1998) Restricted and regulated overexpression reveals calcineurin as a key component in the transition from short-term to long-term memory. Cell 92: 39–49.
21. Ikegami S, Inokuchi K (2000) Antisense DNA against calcineurin facilitates memory in contextual fear conditioning by lowering the threshold for hippocampal long-term potentiation induction. Neuroscience 98: 637–646.
22. Malleret G, Haditsch U, Genoux D, Jones MW, Bliss TV, et al. (2001) Inducible and reversible enhancement of learning, memory, and long-term potentiation by genetic inhibition of calcineurin. Cell 104: 675–686.
23. Escorihuela RM, Vallina IF, Martinez-Cue C, Baamonde C, Dierssen M, et al. (1998) Impaired short- and long-term memory in Ts65Dn mice, a model for Down syndrome. Neurosci Lett 247: 171–174.
24. Dierssen M, Marmol F, Vivas NM, Clos MV, Badia A (1992) Post-train administration of 9-amino-1,2,3,4-tetrahydroacridine enhances passive avoidance retention and decreases beta-adrenoceptor-linked cyclic AMP formation in middle-aged rats. Brain Res 586: 117–120.

Prion Protein Is Decreased in Alzheimer's Brain and Inversely Correlates with BACE1 Activity, Amyloid-β Levels and Braak Stage

Isobel J. Whitehouse[1], J. Scott Miners[2], Elizabeth B. C. Glennon[1], Patrick G. Kehoe[2], Seth Love[2], Katherine A. B. Kellett[1]*, Nigel M. Hooper[1]*

1 School of Molecular and Cellular Biology, Faculty of Biological Sciences, University of Leeds, Leeds, United Kingdom, **2** Dementia Research Group, School of Clinical Sciences, Institute of Clinical Neurosciences, University of Bristol, Bristol, United Kingdom

Abstract

The cellular prion protein (PrP^C) has been implicated in the development of Alzheimer's disease (AD). PrP^C decreases amyloid-β (Aβ) production, which is involved in AD pathogenesis, by inhibiting β-secretase (BACE1) activity. Contactin 5 (CNTN5) has also been implicated in the development of AD by a genome-wide association study. Here we measured PrP^C and CNTN5 in frontal cortex samples from 24 sporadic AD and 24 age-matched control brains and correlated the expression of these proteins with markers of AD. PrP^C was decreased in sporadic AD compared to controls (by 49%, $p = 0.014$) but there was no difference in CNTN5 between sporadic AD and controls ($p = 0.217$). PrP^C significantly inversely correlated with BACE1 activity ($r_s = -0.358$, $p = 0.006$), Aβ load ($r_s = -0.456$, $p = 0.001$), soluble Aβ ($r_s = -0.283$, $p = 0.026$) and insoluble Aβ ($r_s = -0.353$, $p = 0.007$) and PrP^C also significantly inversely correlated with the stage of disease, as indicated by Braak tangle stage ($r_s = -0.377$, $p = 0.007$). CNTN5 did not correlate with Aβ load ($r_s = 0.040$, $p = 0.393$), soluble Aβ ($r_s = 0.113$, $p = 0.223$) or insoluble Aβ ($r_s = 0.169$, $p = 0.125$). PrP^C was also measured in frontal cortex samples from 9 Down's syndrome (DS) and 8 age-matched control brains. In contrast to sporadic AD, there was no difference in PrP^C in the DS brains compared to controls ($p = 0.625$). These data are consistent with a role for PrP^C in regulating Aβ production and indicate that brain PrP^C level may be important in influencing the onset and progression of sporadic AD.

Editor: Sophie Mouillet-Richard, INSERM, UMR-S747, France

Funding: The authors gratefully acknowledge the financial support of the Medical Research Council of Great Britain, www.mrc.ac.uk, (G0802189), Alzheimer's Research UK, www.alzheimersresearchuk.org, (PG2008-2 and PhD2009-1) and BRACE (Bristol Research into Ageing and Care of the Elderly, www.alzheimers-brace.org, (BRACE(8120)). The funders had no role in study design, data collection and analysis, decision to publish, or preparation of the manuscript.

Competing Interests: The authors have declared that no competing interests exist.

* E-mail: n.m.hooper@leeds.ac.uk (NMH); k.a.b.kellett@leeds.ac.uk (KABK)

Introduction

Alzheimer's disease (AD) is the most common form of dementia and its socioeconomic impact is increasing as the population ages [1]. The number of individuals suffering from AD worldwide is predicted to rise to 34 million by 2025 [2]. AD is characterised pathologically by the formation of intracellular neurofibrillary tangles and extracellular amyloid plaques. Neurofibrillary tangles, composed of hyperphosphorylated and aggregated tau [3], initially appear in the entorhinal cortex and hippocampus, before the spread of tau pathology into other regions [4]. Tau pathology is staged in AD using the Braak system, encompassing 6 stages which are distinguished according to the distribution of neurofibrillary tangles [4]. As tau pathology spreads, it is accompanied by neuronal loss, following which the tau may be found in the extracellular space – either in a monomeric form or in an aggregated form where it is assembled in extracellular ghost tangles [5]. Amyloid plaques are composed of the amyloid-β peptide (Aβ). Aβ is derived from the sequential cleavage of the amyloid-β precursor protein (APP) first by the β-secretase, β-site APP cleaving enzyme-1 (BACE1), and then by the γ-secretase complex. A number of rare autosomal dominant mutations in the genes encoding either APP or components of the γ-secretase complex have been identified which cause early-onset, or familial, AD. The majority of AD patients, however, do not have such underlying genetic factors and, although some risk factors have been identified (e.g. ageing and the ε4 allele of the apolipoprotein E gene), the cause of these sporadic AD cases remains unknown.

Relatively little is known about the physiological roles of APP, Aβ and BACE1; several studies have endeavoured to investigate the normal biology of these proteins and to identify other interacting proteins which may be involved in their regulation, trafficking and processing. A study of the APP interactome [6] identified several potential APP-interacting proteins, one of which was from the contactin family of proteins, and a later genome-wide association study (GWAS) identified contactin 5 (CNTN5) as one of 13 genes that showed an association with AD [7]. CNTN5 has also been associated with AD neuroimaging measures such as white matter lesion volume and entorhinal cortex thickness [8]; however, the amount of CNTN5 in the AD or ageing brain has not been reported previously. An even greater effort has been made to establish the proteins interacting with BACE1 as it is the BACE1 cleavage of APP that is the rate-limiting step in Aβ production [9], and BACE1 is a potential therapeutic target for AD. BACE1 activity in the brain is increased in sporadic AD and

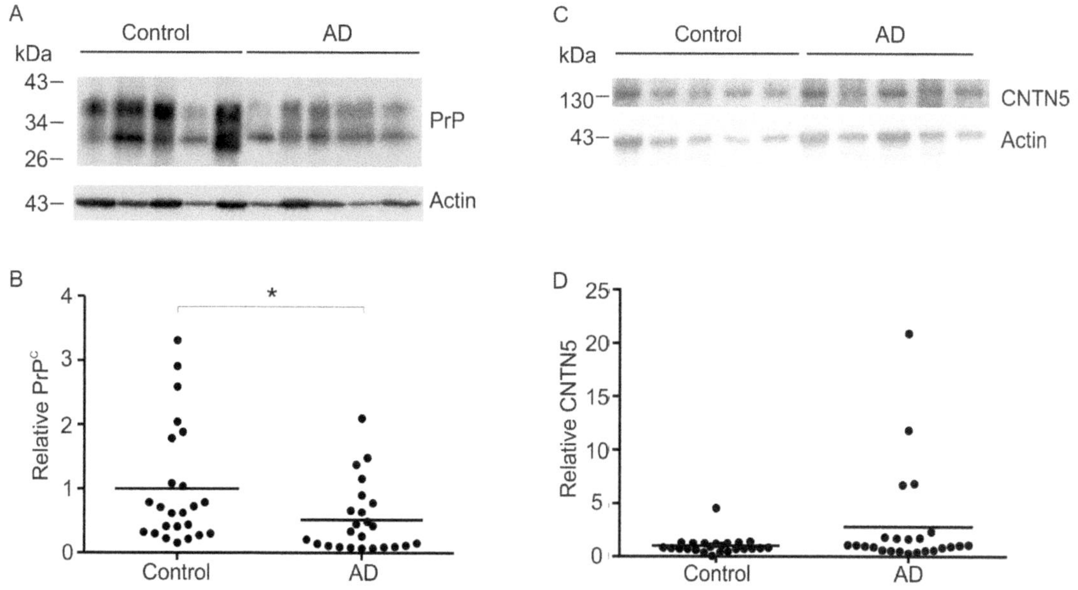

Figure 1. PrP^C, but not CNTN5, is decreased in sporadic AD. Representative immunoblots of PrP^C and actin in temporal cortex samples from sporadic AD patients compared to age-matched controls (A) with densitometric analysis relative to actin levels represented in a grouped scatter plot (B). Representative immunoblots of CNTN5 relative to actin (C) with densitometry analysis (D). Line represents mean, *p<0.05, n = 24 per group.

correlates with increased Aβ load [10,11,12], indicating a disruption in the normal regulation of BACE1 activity. Several proteins regulating BACE1 activity have been identified [13,14], including the cellular form of the prion protein (PrP^C) [15]. PrP^C inhibited the action of BACE1 towards wild type human APP in cellular models and the levels of endogenous murine Aβ were significantly increased in the brain of PrP^C null mice [15], and we proposed that a normal function of PrP^C may be to protect against AD [16], i.e. that BACE1 activity is negatively modulated by PrP^C, which thereby influences Aβ load and the onset and severity of AD. Consistent with this hypothesis, we reported that, in a small cohort, PrP^C was decreased in the hippocampus in sporadic AD [17], although we did not examine the relationship to BACE1 activity and Aβ load.

In this study we measured PrP^C and CNTN5 in frontal neocortex from cases of sporadic AD and age-matched control brain samples. We confirmed our previous finding [17], in a new, larger patient cohort, that PrP^C is decreased in sporadic AD and demonstrate that CNTN5 levels are unchanged in sporadic AD. As PrP^C is decreased [17], and BACE1 activity is increased, in sporadic AD [10,18], and as PrP^C negatively modulates BACE1 activity [15,19], we tested the hypothesis that there is a negative correlation between PrP^C and (i) BACE1 activity, (ii) Aβ and (iii) Braak tangle stage, in human brain tissue. We found that PrP^C did indeed correlate inversely with BACE1 activity, Aβ load, soluble and insoluble Aβ levels, and with the severity of disease, as measured by Braak tangle stage. CNTN5, however, showed no correlation with Aβ load, soluble or insoluble Aβ level.

We previously showed that while PrP^C is decreased in sporadic AD and also declines with age, there is no alteration in PrP^C in familial AD cases [17]. Down's syndrome (DS) is caused by an extra copy of chromosome 21, which results in development abnormalities and neuropathology in the brain that are similar to that seen in AD. APP maps to chromosome 21 and trisomy 21 results in increased APP and Aβ production and early senile plaque formation [20]. Here we demonstrate that PrP^C levels are unchanged in the cortex in DS, compared to age-matched controls.

Results

PrP^C is reduced but CNTN5 is unchanged in sporadic Alzheimer's disease

Quantitative immunoblotting was used to assess PrP^C and CNTN5 in the temporal cortex from sporadic AD individuals in comparison to that in the brain of age-matched cognitively normal individuals. PrP^C was significantly reduced in sporadic AD by a mean of 49% (p = 0.014) compared to the age matched controls (Figure 1A and B, Table 1) but there was no significant difference in CNTN5 between sporadic AD and controls (Figure 1C and D, Table 1). PrP^C is variably glycosylated at two asparagine residues (N181 and N197), so the protein appears on immunoblots as multiple bands corresponding to un-, mono- and diglycosylated species [21]. We previously reported that PrP^C declines with age in the human brain [17] but there was no significant difference in age between the sporadic AD and control cases (mean age ± SEM; 82.5±1.4 years and 76.5±2.7 years, respectively, p = 0.204) (Table 1 and Table S1), indicating that the reduction of PrP^C in individuals with sporadic AD cannot simply be attributed to the effects of age. To ensure age had no effect, the three youngest controls (43, 48 and 53 years) were omitted to give a control mean age of 80.5±1.7 years. PrP^C was still significantly reduced in sporadic AD by a mean of 41% (p = 0.032) compared to age matched controls (Figure S1). In addition, there was no significant difference in the level of neuron-specific enolase (NSE) between the sporadic AD and control samples (Table 1), indicating that the lower PrP^C in the sporadic AD samples was not caused by neuronal loss. The post-mortem delay was also not significantly different between the sporadic AD and control group (Table 1 and Table S1).

Table 1. Summary data of the sporadic AD and age-matched control samples.

Characteristic	Control (n = 24*)	AD (n = 24)	p value
Age (y)	76.46±2.72	82.50±1.44	0.204
PM delay (h)	38.50±6.27	51.08±4.11	0.100
APOE ε4 allele (%)	13%	75%	<0.001
NSE (pg/ml)	0.51±0.05	0.51±0.05	0.992
PrP^C protein (arbitrary units)	1.00±0.19	0.51±0.11	0.014
CNTN5 protein (arbitrary units)	1.00±0.17	2.78±0.96	0.167
BACE1 activity (relative fluorescence units)	2314.79±133.28	2720.45±169.71	0.066
Soluble Aβ (nM)	1.62±0.36	2.54±0.71	0.391
Insoluble Aβ (nM)	20.44±6.56	138.92±16.41	<0.001
Aβ load (%)	0.04±0.04	2.42±0.59	<0.001
Braak stage	1.33±0.23	5.08±0.16	<0.001

All data are mean ± SEM unless stated. *n = 20 for control Aβ load analysis.

PrP^C levels inversely correlate with BACE1 activity, Aβ load and Braak stage

As PrP^C negatively regulates the activity of BACE1 towards APP [15,19], we investigated whether there was a correlation between PrP^C, measured by immunoblotting, and BACE1 activity, measured using a fluorogenic peptide substrate (Table 1). Across the cohort there was a statistically significant inverse correlation between PrP^C and BACE1 activity (Figure 2A) ($r_s = -0.358$, $p = 0.006$), consistent with PrP^C normally acting to inhibit BACE1. We next examined whether the negative modulation of BACE1 activity by PrP^C influenced the Aβ plaque load in an individual. To do this we analysed frontal cortex Aβ levels by immunohistochemical staining of Aβ and measurement of both soluble and insoluble Aβ levels by ELISA and then correlated these data with PrP^C. The Aβ plaque load, as determined by immunohistochemical staining was significantly higher in AD than controls (Table 1) and, in addition, significantly inversely correlated with PrP^C (Figure 2B) ($r_s = -0.456$, $p = 0.001$). Soluble Aβ levels were not statistically different between AD and controls (Table 1), but soluble Aβ did significantly inversely correlate with PrP^C (Figure 2C) ($r_s = -0.283$, $p = 0.026$). Insoluble Aβ was significantly higher in AD compared with controls (Table 1) and significantly inversely correlated with PrP^C (Figure 2D) ($r_s = -0.353$, $p = 0.007$). Finally, as PrP^C correlated inversely with both BACE1 and Aβ load, we went on to examine whether PrP^C correlated with disease severity, as measured by Braak stage (Table 1). This analysis revealed a statistically significant inverse correlation between PrP^C and Braak stage ($r_s = -0.377$, $p = 0.007$) across the cohort (Figure 2E). Again, to ensure age had no effect on the outcome, all correlation analyses were also carried out omitting the three youngest controls (43, 48 and 53 years). PrP^C remained inversely correlated with BACE1 activity, Aβ levels and Braak stage (data not shown).

CNTN5 levels do not correlate with soluble or insoluble Aβ

Although CNTN5 levels are unchanged in sporadic AD this does not rule out a correlation of this protein with markers of disease progression. As CNTN5 has been identified as having an association with AD by GWAS [7], we also examined the relation between CNTN5 and Aβ load. CNTN5 did not correlate with Aβ load (Figure 3A), soluble Aβ (Figure 3B) or insoluble Aβ (Figure 3C).

PrP^C is not reduced in Down's syndrome

PrP^C was also measured in frontal cortex samples from DS and control brains. Frontal cortex samples were immunoblotted for PrP^C and actin (Figure 4A and B). PrP^C was not significantly different in the DS compared to the control brains (Figure 4B and Table 2). BACE1 activity and Aβ levels were also assessed in the DS and control cohort. BACE1 activity, although higher in the DS brains, did not differ significantly from control values ($p = 0.061$, Table 2). Soluble Aβ level, although higher in the DS brain, was not significantly different from controls ($p = 0.179$, Table 2). Insoluble Aβ, however, was significantly increased in the DS brain compared to controls ($p < 0.001$, Table 2). The DS and control cohorts were closely matched in age ($p = 0.226$) (Table 2 and Table S2). The post-mortem delay was not significantly different between the DS and control groups ($p = 0.217$) (Table 2 and Table S2).

Discussion

In this study we have demonstrated a significant inverse correlation between PrP^C and BACE1 activity in cortex from patients with sporadic AD (in whom PrP^C level is lower and BACE1 activity higher than in age-matched controls) but not in Down's syndrome, despite the accumulation of Aβ and the presence of other AD-type pathological abnormalities in the latter. We previously demonstrated that PrP^C negatively modulates the activity of BACE1 [15], in part through an interaction of PrP^C with the prodomain of the immature form of BACE1 within the Golgi, thereby decreasing the amount of BACE1 that is trafficked to the cell surface and endosomes where it cleaves wild type APP [19]. To test our previous hypothesis [16] that PrP^C may function normally to protect against AD by reducing BACE1 activity, we have explored the relationship between PrP^C level and AD pathology in two contexts: first in sporadic AD, and second in Down's syndrome. The latter group provides an opportunity to explore another Aβ-related condition since people with DS also develop abundant AD pathology, but this is attributable to increased production of APP. Previous work has demonstrated that BACE1 activity in the brain increases with age and in

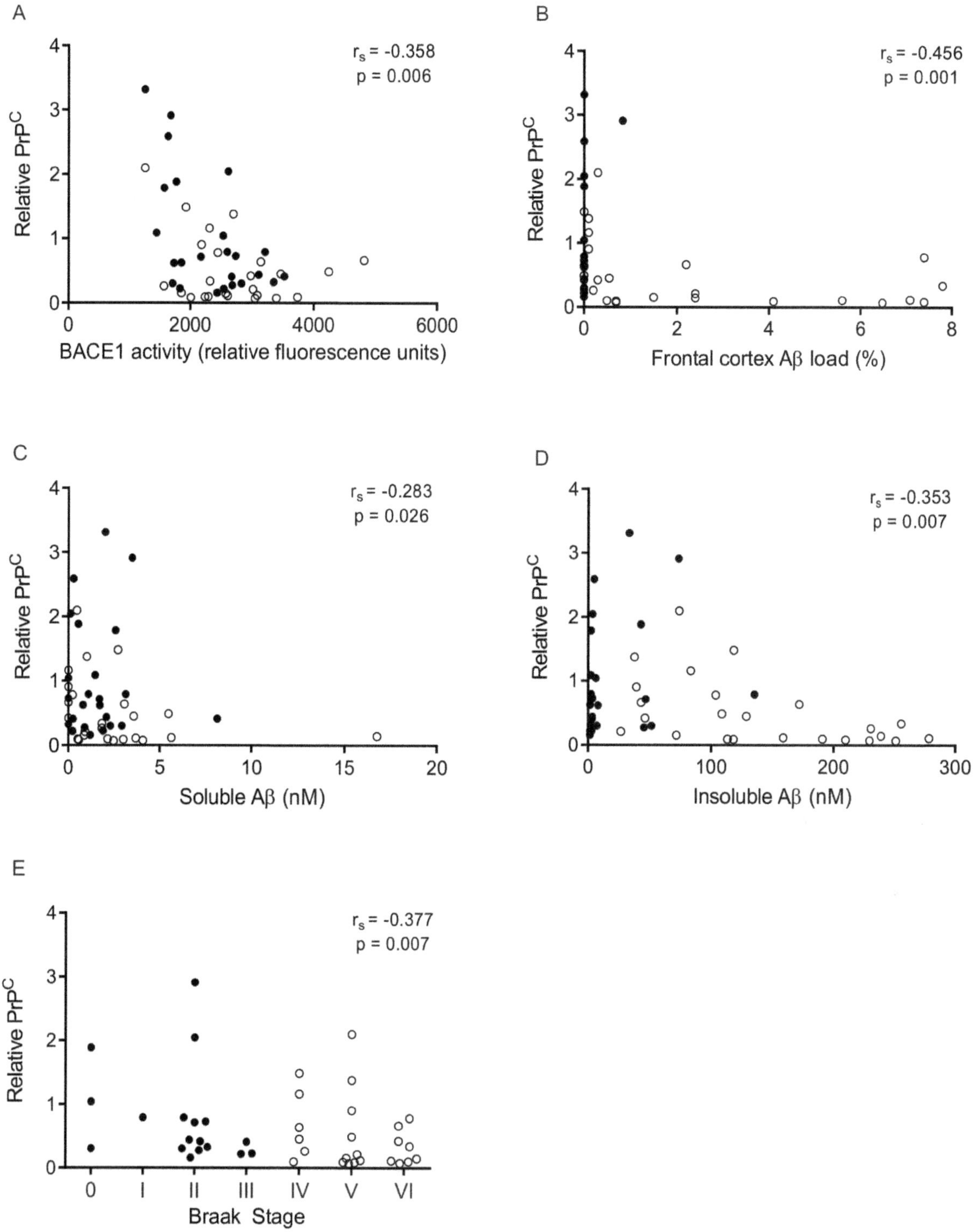

Figure 2. PrP^C inversely correlates with BACE1 activity, Aβ load, soluble and insoluble Aβ and Braak stage. Relative PrP^C protein levels were plotted against BACE1 activity (A), Aβ load (B), soluble Aβ (C), insoluble Aβ (D) and Braak stage (E) for each subject in the cohort (n = 48. Control, filled circles; AD, empty circles). PrP^C significantly inversely correlates with BACE1 activity, Aβ load, soluble Aβ, insoluble Aβ and Braak stage as determined by Spearman's rank correlation coefficient (r_s).

association with Aβ accumulation [10,12,18,22], although the molecular mechanisms underlying this are unclear.

As PrP^C is a negative modulator of BACE1 activity, we hypothesised that it would significantly impact on Aβ levels. Our data revealed a significant inverse relationship between PrP^C and both soluble and insoluble Aβ as well as between PrP^C and Aβ plaque load, indicating that the relationship between PrP^C and BACE1 may have important downstream effects on the develop-

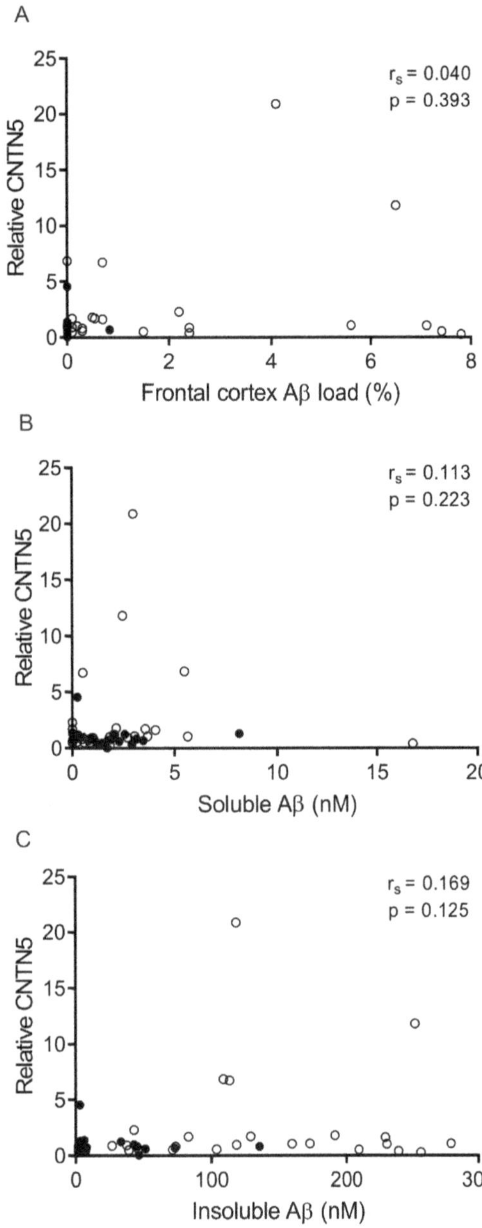

Figure 3. CNTN5 does not correlate with Aβ load, soluble Aβ or insoluble Aβ. Relative CNTN5 protein levels were plotted against Aβ load (A), soluble Aβ (B) and insoluble Aβ (C) for each subject in the cohort (n = 48. Control, filled circles; AD, empty circles). CNTN5 levels did not correlate with Aβ load, soluble Aβ or insoluble Aβ levels as determined by Spearman's rank correlation coefficient (r_s).

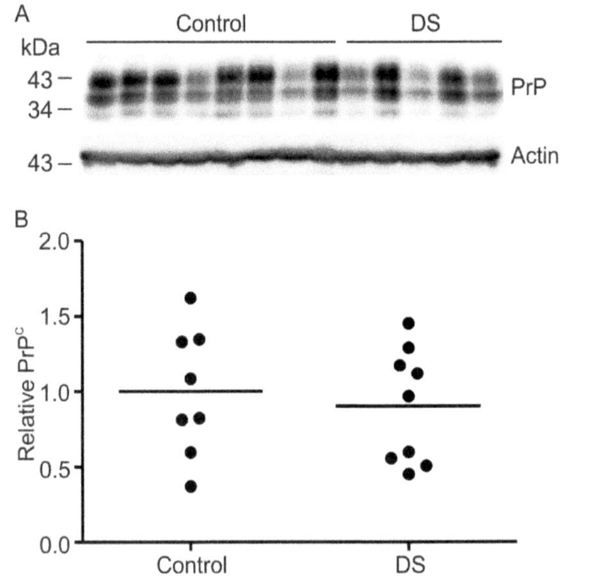

Figure 4. PrP^C is not reduced in DS brains. Representative immunoblots of PrP^C and actin in temporal cortex samples from Down's syndrome patients compared to age-matched controls (A). Densitometric analysis of PrP^C relative to actin levels is represented in grouped scatter plot (B). Line represents mean, *$p<0.05$, n = 8 control group and n = 9 DS group.

ment of AD. In addition, we found a significant inverse correlation between PrP^C and Braak stage, a marker of disease severity or progression. The correlation with Braak stage is likely to be an indirect indicator of the influence of PrP^C on AD progression, as there are no data to support a direct role for PrP^C in preventing neurofibrillary tangle formation. However, taken together these results indicate that PrP^C levels in the brain may be an important factor influencing not only the onset but also the progression of sporadic AD.

Importantly, the correlations extended across the entire cohort (both AD cases and age-matched controls). There was a significant inverse correlation between PrP^C and BACE1 activity, Aβ load, soluble and insoluble Aβ levels and Braak stage, independent of the clinical diagnosis of AD. The symptoms of AD typically progress from mild symptoms of memory loss to severe dementia and it has been suggested that impairment in multiple cognitive domains is observable several years before a clinical diagnosis of AD is made [23]. This observed cognitive dysfunction is not qualitatively different from that seen in normal ageing, and a continuum from normal ageing to preclinical dementia has been proposed [24]. We showed previously that PrP^C decreases with age in the brain [17] and our current data suggest that an inverse correlation between PrP^C and BACE1 activity may anticipate the onset of sporadic AD. Taken together, these findings point towards a decrease in PrP^C in the brain as a primary contributor to the development of disease, at least in some cases of sporadic AD. In addition, the data suggest that the level of PrP^C in the brain may be critical in determining the onset and progression of sporadic AD through its modulation of BACE1 activity.

Down's syndrome (DS) is caused by an extra copy of chromosome 21, which results in developmental abnormalities and also neuropathology in the brain that is similar to that in AD. APP maps to chromosome 21 and trisomy 21 results in increased APP and Aβ production and early plaque formation [20]. Here we demonstrate that the level of PrP^C is unchanged in the cortex in DS, compared to age-matched controls, confirming that the change in PrP^C in sporadic AD is not a secondary consequence of disease. Previous work has implicated the APP intracellular domain (AICD) as a transcription factor regulating PrP^C expression, suggesting that over-expression of APP may increase PrP^C expression [25]. However, in multiple cell lines and two transgenic mouse lines expressing human APP, we could find no evidence for APP-mediated regulation of the expression of PrP^C [26]. Here we have demonstrated that PrP^C is unchanged in brains from DS patients, indicating that the over-expression of APP does not alter PrP^C expression in the human brain. A recent

Table 2. Summary data of the DS and age-matched control samples.

Characteristic	Control (n = 8)	DS (n = 9)	p value
Age (y)	62.63±3.58	59.89±2.18	0.236
PM delay (h)	26.50±6.98	39.22±6.92	0.217
PrP^C protein (arbitrary units)	1.00±0.15	0.90±0.13	0.625
BACE1 activity (relative fluorescence units)	1173.46±75.61	1429.78±98.18	0.061
Soluble Aβ (nM)	4.78±0.42	7.32±1.69	0.179
Insoluble Aβ (nM)	22.38±15.36	288.84±36.82	<0.001

All data are mean ± SEM.

study reported that PrP^C is unchanged in the AD brain [27]. However, while the cohort was well characterised in terms of diagnosis, the authors did not provide any information as to whether the AD cases were familial or sporadic. Previously we reported that PrP^C level was unchanged in the brain in familial AD cases (with mutations in either APP or presenilin-1) [17], indicating that differentiating between the two forms of AD is crucial in evaluating any changes in PrP^C. The decrease in PrP^C protein that we have observed in sporadic AD would be consistent with a recent report of decreased *PRNP* mRNA in AD patients [28].

We have also demonstrated that CNTN5, a protein thought to interact with APP and identified through GWAS [7] as being associated with AD, is unchanged in sporadic AD and does not correlate with Aβ load, soluble Aβ or insoluble Aβ in our cohort. If CNTN5 has a role in the development of AD it appears not to be related to CNTN5 expression level. CNTN5 may, however, contribute to the development of AD without any alteration in its expression level. The subcellular locations of contactin proteins are tightly regulated by their post-translational processing and interactions with contactin-associated proteins [29,30,31]. Cellular trafficking and therefore the subcellular location of CNTN5 may be altered in AD.

Recently, we reported that PrP^C mediates the uptake of extracellular zinc into neuronal cells [32]. Zinc promotes the aggregation of Aβ into toxic oligomeric forms [33] and in an AD mouse model, synaptic zinc was shown to increase insoluble Aβ and its deposition in plaques [34]. In addition, synaptic zinc favours the attachment of Aβ oligomers to the N-methyl-D-aspartate (NMDA) receptor, mediating their excitotoxicity [35]. The reduction in PrP^C in the brain in sporadic AD would be expected to result in decreased zinc uptake. This may result in an increase in the amount of zinc in the synaptic cleft which would promote Aβ aggregation and synaptic targeting, potentially contributing also to the neurodegenerative process in AD.

In conclusion, our data demonstrate that the level of PrP^C is inversely correlated with BACE1 activity and Aβ in the human brain. These findings implicate changes in PrP^C in the pathogenesis of sporadic AD and suggest that modulating PrP^C level may have an impact on the development and course of sporadic AD.

Materials and Methods

Ethics statement

Brain tissue was obtained from the South West Dementia Brain Bank, University of Bristol, UK. The study was conducted with approval from the North Somerset and South Bristol Research Ethics Committee and the Leeds Central Research Ethics Committee.

Study cohorts

All cases had been subjected to detailed neuropathological examination. AD cases had been assessed according to the criteria of the Consortium to Establish a Registry for Alzheimer's Disease (CERAD) [36]. All DS cases had been confirmed genetically. The controls had no history of cognitive decline or dementia, showing the absence of AD (as defined by CERAD) or other neuropathological abnormalities. Total soluble and total guanidine-extracted Aβ levels [37,38], Aβ plaque load [39,40], BACE-1 activity [12,22], and NSE levels [41] had previously been measured in all cases which had also previously been categorised according to the Braak tangle stage [41]. The AD, DS and control groups were matched for post-mortem delay, age-at-death, and gender as presented in Tables 1, 2, S1 and S2.

Tissue Preparation

For measurements of BACE-1 activity, PrP^C protein and NSE, approximately 200 mg of frontal neocortex (Brodmann area 6) was homogenised in 1 ml lysis buffer (0.5% Triton X-100, 20 mM Tris/HCl pH 7.4, 10% (wt/vol) sucrose containing aprotinin (1 μg/ml) and phenylmethane sulfonyl fluoride (PMSF; 10 μM)) (all reagents from Sigma Aldrich, Poole, UK). Brain tissue was homogenized for 30 seconds in a Precellys 24 automated tissue homogenizer (Stretton Scientific, Derbyshire, UK) with 2.3-mm silica beads (Biospec, Thistle Scientific, Glasgow, UK) and total protein was measured using Total Protein kit (Sigma Aldrich). The homogenates were centrifuged at 20 17 *g* for 15 min at 4°C, and aliquots of the supernatant were stored at −80°C until used.

For measurements of Aβ, tissue (200 mg) was allowed to thaw to 4°C, homogenised in 5 volumes (wt: vol) of Tris-buffered saline (TBS) extraction buffer [140 mM NaCl, 3 mM KCl, 25 mM Tris/HCl, pH 7.4, containing 1% Nonidet P-40 (NP40), 5 mM EDTA, 2 mM 1,10-phenanthroline, 10 μM PMSF and 1 μg/ml aprotinin (all reagents from Sigma Aldrich), as detailed in [37,38]. The homogenate was then centrifuged at 20 817 *g* for 15 min at 4 C and the supernatant (soluble fraction) was stored at −80 C until used. The pellet was homogenized in 6.25 M guanidine HCl in 50 mM Tris/HCl, pH 8.0, incubated for 4 h at 25 C and centrifuged at 20 817 *g* for 20 min at 4°C. The resultant supernatant (guanidine-extractable fraction) was stored at −80°C until used.

Immunoblotting of PrP^C and CNTN5

Samples were mixed with an equal volume of SDS dissociation buffer (125 mM Tris/HCl, pH 6.8, 2% (w/v) SDS, 20% (v/v) glycerol, 100 mM dithiothreitol, 0.002% (w/v) bromophenol blue), and boiled for 5 min. Proteins were resolved by SDS polyacrylamide gel electrophoresis using 10% (CNTN5) and

14.5% (PrP^C) polyacrylamide gels. Resolved proteins were transferred to Immobilon P polyvinylidene difluoride membrane (Amersham, Little Chalfont, UK). The membrane was blocked by incubation for 1 h with PBS containing 0.1% (v/v) Tween-20 and 5% (w/v) dried milk powder. Antibody incubations were performed in PBS Tween containing 2% (v/v) bovine serum albumin. Antibody 6D11 (Eurogentec Ltd.) which recognises amino acids 93–109 of human PrP^C was used at 1:5000, antibody AF3030 (R&D Systems, Abingdon, UK) against CNTN5 was used at 1:500 and anti-actin antibody AC15 (Sigma, Poole, UK) was used at 1:5000. Horseradish peroxidase-conjugated secondary antibody was used at 1:4000 in the same buffer. Bound antibody was detected using the enhanced chemiluminescence detection method (Amersham Biosciences, Amersham, UK). Blots were stripped using 100 mM glycine, pH 2.5 for 30 min, blocked by incubation for 1 h with PBS containing 0.1% (v/v) Tween20 and 5% (w/v) dried milk powder, and reprobed using the anti-actin antibody as described above.

Measurement of BACE-1 activity

The fluorogenic substrate (Mca-SEVNLDAEFRK(Dnp)RR-NH_2) containing the Swedish double point mutation of APP (R&D Systems) was used according to the manufacturer's guidelines to measure BACE-1 activity (relative fluorescence units) in brain homogenates as previously reported [12,22]. Each homogenate was assayed in duplicate in the presence and absence of the BACE1 inhibitor III (5 μM) (Millipore, Durham, UK). BACE-1 activity was interpolated from a standard curve generated from serial dilutions of recombinant human BACE-1 after subtraction of the inhibited from the uninhibited value. BACE-1 activity was finally adjusted according to total protein content (measured using the Total Protein Kit; Sigma).

Measurement of total soluble and insoluble (guanidine-extractable) Aβ

The method of ELISA measurement of total soluble and insoluble Aβ was reported previously [37,38]. Soluble and insoluble (guanidine-HCl-extractable) fractions were analysed by sandwich ELISA in which monoclonal anti-Aβ (4G8 clone, raised against amino acids 18–22; Millipore, Watford, UK) was used for the capture step and biotinylated anti-human Aβ monoclonal antibody (10H3 clone) (Thermo Fisher Scientific, Northumberland, UK) for the detection step.

Measurement of neuron-specific enolase

NSE in brain homogenates was measured by a direct ELISA as described previously [41]. Serial dilutions of recombinant human NSE (Biomol, Exeter, UK) were used to construct a best-fit curve, and NSE concentrations were calculated by interpolation. Each sample was assayed in duplicate, and the mean was determined. The NSE concentration was used to provide a proxy measurement of the number of neurons in the tissue samples.

Measurement of Aβ load

Parenchymal Aβ load had previously been measured in all cases [39]. The field fraction (percentage area occupied by Aβ) was measured in an unbiased selection of 10 areas of cortex covering 4 mm^2 with the help of Histometrix software (Kinetic Imaging, Wirral, UK) driving a Leica DM microscope with a motorised stage. Aβ-laden blood vessels were excluded from analysis.

Statistical Analysis

Densitometric analysis was performed using either the advanced image data analyser (AIDA) programme (Raytest Scientific Ltd) or Image J 1.44p (National Institutes of Health, USA). Quantification of PrP^C and CNTN5 was in relation to actin. The distribution of the AD cases compared to their age-matched controls was determined by the Kolmogorov-Smirnov test. Group data were compared using either an Independent T-test for parametric, or a Mann-Whitney U test (with an exact test for ApoE ε4 analysis) for non-parametric data. One-tailed Spearman's rank correlation coefficient was used to assess the correlation of PrP^C and CNTN5 to BACE1 activity, soluble and insoluble Aβ and Braak Stage, $p \leq 0.05$ was considered significant. The data were analysed using the Statistical Package for Social Sciencs (SPSS 17.0) program (Chicago, USA) and GraphPad Prism (version 6) (Graphpad Software Inc , California, USA).

Supporting Information

Figure S1 PrP^C is decreased in Sporadic AD. Densitometric analysis of PrP^C levels relative to actin represented in a grouped scatter plot. Line represents mean, *$p<0.05$, n = 21 control group and n = 24 AD group.

Table S1. Characteristics of the sporadic AD and control subjects used in the study.

Table S2 Characteristics of the Down's syndrome and control subjects used in the study.

Author Contributions

Contributed to finalisation of the submitted manuscript: IJW JSM EBCG PGK SL KABK NMH. Conceived and designed the experiments: IJW JSM EBCG PGK SL NMH. Performed the experiments: IJW JSM EBCG. Analyzed the data: IJW JSM EBCG SL KABK. Wrote the paper: KABK NMH.

References

1. Burns A, Iliffe S (2009) Alzheimer's disease. BMJ 338: b158.
2. Mount C, Downton C (2006) Alzheimer disease: progress or profit? Nat Med 12: 780–784.
3. Iqbal K, Alonso Adel C, Chen S, Chohan MO, El-Akkad E, et al. (2005) Tau pathology in Alzheimer disease and other tauopathies. Biochim Biophys Acta 1739: 198–210.
4. Braak H, Braak E (1991) Neuropathological stageing of Alzheimer-related changes. Acta Neuropathol 82: 239–259.
5. Cras P, Smith MA, Richey PL, Siedlak SL, Mulvihill P, et al. (1995) Extracellular neurofibrillary tangles reflect neuronal loss and provide further evidence of extensive protein cross-linking in Alzheimer disease. Acta Neuropathol 89: 291–295.
6. Bai Y, Markham K, Chen F, Weerasekera R, Watts J, et al. (2008) The in vivo brain interactome of the amyloid precursor protein. Mol Cell Proteom 7: 15–34.
7. Harold D, Abraham R, Hollingworth P, Sims R, Gerrish A, et al. (2009) Genome-wide association study identifies variants at CLU and PICALM associated with Alzheimer's disease. Nat Genet 41: 1088–1093.
8. Biffi A, Anderson CD, Desikan RS, Sabuncu M, Cortellini L, et al. (2010) Genetic variation and neuroimaging measures in Alzheimer disease. Arch Neurol 67: 677–685.
9. Cole SL, Vassar R (2008) The role of amyloid precursor protein processing by BACE1, the beta-secretase, in Alzheimer disease pathophysiology. J Biol Chem 283: 29621–29625.
10. Fukumoto H, Cheung BS, Hyman BT, Irizarry MC (2002) Beta-secretase protein and activity are increased in the neocortex in Alzheimer disease. Arch Neurol 59: 1381–1389.

11. Li R, Lindholm K, Yang LB, Yue X, Citron M, et al. (2004) Amyloid beta peptide load is correlated with increased beta-secretase activity in sporadic Alzheimer's disease patients. Proc Natl Acad Sci USA 101: 3632–3637.
12. Miners JS, van Helmond Z, Kehoe PG, Love S (2010) Changes with age in the activities of beta-secretase and the Abeta-degrading enzymes neprilysin, insulin-degrading enzyme and angiotensin-converting enzyme. Brain Pathol 20: 794–802.
13. He W, Lu Y, Qahwash I, Hu XY, Chang A, et al. (2004) Reticulon family members modulate BACE1 activity and amyloid-beta peptide generation. Nat Med 10: 959–965.
14. Majercak J, Ray WJ, Espeseth A, Simon A, Shi XP, et al. (2006) LRRTM3 promotes processing of amyloid-precursor protein by BACE1 and is a positional candidate gene for late-onset Alzheimer's disease. Proc Natl Acad Sci USA 103: 17967–17972.
15. Parkin ET, Watt NT, Hussain I, Eckman EA, Eckman CB, et al. (2007) Cellular prion protein regulates beta-secretase cleavage of the Alzheimer's amyloid precursor protein. Proc Natl Acad Sci USA 104: 11062–11067.
16. Hooper NM, Turner AJ (2008) A new take on prions: preventing Alzheimer's disease. Trends Biochem Sci 33: 151–155.
17. Whitehouse IJ, Jackson C, Turner AJ, Hooper NM (2010) Prion protein is reduced in aging and in sporadic but not in familial Alzheimer's disease. J Alzheimer's Dis: JAD 22: 1023–1031.
18. Fukumoto H, Rosene DL, Moss MB, Raju S, Hyman BT, et al. (2004) Beta-secretase activity increases with aging in human, monkey, and mouse brain. Am J Pathol 164: 719–725.
19. Griffiths HH, Whitehouse IJ, Baybutt H, Brown D, Kellett KA, et al. (2011) Prion protein interacts with BACE1 protein and differentially regulates its activity toward wild type and Swedish mutant amyloid precursor protein. J Biol Chem 286: 33489–33500.
20. Menendez M (2005) Down syndrome, Alzheimer's disease and seizures. Brain Dev 27: 246–252.
21. Stimson E, Hope J, Chong A, Burlingame AL (1999) Site-specific characterization of the N-linked glycans of murine prion protein by high-performance liquid chromatography/electrospray mass spectrometry and exoglycosidase digestions. Biochem 38: 4885–4895.
22. Miners JS, Morris S, Love S, Kehoe PG (2011) Accumulation of insoluble amyloid-beta in down's syndrome is associated with increased BACE-1 and neprilysin activities. J Alzheimer's Dis 23: 101–108.
23. Matthews FE, McKeith I, Bond J, Brayne C (2007) Reaching the population with dementia drugs: what are the challenges? Int J Ger Psych 22: 627–631.
24. Brayne C (2007) The elephant in the room – healthy brains in later life, epidemiology and public health. Nat Rev Neurosci 8: 233–239.
25. Vincent B, Sunyach C, Orzechowski HD, St George-Hyslop P, Checler F (2009) p53-Dependent transcriptional control of cellular prion by presenilins. J Neurosci 29: 6752–6760.
26. Lewis V, Whitehouse IJ, Baybutt H, Manson JC, Collins SJ, et al. (2012) Cellular prion protein expression is not regulated by the Alzheimer's amyloid precursor protein intracellular domain. PloS one 7: e31754.
27. Saijo E, Scheff SW, Telling GC (2011) Unaltered prion protein expression in Alzheimer disease patients. Prion 5: 109–116.
28. Beyer N, Coulson DT, Heggarty S, Ravid R, Hellemans J, et al. (2012) Zinc Transporter mRNA Levels in Alzheimer's Disease Postmortem Brain. J Alzheimer's Dis 29: 863–873.
29. Peles E, Nativ M, Lustig M, Grumet M, Schilling J, et al. (1997) Identification of a novel contactin-associated transmembrane receptor with multiple domains implicated in protein-protein interactions. EMBO J 16: 978–988.
30. Rios JC, Melendez-Vasquez CV, Einheber S, Lustig M, Grumet M, et al. (2000) Contactin-associated protein (Caspr) and contactin form a complex that is targeted to the paranodal junctions during myelination. J Neurosci 20: 8354–8364.
31. Gollan L, Salomon D, Salzer JL, Peles E (2003) Caspr regulates the processing of contactin and inhibits its binding to neurofascin. J Cell Biol 163: 1213–1218.
32. Watt NT, Taylor DR, Kerrigan TL, Griffiths HH, Rushworth JV, et al. (2012) Prion protein facilitates uptake of zinc into neuronal cells. Nat Ccomm 3: 1134.
33. Bush AI, Pettingell WH, Multhaup G, d Paradis M, Vonsattel JP, et al. (1994) Rapid induction of Alzheimer A beta amyloid formation by zinc. Science 265: 1464–1467.
34. Lee JY, Cole TB, Palmiter RD, Suh SW, Koh JY (2002) Contribution by synaptic zinc to the gender-disparate plaque formation in human Swedish mutant APP transgenic mice. Proc Natl Acad Sci USA 99: 7705–7710.
35. Deshpande A, Kawai H, Metherate R, Glabe CG, Busciglio J (2009) A Role for Synaptic Zinc in Activity-Dependent A{beta} Oligomer Formation and Accumulation at Excitatory Synapses. J Neurosci 29: 4004–4015.
36. Morris JC, Heyman A, Mohs RC, Hughes JP, van Belle G, et al. (1989) The Consortium to Establish a Registry for Alzheimer's Disease (CERAD). Part I. Clinical and neuropsychological assessment of Alzheimer's disease. Neurology 39: 1159–1165.
37. van Helmond Z, Miners JS, Kehoe PG, Love S (2010) Higher soluble amyloid beta concentration in frontal cortex of young adults than in normal elderly or Alzheimer's disease. Brain Pathol 20: 787–793.
38. van Helmond Z, Miners JS, Kehoe PG, Love S (2010) Oligomeric Abeta in Alzheimer's disease: relationship to plaque and tangle pathology, APOE genotype and cerebral amyloid angiopathy. Brain Pathol 20: 468–480.
39. Chalmers K, Wilcock GK, Love S (2003) APOE epsilon 4 influences the pathological phenotype of Alzheimer's disease by favouring cerebrovascular over parenchymal accumulation of A beta protein. Neuropathol Appl Neurobiol 29: 231–238.
40. Ballard CG, Chalmers KA, Todd C, McKeith IG, O'Brien JT, et al. (2007) Cholinesterase inhibitors reduce cortical Abeta in dementia with Lewy bodies. Neurology 68: 1726–1729.
41. Miners JS, Baig S, Tayler H, Kehoe PG, Love S (2009) Neprilysin and insulin-degrading enzyme levels are increased in Alzheimer disease in relation to disease severity. J Neuropathol Expt Neurol 68: 902–914.

Gut Microbiome in Down Syndrome

Elena Biagi[1], Marco Candela[1]*, Manuela Centanni[1], Clarissa Consolandi[2], Simone Rampelli[1], Silvia Turroni[1], Marco Severgnini[2], Clelia Peano[2], Alessandro Ghezzo[3], Maria Scurti[3,4], Stefano Salvioli[3,4], Claudio Franceschi[3,4], Patrizia Brigidi[1]

1 Department of Pharmacy and Biotechnology, University of Bologna, Bologna, Italy, **2** Institute of Biomedical Technologies - Italian National Research Council, Milan, Italy, **3** Department of Experimental, Diagnostic and Specialty Medicine, University of Bologna, Bologna, Italy, **4** Interdepartmental Centre "L. Galvani" (CIG), University of Bologna, Bologna, Italy

Abstract

Background: Premature aging seriously compromises the health status of Down Syndrome (DS) persons. Since human aging has been associated with a deterioration of the gut microbiota (GM)-host mutualism, here we investigated the composition of GM in DS.

Methods: The observational study presented involved 17 adult DS persons. We characterized the GM structure by 454 pyrosequencing of the V4 region of the 16S rRNA gene. DS microbiome was compared with that of age-matched healthy non-trisomic adults enrolled in the same geographic area.

Results and Conclusions: The dominant GM fraction of DS persons showed an overall mutualistic immune-modulatory layout, comparable to that of healthy controls. This makes GM a possible factor counteracting the genetic determined acceleration of immune senescence in DS persons. However, we also found detectable signatures specific for DS among subdominant GM components, such as the increase of *Parasporobacterium* and *Sutterella*. In particular, the abundance of this last microorganism significantly correlated with the Aberrant Behavior Checklist (ABC) total score, allowing us to hypothesize a possible role for this microbial genus in behavioral features in DS.

Editor: Francesco Cappello, University of Palermo, Italy

Funding: The research leading to these results has received funding from the European Union's Seventh Framework Programme (FP7/2007–2011) under grant agreement n. 259679 (IDEAL), and the Italian Ministry of Health, Progetto Ricerca Finalizzata 2008, convenzione 35: "An integrated approach to identify functional, biochemical and genetic markers for diagnostic and prognostic purposes in the elderly, in the centenarians and in people with dementia, Alzheimer's disease, mild cognitive impairment" to CF. The funders had no role in study design, data collection and analysis, decision to publish, or preparation of the manuscript.

Competing Interests: The authors have declared that no competing interests exist.

* Email: marco.candela@unibo.it

Introduction

Resulting from the trisomy of the 21st chromosome, Down Syndrome (DS) represents the most common genetic cause of intellectual disability. The incidence of DS is of 14.47 per 10,000 live births, with higher incidence for increasing maternal age [1]. Even if lifespan of persons with DS is significantly increased in the past decades - from 12 years of age in the 1940s to a mean life expectancy of 60 years today – DS persons exhibit sign of premature aging [2]. Thus, the overall increase in life expectancy in DS comes with a parallel increase of risk for age-related diseases, such as Alzheimer's disease, increased rate of infections, hypertension and obesity [3,4]. This results in a considerable need of medical, rehabilitative and social services, as well as a compromised health status and premature death.

The acceleration of biological aging in DS principally involves the increase in the oxidative stress [5], as well as a premature immunosenescence in the immune system [6]. In particular, adult DS persons show typical signs of immunosenescence which are normally found in much older non-trisomic individuals, including alterations of B and T cell subpopulations [7,8], and they have higher local inflammation with respect to age-matched non-trisomic subjects [9,10]; however it is not clear whether DS is characterized by the age-related increase of pro-inflammatory status - known as inflamm-aging - found in the elderly [11–13].

Human aging and immunosenescence are accompanied by a deterioration of the mutualistic relationship with the gut microbiota (GM) [14–16]. Encompassing the reduction of key immunomodulating groups as members of the butyrate producers *Clostridium* clusters IV and XIVa [17], and the concomitant increase of pro-inflammatory pathobionts [18], age-dependent GM dysbioses result in an overall pro-inflammatory configuration of the ecosystem capable to boost a self-sustained pro-inflammatory loop favoring immunosenescence [14]. In this context, we investigated - to our knowledge for the first time - the GM structure in DS persons, under the hypothesis that the GM structure of these subjects could present alterations typical of an aged-type microbiota which favors immunosenescence.

Autism Spectrum Disorder (ASD) features are also quite common in DS persons, among which behavioral problems are prominent [19]. In particular, higher total score of the Aberrant

Behavior Checklist (ABC), a rating scale specifically designed for individuals with severe intellectual disability [20], occurs in DS persons with ASD [21]. Since in recent years an association between ASD and specific GM genera has been outlined [22,23], the characterization of the GM ecosystem in DS persons allows us to further explore the association between GM and ASD.

Here we characterized the GM structure in 17 adult DS persons by 454 pyrosequencing of the V4 region of the 16S rRNA gene. In order to highlight deviations from a healthy-like GM structure, the gut microbial ecosystem of DS was compared with the previously published GM profiles of 16 age-matching healthy adults [24]. Furthermore, in order to look for any alterations of the DS microbiota ecosystem towards an aged-type configuration, a GM meta-analysis also including elderly and centenarians from Rampelli *et al.* [25] was performed. According to our data, the dominant GM fraction of DS persons showed an overall immune-modulatory layout, comparable to that of healthy adults. However, signatures specific for DS gut microbiome were detectable among the subdominant GM components and associated with the ABC total score. This suggests that such components are correlated to behavioral features in DS as already demonstrated in subjects with diagnosed ASD.

Materials and Methods

Subject enrolment and sample collection

Persons with DS were enrolled prospectively from 2008, in the framework of an open-label study on DS. The study was approved by the local Ethics Committee (S. Orsola Hospital, University of Bologna; ethical clearance #126/2007/U/Tess, released on December 18, 2007). A written informed consent to participate to the study was obtained from DS persons and from their parents or relatives (brothers/sisters). DS persons were recruited with the help of CEPS, OPIMM and ANFFAS, three local non-profit associations dealing with DS persons operating in the eastern part of Emilia-Romagna Region (Bologna and Ferrara provinces). Participation to the study was totally on a voluntary basis, with no reward for the participants or their families. A standard questionnaire to collect information regarding the health status, drugs use, clinical anamnesis, and lifestyle was administered. In order to take account of the dietary habits of DS persons, 24-hour dietary recalls were provided for each of the enrolled subjects for 3 days. Subjects affected by malignant neoplasia and/or in therapy with immunosuppressive drugs like cyclosporin, methotrexate, glucorticoids, anticoagulant drugs, and who recently (at one month) used antibiotics and/or probiotics were excluded from the study. Stool samples from 17 adult DS persons randomly selected from this group were used for this study. Feces were collected and stored at −80°C and analyses were performed within 3 months.

Neuropsychiatric assessment and adaptive behavior assessment

The cognitive level of 13 DS persons was evaluated with Wechsler Scale and resulted to be within the range of Cognitive Impairment (IQ scores below 70), as expected. For the remaining 4 DS persons, the cognitive level was assessed by using the mental age values extrapolated from VABS (see below). DS persons were classified within 4 levels of Cognitive Impairment (mild, moderate, severe and profound) according to DSM IV criteria.

For neuropsychiatric assessment, the ABC (Aberrant Behavior Checklist) [20] test was used. The italian version of ABC was used during verbal interview to care givers (parents and/or siblings, or educational personnel in one case). ABC is a 58-item caregiver report checklist that assesses maladaptive behaviors in individuals with developmental disabilities using a simple four-point rating scale (0–3) with higher scores reflecting more problems. ABC items are grouped into five subscales: (1) Irritability, Agitation, Crying, (2) Lethargy, social withdrawal, (3) Stereotypic behavior, (4) Hyperactivity, non-compliance, and (5) Inappropriate speech.

For adaptive behavior assessment, the Vineland Adaptive Behavior Scales (VABS) [26,27] were used. The test assesses personal autonomy and social responsibility of individuals from birth to adulthood through questions designed to assess the skills actually possessed by the subject at the time of evaluation. The scales are used with both non-disabled and disabled persons. The questionnaire in its complete form consists of 540 items that include the following areas: communication, daily living skills, socialization, motor skills. The questionnaire was directly administered to parents, or whoever takes care of the DS person.

Microbial DNA extraction from feces

Total bacterial DNA from fecal material was extracted using QIAamp DNA Stool Mini Kit (QIAGEN) with a modified protocol [28]. Briefly, 250 milligrams of feces were suspended in 1 mL of lysis buffer (500 mM NaCl, 50 mM Tris-HCl pH 8, 50 mM EDTA, 4% SDS). Four 3-mm glass beads and 0.5 g of 0.1-mm zirconia beads (BioSpec Products) were added, and the samples were treated in FastPrep (MP Biomedicals) at 5.5 movements per second for 1 min for 3 times, with 5-min intervals in ice. Samples were heated at 95°C for 15 min, then centrifuged for 5 min at full speed to pellet stool particles. Supernatants were collected and 260 µL of 10 M ammonium acetate was added, incubated in ice for 5 min and centrifuged at full speed for 10 min. One volume of isopropanol was added to each sample and incubated in ice for 30 min. The precipitated nucleic acids were collected by centrifugation for 15 min at full speed and washed with 70% ethanol. Pellets were resuspended in 100 µL of TE buffer and treated with 2 µL of DNase-free RNase (10 mg/mL) at 37°C for 15 min. Proteins were removed by proteinase K treatment, and DNA was subsequently purified following the manufacturer's instructions. Final DNA concentration was measured by using NanoDrop ND-1000 (NanoDrop Technologies).

16S rRNA gene amplification

For the amplification of the V4 region of the 16S rRNA gene the primer set 520F (5′-AYTGGGYDTAAAGNG-3′) and 802R (5′-TACNVGGGTATCTAATCC-3′) (with Y = C/T, D = A/G/T, N = any base, V = A/C/G) [29] was utilized. Primers included at their 5′ end the adaptor sequence used in the 454-sequencing library preparation protocol, linked to a unique MID tag barcode of 10 bases that allowed the identification of the different samples. PCR mixtures contained 0.5 µM of each forward and reverse primer, 100 ng of template DNA, 2.5 U of GoTaq Flexi Polymerase (Promega), 200 µM of dNTPs and 2 mM of $MgCl_2$ in a final volume of 50 µL. Samples were initially denatured at 95°C for 5 min, followed by 35 cycles of 94°C for 50 s, 40°C for 30 s, and 72°C for 60 s, with a final extension step at 72°C for 5 min [24]. PCR amplifications were carried out in a Biometra Thermal Cycler T Gradient (Biometra).

Pyrosequencing

16S rRNA gene V4 hypervariable region amplicons were purified using MinElute PCR Purification Kit (QIAGEN) and quantified using the Quant-iT PicoGreen dsDNA Kit (Invitrogen). Amplicons were pooled in equal amounts (creating one 9-plex and one 8-plex pools) and again purified by 454-Roche Double Ampure size selection protocol with Agencourt AMPure XP DNA purification beads (Beckman Coulter Genomics GmbH) to remove

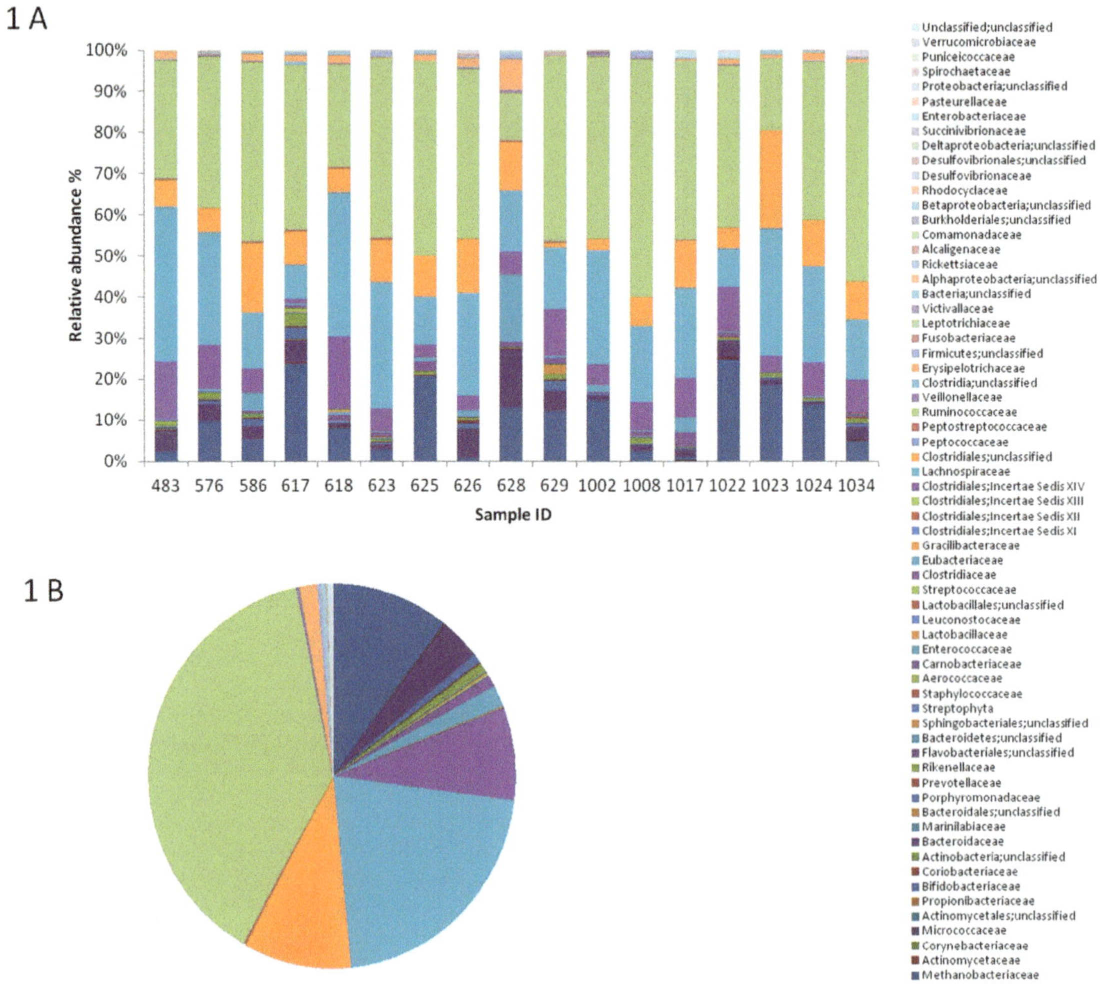

Figure 1. Individual (A) and average (B) gut microbiota profiles of the enrolled DS persons. Relative abundance of family-level assigned OTUs is reported. Colors were assigned for all families detected.

primer dimers, according to the manufacturer's instructions (454 LifeSciences, Roche). Before emulsion PCR, the purified amplicon pools were quantified using a quantitative Real Time PCR (qPCR) by KAPA Library Quant Kits (KAPA Biosystems). Afterwards pools were fixed to microbeads to be clonally amplified by emulsion PCR following the GS-FLX protocol Titanium emPCR LIB-A (454 LifeSciences, Roche). Beads were enriched in order to keep only those carrying identical PCR products on their surface, and loaded onto a picotiter plate for pyrosequencing reactions, following the GS-FLX Titanium sequencing protocol. Each pool was sequenced in one eighth of a plate. Amplicon sequences were deposited in MG-RAST under the project ID 10557 (http://metagenomics.anl.gov/linkin.cgi?project=10557).

Bioinformatic analysis and statistical data analysis

Sequencing reads were analyzed using the QIIME pipeline as described previously [24]. Briefly, V4 sequences were filtered according to the following criteria: (i) read length not shorter than 150 bp and not longer than 350 bp; (ii) no ambiguous bases (Ns); (iii) a minimum average quality score over a 50-bp rolling window of 25; (iv) exact match to primer sequences and maximum 1 error in barcode tags. RDP-classifier (version 2.2) with 50% as confidence value threshold was used for bacterial taxonomy assignment. Trimmed reads were clustered into OTUs at 97% identity level and further filtered for chimeric sequences using ChimeraSlayer (http://microbiomeutil.sourceforge.net/#A_CS). Alpha-diversity and rarefaction plots were computed using Shannon, PD whole tree, Chao1 and observed species metrics. Weighted and unweighted UniFrac distances were used to perform Principal Coordinates Analysis (PCoA). PCoA and heatmap were built using R packages Made4 [30], and Vegan (http://cran.r-project.org/package=vegan).

The R packages Stats and Vegan were used to perform statistical analysis. In particular, to compare the GM structure between DS persons and healthy adults, Wilcoxon signed rank test was used. Data separation in the PCoA was tested using a permutation test with pseudo F-ratios (function Adonis in the Vegan package). Significant differences in phylum- or genus-level abundance between DS persons and healthy controls were assessed by Mann-Whitney U tests, and corrected for multiple comparisons using the Benjamini-Hochberg method when appropriate. PCoA of the Euclidean distances of GM genera between DS persons, 16 healthy Italian adults from Schnorr *et al.* [24], and 5 elderly and 3 centenarians from Rampelli *et al.* [25] was carried out by using Vegan. The Kendall correlation test between ABC score and the relative abundance of genera in DS microbiome was

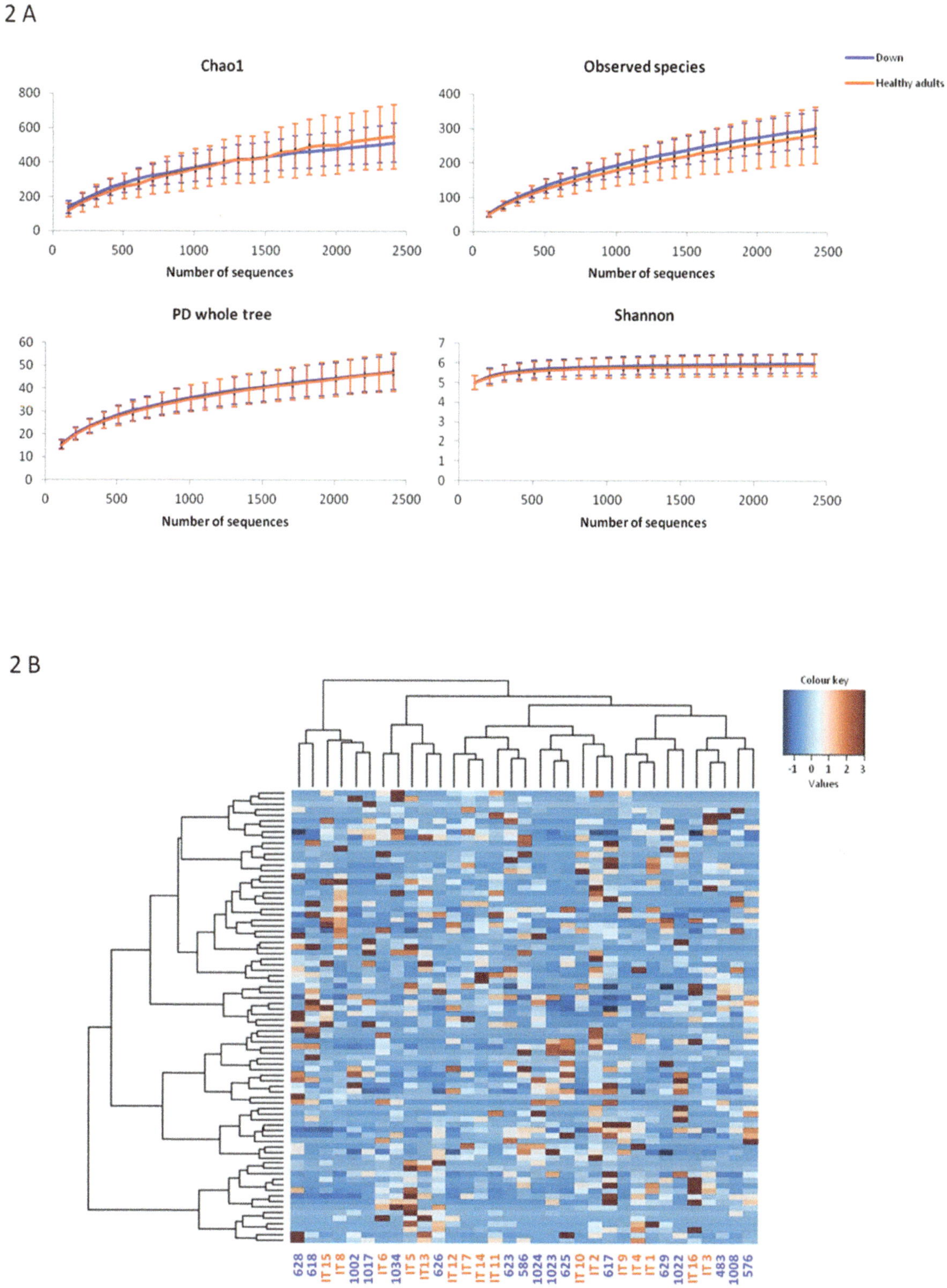

Figure 2. Similarity between the gut microbiota of DS persons and healthy non-trisomic adults for diversity and overall community composition. (A) Superimposition of the rarefaction curves of different α-diversity metrics (Faith's phylogenetic diversity (PD whole tree), observed OTUs, the Chao1 measure of microbial richness, and the Shannon index of biodiversity). (B) Hierarchical Ward-linkage clustering based on the Spearman correlation coefficients of genus proportion, showing no separation between DS persons and healthy adults. Blue, DS persons; red, healthy adults [24].

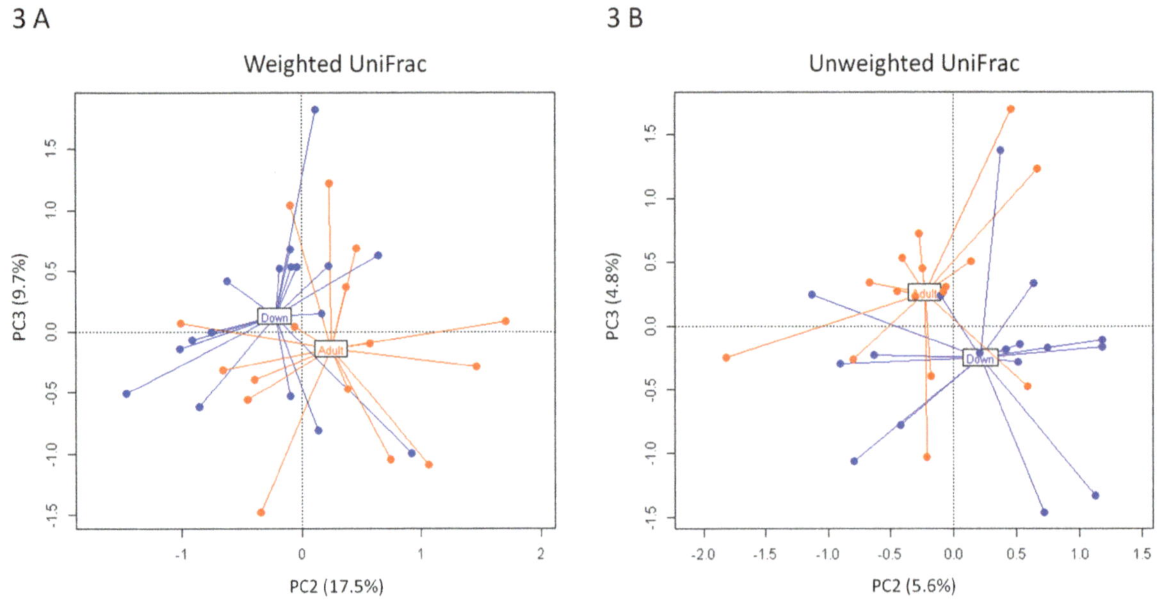

Figure 3. Weighted (A) and unweighted (B) UniFrac distance PCoA of the fecal microbiota of DS persons and healthy non-trisomic adults. Percentage of variance in the dataset shown by the second and third principal component (PC) is reported. Blue, DS persons; red, healthy adults [24].

achieved using function cor.test of the R package Stats. In all statistical tests, $P<0.05$ was considered as statistically significant.

Results

Intestinal microbiota in DS persons

Seventeen adult DS persons (19–35 years, 7 males and 10 females) randomly selected from a larger cohort participated to this study. The main characteristics of these subjects are provided in Table S1. As expected, they were in general overweight (mean BMI 27.05), while problems in alvus or eating were reported for 7 out of 17 subjects (41%). Stools were collected and GM structure was characterized by means of pyrosequencing of the V4 region of the bacterial 16S rRNA gene (Figure 1A). A total of 67,029 high-quality reads were obtained with a mean of 3,943 reads per subject. Reads were clustered in 7,457 operational taxonomic units at 97% of identity. OTU rarefaction curves based on number of unique OTUs were obtained with different phylogenetic diversity metrics, such as Shannon, Chao1, PD whole tree and observed species; curves reached the plateau, approximating the saturation level, after 2,400 reads (see Figure S1).

According to our data, the GM of DS persons was largely dominated by Firmicutes (relative abundance (rel. ab.) 83%±2), Actinobacteria (rel. ab. 9%±1.6) and Bacteroidetes (rel. ab. 8%±1.8). With rel. ab. values below 5%, Proteobacteria, Verrucomicrobia and Fusobacteria were largely subdominant phyla. The most represented families in DS gut microbial communities were *Ruminococcaceae* (rel. ab. 39%±3), *Lachnospiraceae* (rel. ab. 20%±1.4), *Clostridiales* (rel. ab. 9%±1), *Clostridiales Incertae Sedis XIV* (rel. ab. 8%±1.2), *Bifidobacteriaceae* (rel. ab. 8%±1.5) and *Bacteroidaceae* (rel. ab. 5%±1.4) (Figure 1B). Subdominant families showing rel. ab. values below 5% were *Eubacterium*, *Porphyromonadaceae*, *Rikenellaceae*, *Erysipelotrichaceae*, *Veillonellaceae*, *Alcaligenaceae*, and *Verrucomicrobiaceae*.

No separation of the DS microbiota structure according to BMI [31] was found ($P>0.05$) (see Figure S2).

Comparison between GM communities in DS persons and healthy non-trisomic adults

In order to highlight possible GM signatures of DS, the microbiota structure from the 17 DS persons enrolled in the present study was compared with that previously published from 16 healthy young adults aged between 20 and 40 years [24]. To exclude any country- and age-related effect on microbiota structure, as well as biases due to a study effect [32], age-matched Italian adults were selected for comparison. Both DS persons (see Table S2) and healthy adults [24] adhered to the standard Mediterranean diet, abundant in plant foods, fruit, pasta, bread and olive oil, and low-to-moderate in dairy and red meat.

According to our data, DS persons and healthy adults showed comparable levels of GM diversity and an overall similarity in the composition of the GM community (Figure 2). The visualization of community structures using PCoA of weighted UniFrac distances showed only a weak segregation between the two groups ($P=0.28$), confirming the overall similarity of the two GM ecosystems (Figure 3A). However, the PCoA of unweighted UniFrac distances tended to separate the two subject groups (Figure 3B) ($P=0.09$). This suggests that GM differences between DS persons and healthy controls principally involved subdominant GM components. Indeed, within the dominant GM families no significant differences in rel. ab. between the two groups of subjects were detected. Differently, DS persons were characterized by a higher abundance in several subdominant GM genera, such as *Parasporobacterium* ($P=0.036$) and *Sutterella* ($P=0.012$), as well as by a reduction in the rel. ab. of the family *Veillonellaceae* ($P=0.005$).

In order to explore possible alterations of the GM of DS persons matching an aged-type ecosystem, we performed a meta-analysis of the GM structure also including 5 healthy Italian elderly and 3 centenarians from Rampelli *et al.* [25]. The PCoA of the Euclidean distances of the genus-level GM composition in DS persons, healthy adults, elderly (mean age 66.4 years) and centenarians (mean age 100.7 years) is provided as Figure S3.

Data shows that DS persons and heathy adults segregate together, suggesting that the gut microbial ecosystem of DS persons does not show the typical deviations of an aged-type gut microbial community.

Correlation between ABC score and signature genera of DS microbiome

Since microbiota dysbioses have been recently associated with certain neuro-behavioral disorders [33], here we sought Kendall correlations between ABC or VABS total score in DS persons and the three GM groups characterizing DS microbiome: *Parasporobacterium*, *Sutterella* and *Veillonellaceae*. The values of ABC and VABS scores for the enrolled DS persons are reported in Table S3. While no significant correlations were found between signature DS microorganisms and VABS score, which is indicative of the adaptive behavior of DS persons, *Sutterella* was positively correlated with the ABC total score ($tau = 0.40$, $P < 0.05$). On the other hand, no correlation was found between ABC and *Parasporobacterium* as well as *Veillonellaceae*.

Discussion

Hypothesizing that the layout of the GM in DS persons could be of some relevance for their health, here we investigated the GM structure of 17 DS persons. In order to highlight signatures of an aged-type microbiota in DS, the GM profile of DS persons was compared with that of age-matched healthy non-trisomic Italian adults, and healthy Italian elderly and centenarians. According to our finding, DS persons and healthy adults possessed a similar complement of dominant groups in the GM, showing an overall healthy-like microbiota profile without any signs of premature microbiota aging [34].

The GM of DS persons was found to be well forged to provide the host with short-chain fatty acids (SCFA), butyrate, propionate and acetate, from fermentation of indigestible polysaccharides in the gut. Indeed, DS microbiota was largely dominated by the butyrate producers *Ruminococcaceae* (*Clostridium* cluster IV) and *Lachnospiraceae* (*Clostridium* cluster XIVa) [35], propionate-producing Bacteroidetes [36], and the acetate producer *Bifidobacterium* [37,38]. SCFA are pivotal metabolites in the microbiota-host immunological cross-talk, and their specific role as immune system modulators has been recently proved. In particular, butyrate is crucial to promote the extrathymic differentiation of regulatory T cells (Treg), whereas acetate is functional to drive their accumulation in the colon. Propionate exerts a dual function, capable to boost peripheral Treg generation and subsequent homing in the colon [39]. Thus, it is tempting to speculate that - by providing the host with SCFA from dietary polysaccharides - the gut microbiome of DS persons could be strategic to counteract the pro-inflammatory immune defects driving to immunosenescence [40]. This could explain why signs of premature immunosenescence found at the level of lymphocyte subpopulations (decreased B cells and T cells, in particular CD8+ T cells, and increased NK cells) are not apparently paralleled by the other major event of immunosenescence, *i.e.* the increased level of pro-inflammatory molecules. In any case, due to the limited number of DS persons enrolled in the present study, these assumptions need to be taken with extreme caution. Moreover, it is to note that the relatively young age of the subjects studied here (max 35 years) does not allow us to exclude that later on this event takes place anyway. Thus, further studies enrolling more DS persons and including older subjects are needed to prove these hypotheses, however, should it turn to be confirmed, it will make GM a strategic factor to counteract the genetically determined acceleration of the process of immunosenescence of DS persons. Within this context, it will become of extreme relevance to control diet in DS persons, supporting the maintenance of their healthy profile of the dominant GM. For instance, the consumption of a fiber-containing diet, which favors immunomodulating GM actors as *Clostridium* clusters IV and XIVa [41], should be encouraged.

While the general GM structure of DS persons was comparable to the one of healthy subjects, we observed significant differences among the subdominant groups. In particular, according to our findings, DS persons were enriched in *Parasporobacterium* and *Sutterella*, and reduced in *Veillonellaceae*. The increase of *Sutterella* and the reduction of *Veillonellaceae* have been described in autistic children with gastrointestinal symptoms [22,23,42]. In our study, the abundance of *Sutterella* in the GM was positively correlated with the ABC total score in DS persons, suggesting a possible link between this microorganism and ASD in DS [21,43]. As a Gram-negative opportunistic pathogen, *Sutterella* has been proposed to aggravate ASD through LPS-induced inflammation in the brain [44]. Conversely, the connection between *Veillonellaceae* and autistic symptoms was apparently less obvious. However, according to Kang *et al.* [42], the reduction of this group in the gut was more closely linked to the presence of autistic symptoms, rather than to the severity of gastrointestinal symptoms or the specific dietary regimen.

The correlation between the relative abundance of *Sutterella* in the GM and ABC total score in DS persons further strengthens the hypothesis in favor of a possible role for this gut microorganism in maladaptive behavior, opening the way to further investigation on the role of GM dysbioses in adults with ASD.

Supporting Information

Figure S1 Alpha-diversity rarefaction curves for the 16S rRNA V4 region pyrosequencing reads. The OTU table was rarefied up to 2,500 reads per sample and analyzed using various diversity metrics for each enrolled DS person. Metrics used were the Chao1 index of microbial richness, observed species, Faith's phylogenetic diversity index (PD whole tree), and the Shannon index of biodiversity. The individual rarefaction curves are color-coded according to the list of DS persons on the right.

Figure S2 PCoA of the unweighted Unifrac distances of the fecal microbiota of DS persons grouped according to body mass index (BMI). The BMI cutoff point of ≥ 25 kg/m^2 for overweight was used [31]. Green, BMI <25 kg/m^2; yellow, BMI ≥ 25 kg/m^2.

Figure S3 PCoA of the fecal microbiota in DS persons, healthy adults, elderly and centenarians. PCoA was based on the Euclidean distances of the relative abundance of gut microbiota genera in DS persons from the present study (green), healthy adults from Schnorr *et al.* [24] (blue), healthy elderly (red) and centenarians from Rampelli *et al.* [25] (orange).

Table S1 Demographic and clinical features of the enrolled Down Syndrome persons.

Table S2 Percent contribution of food categories to the diet of Down Syndrome persons.

Table S3 Level of cognitive impairment, Aberrant Behavior Checklist (ABC) and Vineland Adaptive Behavior Scale (VABS) scores in the enrolled Down Syndrome persons.

Acknowledgments

The authors are grateful to "ANFFAS", "CEPS" and "OPIMM" no-profit associations and all the DS persons and their families who participated to the study. The authors also acknowledge Dr. Daniela Follo for her precious contribution in contacting DS persons' families.

Author Contributions

Conceived and designed the experiments: CF PB. Performed the experiments: EB M. Centanni CC CP SS AG M. Scurti. Analyzed the data: SR M. Candela M. Severgnini. Contributed reagents/materials/analysis tools: CF PB. Contributed to the writing of the manuscript: M. Candela SS EB ST.

References

1. Parker SE, Mai CT, Canfield MA, Rickard R, Wang Y, et al; National Birth Defects Prevention Network (2010) Updated National Birth Prevalence estimates for selected birth defects in the United States, 2004–2006. Birth Defects Res A Clin Mol Teratol 88(12): 1008–1116.
2. Zigman WB (2013) Atypical aging in Down syndrome. Dev Disabil Res Rev 18(1): 51–67.
3. Nakamura E, Tanaka S (1998) Biological ages of adult men and women with Down's syndrome and its changes with aging. Mech Ageing Dev 105(1–2): 89–103.
4. Bittles AH, Glasson EJ (2004) Clinical, social, and ethical implications of changing life expectancy in Down syndrome. Dev Med Child Neurol 46(4): 282–286.
5. Patterson D, Cabelof DC (2012) Down syndrome as a model of DNA polymerase beta haploinsufficiency and accelerated aging. Mech Ageing Dev 133(4): 133–137.
6. Trotta MB, Serro Azul JB, Wajngarten M, Fonseca SG, Goldberg AC, et al. (2011) Inflammatory and Immunological parameters in adults with Down syndrome. Immun Ageing 8(1): 4.
7. Cossarizza A, Monti D, Montagnani G, Ortolani C, Masi M, et al. (1990) Precocious aging of the immune system in Down syndrome: alteration of B lymphocytes, T-lymphocyte subsets, and cells with natural killer markers. Am J Med Genet Suppl 7: 213–218.
8. Cossarizza A, Ortolani C, Forti E, Montagnani G, Paganelli R, et al. (1991) Age-related expansion of functionally inefficient cells with markers of natural killer activity in Down's syndrome. Blood 77(6): 1263–1270.
9. Griffin WS, Stanley LC, Ling C, White L, MacLeod V, et al. (1989) Brain interleukin 1 and S-100 immunoreactivity are elevated in Down syndrome and Alzheimer disease. Proc Natl Acad Sci U S A 86(19): 7611–7615.
10. Broers CJ, Gemke RJ, Weijerman ME, van der Sluijs KF, van Furth AM (2012) Increased pro-inflammatory cytokine production in Down Syndrome children upon stimulation with live influenza A virus. J Clin Immunol 32(2): 323–329.
11. Franceschi C, Bonafè M, Valensin S, Olivieri F, De Luca M, et al. (2000) Inflamm-aging. An evolutionary perspective on immunosenescence. Ann N Y Acad Sci 908: 244–254.
12. Franceschi C, Capri M, Monti D, Giunta S, Olivieri F, et al. (2007) Inflammaging and anti-inflammaging: a systemic perspective on aging and longevity emerged from studies in humans. Mech Ageing Dev 128(1): 92–105.
13. Franceschi C, Campisi J (2014) Chronic inflammation (inflammaging) and its potential contribution to age-associated diseases. J Gerontol A Biol Sci Med Sci (Suppl 1): S4–S9.
14. Biagi E, Nylund L, Candela M, Ostan R, Bucci L, et al. (2010) Through ageing, and beyond: gut microbiota and inflammatory status in seniors and centenarians. PLoS One 5(5): e10667.
15. Biagi E, Candela M, Franceschi C, Brigidi P (2011) The aging gut microbiota: new perspectives. Ageing Res Rev 10(4): 428–429.
16. Biagi E, Candela M, Turroni S, Garagnani P, Franceschi C, et al. (2013) Ageing and gut microbes: perspectives for health maintenance and longevity. Pharmacol Res 69(1): 11–20.
17. Atarashi K, Tanoue T, Oshima K, Suda W, Nagano Y, et al. (2013) Treg induction by a rationally selected mixture of Clostridia strains from the human microbiota. Nature 500(7461): 232–236.
18. Kamada N, Chen GY, Inohara N, Núñez G (2013) Control of pathogens and pathobionts by the gut microbiota. Nat Immunol 14(7): 685–690.
19. Roizen NJ, Patterson D (2003) Down's syndrome. Lancet 361(9365): 1281–1289.
20. Aman MG, Singh NN, Stewart AW, Field CJ (1985) The aberrant behavior checklist: a behavior rating scale for the assessment of treatment effects. Am J Ment Defic 89: 485–491.
21. Ji NY, Capone GT, Kaufmann WE (2011) Autism spectrum disorder in Down syndrome: cluster analysis of Aberrant Behaviour Checklist data supports diagnosis. J Intellect Disabil Res 55(11): 1064–1077.
22. Williams BL, Hornig M, Parekh T, Lipkin WI (2012) Application of novel PCR-based methods for detection, quantitation, and phylogenetic characterization of Sutterella species in intestinal biopsy samples from children with autism and gastrointestinal disturbances. MBio 3(1). pii: e00261-11.
23. Wang L, Christophersen CT, Sorich MJ, Gerber JP, Angley MT, et al. (2013) Increased abundance of Sutterella spp. and Ruminococcus torques in feces of children with autism spectrum disorder. Mol Autism 4(1): 42.
24. Schnorr SL, Candela M, Rampelli S, Centanni M, Consolandi C, et al. (2014) Gut microbiome of the Hadza hunter-gatherers. Nat Commun 5: 3654.
25. Rampelli S, Candela M, Turroni S, Biagi E, Collino S, et al. (2013) Functional metagenomic profiling of intestinal microbiome in extreme ageing. Aging (Albany NY) 5: 902–912.
26. Sparrow SS, Balla DA, Cicchetti DV (1984) Vineland adaptive behavior scales. Circles Pines, MN: American Guidance Service.
27. Balboni G, Pedrabissi L (2003) Adattamento italiano delle Vineland Adaptive Behavior Scales. Firenze: O.S. Organizzazioni Speciali.
28. Salonen A, Nikkilä J, Jalanka-Tuovinen J, Immonen O, Rajilić-Stojanović M, et al. (2010) Comparative analysis of fecal DNA extraction methods with phylogenetic microarray: effective recovery of bacterial and archaeal DNA using mechanical cell lysis. J Microbiol Methods 81(2): 127–134.
29. Claesson MJ, O'Sullivan O, Wang Q, Nikkila J, Marchesi JR, et al. (2009) Comparative analysis of pyrosequencing and a phylogenetic microarray for exploring microbial community structures in the human distal intestine. PLoS One 4(8): e6669.
30. Culhane AC, Thioulouse J, Perrière G, Higgins DG (2005) MADE4: an R package for multivariate analysis of gene expression data. Bioinformatics 21: 2789–2790.
31. Physical Status: the use and interpretation of anthropometry. Report of a WHO Expert Committee. (1995) World Health Organ Tech Rep Ser 854: 1–452.
32. Lozupone CA, Stombaugh J, Gonzalez A, Ackermann G, Wendel D, et al. (2013) Meta-analyses of studies of the human microbiota. Genome Res 23(10): 1704–1714.
33. Benach JL, Li E, McGovern MM (2012) A microbial association with autism. MBio 14: 3(1).
34. Biagi E, Candela M, Fairweather-Tait S, Franceschi C, Brigidi P (2012) Aging of the human metaorganism: the microbial counterpart. Age (Dordr) 34(1): 247–267.
35. Flint HJ, Bayer EA, Rincon MT, Lamed R, White BA (2008) Polysaccharide utilization by gut bacteria: potential for new insights from genomic analysis. Nat Rev Microbiol 6(2): 121–131.
36. Fischbach MA, Sonnenburg JL (2011) Eating for two: how metabolism establishes interspecies interactions in the gut. Cell Host Microbe 10(4): 336–347.
37. Fukuda S, Toh H, Hase K, Oshima K, Nakanishi Y, et al. (2011) Bifidobacteria can protect from enteropathogenic infection through production of acetate. Nature 469(7331): 543–547.
38. Fanning S, Hall LJ, Cronin M, Zomer A, MacSharry J, et al. (2012) Bifidobacterial surface-exopolysaccharide facilitates commensal-host interaction through immune modulation and pathogen protection. Proc Natl Acad Sci U S A 109(6): 2108–2113.
39. Arpaia N, Campbell C, Fan X, Dikiy S, van der Veeken J, et al. (2013) Metabolites produced by commensal bacteria promote peripheral regulatory T-cell generation. Nature 504(7480): 451–455.
40. Li C, Jin L, Bai Y, Chen Q, Fu L, et al. (2012) Genome-wide expression analysis in Down syndrome: insight into immunodeficiency. PLoS One 7(11): e49130.
41. David LA, Maurice CF, Carmody RN, Gootenberg DB, Button JE, et al. (2014) Diet rapidly and reproducibly alters the human gut microbiome. Nature 505(7484): 559–563.
42. Kang DW, Park JG, Ilhan ZE, Wallstrom G, Labaer J, et al. (2013) Reduced incidence of Prevotella and other fermenters in intestinal microflora of autistic children. PLoS One 8(7): e68322.
43. Carter JC, Capone GT, Gray RM, Cox CS, Kaufmann WE (2007) Autistic-spectrum disorders in Down syndrome: further delineation and distinction from other behavioral abnormalities. Am J Med Genet B Neuropsychiatr Genet 144B (1): 87–94.
44. Adams JB, Romdalvik J, Levine KE, Hu LW (2008) Mercury in first-cut baby hair of children with autism versus typically-developing children. Toxicol Environ Chem 90: 739–753.

The Feasibility Study of Non-Invasive Fetal Trisomy 18 and 21 Detection with Semiconductor Sequencing Platform

Young Joo Jeon[1,2◆], Yulin Zhou[3◆], Yihan Li[4◆], Qiwei Guo[3], Jinchun Chen[4], Shengmao Quan[5], Ahong Zhang[5], Hailing Zheng[5], Xingqiang Zhu[5], Jin Lin[5], Huan Xu[5], Ayang Wu[6], Sin-Gi Park[1,2], Byung Chul Kim[7,8], Hee Jae Joo[1,2], Hongliang Chen[5]*, Jong Bhak[1,2,8,9]*

1 TheragenEtex Bio Institute, Suwon, Republic of Korea, **2** Genome Care, Seoul, South Korea, **3** Molecular Diagnostics Laboratory, Department of Medical Genetics, Prenatal Diagnosis Center, Xiamen Maternal and Child Health Hospital, Xiamen, Fujian, China, **4** Xiamen Hospital of Traditional Chinese Medicine, Fujian University of Traditional Chinese Medicine, Xiamen, Fujian, China, **5** Xiamen Vangenes BioTech, Xiamen, Fujian, China, **6** Zhangzhou Affiliated Hospital of Fujian Medical University, Zhangzhou, Fujian, China, **7** Clinomics, Ulsan, Republic of Korea, **8** Personal Genomics Institute, Genome Research Foundation, Suwon, Republic of Korea, **9** BioMedical Engineering, UNIST, Ulsan, Republic of Korea

Abstract

Objective: Recent non-invasive prenatal testing (NIPT) technologies are based on next-generation sequencing (NGS). NGS allows rapid and effective clinical diagnoses to be determined with two common sequencing systems: Illumina and Ion Torrent platforms. The majority of NIPT technology is associated with Illumina platform. We investigated whether fetal trisomy 18 and 21 were sensitively and specifically detectable by semiconductor sequencer: Ion Proton.

Methods: From March 2012 to October 2013, we enrolled 155 pregnant women with fetuses who were diagnosed as high risk of fetal defects at Xiamen Maternal & Child Health Care Hospital (Xiamen, Fujian, China). Adapter-ligated DNA libraries were analyzed by the Ion Proton™ System (Life Technologies, Grand Island, NY, USA) with an average 0.3× sequencing coverage per nucleotide. Average total raw reads per sample was 6.5 million and mean rate of uniquely mapped reads was 59.0%. The results of this study were derived from BWA mapping. Z-score was used for fetal trisomy 18 and 21 detection.

Results: Interactive dot diagrams showed the minimal z-score values to discriminate negative versus positive cases of fetal trisomy 18 and 21. For fetal trisomy 18, the minimal z-score value of 2.459 showed 100% positive predictive and negative predictive values. The minimal z-score of 2.566 was used to classify negative versus positive cases of fetal trisomy 21.

Conclusion: These results provide the evidence that fetal trisomy 18 and 21 detection can be performed with semiconductor sequencer. Our data also suggest that a prospective study should be performed with a larger cohort of clinically diverse obstetrics patients.

Editor: Sinuhe Hahn, University Hospital Basel, Switzerland

Funding: This work was supported by the Industrial Strategic Technology Development Program, 10040231, 'Bioinformatics platform development for next generation bioinformation analysis' funded by the Ministry of Knowledge Economy (MKE, Korea). Co-authors Young Joo Jeon, Sin-Gi Park, Hee Jae Joo, and Jong Bhak are employed by TheragenEtex Bio Institute. TheragenEtex Bio Institute provided support in the form of salaries for authors YJJ, SGP, HJJ, and JB, but did not have any additional role in the study design, data collection and analysis, decision to publish, or preparation of the manuscript. The specific roles of these authors are articulated in the 'author contributions' section. Co-authors Young Joo Jeon, Sin-Gi Park, Hee Jae Joo, and Jong Bhak are employed by Genome Care. Genome Care provided support in the form of salaries for authors YJJ, SGP, HJJ, and JB, but did not have any additional role in the study design, data collection and analysis, decision to publish, or preparation of the manuscript. The specific roles of these authors are articulated in the 'author contributions' section. Co-authors Shengmao Quan, Ahong Zhang, Hailing Zheng, Xingqiang Zhu, Jin Lin, Huan Xu, and Hongliang Chen are employed by Xiamen Vangenes BioTech. Xiamen Vangenes BioTech provided support in the form of salaries for authors SQ, AZ, HZ, XZ, JL, HX, and HC, but did not have any additional role in the study design, data collection and analysis, decision to publish, or preparation of the manuscript. The specific roles of these authors are articulated in the 'author contributions' section. Co-author Byung Chul Kim is employed by Clinomics. Clinomics provided support in the form of salaries for author BCK, but did not have any additional role in the study design, data collection and analysis, decision to publish, or preparation of the manuscript. The specific roles of this author are articulated in the 'author contributions' section.

Competing Interests: We have the following interests: co-authors Young Joo Jeon, Sin-Gi Park, Hee Jae Joo, and Jong Bhak are employed by TheragenEtex Bio Institute. Co-authors Young Joo Jeon, Sin-Gi Park, Hee Jae Joo, and Jong Bhak are employed by Genome Care. Co-authors Shengmao Quan, Ahong Zhang, Hailing Zheng, Xingqiang Zhu, Jin Lin, Huan Xu, and Hongliang Chen are employed by Xiamen Vangenes BioTech. Co-author Byung Chul Kim is employed by Clinomics. There are no patents, products in development or marketed products to declare.

* Email: hongliangchen@gmail.com (HC); jongbhak@genomics.org (JB)

◆ These authors contributed equally to this work.

Introduction

Prenatal screening and diagnostics for fetal chromosomal aneuploidy are well established worldwide for pregnant women [1,2]. Predictive testing during the first trimester includes a combination of fetal ultrasound and maternal serum biomarkers [3]. Women with fetuses at high risk of defects are also provided opportunities for invasive diagnostic testing, such as chorionic villus sampling (CVS) at 12 weeks of gestation and amniocentesis at 15 weeks of gestation [4,5]. Although these invasive tests are highly accurate, they are associated with iatrogenic pregnancy loss [6].

The prevalence rate of the common aneuploidy, trisomy 21, is around 1 in 500 in the group of women that request screening. In contrast, 1 in 200 women who receive first-trimester screening (FTS) are categorized as increased risk. The main reason that many women avoid testing or screening is because they are aware of the risks associated with invasive testing [7]. Further, FTS has two serious limitations; FTS has a false-negative rate of 10–25% and a restricted time-window of 11–13 gestational weeks [8–12].

After Lo et al. discovered fetal cell-free DNA (cffDNA) floating in maternal blood [13], there have been concerted attempts to perform non-invasive prenatal testing (NIPT) with cffDNA [14]. The cffDNA is originated from apoptotic trophoblasts in the placenta [13]. On average, the amount of cffDNA in plasma from a pregnant woman is approximately 10% during 10–22 weeks of gestation but there is a large variance in the fraction of cffDNA between individuals [15]. The typical cffDNA size is approximately 150 base pairs (bp) [16]. The half-life of cffDNA is very short [17], and fetal DNA fragments of maternal blood are no longer detectable after birth [18]. Despite these limitations, NIPT consists of well-accepted and advanced technologies. NIPT has two key clinical advantages compared with those of invasive prenatal testing; it does not confer a risk of pregnancy loss, and can be performed during early pregnancy. However, NIPT is not currently considered to be fully diagnostic and requires invasive testing to confirm positive results because the discordant NIPT data for detecting chromosomal abnormality have resulted from placental or maternal cell mosaicism [19–21]. To minimize this problem, risk scores and multiple cut-offs have been often used for NIPT services [14].

Recent NIPT technologies are based on next-generation sequencing (NGS) [22–27]. NGS allows rapid and effective clinical diagnostic testing with two commonly used systems, the Illumina and Ion Torrent platforms. Ion Torrent, semiconductor sequencing platform, enables acquisition of sequencing data within 2 to 4 hours, thus the sequencer may provide an alternative clinical sequencing service with a reduced turn-around time. The majority of NIPT technology is associated with Illumina platform. Previous NIPT studies with the Illumina platform report consistent data for common aneuploidies, particularly trisomy 18 and 21; sensitivity and specificity are each higher than 98% [22–26]. A recent study reports the results for non-invasive detection of common fetal trisomy 13, 18, and 21 with Ion Proton, a semiconductor sequencer [27]. The sensitivity and specificity of the common fetal aneuploidies (Trisomy 13, 18, and 21) are each higher than 98% [27]. However, more references of non-invasive fetal aneuploidy detection with semiconductor sequencing platform are required.

In our study, we performed NIPT for fetal trisomy 18 and 21 with Ion Proton. The testing results of semiconductor sequencing platform have rarely been reported as an NIPT technology [27]. Therefore, we investigated whether fetal trisomy 18 and 21 were sensitively and specifically detectable by Ion Proton.

Materials and Methods

Study Subjects

From March 2012 to October 2013, we enrolled 155 pregnant women with fetuses who were diagnosed as high risk of fetal defects at Xiamen Maternal & Child Health Care Hospital (Xiamen, Fujian, China). 28 pregnant women (18.1%) were 12–16 weeks of gestation, 86 women (55.5%) were 17–21 weeks of gestation, and 41 women with fetuses (26.5%) were more than 22 weeks of gestation. Pregnant women who were scheduled to receive invasive diagnostic testing (Amniocentesis) for fetal karyotyping were asked to donate a blood sample before having the invasive test. Women who gave written informed consent participated in the study if they were ≥ 19 years old and had a singleton pregnancy with a gestational age of at least 12 weeks. The institutional review board at Xiamen Maternal & Child Health Care Hospital approved this study.

We used the results of standard prenatal aneuploidy screening with individual risk scores and interpretations produced by accredited clinical laboratories for sorting out high risk group of fetal defects. First-trimester serum markers included pregnancy-associated plasma protein A (PAPP-A) and free beta subunit or total human chorionic gonadotropin (hCG). Second-trimester serum markers included maternal serum alpha-fetoprotein (MSAFP), hCG, unconjugated estriol, and inhibin A. First-trimester serum markers were used in combination with sonographic measurement of fetal nuchal translucency (combined FTS test) to categorize patients into high or low risk groups. Second-trimester serum values were evaluated alone (quadruple screening test) or in combination with FTS results to define aneuploidy risk. To determine fetal karyotypes, fetal cells from amniotic fluid were cultured to test for chromosomal abnormalities by the method of Barch et al [28]. Cytogenetic analysis performed on all 155 fetal cells indicated that 139 (89.7%) were chromosomally normal, 5 (3.2%) were trisomy 18, and 11 (7.1%) were trisomy 21.

Cell-free DNA Preparation and Sequencing

Eligible subjects were asked to participate in the study after receiving counseling about the invasive diagnostic test. Approximately 10 mL of whole blood was collected from each subject and placed in a Cell-Free DNA BCT™ tube (Streck, Omaha, NE, USA) before the invasive procedure. Within 6 hours of collection, the maternal blood samples were centrifuged first at 1,200×g for 15 min at 4°C. Plasma was transferred to microcentrifuge tubes, centrifuged again at 16,000×g for 10 min at 4°C to remove residual cells, transferred to fresh tubes, and stored at −80°C. For each sample, plasma cfDNA was extracted from 1 mL of plasma using the QIAamp Circulating Nucleic Acid Kit from Qiagen (Hilden, Germany). The resulting plasma cfDNA was used as input DNA to make a library for sequencing. End-repair of the plasma cfDNA was performed with T4 DNA polymerase, Klenow DNA polymerase, and T4 polynucleotide kinase. The adapter-ligated DNA libraries were analyzed with the Ion Proton™ System (Life Technologies, Grand Island, NY, USA) with an average 0.3×sequencing coverage per nucleotide. Ion PI™ Chip Kit version 2.0 (Life Technologies) was used for cfDNA sequencing and 10 cfDNA samples per chip were analyzed. Average total raw reads per sample was 6.5 million and mean rate of uniquely mapped reads was 59.0%.

Data Analysis

Raw reads with different lengths acquired from the Ion Torrent Suite software trimmed from the 3′ end by sequencing quality

Table 1. Demographic characteristics of study subjects.

Demographic characteristics	Euploid (n = 139)	T18 (n = 5)	T21 (n = 11)	Total (n = 155)
Maternal age, years, mean±SD	30.61±5.01	27.60±5.50	33.64±3.29	30.73±4.99
≥ 35 years (%)	36 (25.9)	1 (20.0)	5 (45.5)	42 (27.1)
NIPT during 12–16 gestational weeks (%)	25 (18.0)	1 (20.0)	2 (18.2)	28 (18.1)
NIPT during 17–21 gestational weeks (%)	78 (56.1)	4 (80.0)	4 (36.4)	86 (55.5)
NIPT ≥ 22 gestational weeks (%)	36 (25.9)	0 (0.0)	5 (45.5)	41 (26.5)
Male fetus (%)	65 (46.8)	4 (80.0)	9 (81.8)	78 (50.3)
Female fetus (%)	74 (53.2)	1 (20.0)	2 (18.2)	77 (49.7)
Z-score of chr18 (min, max)	−3.184, 2.459	4.017, 10.193	−1.730, 1.592	−3.184, 10.193
Z-score of chr21 (min, max)	−3.080, 2.566	−1.449, 0.387	4.693, 30.943	−3.080, 30.943

T18, Trisomy 18; T21, Trisomy 21; SD, standard deviation; NIPT, non-invasive prenatal testing.

value of >15, and filtered by read length (<50 bp) and GC contents (35%–45%). Duplicate reads were identified by Picard (http://picard.sourceforge.net/) with the default parameters and removed by in-house python script. The sequences were binned for each sample according to the index and mapped to the unmasked human genome sequence (hg19). We tested several mapping software programs, including BWA [29], Bowtie [30], and SOAP2 [31]. The results in this study were derived from the BWA mapping analysis. All chromosomes were divided into segments with a bin size of 300 kb to calculate z-score for fetal trisomy 18 and 21 detection. For the 155 samples, we calculated the z-score for each chromosome of each sample to examine fetal aneuploidy with mapped reads for each sample, and mean mapped reads and standard deviation (SD) of 139 euploid samples. For example, the z-score of case 1 for chr21 could be calculated as follows: $\text{z-score}_{chr21\_case1}$ = (mapped reads of $chr21_{case1}$ − mean mapped reads of $chr21_{euploid\ group}$)/(SD for mean mapped reads of $chr21_{euploid\ group}$). The minimal z-scores to classify negative versus positive cases of trisomy based on interactive dot diagrams were > 2.459 for fetal trisomy 18 and >2.566 for fetal trisomy 21. Sequence data has been deposited in the NIH short read archive (SRA) with the following BioProject accession number: SRP044689.

Statistical Analysis

Categorical variables were summarized with the number and percentage of subjects. Continuous variables were described as means with SD. Positive predictive value (PPV) and negative predictive value (NPV) were calculated with standard formulas for binomial distributions. Wilson's interval method was used to calculate 95% confidence intervals (CI). Interactive dot diagrams were used to assign classifications according to the presence of fetal aneuploidy. Analyses were performed with MedCalc version 12.1.4 (MedCalc Software bvba, Ostend, Belgium).

Results

Table 1 shows the demographic characteristics of the enrolled participants in this study. The mean maternal age of this study cohort was 30.73±4.99 years (range 19–43 years). 28 pregnant women (18.1%) received NIPT during 12–16 weeks of gestation, 86 women (55.5%) received testing during 17–21 weeks of gestation, and 41 women with fetuses (26.5%) who were more than 22 weeks of gestation received testing. The ratio of male (50.3%) to female (49.7%) fetuses was nearly 1:1; however, in aneuploidies, the ratio of male (81.3%) to female fetuses (13.8%) was 13:3.

Figure 1 presents interactive dot diagrams for fetal trisomy 18 and 21 showed the minimal z-score values of 100% PPV and NPV. For fetal trisomy 18, the minimal z-score value of 2.459

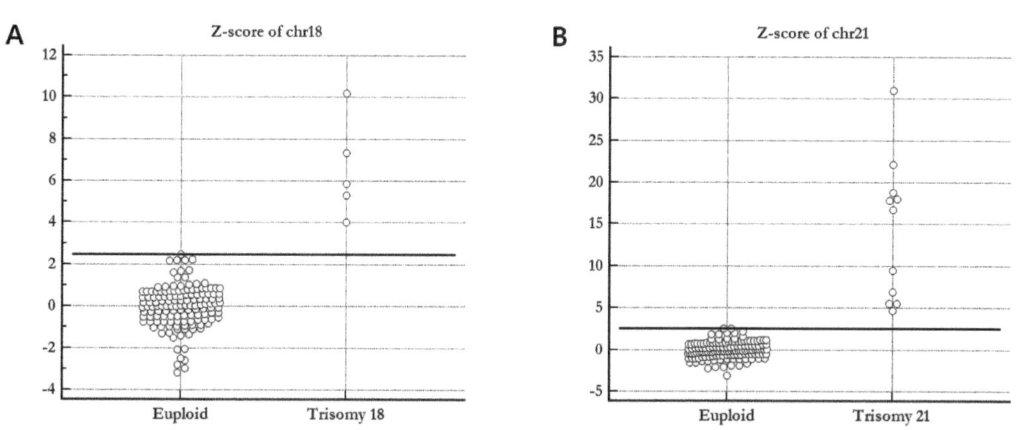

Figure 1. Interactive dot diagrams of trisomy 18 and 21. (A) Interactive dot diagram of trisomy 18. (B) Interactive dot diagram of trisomy 21.

Table 2. Positive predictive and negative predictive values in this study.

Aneuploidy	Positive predictive value (95% CI)	Negative predictive value (95% CI)
T18 (n = 5)	100.0% (47.8%–100.0%)	100.0% (97.6%–100.0%)
T21 (n = 11)	100.0% (71.5%–100.0%)	100.0% (97.5%–100.0%)
Combined detection (n = 16)	100.0% (79.4%–100.0%)	100.0% (97.4%–100.0%)

T18, trisomy 18; T21, trisomy 21.

showed 100% PPV and NPV. The minimal z-score of 2.566 was used to classify negative versus positive cases of fetal trisomy 21.

Table 2 summarizes the PPVs and NPVs of the NIPT results for fetal trisomy 18 and 21. For fetal trisomy 18, the PPV (95% CI: 47.8%–100.0%) and NPV (95% CI: 97.6%–100.0%) were 100%. The PPV (95% CI: 71.5%–100.0%) and NPV (95% CI: 97.5%–100.0%) for detecting fetal trisomy 21 were also 100%. On the whole, the PPV (95% CI: 79.4%–100.0%) and NPV (95% CI: 97.4%–100.0%) of combined detection of fetal trisomy 18 and 21 were 100%.

Discussion

We have examined the feasibility of NIPT using cffDNA in a predominantly high-risk obstetrics population using the semiconductor sequencing system: Ion Proton. Fetal trisomy 18 and 21 were non-invasively detectable with 100% PPV and NPV. The results of present study provide the evidence that non-invasive fetal trisomy 18 and 21 detection can be performed with semiconductor sequencing platform. However, our test is still far away from a clinically validated test because there was not consideration for plasma fetal DNA fraction.

According to previous reports, the Ion Torrent sequencer shows equivalent performance to the Illumina platform [32–34]. Quail et al. [32] measured Ion Torrent PGM data against Illumina HiSeq2000 and MiSeq results, and found that the error rate of Ion Torrent PGM data was 1.78%. In contrast, Illumina HiSeq2000 and MiSeq platforms demonstrated error rates ranging from 0.26% to 0.80%, and the rates of true single nucleotide polymorphisms (SNPs) were higher for Ion Torrent PGM analysis compared to that of the Illumina HiSeq2000 and MiSeq analysis [32]. Boland et al. [33] demonstrated that Ion Proton genotyping data were nearly concordant with SNP microarray data; further, the concordance rates were similar to those of the Illumina HiSeq2000 results. Chen et al. [34] compared the performances of the Ion Proton and Illumina MiSeq systems for ultra-low coverage sequencing. Ion Proton and Illumina MiSeq platforms present similar coverage for relative depth (RD) at each 1-Mbp of sequencing for GC-content. Both sequencing systems correctly detected fetal tissue aneuploidies [34]. Ion Proton system can construct ~80 million raw reads in 3–4 hours, which allows chromosomal abnormality detection within 1–2 working days, is advantageous for applications that require precise turn-around times, such as prenatal genetic screening [34].

Conventional noninvasive aneuploidy screening tests are not straight forward. None of the screening tests are ideal, because detection rates for chromosomal abnormalities are less than 100%. By definition, the false-positive rate is 5% if modeled for a common obstetrics population. Maternal serum marker and ultrasound screening tests have been performed widely for over a decade. These have been popular but have limitations. Henry et al. [35] analyzed the birth of Down's syndrome after routine noninvasive screening largely replaced age-related invasive procedures in Colorado from 1989 to 2005. Despite the increase in prenatal screening, neonates with trisomy 21 increased in women over 35 years of age. One explanation is that women did not receive the recommended protocol, perhaps incorrectly assuming that a single blood test would definitively detect abnormalities.

Serum biomarker analysis and ultrasound sonography do not definitively detect chromosomal aneuploidy. A positive screen result must be followed up with an invasive prenatal test (CVS or amniocentesis) to determine whether fetal aneuploidy is truly present. Previous studies of NIPT with cffDNA report consistently accurate results for detecting common aneuploidies, particular trisomy 18 and 21 [22–27]. However, the cost of the test is a major issue. Currently, the cost of a plasma cffDNA test ranges from about $800 to $2,000 in the US and from $500 to $1,500 in other countries [14]. Two previously published reports have estimated costs when the cfDNA test is applied to women with positive conventional screening results [36,37]. They concluded that applying the cfDNA test was connected to a net cost reduction in comparison with CVS or amniocentesis [36,37].

In summary, we investigated whether fetal trisomy 18 and 21 could be detected by noninvasive Ion Torrent sequencing as has previously been published for Illumina sequencing. However, the present study has several limitations. First, our sample size was smaller than other obstetrics populations in previous reports [22–27]. The lower 95% CIs for NPV were almost 97.0% in our study, whereas other studies usually demonstrate >98.0% of the lower 95% CIs for specificity. More than 400 high-risk pregnant women will need to be enrolled in future studies to estimate >98.0% of the lower 95% CIs for NPV or specificity with Wilson's interval method. Second, we did not find any positive cases for rare chromosomal abnormalities, such as trisomy 9, trisomy 13, and sex chromosome aneuploidies. Third, the participation rates for low-risk pregnant women after serum biomarker testing and ultrasound sonography did not reach expected levels. Fourth, we could not measure Ion Proton sequencing data against data that were analyzed by Illumina HiSeq or MiSeq due to insufficient quantities of blood samples. Although the results of our study provide initial evidence for NIPT of fetal trisomy 18 and 21 using the semiconductor sequencing system, a prospective study on a larger cohort of clinically diverse obstetrics participants is warranted to validate these findings.

Author Contributions

Conceived and designed the experiments: YJJ YZ YL HC JB. Performed the experiments: SQ AZ HZ XZ JL HX. Analyzed the data: YJJ SGP JB. Contributed reagents/materials/analysis tools: YZ YL QG JC AW BCK HJJ HC. Contributed to the writing of the manuscript: YJJ YZ YL HC JB.

References

1. Morgan S, Delbarre A, Ward P (2013) Impact of introducing a national policy for prenatal Down syndrome screening on the diagnostic invasive procedure rate in England. Ultrasound Obstet Gynecol 41: 526–529.
2. ACOG Committee on Practice Bulletins (2007) ACOG Practice Bulletin No. 77: screening for fetal chromosomal abnormalities. Obstet Gynecol 109: 217–227.
3. Nicolaides KH (2011) Screening for fetal aneuploidies at 11 to 13 weeks. Prenat Diagn 31: 7–15.
4. Fortuny A, Borrell A, Soler A, Casals E, Costa D, et al. (1995) Chorionic villus sampling by biopsy forceps. Results of 1580 procedures from a single centre. Prenat Diagn 15: 541–550.
5. Crandall BF, Kulch P, Tabsh K (1994) Risk assessment of amniocentesis between 11 and 15 weeks: comparison to later amniocentesis controls. Prenat Diagn 14: 913–919.
6. Tabor A, Alfirevic Z (2010) Update on procedure-related risks for prenatal diagnosis techniques. Fetal Diagn Ther 27: 1–7.
7. van den Berg M, Timmermans DR, Kleinveld JH, Garcia E, van Vugt JM, et al. (2005) Accepting or declining the offer of prenatal screening for congenital defects: test uptake and women's reasons. Prenat Diagn 25: 84–90.
8. Borrell A, Casals E, Fortuny A, Farre MT, Gonce A, et al. (2004) First-trimester screening for trisomy 21 combining biochemistry and ultrasound at individually optimal gestational ages. An interventional study. Prenat Diagn 24: 541–545.
9. Kagan KO, Wright D, Baker A, Sahota D, Nicolaides KH (2008) Screening for trisomy 21 by maternal age, fetal nuchal translucency thickness, free beta-human chorionic gonadotropin and pregnancy-associated plasma protein-A. Ultrasound Obstet Gynecol 31: 618–624.
10. Berktold L, von Kaisenberg CS, Hillemanns P, Vaske B, Schmidt P (2013) Analysis of the impact of PAPP-A, free β-hCG and nuchal translucency thickness on the advanced first trimester screening. Arch Gynecol Obstet 287: 413–420.
11. Muñoz-Cortes M, Arigita M, Falguera G, Seres A, Guix D, et al. (2012) Contingent screening for Down syndrome completed in the first trimester: a multicenter study. Ultrasound Obstet Gynecol 39: 396–400.
12. Sainz JA, Serrano R, Borrero C, Turmo E (2012) First trimester contingent test as a screening method for Down's syndrome. A prospective study in the general population. J Matern Fetal Neonatal Med 25: 2221–2224.
13. Lo YM, Corbetta N, Chamberlain PF, Rai V, Sargent IL, et al. (1997) Presence of fetal DNA in maternal plasma and serum. Lancet 350: 485–487.
14. Benn P, Cuckle H, Pergament E (2013) Non-invasive prenatal testing for aneuploidy: current status and future prospects. Ultrasound Obstet Gynecol 42: 15–33.
15. Norton ME, Brar H, Weiss J, Karimi A, Laurent LC, et al. (2012) Non-Invasive Chromosomal Evaluation (NICE) Study: results of a multicenter prospective cohort study for detection of fetal trisomy 21 and trisomy 18. Am J Obstet Gynecol 207: 137.e1–8.
16. Chan KC, Zhang J, Hui AB, Wong N, Lau TK, et al. (2004) Size distributions of maternal and fetal DNA in maternal plasma. Clin Chem 50: 88–92.
17. Lo YM, Zhang J, Leung TN, Lau TK, Chang AM, et al. (1999) Rapid clearance of fetal DNA from maternal plasma. Am J Hum Genet 64: 218–224.
18. Smid M, Galbiati S, Vassallo A, Gambini D, Ferrari A, et al. (2003) No evidence of fetal DNA persistence in maternal plasma after pregnancy. Hum Genet 112: 617–618.
19. Grati FR, Malvestiti F, Ferreira JC, Bajaj K, Gaetani E, et al. (in press) Fetoplacental mosaicism: potential implications for false-positive and false-negative noninvasive prenatal screening results. Genet Med DOI: 10.1038/gim.2014.3.
20. McNamara CJ, Limone LA, Westover T, Miller RC (2014) Maternal source of false-positive fetal sex chromosome aneuploidy in noninvasive prenatal testing. Obstet Gynecol 123: 69S–70S.
21. Wang Y, Chen Y, Tian F, Zhang J, Song Z, et al. (2014) Maternal mosaicism is a significant contributor to discordant sex chromosomal aneuploidies associated with noninvasive prenatal testing. Clin Chem 60: 251–259.
22. Bianchi DW, Parker RL, Wentworth J, Madankumar R, Saffer C, et al. (2014) DNA sequencing versus standard prenatal aneuploidy screening. N Engl J Med 370: 799–808.
23. Sparks AB, Struble CA, Wang ET, Song K, Oliphant A (2012) Noninvasive prenatal detection and selective analysis of cell-free DNA obtained from maternal blood: evaluation for trisomy 21 and trisomy 18. Am J Obstet Gynecol 206: 319.e1–9.
24. Lau TK, Cheung SW, Lo PS, Pursley AN, Chan MK, et al. (2014) Non-invasive prenatal testing for fetal chromosomal abnormalities by low-coverage whole-genome sequencing of maternal plasma DNA: review of 1982 consecutive cases in a single center. Ultrasound Obstet Gynecol 43: 254–264.
25. Ehrich M, Deciu C, Zwiefelhofer T, Tynan JA, Cagasan L, et al. (2011) Noninvasive detection of fetal trisomy 21 by sequencing of DNA in maternal blood: a study in a clinical setting. Am J Obstet Gynecol 204: 205.e1–11.
26. Ashoor G, Syngelaki A, Wagner M, Birdir C, Nicolaides KH (2012) Chromosome-selective sequencing of maternal plasma cell-free DNA for first-trimester detection of trisomy 21 and trisomy 18. Am J Obstet Gynecol 206: 322.e1–5.
27. Liao C, Yin AH, Peng CF, Fu F, Yang JX, et al. (2014) Noninvasive prenatal diagnosis of common aneuploidies by semiconductor sequencing. Proc Natl Acad Sci U S A 111: 7415–7420.
28. Barch MJ, Knutsen T, Spurbeck JL (1997) The AGT Cytogenetics Laboratory Manual, 3rd edn. New York: Lippincott-Raven publishers.
29. Li H, Durbin R (2009) Fast and accurate short read alignment with Burrows-Wheeler transform. Bioinformatics 25: 1754–1760.
30. Langmead B, Trapnell C, Pop M, Salzberg SL (2009) Ultrafast and memory-efficient alignment of short DNA sequences to the human genome. Genome Biol 10: R25.
31. Li R, Yu C, Li Y, Lam TW, Yiu SM, et al. (2009) SOAP2: an improved ultrafast tool for short read alignment. Bioinformatics 25: 1966–1967.
32. Quail MA, Smith M, Coupland P, Otto TD, Harris SR, et al. (2012) A tale of three next generation sequencing platforms: comparison of Ion Torrent, Pacific Biosciences and Illumina MiSeq sequencers. BMC Genomics 13: 341.
33. Boland JF, Chung CC, Roberson D, Mitchell J, Zhang X, et al. (2013) The new sequencer on the block: comparison of Life Technology's Proton sequencer to an Illumina HiSeq for whole-exome sequencing. Hum Genet 132: 1153–1163.
34. Chen S, Li S, Xie W, Li X, Zhang C, et al. (2014) Performance Comparison between Rapid Sequencing Platforms for Ultra-Low Coverage Sequencing Strategy. PLoS One 9: e92192.
35. Henry GP, Britt DW, Evans MI (2008) Screening advances and diagnostic choice: the problem of residual risk. Fetal Diagn Ther 23: 308–315.
36. Palomaki GE, Kloza EM, Lambert-Messerlian GM, Haddow JE, Neveux LM, et al. (2011) DNA sequencing of maternal plasma to detect Down syndrome: an international clinical validation study. Genet Med 13: 913–920.
37. Song K, Musci TJ, Caughey AB (2013) Clinical utility and cost of non-invasive prenatal testing with cfDNA analysis in high-risk women based on a US population. J Matern Fetal Neonatal Med 26: 1180–1185.

6

Alzheimer's Disease Amyloid-β Links Lens and Brain Pathology in Down Syndrome

Juliet A. Moncaster[1], Roberto Pineda[2], Robert D. Moir[3], Suqian Lu[1], Mark A. Burton[1], Joy G. Ghosh[1], Maria Ericsson[4], Stephanie J. Soscia[3], Anca Mocofanescu[1], Rebecca D. Folkerth[5], Richard M. Robb[6], Jer R. Kuszak[7], John I. Clark[8], Rudolph E. Tanzi[3], David G. Hunter[6], Lee E. Goldstein[1]*

1 Molecular Aging & Development Laboratory, Department of Surgery, Brigham and Women's Hospital, Harvard Medical School, Boston, Massachusetts, United States of America, **2** Department of Ophthalmology, Massachusetts Eye and Ear Infirmary, Harvard Medical School, Boston, Massachusetts, United States of America, **3** Genetics and Aging Research Unit, Department of Neurology, Massachusetts General Hospital, Harvard Medical School, Charlestown, Massachusetts, United States of America, **4** Electron Microscopy Facility, Department of Cell Biology, Harvard Medical School, Boston, Massachusetts, United States of America, **5** Department of Pathology, Brigham and Women's Hospital, Harvard Medical School, Boston, Massachusetts, United States of America, **6** Department of Ophthalmology, Children's Hospital Boston, Harvard Medical School, Boston, Massachusetts, United States of America, **7** Departments of Ophthalmology and Pathology, Rush University Medical Center, Chicago, Illinois, United States of America, **8** Departments of Biological Structure and Ophthalmology, University of Washington, Seattle, Washington, United States of America

Abstract

Down syndrome (DS, trisomy 21) is the most common chromosomal disorder and the leading genetic cause of intellectual disability in humans. In DS, triplication of chromosome 21 invariably includes the *APP* gene (21q21) encoding the Alzheimer's disease (AD) amyloid precursor protein (APP). Triplication of the *APP* gene accelerates APP expression leading to cerebral accumulation of APP-derived amyloid-β peptides (Aβ), early-onset AD neuropathology, and age-dependent cognitive sequelae. The DS phenotype complex also includes distinctive early-onset cerulean cataracts of unknown etiology. Previously, we reported increased Aβ accumulation, co-localizing amyloid pathology, and disease-linked supranuclear cataracts in the ocular lenses of subjects with AD. Here, we investigate the hypothesis that related AD-linked Aβ pathology underlies the distinctive lens phenotype associated with DS. Ophthalmological examinations of DS subjects were correlated with phenotypic, histochemical, and biochemical analyses of lenses obtained from DS, AD, and normal control subjects. Evaluation of DS lenses revealed a characteristic pattern of supranuclear opacification accompanied by accelerated supranuclear Aβ accumulation, co-localizing amyloid pathology, and fiber cell cytoplasmic Aβ aggregates (~5 to 50 nm) identical to the lens pathology identified in AD. Peptide sequencing, immunoblot analysis, and ELISA confirmed the identity and increased accumulation of Aβ in DS lenses. Incubation of synthetic Aβ with human lens protein promoted protein aggregation, amyloid formation, and light scattering that recapitulated the molecular pathology and clinical features observed in DS lenses. These results establish the genetic etiology of the distinctive lens phenotype in DS and identify the molecular origin and pathogenic mechanism by which lens pathology is expressed in this common chromosomal disorder. Moreover, these findings confirm increased Aβ accumulation as a key pathogenic determinant linking lens and brain pathology in both DS and AD.

Editor: Leonard Petrucelli, Mayo Clinic, United States of America

Funding: National Institutes of Health, Bethesda, MD (R01GM75986 and K23AG024792, LEG); American Federation for Aging Research, New York, NY (LEG); Alzheimer's Association, Chicago, IL (LEG); American Health Assistance Foundation, Clarksburg, MD (LEG); Anonymous Foundation (LEG); Cure Alzheimer's Fund, Wellesley Hills, MA (RDM); Boston University School of Medicine, Boston, MA (LEG); and Boston University Alzheimer's Disease Center, Boston, MA (NIH ADCC grant P30AG13846). The funding sponsors had no role in study design, data collection, data analysis, data interpretation, or writing of the report. The senior corresponding author (LEG) has full access to all study data and takes final responsibility for the decision to submit the results of the study for publication.

Competing Interests: Authors Moncaster, Pineda, Lu, Burton, Ghosh, Ericsson, Soscia, Mocofanescu, Folkerth, Robb, Kuszak, Clark, and Hunter report no conflict of interest. The following authors reported consultant activity during the course of this study: Drs. Tanzi and Goldstein, Neuroptix Corp, Acton, MA; Drs. Moir, Tanzi, and Goldstein, Covance, Dedham, MA. No financial support was provided by any commercial entity for this study.

* E-mail: LGOLD@BU.EDU

These authors contributed equally to this work.

Introduction

Down syndrome (DS, [1]) is the leading genetic cause of intellectual disability and the most common chromosomal disorder compatible with human survival [2,3,4,5]. DS affects approximately 1 in 700 live births and an estimated 220,000 newborns each year [6]. In the majority of cases, the disorder arises from sporadic non-disjunction of chromosome 21 (HSA21) and triplication of the entire chromosome [7,8,9], or infrequently, from partial aneuploidy due to unbalanced chromosomal translocation [10,11,12,13]. In most cases, DS aneuploidy disrupts gene-dose equilibrium in all somatic cells, whereas a minority of cases demonstrates mosaicism [14]. Chromosomal triplication invariably includes the *APP* gene (21q21) that encodes the amyloid precursor protein, APP [15,16]. Endoproteolytic cleavage of APP yields the pathogenic amyloid-β peptides (Aβ) that progressively accumulate in the brain as the diffuse and neuritic plaques of Alzheimer's disease (AD). In DS, cerebral Aβ accumulation is greatly accelerated [17] and leads to invariant early-onset AD neuropathology and age-dependent neurocognitive sequelae [18,19].

Lens abnormalities in subjects with clinical features of DS were first reported over a century ago [20,21] followed by numerous confirmatory reports since [20,22,23,24]. The distinctive DS lens phenotype clinically manifests as cerulean "blue dot" opacities that often emerge in the first decade of life, and in some cases, may be evident at birth [22,25,26,27]. DS cataracts typically localize to the supranuclear region and are histologically characterized by granular material of uncertain composition [20,24,25]. The molecular origin and pathogenic mechanisms by which the DS aneuploidy is expressed as a distinctive age-dependent lens phenotype are unknown.

We previously reported disease-linked supranuclear cataracts that correlate with pathogenic Aβ accumulation, classical amyloid pathology, and co-localizing pathology in lenses obtained from subjects with Alzheimer's disease (AD) but not in those with other neurodegenerative disorders nor in normal aged controls [28]. In AD lenses, Aβ accumulates as electron-dense cytosolic aggregates (longest axial dimension, ~5 nm to ~200 nm) that distribute heterogeneously within the cytoplasm of supranuclear and deep cortical lens fiber cells. AD-linked Aβ aggregates in the lens qualify as Raleigh scattering centers that clinically manifest as supranuclear opacities that ultimately progress to frank cataracts. These AD-linked supranuclear cataracts are phenotypically, anatomically, ultrastructurally, and biochemically distinguishable from common age-related nuclear cataracts. Given the association between Aβ amyloid lens pathology in AD [28], we hypothesized that subjects with DS would also demonstrate age-related Aβ amyloid pathology in the lens. The aim of the present study was to test the hypothesis that DS-linked lens pathology reflects accelerated Aβ accumulation and co-localizing amyloid pathology that clinically manifests as the characteristic supranuclear cataract phenotype associated with this common chromosomal disorder.

Methods

Subjects and Specimens

Lens specimens were obtained from the following sources: (i) subjects with DS requiring cataract surgery (n = 3 males: 36, 46, and 47 years of age) at the Massachusetts Eye and Ear Infirmary; (ii) postmortem specimens from donors with DS (n = 12 total; n = 9 males: 2 to 69 years of age; n = 3 females: 42, 47, and 61 years of age) and normal controls (n = 34 total; n = 20 males: 7 months to 88 years of age; n = 14 females: 2 to 82 years of age) procured through national tissue networks (National Disease Registry Interchange, Philadelphia; PA; Florida Lion's Eye Bank, Miami, FL; Sun Health Research Institute, Sun City, AZ); and (iii) archival lens specimens generously provided by Dr. Richard Robb, Children's Hospital, Harvard Medical School, Boston, MA (DS, n = 4 total; n = 3 males: 1 day, 3 weeks, and 22 years of age; n = 1 female: 7 months of age. Normal controls, n = 3 total; n = 2 males, 1 day and 21 years of age; n = 2 females, 2 days and 4 months of age). An earlier histochemical analysis of lenses from this archival collection was reported in 1978 [24]. Postmortem brain specimens (superior temporal cortex) were obtained from the Massachusetts Alzheimer's Disease Research Center Brain Bank (Massachusetts General Hospital, Boston, MA, USA), and included the following donor groups: AD (CERAD criteria) n = 3 total; n = 1 male: 86 years of age; n = 2 females: 76 and 81 years of age); DS (karyotype confirmed) n = 4 total; n = 4 males: 56, 57, 58, and 60 years of age); normal controls (n = 3 total; n = 1 male: 86 years of age; n = 2 females: 72 and 88 years of age). Clinical information regarding cytogenetic microanalysis and chromosomal subtyping was not available. Lenses obtained from intact postmortem eyes were the only specimens used for biochemical analysis. All lenses obtained from intact, non-traumatic globes were included in the study and assigned to cohorts based on available clinical information. No other selection criteria were applied.

Ethical review and permission to conduct this investigation were approved by Harvard Medical School, Brigham and Women's Hospital, Massachusetts Eye and Ear Infirmary, and Children's Hospital Boston. This study conforms to applicable regulatory guidelines at Harvard Medical School and principles of human research subject protection in the Declaration of Helsinki. Patients were informed, consent forms signed, and patient samples collected and signed in accordance with an approved IRB protocol (02-08-053X) at the Massachusetts Eye and Ear Infirmary, Boston, MA, USA.

Slit Lamp Biomicroscopy

Clinical ophthalmological examinations included slit lamp stereophotomicroscopy and microvideography following routine pupillary dilation. In three DS cases (n = 3 males: 36, 46, and 47 years of age), slit lamp photomicrographs were obtained in conjunction with cataract surgery. Patients were informed and signed consent forms in accordance with an approved IRB protocol at the Massachusetts Eye and Ear Infirmary, Boston, MA, USA. Stereophotomicroscopic analysis of dissected intact human lenses was performed on postmortem specimens obtained from enucleated eyes procured through national tissue bank resources (National Disease Registry Interchange, Philadelphia; PA; Florida Lion's Eye Bank, Miami, FL). Harvested lenses were bathed in buffered artificial aqueous humor (295 mOsm, pH 7.20) at 37°C, visualized with a custom-adapted surgical slit lamp stereophotomicroscope (Carl Zeiss, Thornwood, NY) equipped with a stereo beamsplitter (Urban Engineering, Burbank, CA) and side-arm digital camera assembly (Nikon, Melville, NY).

Histopathology, Immunohistochemistry, Light and Electron Microscopy

A portion of the present study included re-analysis of lens specimens from an archival collection generously provided by co-author Richard Robb, M.D., Department of Ophthalmology, Children's Hospital Boston, Harvard Medical School, Boston, MA. Paraffin-embedded specimens in this collection date back to the 1960's and have been previously described [24]. Original paraffin blocks in this archival collection were highly friable and required re-embedding in fresh paraffin prior to histological processing. For all histological studies, routine tissue sections (8 μm) were obtained by microtomy, immunostained with Aβ monoclonal antibody 6E10 directed against $A\beta_{3-8}$ or 4G8 directed against $A\beta_{18-22}$ (generously provided by Joseph Bertelsen, Signet Laboratories, Covance, Dedham, MA), and processed by conventional immunohistochemistry using a commercial kit (Vector Laboratories, Burlingame, CA) according to the manufacturer's instructions. Bennhold's modified Congo red staining method [29] was used for amyloid histopathology. Brightfield and cross-polarization photomicroscopy were conducted using a Nikon Eclipse E600 upright microscope (Nikon USA, Melville, NY) equipped with a Spot Slider RT digital CCD photomicroscope camera and proprietary image acquisition software (Diagnostic Instruments, Sterling Heights, MI).

Immunogold Electron Microscopy

Immunogold electron microscopy (IEM) was conducted as previously described using ultra-thin cryosections without plastic embedding [28]. For IEM analyses, specimens were adsorbed to a carbon-coated grid, blocked for 10 min in 1% BSA, immunolabeled with the first detection antibody using anti-Aβ monoclonal antibody 4G8 (Signet Laboratories, Covance, Dedham, MA), then incubated with rabbit anti-mouse bridging antibody followed by incubation with 10 nm immunogold-conjugated Protein A (Jan Slot, Utrecht, Netherlands). Grids were fixed briefly in 1% glutaraldehyde, floated on 4 drops of 0.02M glycine/PBS to quench free aldehyde groups, then immunolabeled with the second detection antibody using a rabbit anti-αB-crystallin polyclonal antibody (Dr. Jack Liang, Brigham & Women's Hospital, Boston, MA, USA) or normal rabbit serum control. Specimens were then exposed to 15 nm immunogold-conjugated Protein A (Jan Slot, Utrecht, Netherlands), negatively stained with uranyl acetate, and examined on a JEOL 1200EX transmission electron microscope at the Electron Microscope Facility, Harvard Medical School. All immunohistochemical analyses included specificity controls in which identically processed specimens were incubated with detection antibody that was immunodepleted by pre-absorption with synthetic antigen (human Aβ42, Keck Laboratory, Yale University, New Haven, CT) as previously described[28].

Tryptic Digest Tandem Mass Spectrometry Protein Sequencing

Lens specimens were homogenized in 70% formic acid, ultracentrifuged at 100,000×*g* for 1 h at 4°C, and fractions separately retained for biochemical analysis. Supernatant was concentrated by nitrogen stream, neutralized with NaOH, and diluted 50-fold in TBS containing 10 μg anti-Aβ monoclonal antibody 6E10 (Signet Laboratories, Covance, Dedham, MA). Immunocomplexes were precipitated with magnetic beads covalently coupled to sheep anti-mouse antibody (Invitrogen, Carlsbad, CA), separated from unbound material by exposure to a magnetic field, and released by acidification in 100 mM glycine at pH 3. Samples were then subjected to reverse phase HPLC on a ZORBAX SB-C8 column (Agilent, Santa Clara, CA) and eluted under isocratic conditions (0.1% TFA; 30.5% acetonitrile) at 1 ml/min at 80°C. Elution times were determined by comparison to chromatographic profiles of synthetic human Aβ (Keck Laboratory, Yale University, New Haven, CT). Isolated fractions were dried by vacuum centrifugation, digested with trypsin, and fractionated by reverse phase HPLC. Post-digest eluates were subjected to electrospray ionization and ESI-tandem MS/MS LCQ-DECA ion-trap mass spectrometry (ThermoFinnigan, San Jose, CA) at the Taplin Mass Spectrometry Facility, Harvard Medical School. Peptide sequences were identified by computer-assisted search program (Sequest, Thermo Fisher Scientific, Waltham, MA).

Aβ Fluoro-ELISA and Aβ Immunoblotting

Analytical quantification of human Aβ40 and human Aβ42 was accomplished using two commercially available human Aβ specific ELISA kits (BetaMark, Covance, Dedham, MA; BioSource, Invitrogen, San Diego, CA). For experiments utilizing SDS extracted tissue, we used a commercially available human Aβ ELISA kit (BetaMark, Covance, Dedham, MA) that is resistant to interference from detergent. This ELISA assay system is compatible with tissue extracts containing SDS with minimal loss in sensitivity. Samples containing SDS were diluted to a final detergent concentration of less than 0.1%. For experiments utilizing formic acid extracted tissue, we used a second commercially available Aβ ELISA kit (BioSource, Invitrogen, San Diego, CA). For immunoblotting analysis, lens subcellular fractions were normalized for protein concentration and analyzed as previously described [28]. Blots were probed with human Aβ-specific monoclonal antibody WO2 (Genetics Company, Zurich, Switzerland) directed against human $A\beta_{4-10}$ or monoclonal antibody 6E10 (Signet Laboratories, Covance, Dedham, MA) directed against human $A\beta_{3-8}$.

Quasi-Elastic Light Scattering Analysis of Human Lens Protein Suspensions

Quasi-elastic light scattering (QLS) experiments were conducted using a custom laboratory instrument (Neuroptix Corporation, Acton, MA) that delivers linearly polarized continuous wave near-infrared laser light ($\lambda = 780$ nm; focused beam diameter, 30–35 μm; power output = 0.3 mW). The instrument incorporates a rigidly positioned pinhole mirror (aperture diameter = 100 μm) for selective detection of backscattered photons at a fixed scattering angle ($\theta = 120$ degrees). Signal detection and analysis of backscattered light intensity was accomplished with an avalanche photodiode, integrated 256-channel multi-tau digital autocorrelator ($\tau = 480$ ns), and custom software analysis package. Analyses involving aqueous suspensions of water-soluble lens proteins were conducted in cylindrical optical glass specimen vials positioned in a rigid holder mounted to the instrument. Three series of five independent measurements (each 1.3 seconds in duration) were performed for a total of fifteen measurements comprising each averaged test point. To investigate the interaction of Aβ peptides with other cytosolic lens proteins, a membrane-free water-soluble protein extract was prepared from freshly dissected human lenses obtained from postmortem donor eyes (National Disease Registry Interchange, Philadelphia; PA; Florida Lion's Eye Bank, Miami, FL). Dissected lenses were mechanically homogenized, ultracentrifuged at 100,000×g for 1 h at 4°C, and diluted to 1 mg/ml in phosphate buffered saline, pH 7.20. This aqueous lens protein extract is predominantly composed of water-soluble proteins in the cytoplasm of lens fiber cells. Purified synthetic human Aβ42 or Aβ40 (Keck Laboratories, Yale University, New Haven, CT) was added to freshly prepared human lens protein extract and incubated in siliconized Eppendorf tubes in a humidified 37°C 5% CO_2-balanced tissue culture chamber prior to light scattering analysis. All samples were incubated in the dark to reduce photodynamic effects. For microscopic visualization, aliquots of the incubated samples were placed on a microscope slide as wet-mount preparations and visualized by conventional photomicroscopy under brightfield and cross-polarized illumination. Immunogold electron microscopic analysis of incubated material was conducted as detailed above.

Results

Supranuclear Cataract Pathology in Down Syndrome Lenses

Slit lamp examination of subjects with karyotype-confirmed DS revealed classical cerulean "blue dot" cataracts (Fig *1A*) with a characteristic subequatorial supranuclear distribution (Fig. *1B,C*) and corresponding increased localized static light scattering (Fig. *1D*). The anatomical localization of the diffuse opacities observed by indirect ophthalmoscopy (Fig. *1A*) correspond to a distinctly annular supranuclear distribution as revealed by retro-illumination (Fig. *1B,C*) and confirmed by scattering densitometry (Fig. *1D*) of the same lens. The lens from a 2-year-old male with DS demonstrated grossly normal transparency without evidence of clinically detectable lenticular pathology (Fig. *1E*). By contrast, the DS supranuclear cataract phenotype was identified in all adult DS patients clinically examined and in all postmortem lens specimens from adult DS donors. Lenses from mature DS subjects

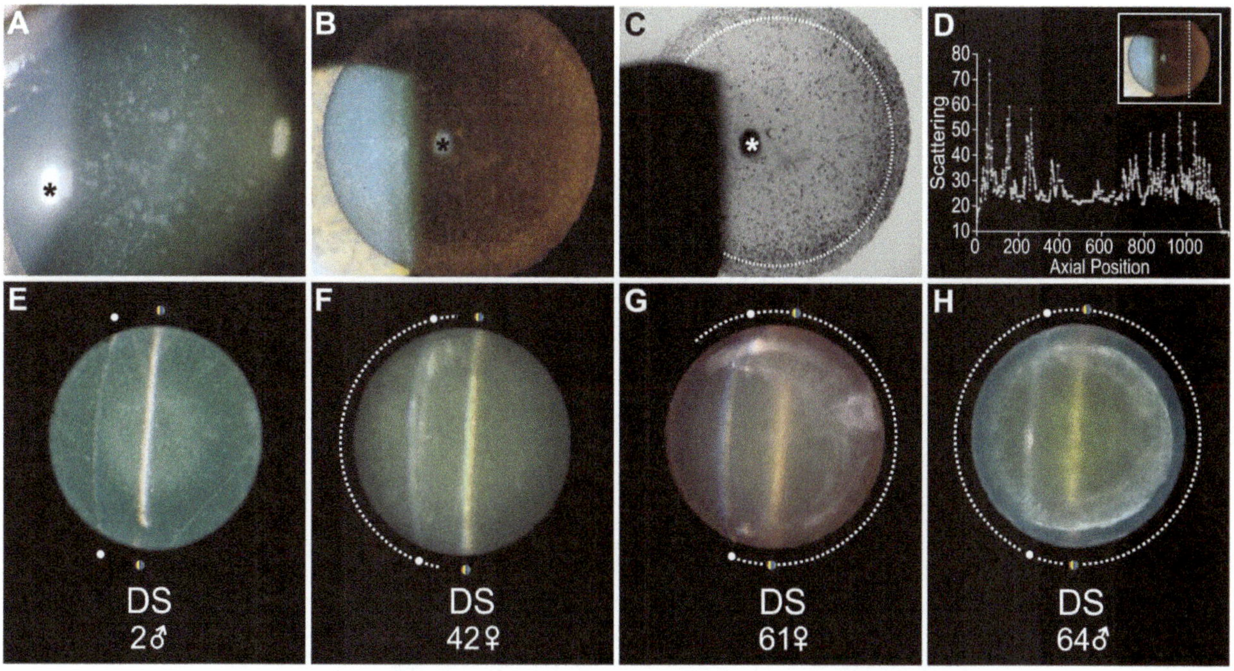

Figure 1. Phenotypic expression of representative supranuclear cataracts in Down syndrome. (**A-C**) Representative supranuclear cataract in a 46-year-old male with Down syndrome observed by slit lamp biomicroscopy. (**A**) Broad-beam illumination demonstrates numerous cerulean coronary "blue dot" lens opacities. Asterisk denotes first Purkinje image (corneal specular reflection). (**B**) Retro-illumination reveals a distinctive peripheral ring of opacification in the subequatorial supranuclear subregion of the lens. Red reflex is imparted by retinal reflection. Corneal Purkinje image is evident centrally (asterisk). (**C**) Inverted grayscale rendering of the retro-illumination image highlights the circumferential subequatorial supranuclear opacification (dashed circle) that characterizes the distinctive Down syndrome cataract phenotype. Corneal Purkinje image is evident centrally (asterisk). (**D**) Static light scattering intensity plotted as a function of anatomical position within the lens. Axial location is referenced to the dashed line and anatomical orientation axes represented in the inset. (**E-H**) Representative stereophotomicroscopic images of *ex vivo* lenses from subjects with Down syndrome of indicated ages and gender. Colored dots indicate superior and inferior extent of the slit beam ribbon defining the posterior surface of each imaged lens. White dots indicate superior and inferior extent of the light reflex on the anterior aspect of each imaged lens. (**E**) Lens from a 2-year-old male with Down syndrome. Slit beam photomicroscopy demonstrates a grossly normal transparent lens. (**F**) Lens from a 42-year-old female with Down syndrome. Supranuclear opacification is evident in a semicircular arc (dashes) with prominent cortical spokes and moderate lenticular brunescence. (**G**) Lens from a 61-year-old female with Down syndrome. Distinctive supranuclear opacification describes an incomplete supranuclear arc (dashes). Cortical spokes and moderate lenticular brunescence are present. (**H**) Lens from a 64-year-old male with Down syndrome. Prominent circumferential opacification is present as a subequatorial supranuclear ring cataract (dashed circle). This cataract describes an annular half torroid that follows the anteroposterior orientation of the supranuclear fiber cells enveloping the peripheral extent of the embryonic nucleus. Cortical spokes and moderate lenticular brunescence are evident. This same lens is presented as a stereo image pair with and without intact zonule fibers (Fig. S1 and Fig. 2, respectively). See text for details.

demonstrated apparent age-dependent supranuclear lens pathology (Fig. *1E-H*) that was phenotypically indistinguishable from that previously reported in late-onset sporadic AD (Fig. 1*F-H*) [*28*].

A representative stereo image of a lens from a 64-year-old male with DS (Fig. 2*A*) illustrates an advanced circumferential supranuclear cataract characteristic of the DS phenotype. The phenotypic features of this distinctive cataract phenotype are demonstrated in the same lens observed by slit lamp photomicroscopy (Fig. 1*H*) and as a stereo image pair with intact zonule fibers (Fig. S1). The cataract phenotype observed in DS was strikingly similar to the mature subequatorial supranuclear cataracts previously reported in advanced AD (Fig. *2B;* [28]). This distinctive DS-associated cataract was not present in age-matched normal control subjects nor was this focal lens pathology associated with global swelling, diffuse opacification, or capsular disruption indicative of postmortem tissue injury.

Histochemical and Ultrastructural Analyses

The phenotypic correspondence of the distinctive cataracts in DS and AD encouraged us to investigate the possibility of Aβ pathology in DS lenses. Orientation to the anatomy of the adult human lens is shown (Fig. *3A,B*) and compared to an historical drawing (Fig. 3*C*) illustrating the distinctive localized supranuclear lens pathology in a 37-year-old subject with clinical features consistent with Down syndrome [23]. Amyloid histochemical analysis of DS lenses in the present study demonstrated Congo red staining (Fig. 3*D*) and intense apple-green birefringence (Fig. *3E*) under cross-polarized illumination, findings consistent with the tinctorial requirements for designation as amyloid pathology [30,31]. Amyloid histopathology was not evident in a lens from an age- and sex-matched normal control donor (Fig. 3*F*) and co-localized with lens pathology and Aβ immunoreactivity as demonstrated by specific Aβ immunoreactivity in the deep cortical, supranuclear, and anterior epithelial subregions (Fig. 3*G*). Anti-Aβ immunoreactivity was not detected in adjacent control sections probed with immunodepleted detection antibody (Fig. 3*H*) or in lens specimens from age- and sex-matched normal control donors (Fig. 3*I*). Anti-Aβ immunogold electron microscopy revealed immunoreactive aggregates (~5–50 nm) that localized to the cytoplasm of supranuclear fiber cells in DS lenses (Fig. 3*J,K*) but was not observed in adjacent control sections probed with

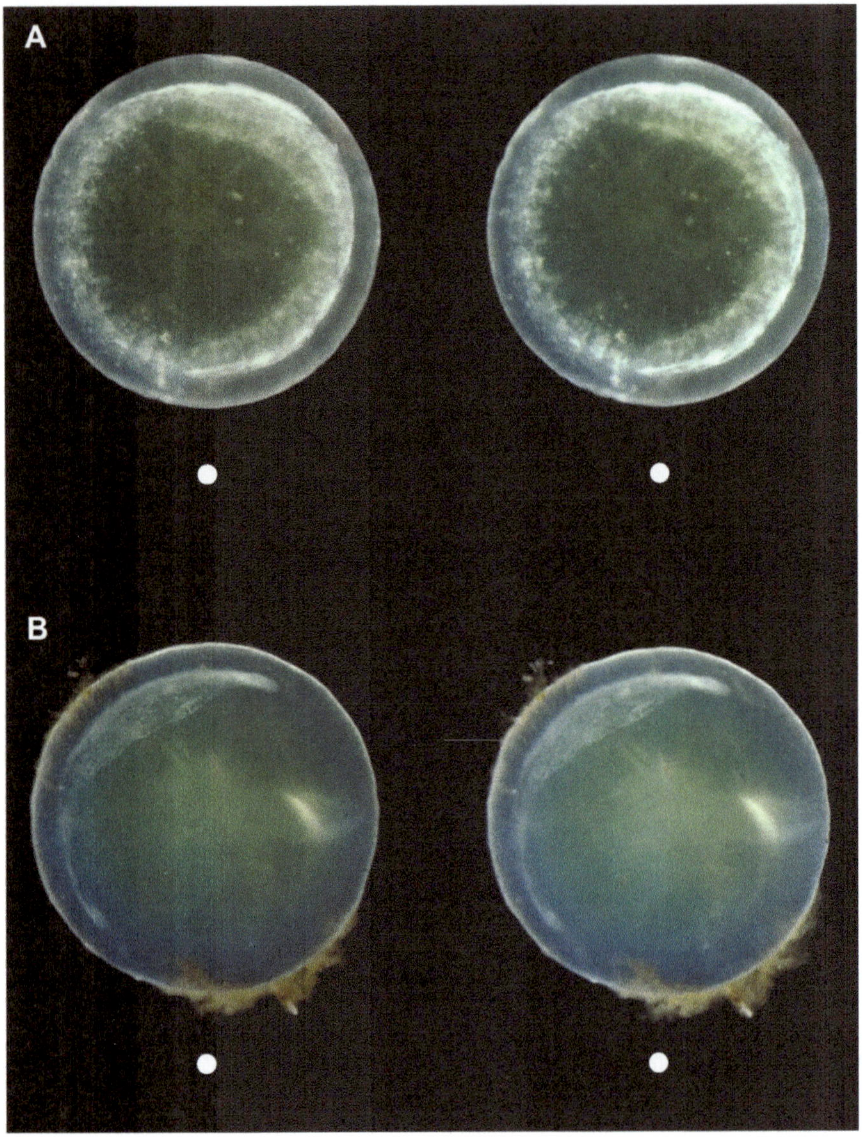

Figure 2. Stereo images demonstrating mature supranuclear lens pathology in Down syndrome and Alzheimer's Disease. (**A**) Characteristic circumferential supranuclear cataract in the lens of a 64-year-old male subject with Down syndrome. This distinctive cataract is evident as an annular half-toroid band of opacification in the deep cortical and supranuclear subregions of the lens. This same lens specimen is presented as a slit lamp biomicrocopic image (Fig. 1H) and as a stereo image pair (with intact zonule fibers, Fig. S1). This dramatic Down syndrome cataract is phenotypically comparable to the incomplete subequatorial supranuclear cataract observed in the lens of a 76-year-old male subject with advanced Alzheimer's disease (**B**). These distinctive supranuclear cataracts are not observed in age-normal control subjects. See text for details.

immunodepleted detection antibody (Fig. 3*L*). These histopathological findings are identical to those previously described for lens pathology in late-onset sporadic AD [28].

Identification and Biochemical Characterization of Aβ in Down Syndrome Lens

Definitive identification of human Aβ in DS lens was accomplished by tryptic digest tandem mass spectrometry peptide sequencing. Biochemical sequencing analysis was conducted on small molecular weight eluates derived from HPLC fractionation of human DS lens protein extract (Fig. 4). In positive electrospray mode, the LC-MS/MS spectrum detected two tryptic peptide signals corresponding to $_{17}$LVFFAEDVGSNK$_{28}$ and $_{6}$HDSGYEVHHQK$_{16}$ that uniquely identify human Aβ. The detected fragments did not derive from the larger amyloid precursor protein (APP) as sequencing was performed on eluates with retention times corresponding to monomeric Aβ (~4 kDa). In order to establish the tissue concentration of Aβ in the lens, we first investigated the relative efficiency of sodium dodecyl sulfate compared to formic acid extraction performed on protein extracts obtained from human lens homogenates (Fig. 5). Formic acid demonstrated a far superior extraction profile relative to sodium dodecyl sulfate for both Aβ1-40 and Aβ1-42. ELISA results (Fig. 6*A*,*B*) demonstrated elevated lens and brain tissue levels of the major human Aβ isoforms (Aβ_{40} and Aβ_{42}) and total Aβ that were consistently elevated in DS compared to normal controls and comparable to the values previously reported in AD [28]. Immunoblot analysis of DS lens extract (Fig. 6*C*) revealed a prominent Aβ-immunoreactive band that migrated with an apparent

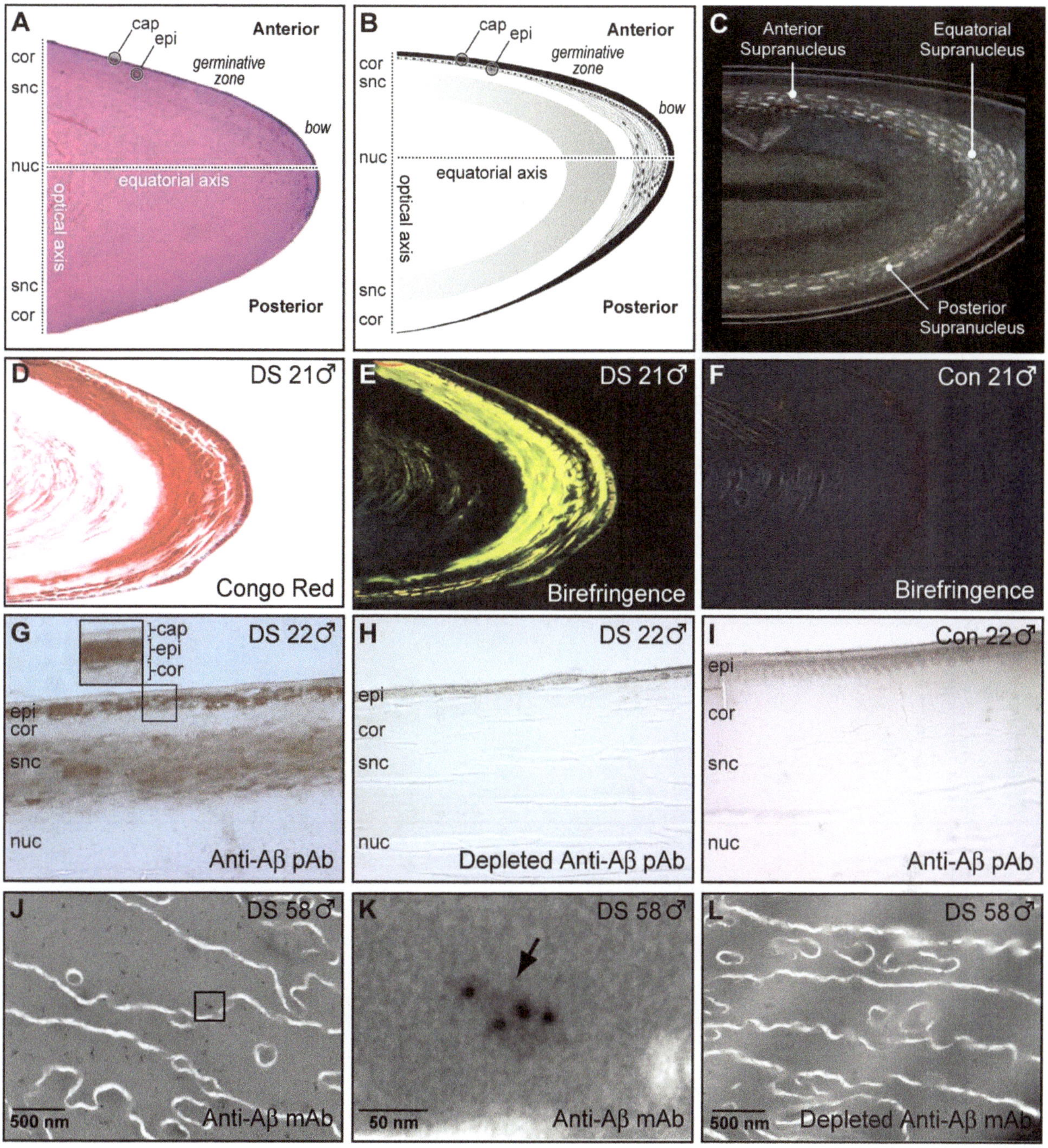

Figure 3. Alzheimer's disease amyloid-β (Aβ) pathology in Down syndrome lens. (**A**) Histological section of a human lens obtained from a 21-year-old male subject with Down syndrome. Hematoxylin and eosin. (**B**) Schematic diagram identifying anatomical regions of the human lens (adapted from *Histology of the Human Eye: An Atlas and Textbook* [52]). (**C**) Archival rendering of classical coronary cerulean "flake" arcuate cataracts in a 40-year-old male with presumptive Down syndrome (from Lowe, 1949 [23]). This historical folio drawing illustrates the mature Down syndrome supranuclear cataract phenotype with dominant subequatorial localization and anteroposterior extension. (**D-F**) Congo red amyloid histochemical analysis of lenses from a 21-year-old male with Down syndrome and age-matched normal male control. (**D**) Congophilia in the cortex and supranuclear subregion of the lens from a 21-year-old male with Down syndrome. (**E**) Intense co-localizing apple-green birefringence in the corresponding cortical and supranuclear subregions of the same Congo red-stained Down syndrome lens imaged with cross-polarized illumination. (**F**) Amyloid histochemical analysis of a lens from a 21-year-old normal control subject did not demonstrate Congophilia nor classical apple-green birefringence under identical cross-polarized illumination. (**G**) Aβ immunoreactivity in the epithelium, deep cortex, and supranuclear regions in a lens from a 22-year-old male with Down syndrome. Inset, magnified detail of the anterior lens (box). *Cap*, capsule; *epi*, epithelium; *cor*, cortex; *snc*, supranucleus; *nuc*, nucleus. (**H**) Confirmation of anti-Aβ antibody specificity in the same Down syndrome lens by immunodepletion of the detection antibody with synthetic human Aβ. Adjacent section of the same Down syndrome lens in Fig. 3G (**I**) Absence of Aβ immunoreactivity in the lens of a normal 22-year-old male control subject. (**J**) Anti-Aβ immunogold electron microscopic analysis of lens from a 58-year-old male with Down syndrome. Heterogeneously distributed anti-Aβ immunoreactive protein aggregates of dimensions ~5–200 nm localize heterogeneously within the lens fiber cell cytoplasm. Aβ immunoreactivity was not detected at the plasmalemma. Boxed region denotes magnified area shown in Fig. 3*k*. Scale

bar = 500 nm. (**K**) High-magnification electron micrograph of a single Aβ-immunoreactive cytoplasmic protein aggregate (arrow) in a lens fiber cell from same Down syndrome lens section shown in Fig. 3*J*. Multiple immunogold particles detect a single cytoplasmic protein aggregate with longest axial cross-section ~50 nm. Scale bar = 50 nm. (**L**) Confirmation of anti-Aβ antibody specificity. Anti-Aβ immunostaining was not detected in Down syndrome lens when probed with immunodepleted anti-Aβ antibody.

molecular weight of ~4 kDa corresponding to monomeric Aβ that was also detected in homogenate of AD brain. The apparent Aβ monomer bands detected in DS and AD lens and brain homogenate migrated with the same electrophoretic mobility observed in the single band detected in a sample of purified synthetic human Aβ40. Aβ monomer and apparent oligomeric species were also detected as weak but distinct bands in normal control lens. Total Aβ immunoreactive material detected in the lens of a 2-year-old DS subject was comparable to that detected in lenses from a 57-year-old subject with familial AD and an 85-year-old subject with neuropathologically-confirmed late-onset AD (Fig. 6*C*). The results of the immunoblot analysis provide confirmatory evidence supporting the finding of Aβ in DS lenses and also demonstrate an apparent increase in oligomeric Aβ and corresponding decrease in monomeric Aβ in the lens as a function of advancing age.

Down Syndrome Aβ Lens Pathology Recapitulated in a Model Lens Protein System *In Vitro*

These data indicate that Aβ accumulates in the cytoplasm of supranuclear lens fiber cells in individuals with DS. We previously showed that Aβ binds (Kapp ~20 nmol/L) and co-aggregates with αB-crystallin (HspB5) [28], a prototypic molecular chaperone and small heat shock protein [32] that is abundantly present in the lens

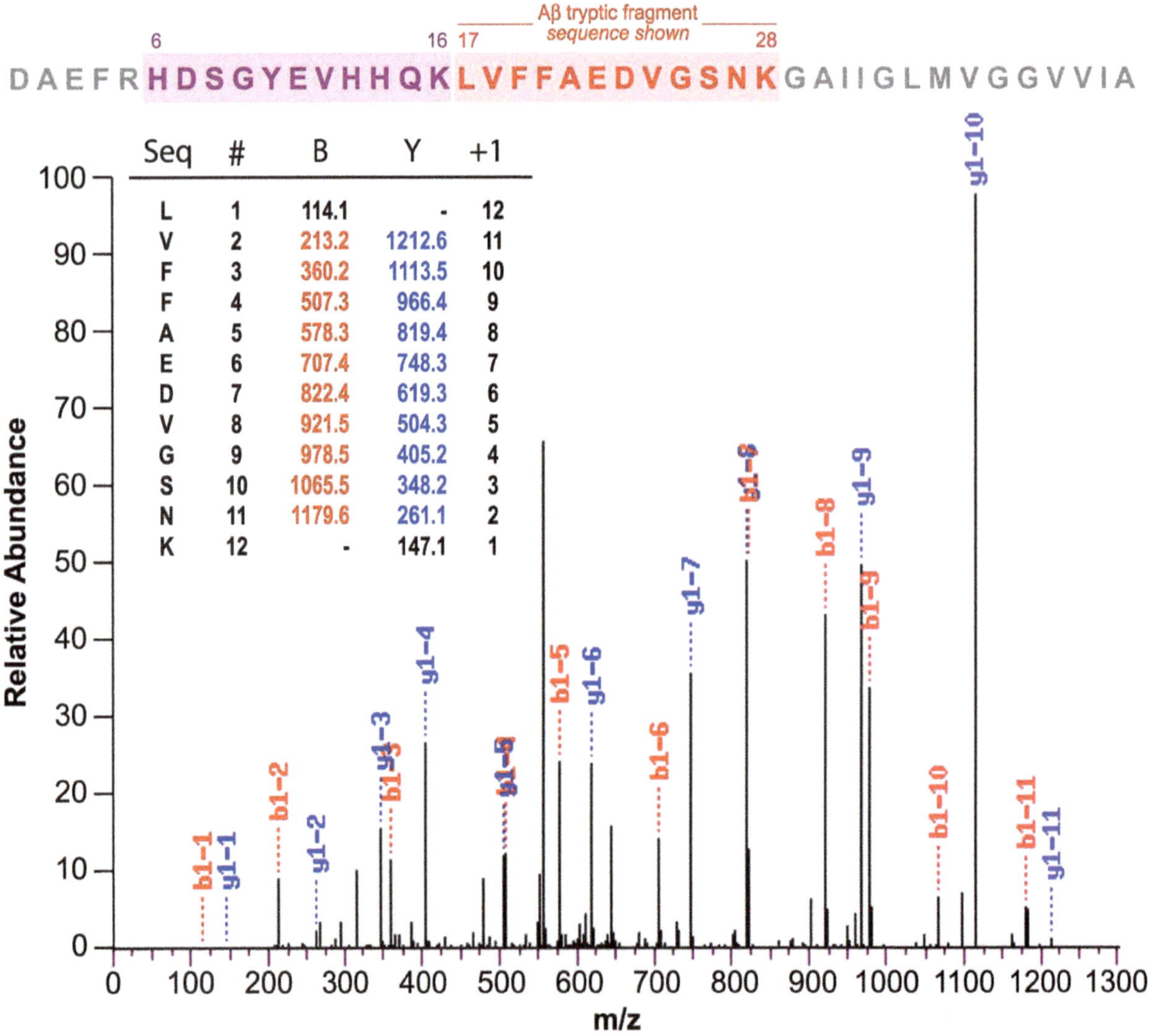

Figure 4. Peptide sequencing of human Aβ from Down syndrome lens. Tryptic digest tandem mass spectrometry sequencing of a ~4 kDa HPLC eluate derived from human Down syndrome lens protein extract. The retention time of the immunopurified HPLC eluate used for sequencing was identical to synthetic human Aβ. The red shade box denotes the detected 12-residue internal tryptic peptide sequence ${}_{17}$LVFFAEDVGSNK${}_{28}$ that uniquely identifies human Aβ. We detected a second unique tryptic peptide ${}_{6}$HDSGYEVHHQK${}_{16}$ in another analysis (purple underline).

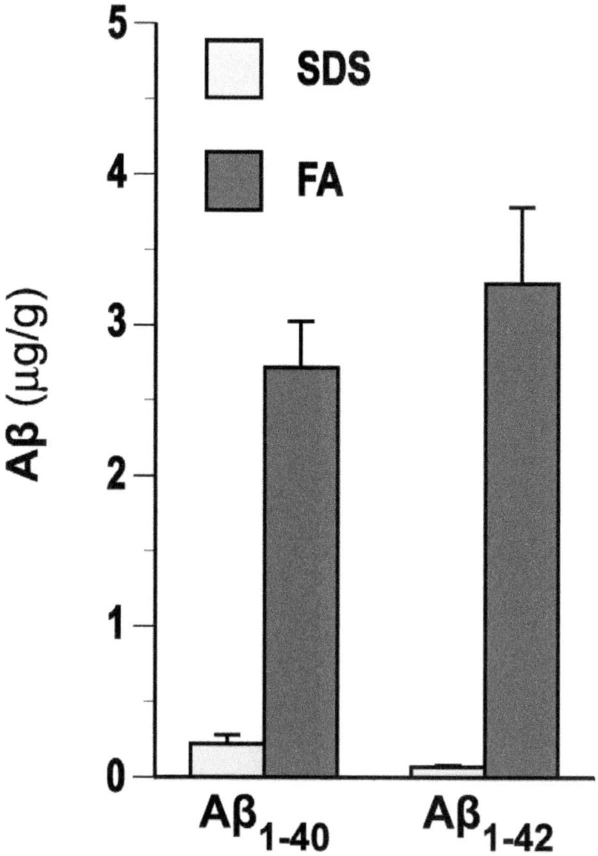

Figure 5. Lens Aβ extraction efficiency in sodium dodecyl sulfate and formic acid. See text for details.

fiber cell cytoplasm and upregulated in AD brain [33]. We hypothesized that accumulation of amyloidogenic Aβ peptides in the lens fiber cell would potentiate cytosolic lens protein aggregation and increase Rayleigh light scattering. To investigate this hypothesis, we incubated synthetic Aβ with human lens protein extract. Addition of Aβ to human lens protein extract generated birefringent congophilic aggregates consistent with amyloid (Fig. 7*A,B*). Double immunogold electron microscopic analysis revealed electron-dense aggregates that co-immunostained for Aβ and αB-crystallin (Fig. 7*C*). These hetero-oligomeric aggregates demonstrated comparable size, morphology, and immunoreactivity relative to the cytosolic protein aggregates identified in postmortem DS lens specimens. Significantly, the dimensions of these Aβ-containing protein aggregates (~5pone.0010645 pone.0010646 200 nm in longest axial cross-section) describe classical Rayleigh light scattering centers. Therefore, we sought to determine whether Aβ potentiated lens protein aggregation as assessed by quasi-elastic light scattering (QLS) analysis. Addition of synthetic human Aβ to human lens protein extract resulted in dose- and time-dependent increases in backscatterd light intensity that was not observed in control lens protein extracts without added human Aβ (Fig. 7*D*). These findings are consistent with Aβ-potentiated lens protein aggregation.

Discussion

In this report, we identify the origin and pathogenic mechanism of cataractogenesis in DS, establish the distinctive lens phenotype in DS as a genetic cataract, and define the molecular correspondence of DS-associated pathology in the lens and brain. Taken together with our previous findings of supranuclear Aβ lens pathology in late-onset sporadic AD [28], these results also establish the pathogenic relationship linking Aβ pathology in the lens and brain in both DS and AD.

AD neuropathology is an invariant feature of DS in subjects over the age of 30 [18,19] but may emerge as early as the first decade [18,34]. A critical factor contributing to the association of DS and AD Aβ pathology is the locus of the amyloid precursor protein gene (*APP*, 21q21) on the long arm of chromosome 21 [16,35,36]. Chromosome 21 triplication leads to increased dosage of the *APP* gene, accelerated cerebral Aβ accumulation, progressive AD neuropathology, and age-dependent cognitive sequelae [18,37,38,39,40]. With the exception of a single reported case of an individual with an atypical DS karyotype involving a specific chromosome 21 micro-deletion in the *APP* gene locus [41], all subjects with Down syndrome (including the rare cases involving Robertsonian translocation, partial duplications, or trisomic mosaicism) demonstrate triplication of the *APP* gene locus (21q21), overexpress amyloid precursor protein (APP) in affected somatic cells, accumulate β-amyloid peptides (Aβ) in the brain, and reveal evidence of early-onset Alzheimer's disease (AD) neuropathology [18,19,34,40,42].

In this report, we hypothesize and confirm that this genotype-phenotype concordance extends to Aβ-linked molecular pathology in the supranucleus and deep cortex of the lens. The characteristic cataract phenotype associated with Aβ lens pathology has been identified in only two clinical disorders, Alzheimer's disease [28] and as reported here, Down syndrome. This distinctive supranuclear cataract phenotype has not been reported in normal individuals, and is not observed in other non-AD neurodegenerative diseases, nor in normal aged controls [28]. The classical cerulean "blue dot" cataracts characteristic of DS initially emerge at the equatorial periphery of the lens, and over time, encompass progressively larger areas of the supranucleus and deep cortex (Fig. 8). While lens pathology observed in both infantile and mature DS lenses reveal opaque regions that are clinically described as supranuclear, the ages of the corresponding fiber cells comprising these regions are different (Fig 8). In this respect, it is important to note that the lens pathology in DS lenses does not implicate involvement of lens fibers cells in the fetal nucleus.

Distinctive lens pathology is recognized as a characteristic early-onset ocular phenotype in subjects with DS that may be clinically detectable early in life, and in some cases, at birth [20,22,23,24,26,43,44]. By contrast, DS neuropathology and cognitive sequelae typically emerge in the third decade of life and age-dependently progress thereafter [18,19,37,38,39,40]. In the present study, early-onset lens pathology is histochemically documented in illustrative cases of two young adults (21 and 22 years of age) with DS. Lenses obtained from these donors revealed marked Aβ amyloid lens pathology that was evident not only in the supranuclear subregion, but also throughout the anterior and equatorial cortex and epithelium. Aβ biochemical analysis of DS and normal control lenses indicates that increased Aβ expression in the lenses of people with DS may be evident very early in life. In one case included in this study, we detected abnormally high tissue levels of Aβ in the lens of a DS subject at 2 years of age. Although visual impairment may not become clinically apparent due to the peripheral distribution of these lenticular lesions relative to the iris, it is certainly the case that Aβ molecular pathology in the lens may be amongst the earliest expressed age-dependent phenotypes in Down syndrome.

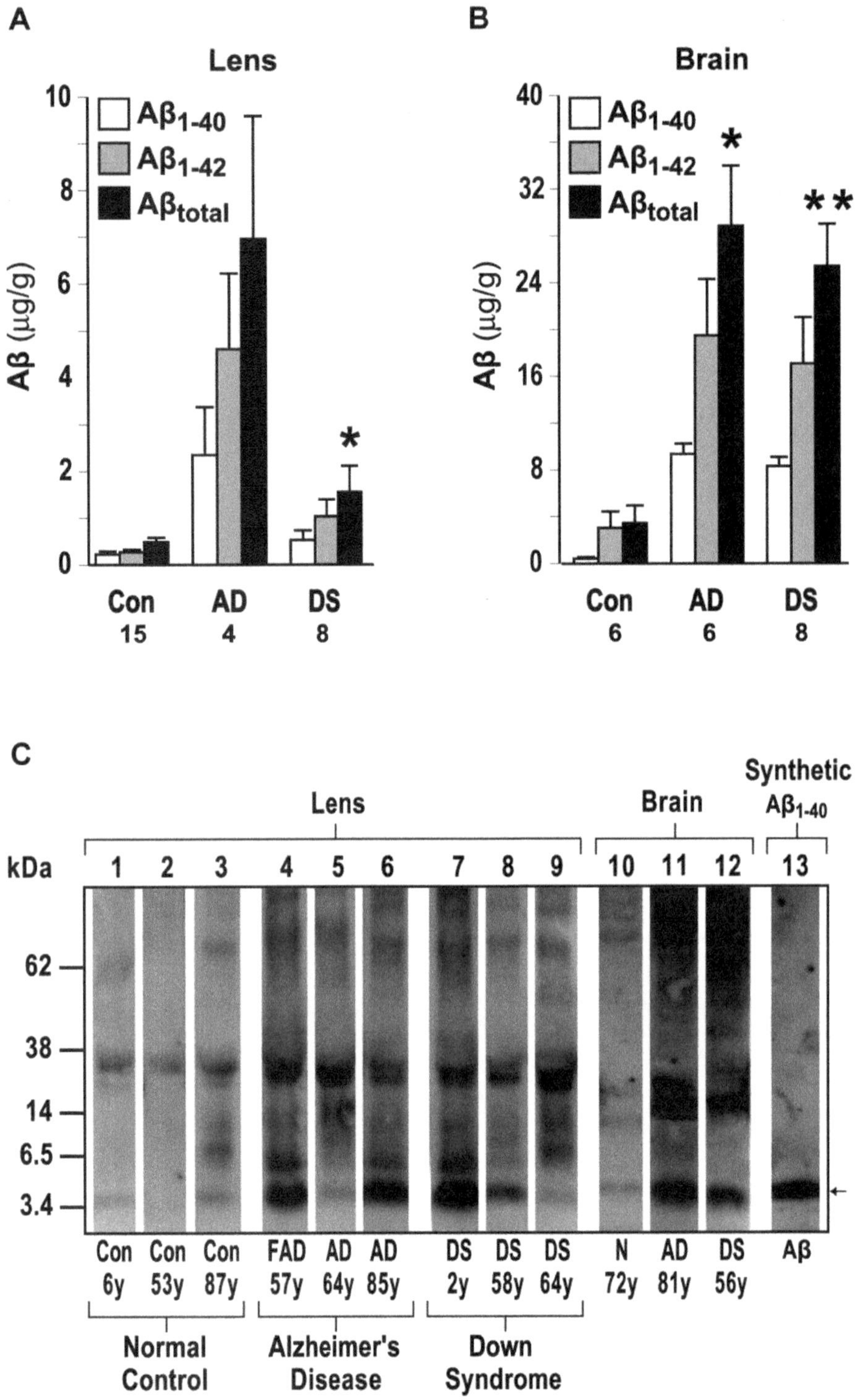

Figure 6. Increased Aβ expression in Down syndrome lens and brain. (**A-D**) Anti-Aβ ELISA analysis of human lens (**A**) and brain (**B**) fractionated by Aβ isoform. (**A**) Lens homogenates demonstrate elevated lens Aβ in subjects with Down syndrome ($n = 8$; $p = 0.027$) compared to normal controls ($n = 15$). (**B**) Brain homogenates demonstrate elevated Aβ in subjects with Down syndrome ($n = 8$; $p = 0.007$) and Alzheimer's disease ($n = 6$; $p = 0.026$) compared to normal controls ($n = 6$). (**C**) Immunoblot analysis of Down syndrome lens and brain homogenates reveals an intense Aβ-immunoreactive band that migrated with an apparent molecular weight of ~4kDa corresponding to synthetic human Aβ monomer (arrow). Note strong band corresponding to Aβ monomer in the 2-year-old Down syndrome lens (lane 7) and apparent shift from lower- to higher-order oligomeric Aβ in Down syndrome lenses with advancing age (lanes 7–9). Protein loading was normalized in each lane.

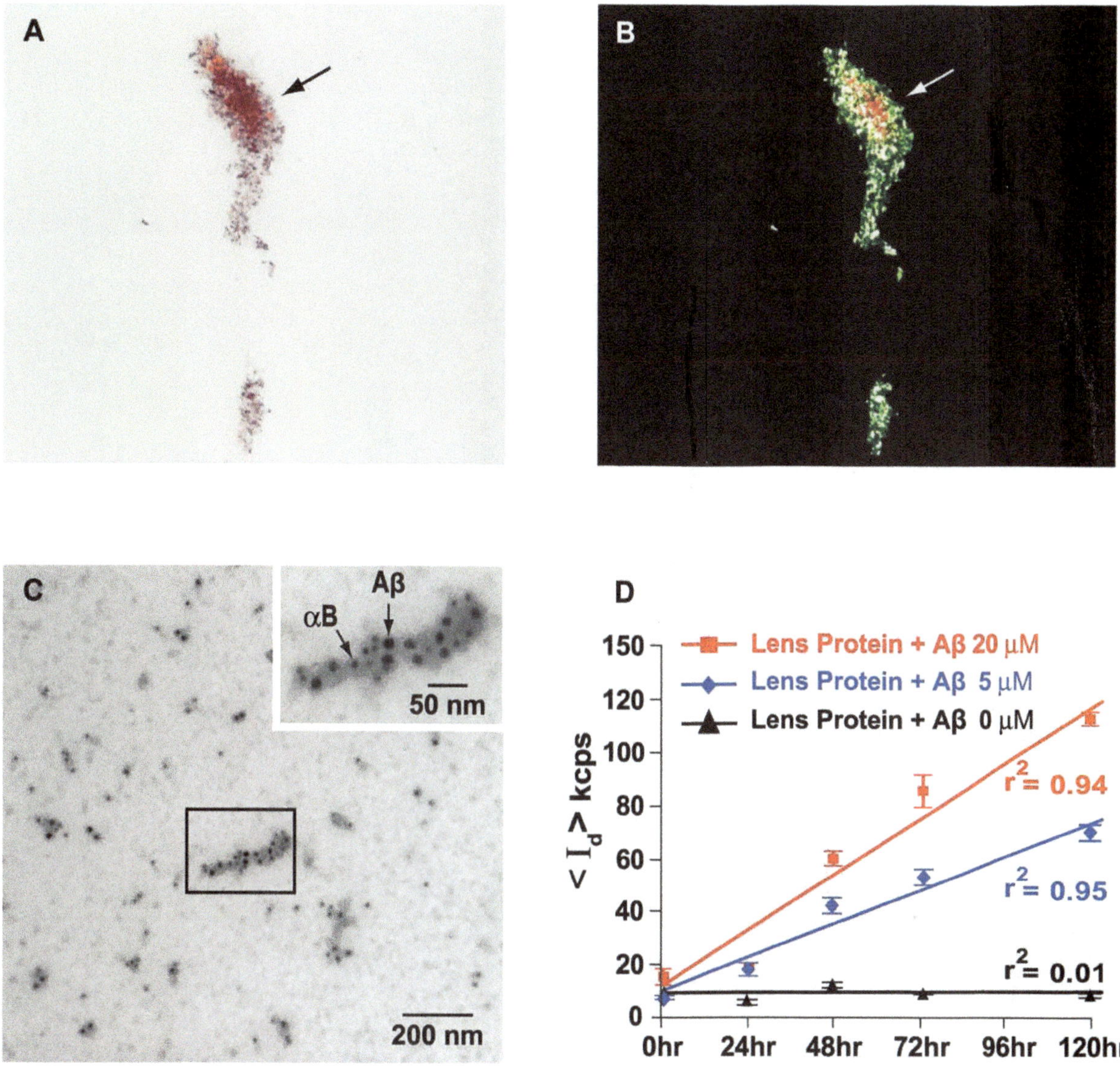

Figure 7. Aβ potentiates lens protein aggregation and Rayleigh light scattering *in vitro.* (**A**) Brightfield photomicroscopic image of a Congo red-stained protein aggregate (arrow) formed during incubation of human lens protein extract with synthetic human Aβ. (**B**) Same Congo red-stained lens protein aggregate demonstrating classical amyloid birefringence under cross-polarized illumination. (**C**) Anti-Aβ/anti-αB-crystallin double immunogold electron microscopic analysis of protein aggregates formed during incubation of human lens protein with synthetic human Aβ. Larger immunogold particles (15 nm diameter) detect Aβ. Smaller immunogold particles (10 nm diameter) detect αB-crystallin. Box indicates region of detail highlighted in Fig. 7*D*. Scale bar = 200 nm. Inset, hetero-oligomeric composition noted in a single protein aggregate demonstrated by double immunogold (anti-Aβ and anti-αB-crystallin) electron microscopy. Analysis was performed on human lens protein incubated with synthetic human Aβ. Larger immunogold particles (15 nm diameter) detect Aβ (black arrow). Smaller immunogold particles (10 nm diameter) detect αB-crystallin (white arrow). Scale bar = 50 nm. (**D**) Quasi-elastic light scattering (QLS) analysis detects increased backscattered light due to concentration-and time-dependent protein aggregation during incubation of human lens protein with synthetic human Aβ. Experimental samples studied by QLS were analyzed by amyloid histochemistry (Fig. 7A,B) and double (anti-Aβ and anti-αB-crystallin) immunogold electron microscopy (Fig. 7C).

The DS-associated cataract phenotype is not observed in other non-AD neurodegenerative diseases, nor in normal aged controls. In this context, it is important to note that DS-associated cataracts are phenotypically distinct from age-related cataracts (ARC) that commonly emerge starting in the fifth decade of life and typically localize in the central nuclear region. In contrast to the lens pathology in ARC, the DS lens phenotype is often clinically detectable early in life, and in some cases, may be present at birth [20,22,23,24,26,43,44]. The distinctive lens phenotype associated with DS is further distinguished from ARC by supranuclear Aβ histopathology, a pathological feature shared with late-onset AD [28].

The results of the present study support a DS-associated pathogenic pathway linking progressive age-dependent Aβ accumulation in the lens and supranuclear cataractogenesis with corresponding cerebral Aβ accumulation and neuropathology in the brain. We propose the following mechanistic pathway leading to expression of the characteristic lens and brain phenotypes associated with DS (Fig. 9). Increased *APP* gene dosage resulting from chromosome 21 triplication (*APP*, 21q21) leads to increased expression of the amyloid precursor protein (APP) and elevated levels of the pathogenic Aβ cleavage peptides in affected tissues. In the brain, Aβ accumulation leads to early-onset neuropathology and progressive age-dependent neurocog-

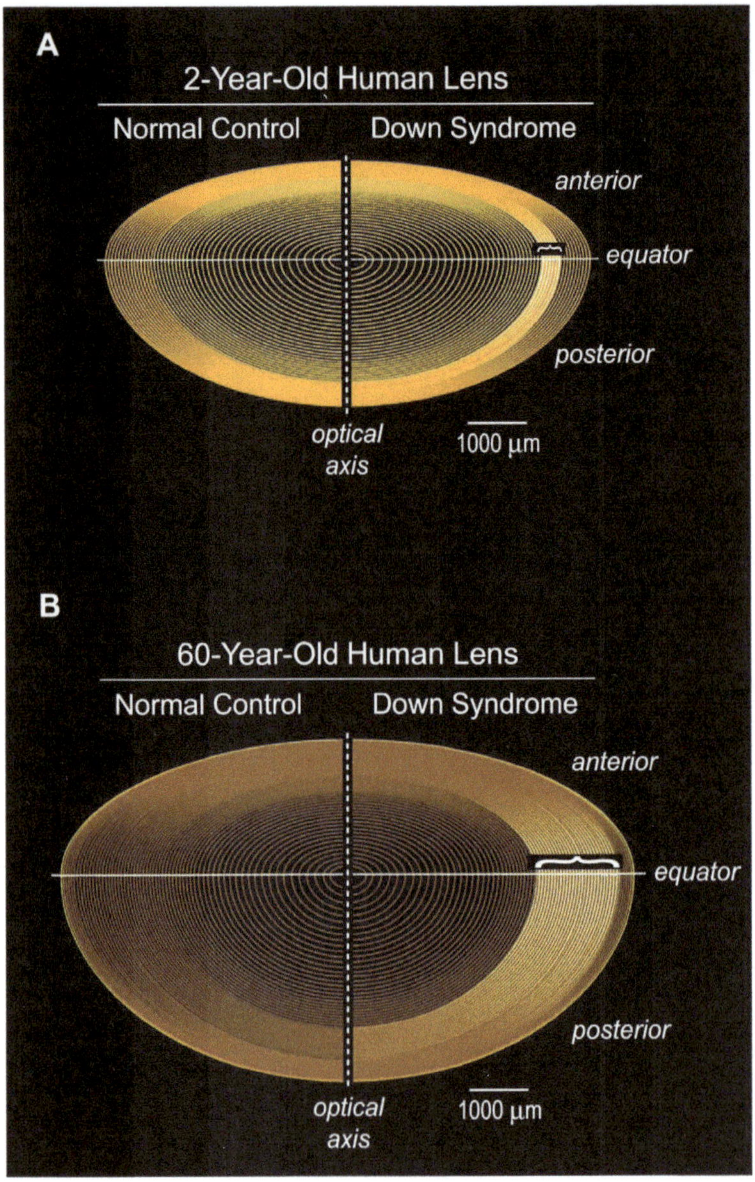

Figure 8. Age-dependent supranuclear cataractogenesis in Down syndrome. The anatomical localization of the characteristic Down syndrome cataract phenotype (white shading) reflects the temporal origin and natural history of the underlying lens pathology. Fetal lens fiber cells are not involved in this pathogenic process. Parentheses indicate equatorial axial extent of age-dependent disease-linked Aβpathology in the supranuclear subregion of Down syndrome lenses. See text for details.

nitive sequelae. With respect to the lens, the present investigation supports the hypothesis that increased expression of Aβ in the lens leads to amyloidogenic interactions with other structural proteins (e.g., αB-crystallin) within the cytoplasm of supranuclear lens fiber cells. This pathogenic cascade leads to increased lens protein aggregation, light scattering, opacification, and ultimately, disease-linked cataracts [45]. Given the fact that the long-lived lens fiber cells are metabolically sluggish and demonstrate limited capacity to catabolize aggregated protein, we speculate that DS-linked Aβ amyloid pathology in the lens may precede corresponding Aβ pathology in the brain. Regardless, the proposed pathogenic model for Aβ pathology in both tissue compartments (brain and lens) is in general agreement with a broad conception of the amyloid cascade hypothesis [16,46,47].

We hypothesize that the Aβ detected in DS lenses is generated endogenously. The human lens expresses the full complement of enzymes and precursor proteins necessary to generate and process Aβ [28,48,49,50]. In the present study, this hypothesis is supported by the finding of intense Aβ immunoreactivity in DS lens epithelial cells. Our finding that lens fiber cell Aβ is exclusively cytoplasmic suggests that this amyloidogenic peptide may be released from intracellular processing compartments during organelle disintegration accompanying epithelial-to-fiber cell terminal differentiation. This model points to the lens as an appropriate target for ascertaining the temporal origin and natural history of AD-linked molecular pathology *in vivo*.

Our findings suggest an apparent temporal discordance in DS with respect to phenotype expression in the lens and brain, with pathology in the former preceding that in the latter. However, we also observed variability in age-dependent phenotypic expression of Aβ molecular pathology in the lens that comports with analogous variability in the brain of subjects with DS [34,51].

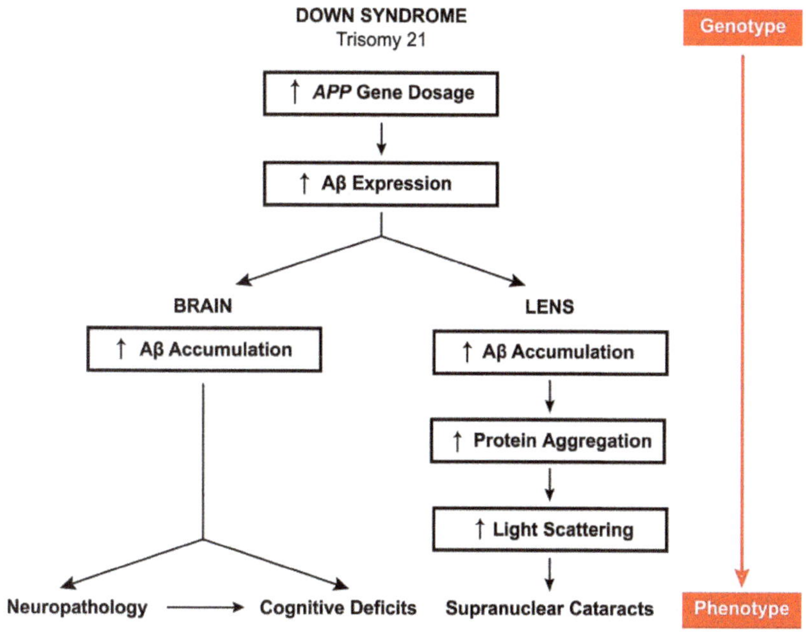

Figure 9. Model pathogenic pathways in Down syndrome brain and lens. Triplication of human chromosome 21 in Down syndrome results in increased dosage of the *APP* gene (21q21), overexpression of the Alzheimer's disease amyloid-β precursor protein (APP), and progressive accumulation of amyloidogenic amyloid-β peptides (Aβ) in the brain and lens. Deposition of Aβ in both anatomical compartments results in age-dependent Aβ amyloid pathology and disease-linked tissue-specific phenotypes in both Down syndrome and Alzheimer's disease. See text for details.

The significance and natural history of variability in Aβ tissue concentration in the lens and its possible relationship to the brain in DS are subjects of ongoing investigation.

In this study, we identify Aβ amyloid pathology as the shared molecular etiology of two defining features of DS, namely, supranuclear cataracts in the lens and AD neuropathology in the brain. The proximal pathogenesis of both pathologies likely derives from the primary chromosomal disorder and associated *APP* gene-dosage imbalance (Fig. 9). The results reported here support a testable pathogenic mechanism by which the primary chromosomal disorder in DS may be translated into a distinctive phenotype expressed in the lens. In this regard, the phenotypic concordance of Aβ lens pathology in both diseases, DS and AD, is striking. Given that DS-linked pathology may be indicative of aberrant Aβ accumulation in both compartments, the lens may provide an optically accessible target tissue for early detection and longitudinal assessment of early Aβ molecular pathology in DS and AD. Future clinical studies will be required to systematically evaluate the frequency of this supranuclear phenotype in DS patients. Quasi-elastic light scattering instrumentation or other techniques may provide a practical approach for quantitative assessment of specific lens pathology throughout the course of the disease.

Supporting Information

Figure S1 Stereo image pair demonstrating mature supranuclear pathology in the lens (with intact zonule fibers) from a subject with Down syndrome. Characteristic circumferential supranuclear cataract in the lens of a 64-year-old male subject with Down syndrome. This distinctive cataract is evident as an annular half-toroid band of opacification in the deep cortical and supranuclear subregions of the lens (shown with intact zonules). This same lens specimen is presented as a slit lamp image (Fig. 1H) and as a stereo image pair (without zonules, Fig. 2A). This dramatic Down syndrome cataract is phenotypically comparable to the subequatorial supranuclear cataract observed in advanced Alzheimer's disease. These distinctive supranuclear cataracts are not observed in age-normal control subjects. See text for details.

Acknowledgments

We thank Mr. Joseph Bertelsen (Signet Laboratories, Covance, Dedham, MA) for generously providing 6E10 and 4G8 monoclonal antibodies. We gratefully acknowledge the National Disease Registry Interchange, Sun Health Research Institute, and the Florida Lion's Eye Bank for their assistance with tissue procurement. We would like to thank the many patients and families who made this work possible.

Author Contributions

Conceived and designed the experiments: JAM RP RDM RMR JIC RET DGH LEG. Performed the experiments: JAM RDM SL MAB JGG ME SJS AM. Analyzed the data: JAM RP RDM MAB ME JK JIC RET DGH LEG. Contributed reagents/materials/analysis tools: JAM RP RDM SL MAB ME RF RMR JK RET DGH LEG. Wrote the paper: JAM RP RDM DGH LEG. Revised the manuscript: JGG AM RF RMR JK JIC RET.

References

1. Down JLH (1866) Observations on an ethnic classification of idiots. London Hosp Clin Lect Rep 3: 259.
2. Epstein CJ (1989) Down syndrome, trisomy 21. In: Scriver CR, Beaudet AL, Sly WS, Valle D, eds. Metabolic Basis of Inherited Disease. New York: McGraw-Hill. pp 291–326.
3. Online Mendelian Inheritance in Man - Down Syndrome. Available: http://www.ncbi.nlm.nih.gov/entrez/dispomim.cgi?id = 190685. Accessed 25 April 2010.
4. Pueschel SM (1990) Clinical aspects of Down syndrome from infancy to adulthood. Am J Med Genet Suppl 7: 52–56.
5. Roizen NJ, Patterson D (2003) Down's syndrome. The Lancet 361: 1281–1289.

6. March of Dimes Birth Defects Foundation (2006) March of Dimes Global Report on Birth Defects: The Hidden Toll of Dying and Disabled Children. White Plains, NY: March of Dimes Birth Defects Foundation. Available: http://www.marchofdimes.com/MOD-Report-PF.pdf. Accessed April 2010.
7. Lejeune J, Gautier M, Turpin R (1959) Etude des chromosomes somatiques de neuf enfants mongoliens. C R Acad Sci 248: 1721–1722.
8. Antonarakis SE, Lyle R, Dermitzakis E, Reymond A, Deutsch S (2004) Chromosome 21 and down syndrome: from genomics to pathophysiology. Nat Rev Genet 5: 725–738.
9. Epstein CJ (2001) Down syndrome (trisomy 21). In: Scriver CR, Beaudet AL, Sly WS, Valle D, eds. The metabolic and molecular bases of inherited disease 8th ed. New York: McGraw Hill. pp 1223–1256.
10. Thuline HC, Pueschel SM (1982) Cytogenetics in Down syndrome. In: Pueschel SM, Rynders JE, eds. Down Syndrome: Advances in Biomedicine and the Behavioral Sciences. Cambridge: Ware Press. 133 p.
11. Hook EB, Cross PK, Schreinemachers DM (1983) Chromosomal abnormality rates at amniocentesis and in live-born infants. J A M A 249: 2034–2038.
12. Korenberg JR, Chen XN, Schipper R, Sun Z, Gonsky R, et al. (1994) Down syndrome phenotypes: the consequences of chromosomal imbalance. Proc Natl Acad Sci USA 91: 4997–5001.
13. Lyle R, Bena F, Gagos S, Gehrig C, Lopez G, et al. (2008) Genotype-phenotype correlations in Down syndrome identified by array CGH in 30 cases of partial trisomy and partial monosomy chromosome 21. Eur J of Hum Gen. pp 1–13.
14. Mikkelsen M (1977) Down's syndrome cytogenetic epidemiology. Hereditas 86: 45–50.
15. Online Mendelian Inheritance in Man - Amyloid Beta A4 Precursor Protein. Available: http://www.ncbi.nlm.nih.gov/entrez/dispomim.cgi?id = 104760. Accessed 24 April 2010.
16. Tanzi RE, Gusella J, Watkins P, Bruns G, George-Hyslop PS, et al. (1987) Amyloid beta protein gene: cDNA, mRNA distribution, and genetic linkage near the Alzheimer locus. Science 235: 880–884.
17. Beyreuther K, Pollwein P, Multhaup G, Monning U, Konig G, et al. (1993) Regulation and expression of the Alzheimer's beta/A4 amyloid protein precursor in health, disease, and Down's syndrome. Ann N Y Acad Sci 695: 91–102.
18. Wisniewski KE, Wisniewski HM, Wen GY (1985) Occurrence of neuropathological changes and dementia of Alzheimer's disease in Down's syndrome. Ann Neurol 17: 278–282.
19. Lott IT, Head E (2005) Alzheimer disease and Down syndrome: factors in pathogenesis. Neurobiol Aging 26: 383–389.
20. Pearce FH, Rankine R, Ormond AK (1910) Notes on twenty-eight cases of Mongolian Imbeciles: with special reference to their ocular condition. British Medical Journal 2: 186–190.
21. Oliver CA (1891) A clinical study of the ocular symptoms found in the so-called Mongolian type of idiocy. Trans Am Ophthalmol Soc 6: 140–148.
22. Igersheimer J (1951) The Relationship of Lenticular Changes to Mongolism. Trans Am Ophthalmol Soc 49: 595–624.
23. Lowe RF (1949) The eyes in Mongolism. Brit, J Ophthal 33: 131–174.
24. Robb RM, Marchevsky A (1978) Pathology of the Lens in Down's syndrome. Arch Ophthalmol 96: 1039–1042.
25. Da Cunha RP, Moreira JB (1996) Ocular findings in Down's syndrome. Am J Ophthalmol 122: 236–244.
26. Creavin AL, Brown RD (2009) Ophthalmic abnormalities in children with Down's syndrome. J Pediatr Ophthalmol Strabismus 46: 76–82.
27. Kallen B, Mastroiacovo P, Robert E (1996) Major congenital malformations in Down's syndrome. Am J Med Genet 65: 160–166.
28. Goldstein LE, Muffat JA, Cherny RA, Moir RD, Ericsson MH, et al. (2003) Cytosolic beta-amyloid deposition and supranuclear cataracts in lenses from people with Alzheimer's disease. Lancet 361: 1258–1265.
29. Armed Forces Institute of Pathology US (1992) Congo red (Bennhold's) method for amyloid. In: Prophet, Mills, Arrington, Sobin, eds. Laboratory Methods in Histotechnology. Washington, D.C.: American Registry of Pathology. 168 p.
30. Merlini G, Ikeda S, Benson MD, Saraiva MJ, Westermark P, et al. Report of the Nomenclature Committee. In: Skinner M, Berk JL, Connors LH, eds. 2006 November 5-9; Marine Biological Laboratory, Woods Hole, MA. CRC Press (Taylor & Francis Group, LLC). pp xxiii–xxiv.
31. Westermark P, Benson MD, Buxbaum JN, Cohen AS, Frangione B, et al. (2007) A primer of amyloid nomenclature. Amyloid 14: 179–183.
32. Horwitz J (2000) The function of alpha-crystallin in vision. Semin Cell Dev Biol 11: 53–60.
33. Lowe J, Errington DR, Lennox G, Pike I, Spendlove I, et al. (1992) Ballooned neurons in several neurodegenerative diseases and stroke contain alpha B-crystallin. Neuropathol Appl Neurobiol 18: 341–350.
34. Leverenz JB, Raskind MA (1998) Early amyloid deposition in the medial temporal lobe of young Down syndrome patients: a regional quantitative analysis. Exp Neurol 150: 296–304.
35. Goldgaber D, Lerman MI, McBride OW, Saffiotti U, Gajdusek DC (1987) Characterization and chromosomal localization of a cDNA encoding brain amyloid of Alzheimer's disease. Science 235: 877–880.
36. Robakis NK, Wisniewski HM, Jenkins EC, Devine-Gage EA, Houck GE, et al. (1987) Chromosome 21q21 sublocalisation of gene encoding beta-amyloid peptide in cerebral vessels and neuritic (senile) plaques of people with Alzheimer disease and Down syndrome. Lancet 1: 384–385.
37. Oyama F, Cairns N, Shimada H, Oyama R, Titani K, et al. (1994) Down's syndrome: up-regulation of beta-amyloid protein precursor and tau mRNAs and their defective coordination. J Neurochem 62: 1062–1066.
38. Rovelet-Lecrux A, Hannequin D, Raux G, Le Meur N, Laquerriere A, et al. (2006) APP locus duplication causes autosomal dominant early-onset Alzheimer disease with cerebral amyloid angiopathy. Nat Genet 38: 24–26.
39. Wavrant-De Vrièze F, Crook R, Holmans P, Kehoe P, Owen MJ, et al. (1999) Genetic variability at the amyloid-[beta] precursor protein locus may contribute to the risk of late-onset Alzheimer's disease. Neurosci Lett 269: 67–70.
40. Zigman WB, Lott IT (2007) Alzheimer's disease in Down syndrome: neurobiology and risk. Ment Retard Dev Disabil Res Rev 13: 237–246.
41. Prasher VP, Farrer MJ, Kessling AM, Fisher EM, West RJ, et al. (1998) Molecular mapping of Alzheimer-type dementia in Down's syndrome. Ann Neurol 43: 380–383.
42. Schupf N, Sergievsky GH (2002) Genetic and host factors for dementia in Down's syndrome. Br J Psychiatry 180: 405–410.
43. Cogan DG, Kuwabara T (1962) Pathology of cataracts in mongoloid idiocy. A new concept of the pathogenesis of cataracts of the coronary-cerulean type. Doc Ophthalmol 16: 73–80.
44. Haargaard B, Fledelius HC (2006) Down's syndrome and early cataract. Br J Ophthalmol 90: 1024–1027.
45. Costello MJ, Johnsen S, Gilliland KO, Freel CD, Fowler WC (2007) Predicted light scattering from particles observed in human age-related nuclear cataracts using mie scattering theory. Invest Ophthalmol Vis Sci 48: 303–312.
46. Hardy JA, Higgins GA (1992) Alzheimer's disease: the amyloid cascade hypothesis. Science 256: 184–185.
47. Hardy J, Selkoe DJ (2002) The amyloid hypothesis of Alzheimer's disease: progress and problems on the road to therapeutics. Science 297: 353–356.
48. Frederikse PH, Garland D, Zigler JSJ, Piatigorsky J (1996) Oxidative stress increases production of beta-amyloid precursor protein and beta-amyloid (Abeta) in mammalian lenses, and Abeta has toxic effects on lens epithelial cells. J Biol Chem 271: 10169–10174.
49. Frederikse PH, Zigler JS (1998) Presenilin expression in the ocular lens. Curr Eye Res 17: 947–952.
50. Li G, Percontino L, Sun Q, Qazi AS, Frederikse PH (2003) Beta-amyloid secretases and beta-amyloid degrading enzyme expression in lens. Mol Vis 9: 179–183.
51. Lemere CA, Blusztajn JK, Yamaguchi H, Wisniewski T, Saido TC, et al. (1996) Sequence of deposition of heterogeneous amyloid beta-peptides and APO E in Down syndrome: implications for initial events in amyloid plaque formation. Neurobiol Dis 3: 16–32.
52. Hogan MJ, Alvarado JA, Weddell JE (1971) Histology of the Human Eye: An Atlas and Textbook. Philadelphia: W.B. Saunders Company. 687 p.

Gene Expression Profiling in a Mouse Model Identifies Fetal Liver- and Placenta-Derived Potential Biomarkers for Down Syndrome Screening

Jeroen L. A. Pennings[1*⁹], Wendy Rodenburg[1⁹], Sandra Imholz[1], Maria P. H. Koster[2], Conny T. M. van Oostrom[1], Timo M. Breit[3], Peter C. J. I. Schielen[2], Annemieke de Vries[1]

1 Laboratory for Health Protection Research (GBO), National Institute for Public Health and the Environment (RIVM), Bilthoven, The Netherlands, **2** Laboratory for Infectious Diseases and Perinatal Screening (LIS), National Institute for Public Health and the Environment (RIVM), Bilthoven, The Netherlands, **3** MicroArray Department (MAD), University of Amsterdam (UvA), Amsterdam, The Netherlands

Abstract

Background: As a first step to identify novel potential biomarkers for prenatal Down Syndrome screening, we analyzed gene expression in embryos of wild type mice and the Down Syndrome model Ts1Cje. Since current Down Syndrome screening markers are derived from placenta and fetal liver, these tissues were chosen as target.

Methodology/Principal Findings: Placenta and fetal liver at 15.5 days gestation were analyzed by microarray profiling. We confirmed increased expression of genes located at the trisomic chromosomal region. Overall, between the two genotypes more differentially expressed genes were found in fetal liver than in placenta. Furthermore, the fetal liver data are in line with the hematological aberrations found in humans with Down Syndrome as well as Ts1Cje mice. Together, we found 25 targets that are predicted (by Gene Ontology, UniProt, or the Human Plasma Proteome project) to be detectable in human serum.

Conclusions/Significance: Fetal liver might harbor more promising targets for Down Syndrome screening studies. We expect these new targets will help focus further experimental studies on identifying and validating human maternal serum biomarkers for Down Syndrome screening.

Editor: Gisela Nogales-Gadea, University Hospital Vall d'Hebron, Spain

Funding: This work was carried out as part of the Strategic Research Program of the authors' institute. No external financial support was provided for this study. Only the authors had influence on the collection, analysis, and interpretation of the data, and on the preparation of the manuscript.

Competing Interests: The authors have declared that no competing interests exist.

* E-mail: Jeroen.Pennings@rivm.nl

⁹ These authors contributed equally to this work.

Introduction

Prenatal screening for Down Syndrome (DS) has been routinely available for two decades. Typically, such screening procedures consist of a risk calculation based on maternal age, nucal translucency and serum biomarker measurements, after which women with a high predicted risk can opt for invasive testing such as amniocentesis or chorionic villus sampling. Initially, the most commonly used method for risk calculation was the second trimester triple test, which combines serum levels for alpha-fetoprotein (AFP), unconjugated estriol (uE3), and the free β subunit of human chorion gonadotrophin (fβ-hCG) with maternal age [1,2]. Currently, many countries including the Netherlands, have replaced this by the first trimester combined test, which is based on fβ-hCG and pregnancy-associated plasma protein A (PAPP-A) serum concentrations, ultrasound nuchal translucency (NT) measurements and maternal age [3]. This latter test has a Detection Rate (DR) of 75–85% at a 5% false positive rate (FPR) [4–6]. Although the reliability of the first trimester combined test is better than the triple test, both the DR and the FPR are still in need for improvement, and a lot of international effort has been put in improving both kinds of prenatal tests.

A promising approach to improve DS screening is by adding multiple biochemical markers to the serum analysis. By means of innovative proteomics, genomics, and bioinformatics approaches, novel discriminative markers can be identified that, when added to the current serum assays, can improve the DR and FPR [7–12].

Serum markers used in these two routinely used screening tests essentially originate from two tissues, namely fetal liver (AFP) and the placenta (fβ-hCG, PAPP-A), whereas the non-protein serum biomarker uE3 is produced by the placenta from its precursor dehydroepiandrosterone sulfate produced by the fetal liver and adrenal glands. We therefore hypothesize that placenta and fetal liver harbor additional biomarkers suitable for improving DS screening, and have set up a research strategy to identify them. Availability of fetal human material for DS cases or controls is limited and therefore existing human studies are restricted to placenta or cultured trophoblasts [13–16]. Additionally, when human material is available, genomics and proteomics studies are inevitably complicated by sources of variation from maternal, fetal, and clinical origin.

A possibility to overcome such limitations is the use of inbred animal models. For ethical and practical reasons, mouse models are preferable for such studies, and fortunately several mouse models are available mimicking human Down syndrome [17–24]. In this study we used the Ts1Cje mouse strain [21], which contains a segmental trisomy of mouse chromosome 16 (Mmu16) distal of the *Sod1* gene, including a region orthologous to the region of human chromosome 21 commonly associated with Down Syndrome: the "Down Syndrome critical region" [21]. We selected a mouse model in which the Mmu16 trisomic region extends beyond the DSCR, as comparative genetic studies [25,26] have indicated that trisomy for only the DSCR is not sufficient for a complete DS phenotype. Ts1Cje mice have been shown to display a recognizable DS phenotype which consists of craniofacial malformations including a smaller cerebellum volume, as well as learning and behavioral abnormalities [17,21,27].

In this study, fetuses were obtained from wild type mothers bred with either wild type or Ts1Cje males. Gene expression profiles in fetal liver and placenta of wild type and Ts1Cje fetuses were compared and for differentially expressed genes it was examined if they code for blood detectable proteins and/or are involved in clinically involved processes. With this strategy, we have identified a number of targets with potential for further studies ultimately aimed at biomarker application in human prenatal DS screening.

Materials and Methods

Ethics statement

This study was agreed upon by the Animal Experimentation Ethical Committee of our institute under permit number 200900176. Animal handling in this study was carried out in accordance with relevant Dutch national legislation, including the 1997 Dutch Act on Animal Experimentation.

Animal studies

The trisomic B6EiC3Sn-Ts(16C-tel)1Cje1 mice, also named Ts1Cje, contain an additional copy of distal chromosome 16 [21]. Trisomic B6EiC3Sn-Ts(16C-tel)1Cje1 mice (genotype Ts/+) and wild type hybrid background B6EiC3SnF1/J mice (genotype +/+) were purchased from the Jackson laboratory (Bar Harbor, ME, USA).

To obtain Ts1Cje and wild type fetuses for RNA isolation, male +/+ mice (control group) or male Ts/+ mice (Down group) were bred with female breeding mice of the C3H/HeNHsd strain (Harlan, Horst, the Netherlands) at 8–10 weeks of age. After mating, females were separated and pregnant females were identified through scoring of vaginal plugs (embryonic time point E0.5 in days). Females were sacrificed on E15.5 using CO_2/O_2. From pregnant mice all embryos were collected and every single embryo was processed further. Placenta and fetal liver were collected for RNA extraction and paws were collected for DNA extraction and genotyping. All tissues were immediately frozen in liquid nitrogen and stored at −80°C until further processing.

DNA extraction, embryo genotyping and sex determination

Genomic DNA was extracted from embryo paws. Genotyping and sex determination on mice embryos were both performed by multiplex PCR using primer sequences given in Supporting Dataset S1. Each PCR contained 5 µl 2× Hotstar Master Mix (Qiagen), 0.5 µM of each primer and 10–50 ng genomic DNA, in a total volume of 10 µl. PCR reactions were carried out in a Perkin-Elmer 9600 thermal cycler under the following conditions: 95°C for 15 min; 30 cycles of 94°C for 30 sec, 55°C for 30 sec, 72°C for 1 min; followed by 72°C for 10 min.

RNA isolation, yield and quality

RNA was extracted from placenta and fetal liver using the miRNeasy kit (Qiagen). RNA concentrations were measured using a NanoDrop spectrophotometer (NanoDrop Technologies, Wilmington, DE, USA). The integrity of the RNA samples was determined with the BioAnalyzer (Agilent Technolgies, Amstelveen, The Netherlands) using the RNA nano 6000 kit (Agilent Technologies) yielding RIN-values ≥9.6. For placenta and fetal liver, microarray analysis was carried out using RNA samples of 24 individual embryos, *i.e.* six male and six female embryos from both genotypes.

Amplification and labeling protocol

Per sample, 500 ng total RNA was amplified according to the Agilent QuickAmp kit manual (Agilent technologies). Amino-allyl modified nucleotides were incorporated during the aRNA synthesis (2.5 mM rGAU (GE Healthcare), 0.75 mM rCTP (GE Healthcare), 0.75 mM AA-rCTP (TriLink Biotechnologies). Synthesized aRNA was purified with the E.Z.N.A. MicroElute RNA Clean Up Kit (Omega Bio-Tek). Test samples were labeled with Cy3 and a Reference sample (made by pooling equimolar amounts of RNA from Test samples) was labeled with Cy5. Next, 5 µg of aRNA was dried down and dissolved in 50 mM carbonate buffer pH 8.5. Individual vials of Cy3/Cy5 from the mono-reactive dye packs (GE Healthcare) were dissolved in 200 µl DMSO. To each sample, 10 µl of the appropriate CyDye dissolved in DMSO was added and the mixture was incubated for 1 h. Reactions were quenched with the addition of 5 µl 4 M hydroxylamine (Sigma-Aldrich). The labeled aRNA was purified with the E.Z.N.A. MicroElute RNA Clean Up Kit. The yields of aRNA and CyDye incorporation were measured on the NanoDrop ND-1000.

Microarray hybridization, scanning & data processing

Each hybridization mixture consisted of 1.1 µg Test (Cy3) and 1.1 µg Reference (Cy5) sample. Samples were dried and 1.98 µl of the appropriate sample tracking control (STC, Roche Nimblegen) was added. The hybridization cocktail was made according to the manufacturer's instructions (Nimblegen Arrays User's Guide – Gene Expression Arrays Version 5.0, Roche Nimblegen). From this mix, 5.22 µl was added to each sample. The samples were incubated for 5 min at 95°C and 5 min at 42°C prior to loading. Hybridization samples were loaded onto a 12×135 k *Mus musculus* microarray (Catalog no. 05543797001, Design 090901 MM9 EXP HX12) containing probes for 44,170 genes with 3 spots per target probe. Microarrays were hybridized for 20 hours at 42°C with the NimbleGen Hybridization System 4 (Roche Nimblegen). Afterwards, the slides were washed according to the Nimblegen Arrays User's Guide – Gene Expression Arrays Version 5.0 and scanned in an ozone-free room with a Agilent DNA microarray scanner G2565CA (Agilent Technologies). Feature extraction was performed with NimbleScan v2.5 (Roche Nimblegen). Each microarray corresponded to labeled RNA from one individual embryo.

Data analysis

Complete raw and normalized microarray data and their MIAME compliant metadata have been deposited at GEO (www.ncbi.nlm.nih.gov/geo) under accession number GSE24272.

Raw microarray signal data were normalized in R (www.r-project.org), using a four step approach [28]: (1) natural log-transformation, (2) quantile normalization of all scans, (3) correcting the sample spot signal for the corresponding reference spot signal and (4) averaging data from replicate probe spots. Normalized data for the resulting 44170 probes were further analyzed in R and Microsoft Excel.

For both placenta and liver, gene expression differences between either sex or genotype were compared with an ANOVA. Obtained p-values were corrected for multiple testing by calculating the false discovery rate (FDR) according to Benjamini and Hochberg [29]. Probes with a False Discovery Rate (FDR)<0.05 were considered significant. When multiple probes corresponding to the same gene were significant, their data were averaged to remove redundancy in further analysis. Probes with significant expression differences between male and female embryos were excluded from the analysis on genotype differences.

Hierarchical clustering analysis was performed using GeneMaths XT (Applied Maths, St-Martens-Latem, Belgium) using Euclidean distance and Ward linkage. Functional Annotation and Gene Ontology (GO) term enrichment were examined with the DAVID Bioinformatics Resource (http://david.abcc.ncifcrf.gov) [30]. Enrichment for tissue-specific or literature-based functional gene sets was determined in R using an in-house developed algorithm based on the DAVID methodology. Tissue- or lineage-specific gene sets were obtained from data downloaded from the BioGPS website (http://biogps.gnf.org) [31,32] as well as other relevant literature sets [33–35].

Groupwise regulation of Gene Ontology categories and above-mentioned custom gene sets were determined by Gene Set Enrichment Analysis (GSEA) [35] using default analysis parameters. Gene sets were considered regulated if the GSEA p-value was<0.05 and the FDR was <0.10.

To determine which genes code for proteins detectable in human serum, we determined which proteins are annotated in Gene Ontology as extracellular, in UniProt as secreted, or have been experimentally detected in the Human Plasma Proteome project [36].

Quantitative RT-PCR

Microarray results were for a subset of genes verified by quantitative RT-PCR analysis on RNA from 12 Ts1Cje versus 12 WT samples. For this, all reagents, methods and equipment were obtained from Applied Biosystems. TaqMan gene expression assays used are given in Supplementary Dataset S2. Assays for *Hprt* and *Polr2a* were custom-made and included as endogenous controls. After RNA samples were reverse transcribed to cDNA, qPCR was performed on 125 ng of cDNA using the 7500 Fast real-time PCR system. Threshold cycles were automatically derived from the amplification plots constructed of the ROX-normalized fluorescence signals by 7500 Fast system SDS software v1.3. The average of the *Hprt* and *Polr2a* level per cDNA sample was used to normalize the expression of the other genes. Relative quantification of the mRNA copies in the Ts1Cje samples compared to that of the WT samples was performed by the comparative threshold cycle method using Microsoft Excel.

Results

Genotype confirmation

To validate the use of a mouse model for DS in a transcriptomics study, we first compared the expression ratio between Ts1Cje and WT embryos for genes located on chromosome Mmu16. Plotting the gene expression ratio against the chromosomal position (Fig. 1) reveals an increased expression for genes in the segmental trisomic locus in both fetal liver and placenta.

Sex-specific gene regulation

Comparing differences in expression levels between male and female embryos of either genotype revealed 31 significant probes (12 genes) in fetal liver and 25 significant probes (11 genes) in placenta. When combined, this resulted in 16 genes for which corresponding probes were excluded from the analysis of genotype differences. Briefly, 7 genes were male-specific genes and 9 female-

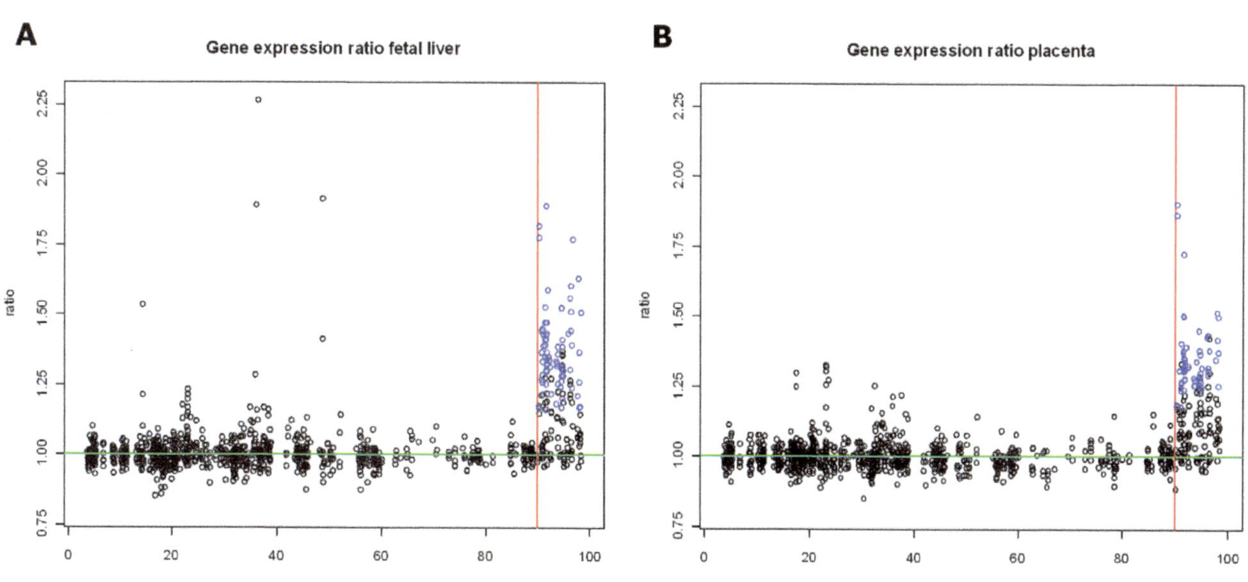

Figure 1. Chromosome plot of Mmu16 with gene expression ratios between Ts1Cje and wild type mice. Significant genes (FDR 5%) are indicated in blue. The border of the trisomic locus is indicated with a vertical red line.

specific, and only 3 out of these 16 genes were not located on either of the sex chromosomes.

Genotype-specific gene expression in fetal liver

For fetal liver, we found significant genotype-related expression changes for 152 probes, corresponding to 109 genes (Supporting Dataset S3). As indicated in the heatmap in Fig. 2, the majority of these (95 genes) are induced in fetal livers of Ts1Cje mice of either sex, with the other 14 being suppressed. Of these, 51 are mapped on the corresponding trisomic locus (Fig. 1).

Functional overrepresentation analysis shows that among the genes with differential expression, there is enrichment for genes involved in immunology and hematopoiesis, including such genes as the calgranulin A and B subunits (*S100a8*, *S100a9*), lacto-

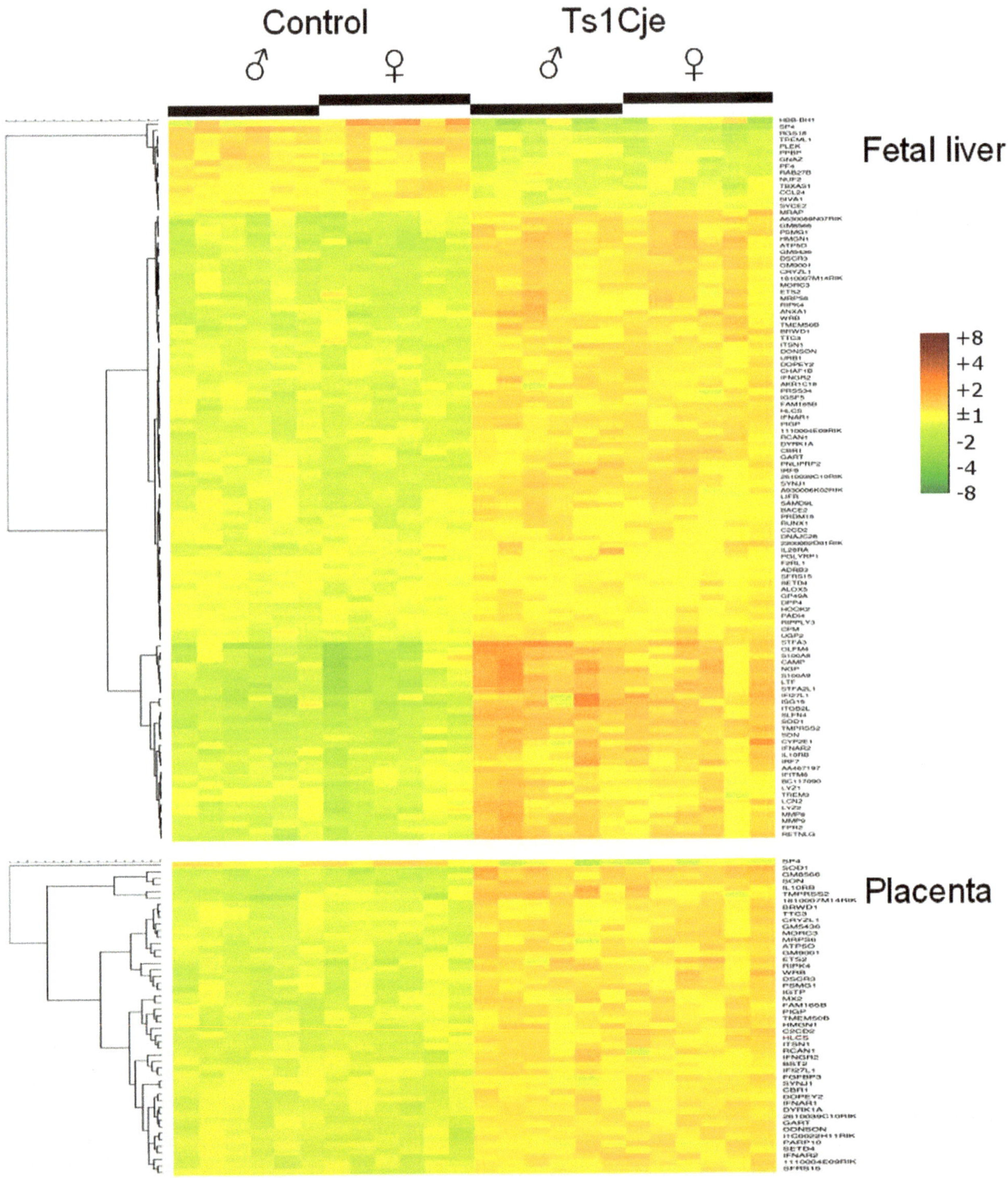

Figure 2. Heatmap for fetal liver and placenta.

transferrin (*Ltf*), matrix metallopeptidase 8 and 9 (*Mmp8, Mmp9*), platelet factor 4 (*Pf4*), pleckstrin (*Plek*), pro-platelet basic protein (*Ppbp*), and the gene for the zeta hemoglobin chain (*Hbb-bh1*). This enrichment is especially strong among genes that are induced in Ts1Cje mice but are not located on the trisomic locus. Among these non-locus genes, significantly enriched gene sets are mainly associated with the myeloid and neutrophil lineages. Among genes with lower expression in Ts1Cje fetal liver, there is significant overrepresentation of genes associated with or expressed in the platelet lineage.

Threshold-free pathway analysis using GSEA indicated that Ts1Cje mice have increased pathway activity in several GO-terms related to hematopoiesis (*e.g.* leukocyte differentiation, response to virus, response to biotic stimulus) and metabolism (alcohol metabolic process, glycerolipid metabolism, glycolysis and gluconeogenesis). Several custom gene sets related to interferon response, myeloid lineage, and (neutrophilic) granulocytes were induced in Ts1Cje whereas the opposite effect was found for terms related to platelets and (B- and T-) lymphocytes. Excluding the trisomic locus from the data used in the analysis did not significantly change these findings.

Among the 95 genes with significant expression differences in liver, there are 24 that encode for proteins potentially detectable in human blood (Supporting Dataset S3, Table 1). Of these, only 7 are located at the trisomic locus. Many of the other blood-detectable proteins are associated with either neutrophils or platelets.

Genotype-specific gene expression in placenta

Gene expression profiling for placental RNA revealed 75 probes with statistical significance, corresponding to 48 genes (Fig. 2, Supporting Dataset S3). For this tissue, induced expression in the Ts1Cje placentas was found for 47 genes, 41 of which are located on the trisomic locus (Fig. 1). Only one gene (*Sp4*) was suppressed in Ts1Cje mice. No significant overrepresentation for pathways or other gene sets was found among placenta-regulated genes.

GSEA found no significant pathway-level effect among GO-terms, and among the custom gene sets included, significant scores were only observed for leukocytes, especially neutrophils. However, significance was less pronounced than in fetal liver and excluding the trisomic locus further reduced the extent of this effect.

Among the genes regulated in placenta, 8 have human homologs that are blood- detectable at the protein level (Supporting Dataset S3, Table 1). With the exception of *Fgfbp3*, these are the same 7 markers located on the trisomic locus as for the fetal liver.

Table 1. Potential blood-detectable biomarkers regulated in fetal liver or placenta.

Gene symbol	Ratio fetal liver	Ratio placenta	Chromosome
Induced in Ts1Cje mice (at DS locus)			
C2cd2	1.173	1.370	16
Dyrk1a	1.290	1.282	16
Ifnar2	1.525	1.375	16
Morc3	1.372	1.340	16
Sfrs15	1.166	1.185	16
Sod1	1.796	1.881	16
Tmprss2	1.629	1.514	16
Induced in Ts1Cje mice (outside DS locus)			
Camp	1.724	NS	9
Dpp4	1.178	NS	2
Isg15	1.947	NS	4
Lcn2	1.486	NS	2
Lifr	1.238	NS	15
Ltf	1.981	NS	9
Mmp8	1.532	NS	9
Mmp9	1.469	NS	2
Olfm4	1.895	NS	14
Pglyrp1	1.124	NS	7
Pnliprp2	1.345	NS	19
S100a8	1.769	NS	3
S100a9	1.922	NS	3
Fgfbp3	NS	1.178	19
Suppressed in Ts1Cje mice			
Ccl24	−1.221	NS	5
Pf4	−1.259	NS	5
Plek	−1.346	NS	11
Ppbp	−1.336	NS	5

NS: not significant.

Overlap

The overlap between regulated genes in placenta and fetal liver comprises 42 genes. Of these, 40 are located in the trisomic region, of which 7 genes encode for potentially blood-detectable proteins (*C2cd2, Dyrk1a, Ifnar2, Morc3, Sfrs15, Sod1, Tmprss2*). Of the two genes that are not located on the trisomic locus, *Ifi27l1* was increased and *Sp4* had decreased expression in Ts1Cje mice compared to WT mice. For neither of these two genes there is evidence for protein detectability in human blood.

Quantitative RT-PCR verification

For two genes with increased expression in Ts1Cje placenta as well as fetal liver (*Sod1* and *Dyrk1a*) and four with differential expression in Ts1Cje fetal liver (*Pf4, Ppbp, S100a8, S100a9*) we performed quantitative RT-PCR (Supporting Dataset S2). For all of these six genes, we confirmed their differential expression as well as their significance at $p<0.05$. The direction of change was in agreement for all assays. Expression changes measured by PCR were comparable to those measured by microarray, with the median difference between microarray versus RT-PCR ratios being 11% (Supporting Dataset S2).

Discussion

Gene expression profiling in animal models has been previously successfully applied to gain insight and discover novel protein biomarkers for detection of human diseases [37–39]. For DS, several mouse models have been developed to study the effect of trisomy in single or multiple genes on DS phenotype and development (reviewed in [17,18]). Of these models, the Ts1Cje and Ts65Dn mice have so far been used most for gene expression analysis on brain tissue [40–44] and to a lesser extent on other adult tissues [45,46]. In this study, we describe for the first time gene expression analysis on fetal tissue of DS model mice with the ultimate goal to identify potential biomarkers applicable for prenatal serum screening. Although over a dozen mouse models for DS have been described in the literature, not all of these are equally useful for DS screening biomarker discovery by gene expression comparisons during fetal development. In mouse models with trisomies for only single genes, the phenotype is less pronounced whereas, on the other hand, mouse models with trisomies for larger segments or even an entire chromosome tend to suffer from male infertility or fetal death. The Ts1Cje mouse shows a recognizable DS phenotype while still allowing for breeding, and was consequently chosen as a model in this study. Gene expression data were compared in fetal liver and placenta between Ts1Cje and wild type embryos of both sexes at gestational age 15.5 days. This age corresponds to the developmental phase at the end of the first trimester in humans (Carnegie stage 22). Because the combined first trimester test is carried out at this time point, the corresponding mouse gestational age was chosen as the optimal time point for DS biomarker discovery.

As expected, gene expression data showed an increased expression of genes located in the trisomic locus (Fig. 1). This is in agreement with the gene dosage effect described earlier in human DS as well as mouse models [41–43,45–47]. In addition, in each tissue we observed sex-specific expression differences for some genes, most of which were located on either the X or Y chromosome. However, for eventual human implementation in a pregnancy screening program, markers should not show sex-specific differences. Firstly, because the accuracy of the screening program (DR and FPR) will benefit most from DS-markers that are applicable to both male and female embryos. Additionally, if sex-specific markers were to be included in a blood test, this would complicate the counseling to pregnant women. Therefore, in this study, these sex-specific markers were primarily identified in order to be excluded from the main analysis.

Comparing fetal liver RNA from Ts1Cje with wild type embryos, we found differential expression for 109 genes, of which slightly more than half (58 genes) were outside the trisomic locus. Remarkably, functional enrichment is stronger among these 58 genes than among the 109 genes as a whole. This indicates that although a large fraction of the differentially expressed genes are located in the same chromosomal regions, the main functional effect is due to genes from multiple other chromosomes. Functional enrichment analysis provided evidence that in Ts1Cje fetal liver there was an increased expression in immune- en hematopoiesis-related genes, more specifically of those expressed in the (early) myeloid and neutrophil lineages, with a concurrent lower expression of platelet-associated genes. As the fetal liver represents the major organ of hematopoietic development during the fetal period in mice as well as in humans, these findings indicate a disturbed hematopoiesis in fetal Ts1Cje mice. Humans with DS also suffer from various hematological abnormalities, including thrombocytopenia, neutrophilia, and macrocytosis. For example, around 10% of human DS newborns have transient megakaryoblastic leukemia. This disease is unique to DS and constitutes proliferation of immature megakaryoblasts. In most cases, this disorder resolves later in life, but in 20–30% it develops into acute megakaryocytic leukemia [48]. Carmichael *et al.* described that although Ts1Cje mice do not develop either of the two leukemic disorders, fetal liver hematopoiesis is nevertheless perturbed in Ts1Cje mice [49], with the main defects in the hematopoietic stem cell and myeloid progenitor cell compartments [49]. Their findings are reflected in the gene expression data described in this study and the functional parallels between murine and human fetal hematopoiesis abnormalities indicates that these markers can be prioritized with regard to human follow-up studies.

Placental gene expression data show differential expression for 48 genes. Most of these genes can be ascribed to gene dosage effects of the trisomic locus at Mmu16. Functionally, there is no significant overrepresentation of functional categories among the differentially expressed genes, although GSEA indicates increased levels of neutrophil-associated genes. In light of the data found for fetal liver, this probably does not indicate an effect occurring primarily in the placenta, but rather results from an increased neutrophil count throughout the embryos as a whole, being detected in the placenta as this tissue is rich in blood vessels. Increased levels in the placenta could lead to increased fetal-maternal exchange of the associated proteins, which could be detected in a screening assay provided they exceed the background variation in maternal blood.

We detected only a small number of non-trisomic genes differentially regulated in placenta. Furthermore, we could not detect a significant effect in *Pappa* (*Papp-a*, ratio −1.01, $p = 0.627$) or in other placental genes that have been described as biomarkers for DS (e.g. *Adam12*: ratio = −1.01, $p = 0.397$; *Inha*: ratio = −1.00, $p = 0.271$; *Pgf* (*Plgf*): ratio = 1.02, $p = 0.648$). It should be noted here that mice lack the genes corresponding to β-hCG or PP13 and therefore these particular comparisons cannot be made. Although it should not be taken for granted that Ts1Cje mice are a suitable model for serum biomarker discovery regarding human DS screening, our finding does not stand on its own. Comparable studies using human placental(-) samples also could not verify gene expression changes for known screening biomarkers [13–16]. A possible explanation might be that the regulation of some biomarker serum levels does not primarily occur at the gene expression levels but at one of several post-transcriptional stages. Alternatively, it needs to be considered that placenta is a relatively heterogeneous tissue, consisting of various cell types from the embryo as well as the mother. Therefore, only a small percentage of placental cells might produce the specific serum biomarkers, so that gene expression measurement in placenta as a whole will give attenuated responses that are statistically more difficult to detect.

A comparison between placenta and fetal liver showed there were two genes (*Ifi27l1* and *Sp4*) regulated in a similar manner in both tissues, but not located on the trisomic locus or sex chromosomes. Concerning the latter, it must be noted that Laffaire *et al.* recently described high resolution comparative genomic hybridization data that show how the translocation of the distal part of Mmu16 to the telomeric part of Mmu12 in Ts1Cje mice results in a deletion of a 2 Mb part containing 5 genes (*Dnahc11*, *Sp4*, *Sp8*, *Abcb5* and *Itgb8*) [43]. Because Ts1Cje mice are monosomic for this fragment, the lower *Sp4* expression found in both fetal liver and placenta of Ts1Cje mice can therefore probably be also attributed to a gene dosage effect. When gene expression data for the other genes in this monosomic locus were compared, we found that they are not expressed at detectable levels in either fetal liver or placenta, which explains why there is no differential expression found for these genes. *Ifi27l1* is also located on chromosome 12, but in an unaffected region, and therefore its differential expression is presumably independent from gene dosage effects. However, because *Ifi27l1* codes for a protein that is not located extracellularly, it is not likely to be useful as a serum biomarker.

An overall comparison between the data obtained for fetal liver and placenta found that more differentially expressed genes were found in fetal liver than in placenta, and that the findings in fetal liver can also be better matched to the pathological features observed in mice and humans. Although current searches for new serum biomarkers that can improve the DS screening accuracy are very much focused on the role of the placenta [50], this study suggests that fetal liver might nevertheless still be of sufficient value in this respect to warrant further studies. Indeed, of the fetal liver hematopoiesis-associated genes, 4 have been suggested as potential biomarkers in a literature data mining study from our laboratory [10]. Two of these (*Pf4*, *Ppbp*) were decreased, whereas both *S100a8* and *S100a9* were increased in Ts1Cje mice. We are aware that any maternal serum level changes in one of these individual markers might originate in changes in the maternal immune or hematopoietic system. Therefore, we put forward that follow-up studies should first determine background levels and variation in maternal blood, and additionally should not focus on single proteins, but rather on concurrent changes in these four markers [38].

In addition to these affected genes shared between both tissues, we also found 7 trisomic genes that are significantly regulated in both mouse tissues and potentially detectable in human serum. These include *Sod1* and *Dyrk1a*, which have been described to be associated with DS pathogenesis in the literature [17,18,51,52]. The corresponding proteins for these genes might therefore also provide potential targets for further study in human maternal serum. Measurement of biomarkers originating in the DS trisomic genotype can have an extra benefit compared to other potential markers. DS screening biomarkers that are currently used, or considered as candidates, are not located on human chromosome 21 and are also predictive for other aneuploidies such as Edwards syndrome (trisomy 18) and Patau syndrome (trisomy 13). It can be expected that markers located on the DS region are not only informative to distinguish DS from normal pregnancies, but also to differentiate between DS from other kinds of fetal chromosomal aberrations. This added information might be an additional reason to include such markers in as screening test.

In DS screening research, the use of omics methods has in recent years contributed to the identification of several markers that have the potential to improve DS screening accuracy [7–12]. However, human cohort serum studies are restricted by limited sample availability, large clinical variations, and additionally substantial costs in terms of laboratory equipment and reagents. In several other research fields, animal models are used to partially overcome such limitations. In this study, we report on the first use of a mouse model to identify a set of potential targets aimed at supporting human biomarker studies by providing a more focused starting position. Altogether, based on our gene expression analysis we describe 25 targets for DS screening studies (Table 1), 6 of which (*Pf4*, *Ppbp*, *S100a8*, *S100a9*, *Sod1*, *Dyrk1a*) have been described earlier to be associated with DS [10,17,18,51,52]. For these latter 6 targets, we confirmed their differential expression by quantitative RT-PCR (Supporting Dataset S2). Evidently, since we identified these new targets in a gene expression study, it still needs to be determined if the changes in RNA levels result in changes at the serum protein level that exceed maternal background levels at a time point suitable for screening. To this end, identification and validation of these targets at the protein level in human serum from pregnant women carrying normal and DS fetuses still has to be performed. As there is ongoing interest [53–55] in how determining fetal RNA and/or (methylated) DNA in maternal plasma can detect DS or other aneuploidies, in such further human studies it might be worth while to find out if such methodology is applicable to these 25 or even other regulated genes (Supporting Dataset S3). However, this study, to our opinion, narrows down the list of potential serum targets to be studied in subsequent case-control biomarker discovery experiments, which is extremely important given the enormous labor and financial efforts associated with the identification and validation of potential biomarkers. In this light, it can also be noted that in order to efficiently perform further human case-control experiments on identified targets, the serum measurements should preferentially be performed by means of a multiplexed assay to keep the workflow and the amount of required serum within reasonable limits. In further, more focused studies, assessing the feasibility of determining serum levels of these 6 targets combined with the currently used markers in a multiplexed assay format will therefore have high priority.

Supporting Information

Dataset S1 Primers used for sex and genotype determination (Microsoft Word document).

Dataset S2 QPCR validation (Microsoft Excel document).

Dataset S3 Regulated genes for fetal liver and placenta (Microsoft Excel document).

Acknowledgments

We thank Wim Vos and Stephane Nooijen at the Central Animal Facility Laboratory for their skilful (bio)technical support.

Author Contributions

Conceived and designed the experiments: JLAP WR SI CTMvO AdV. Analyzed the data: JLAP. Wrote the paper: JLAP WR SI AdV. Performed animal experiments: WR SI MPHK CTMvO. Performed molecular biological experiments: SI. Microarray support: TMB. Interpreted the data: JLAP WR MPHK PCJIS AdV.

References

1. Cuckle HS, Wald NJ, Thompson SG (1987) Estimating a woman's risk of having a pregnancy associated with Down's syndrome using her age and serum alpha-fetoprotein level. Br J Obstet Gynaecol 94: 387–402.
2. Wald NJ, Cuckle HS, Densem JW, Nanchahal K, Royston P, et al. (1988) Maternal serum screening for Down's syndrome in early pregnancy. BMJ 297: 883–887.
3. Wald NJ, Hackshaw AK (1997) Combining ultrasound and biochemistry in first-trimester screening for Down's syndrome. Prenat Diagn 17: 821–829.
4. Cuckle H, Benn P, Wright D (2005) Down syndrome screening in the first and/or second trimester: model predicted performance using meta-analysis parameters. Semin Perinatol 29: 252–257.
5. Schielen PC, Leeuwen-Spruijt M, Belmouden I, Elvers LH, Jonker M, et al. (2006) Multi-centre first-trimester screening for Down syndrome in the Netherlands in routine clinical practice. Prenat Diagn 26: 711–718.
6. Wortelboer EJ, Koster MP, Stoutenbeek P, Elvers LH, Loeber JG, et al. (2009) First-trimester Down syndrome screening performance in the Dutch population; how to achieve further improvement? Prenat Diagn 29: 588–592.
7. Kolialexi A, Tsangaris GT, Papantoniou N, Anagnostopoulos AK, Vougas K, et al. (2008) Application of proteomics for the identification of differentially expressed protein markers for Down syndrome in maternal plasma. Prenat Diagn 28: 691–698.
8. Nagalla SR, Canick JA, Jacob T, Schneider KA, Reddy AP, et al. (2007) Proteomic analysis of maternal serum in down syndrome: identification of novel protein biomarkers. J Proteome Res 6: 1245–1257.
9. Koster MP, Pennings JL, Imholz S, Rodenburg W, Visser GH, et al. (2009) Bead-based multiplexed immunoassays to identify new biomarkers in maternal serum to improve first trimester Down syndrome screening. Prenat Diagn 29: 857–862.
10. Pennings JL, Koster MP, Rodenburg W, Schielen PC, de Vries A (2009) Discovery of novel serum biomarkers for prenatal Down syndrome screening by integrative data mining. PLoS One 4: e8010.
11. Cho CK, Smith CR, Diamandis EP (2010) Amniotic fluid proteome analysis from Down syndrome pregnancies for biomarker discovery. J Proteome Res 9: 3574–3582.
12. Kolla V, Jeno P, Moes S, Tercanli S, Lapaire O, et al. (2010) Quantitative proteomics analysis of maternal plasma in Down syndrome pregnancies using isobaric tagging reagent (iTRAQ). J Biomed Biotechnol 2010: 952047.
13. Gross SJ, Ferreira JC, Morrow B, Dar P, Funke B, et al. (2002) Gene expression profile of trisomy 21 placentas: a potential approach for designing

noninvasive techniques of prenatal diagnosis. Am J Obstet Gynecol 187: 457–462.
14. Rozovski U, Jonish-Grossman A, Bar-Shira A, Ochshorn Y, Goldstein M, et al. (2007) Genome-wide expression analysis of cultured trophoblast with trisomy 21 karyotype. Hum Reprod 22: 2538–2545.
15. Chou CY, Liu LY, Chen CY, Tsai CH, Hwa HL, et al. (2008) Gene expression variation increase in trisomy 21 tissues. Mamm Genome 19: 398–405.
16. Chung IH, Lee SH, Lee KW, Park SH, Cha KY, et al. (2005) Gene expression analysis of cultured amniotic fluid cell with Down syndrome by DNA microarray. J Korean Med Sci 20: 82–87.
17. Delabar JM, Aflalo-Rattenbac R, Creau N (2006) Developmental defects in trisomy 21 and mouse models. ScientificWorldJournal 19: 1945–1964.
18. Seregaza Z, Roubertoux PL, Jamon M, Soumireu-Mourat B (2006) Mouse models of cognitive disorders in trisomy 21: a review. Behav Genet 36: 387–404.
19. Gropp A, Kolbus U, Giers D (1975) Systematic approach to the study of trisomy in the mouse. II. Cytogenet Cell Genet 14: 42–62.
20. Davisson MT, Schmidt C, Akeson EC (1990) Segmental trisomy of murine chromosome 16: a new model system for studying Down syndrome. Prog Clin Biol Res 360: 263–280.
21. Sago H, Carlson EJ, Smith DJ, Kilbridge J, Rubin EM, et al. (1998) Ts1Cje, a partial trisomy 16 mouse model for Down syndrome, exhibits learning and behavioral abnormalities. Proc Natl Acad Sci U S A 95: 6256–6261.
22. Shinohara T, Tomizuka K, Miyabara S, Takehara S, Kazuki Y, et al. (2001) Mice containing a human chromosome 21 model behavioral impairment and cardiac anomalies of Down's syndrome. Hum Mol Genet 10: 1163–1175.
23. Altafaj X, Dierssen M, Baamonde C, Marti E, Visa J, et al. (2001) Neurodevelopmental delay, motor abnormalities and cognitive deficits in transgenic mice overexpressing Dyrk1A (minibrain), a murine model of Down's syndrome. Hum Mol Genet 10: 1915–1923.
24. Gahtan E, Auerbach JM, Groner Y, Segal M (1998) Reversible impairment of long-term potentiation in transgenic Cu/Zn-SOD mice. Eur J Neurosci 10: 538–544.
25. Olson LE, Richtsmeier JT, Leszl J, Reeves RH (2004) A chromosome 21 critical region does not cause specific Down syndrome phenotypes. Science 306: 687–690.
26. Olson LE, Roper RJ, Sengstaken CL, Peterson EA, Aquino V, et al. (2007) Trisomy for the Down syndrome 'critical region' is necessary but not sufficient for brain phenotypes of trisomic mice. Hum Mol Genet 16: 774–782.
27. Richtsmeier JT, Zumwalt A, Carlson EJ, Epstein CJ, Reeves RH (2002) Craniofacial phenotypes in segmentally trisomic mouse models for Down syndrome. Am J Med Genet 107: 317–324.
28. Baken KA, Pennings JL, de Vries A, Breit TM, van Steeg H, et al. (2006) Gene expression profiling of Bis(tri-n-butyltin)oxide (TBTO)-induced immunotoxicity in mice and rats. J Immunotoxicol 3: 227–244.
29. Benjamini Y, Hochberg Y (1995) Controlling the false disovery rate: a practical and powerful approach to multiple testing. J R Stat Soc B 57: 289–300.
30. Huang dW, Sherman BT, Lempicki RA (2009) Systematic and integrative analysis of large gene lists using DAVID bioinformatics resources. Nat Protoc 4: 44–57.
31. Wu C, Orozco C, Boyer J, Leglise M, Goodale J, et al. (2009) BioGPS: an extensible and customizable portal for querying and organizing gene annotation resources. Genome Biol 10: R130.
32. Lattin JE, Schroder K, Su AI, Walker JR, Zhang J, et al. (2008) Expression analysis of G Protein-Coupled Receptors in mouse macrophages. Immunome Res 4: 5.
33. Chaussabel D, Quinn C, Shen J, Patel P, Glaser C, et al. (2008) A modular analysis framework for blood genomics studies: application to systemic lupus erythematosus. Immunity 29: 150–164.
34. Palmer C, Diehn M, Alizadeh AA, Brown PO (2006) Cell-type specific gene expression profiles of leukocytes in human peripheral blood. BMC Genomics 7: 115.
35. Subramanian A, Tamayo P, Mootha VK, Mukherjee S, Ebert BL, et al. (2005) Gene set enrichment analysis: a knowledge-based approach for interpreting genome-wide expression profiles. Proc Natl Acad Sci U S A 102: 15545–15550.
36. Anderson NL, Polanski M, Pieper R, Gatlin T, Tirumalai RS, et al. (2004) The human plasma proteome: a nonredundant list developed by combination of four separate sources. Mol Cell Proteomics 3: 311–326.
37. Kudo LC, Parfenova L, Vi N, Lau K, Pomakian J, et al. (2010) Integrative gene-tissue microarray-based approach for identification of human disease biomarkers: application to amyotrophic lateral sclerosis. Hum Mol Genet 19: 3233–3253.
38. Faca VM, Song KS, Wang H, Zhang Q, Krasnoselsky AL, et al. (2008) A mouse to human search for plasma proteome changes associated with pancreatic tumor development. PLoS Med 5: e123.
39. Pepe MS, Etzioni R, Feng Z, Potter JD, Thompson ML, et al. (2001) Phases of biomarker development for early detection of cancer. J Natl Cancer Inst 93: 1054–1061.
40. Dauphinot L, Lyle R, Rivals I, Dang MT, Moldrich RX, et al. (2005) The cerebellar transcriptome during postnatal development of the Ts1Cje mouse, a segmental trisomy model for Down syndrome. Hum Mol Genet 14: 373–384.
41. Amano K, Sago H, Uchikawa C, Suzuki T, Kotliarova SE, et al. (2004) Dosage-dependent over-expression of genes in the trisomic region of Ts1Cje mouse model for Down syndrome. Hum Mol Genet 13: 1333–1340.
42. Hewitt CA, Ling KH, Merson TD, Simpson KM, Ritchie ME, et al. (2010) Gene Network Disruptions and Neurogenesis Defects in the Adult Ts1Cje Mouse Model of Down Syndrome. PLoS One 5: e11561.
43. Laffaire J, Rivals I, Dauphinot L, Pasteau F, Wehrle R, et al. (2009) Gene expression signature of cerebellar hypoplasia in a mouse model of Down syndrome during postnatal development. BMC Genomics 10: 138.
44. Potier MC, Rivals I, Mercier G, Ettwiller L, Moldrich RX, et al. (2006) Transcriptional disruptions in Down syndrome: a case study in the Ts1Cje mouse cerebellum during post-natal development. J Neurochem 97 Suppl 1: 104–109.
45. Kahlem P, Sultan M, Herwig R, Steinfath M, Balzereit D, et al. (2004) Transcript level alterations reflect gene dosage effects across multiple tissues in a mouse model of down syndrome. Genome Res 14: 1258–1267.
46. Lyle R, Gehrig C, Neergaard-Henrichsen C, Deutsch S, Antonarakis SE (2004) Gene expression from the aneuploid chromosome in a trisomy mouse model of down syndrome. Genome Res 14: 1268–1274.
47. Mao R, Wang X, Spitznagel EL, Jr., Frelin LP, Ting JC, et al. (2005) Primary and secondary transcriptional effects in the developing human Down syndrome brain and heart. Genome Biol 6: R107.
48. Hitzler JK, Zipursky A (2005) Origins of leukaemia in children with Down syndrome. Nat Rev Cancer 5: 11–20.
49. Carmichael CL, Majewski IJ, Alexander WS, Metcalf D, Hilton DJ, et al. (2009) Hematopoietic defects in the Ts1Cje mouse model of Down syndrome. Blood 113: 1929–1937.
50. Koster MP, Heetkamp KM, Pennings JL, de Vries A, Visser GH, et al. (2010) Down syndrome screening: imagining the screening test of the future. Expert Rev Mol Diagn 10: 445–457.
51. Patterson D, Costa AC (2005) Down syndrome and genetics - a case of linked histories. Nat Rev Genet 6: 137–147.
52. Gardiner K, Costa AC (2006) The proteins of human chromosome 21. Am J Med Genet C Semin Med Genet 142C: 196–205.
53. Oudejans CB, Go AT, Visser A, Mulders MA, Westerman BA, et al. (2003) Detection of chromosome 21-encoded mRNA of placental origin in maternal plasma. Clin Chem 49: 1445–1449.
54. Chim SS, Jin S, Lee TY, Lun FM, Lee WS, et al. (2008) Systematic search for placental DNA-methylation markers on chromosome 21: toward a maternal plasma-based epigenetic test for fetal trisomy 21. Clin Chem 54: 500–511.
55. Tsui DW, Lam YM, Lee WS, Leung TY, Lau TK, et al. (2010) Systematic identification of placental epigenetic signatures for the noninvasive prenatal detection of edwards syndrome. PLoS One 5: e15069.

8

Influence of the Environment on Participation in Social Roles for Young Adults with Down Syndrome

Kitty-Rose Foley[1,7], Sonya Girdler[2], Jenny Bourke[1], Peter Jacoby[1], Gwynnyth Llewellyn[3], Stewart Einfeld[3,4], Bruce Tonge[5], Trevor R. Parmenter[6], Helen Leonard[1]*

1 Telethon Kids Institute, University of Western Australia, Perth, Australia, 2 School of Occupational Therapy and Social Work, Curtin University, Perth, Australia, 3 Faculty of Health Sciences, University of Sydney, Sydney, Australia, 4 Brain and Mind Research Institute, University of Sydney, Sydney, Australia, 5 Centre for Developmental Psychiatry and Psychology, Monash University, Melbourne, Australia, 6 Sydney Medical School, University of Sydney, Sydney, Australia, 7 Department of Developmental Disability Neuropsychiatry, School of Psychiatry, The University of New South Wales, Sydney, Australia

Abstract

Background: The concept of disability is now understood as a result of the interaction between the individual, features related to impairment, and the physical and social environment. It is important to understand these environmental influences and how they affect social participation. The purpose of this study is to describe the social participation of young adults with Down syndrome and examine its relationship with the physical and social environment.

Methods: Families ascertained from the Down syndrome 'Needs Opinion Wishes' database completed questionnaires during 2011. The questionnaires contained two parts, young person characteristics and family characteristics. Young adults' social participation was measured using the Assessment of Life Habits (LIFE-H) and the influences of environmental factors were measured by the Measure of the Quality of the Environment (MQE). The analysis involved descriptive statistics and linear and logistic regression.

Results: Overall, participation in daily activities was higher (mean 6.45) than in social roles (mean 5.17) (range 0 to 9). When the physical and/or social environment was reported as a facilitator, compared to being no influence or a barrier, participation in social roles was greater (coef 0.89, 95%CI 0.28, 1.52, coef 0.83, 95%CI 0.17, 1.49, respectively). The relationships between participation and both the physical (coef 0.60, 95% CI −0.40, 1.24) and social (coef 0.20, 95%CI −0.47, 0.87) environments were reduced when age, gender, behavior and functioning in ADL were taken into account.

Conclusion: We found that young adults' participation in social roles was influenced more by the physical environment than by the social environment, providing a potentially modifiable avenue for intervention.

Editor: Tricia A. Thornton-Wells, Vanderbilt University, United States of America

Funding: The study was funded by an Australian Research Council Linkage Project LP0989847. The funders had no role in study design, data collection and analysis, decision to publish, or preparation of the manuscript.

Competing Interests: The authors have declared that no competing interests exist.

* Email: Helen.Leonard@telethonkids.org.au

Introduction

According to the World Health Organisation (WHO), the physical, social and attitudinal factors are important aspects of the environment in which people live and conduct their lives [1]. The experience of disability has been described as an outcome of the interaction between a person's health or functional impairment and environmental factors. It is now recognised that characteristics of the impairment as well as social and physical factors are important to consider in the understanding of disability [2].

The International Classification of Functioning, Disability and Health (ICF) provides an internationally recognized framework for describing health conditions, health-related states and health outcome measurement [1]. Components of the ICF include body functions and structures, activity, participation and contextual components which include environmental and personal factors. When we recently reviewed factors affecting the transition from school to post-school for young adults with intellectual disabilities we found little information on the impact of environmental factors [3]. Our review employed the ICF as a guiding framework and demonstrated that the ICF is a useful tool for framing transition research.

A large scale longitudinal study investigating influence of environmental factors on participation and quality of life of children and adolescents with cerebral palsy across nine European regions has been undertaken by the SPARCLE group [4,5]. Levels of participation for children with cerebral palsy were considerably lower than that of the general population and particularly so for those with severe motor impairment and more impairments in general. The attitudinal environment, reflected by environmental law, regulation and physical and social environment, also varied considerably across the European Union countries included in the study [6]. The SPARCLE group employed the Measure of the Quality of the Environment (MQE), which identifies factors that are facilitators or barriers to participation [7]. It is now recognised that measures of the environment should include not only assistive technology and access to and availability of services but also other factors such as access to benefits, friendships and social integration, and attitudes of others and social inclusion [8]. The Measure of the Quality of the Environment (MQE) is an instrument which includes domains addressing these additional factors and can be matched to the ICF categories [9]. Additionally, the MQE domains can be matched to the domains of the Assessment of Life Habits (LIFE-H) a measure of social participation used by the SPARCLE group [5,10].

The contribution of environmental factors to the disability of individuals with Down syndrome has not been explored previously. Once these contextual factors have been identified, there may be scope to modify them and therefore lessen the experience of disability for young people with Down syndrome and for those with similar intellectual impairments [2]. Therefore, the aims of this research were to use a population-based data source to describe the social participation of young adults with Down syndrome from a parental perspective and to explore the relationship between levels of social participation and the physical and social environment.

Methods

In 2011 parent report questionnaires were administered to families of young people aged between 16 and 32 years in the Western Australian Down syndrome 'Needs Opinions Wishes' (NOW) population-based database [11,12]. Paper copies of the questionnaires were mailed to families in the Down syndrome NOW database and families were given the option to complete the questionnaire on paper, on the internet or via phone interviews. All families were phoned within a few days of sending out the questionnaires in order to achieve personal contact, provide clear explanation of the study and encourage families to participate. Prior to mailing questionnaires to participants all families were sent a summary booklet of the findings from the previous wave of questionnaires administered in 2009 [11,13].

The parent report questionnaires contained two parts; part one described young person characteristics including demographic information, presence of medical conditions, health service use and emotional and behavioural problems, as well as information about everyday functioning in activities of daily living, social relationships and day occupations. Part two contained information about family characteristics including family communication, support, informal assistance needs, availability of time and family quality of life. Detailed description of data collection methods has been previously reported [11,12]. Ethics approval for this study was obtained through the Ethics Committee of the Women's and Children's Health Services in Western Australia (Registration number 1715/EP).

Measures

Participation: Assessment of Life Habits (LIFE-H). The Assessment of Life Habits (LIFE-H) is a measure of social participation and includes twelve life domains (nutrition, fitness, personal care, communication, housing, mobility, responsibilities, employment, education, relationships, community life and recreation). It is also possible to calculate daily activities and social roles accomplishment sub scores [14]. The LIFE-H has been employed in populations of people with spinal cord injury, stroke, traumatic brain injury, children and older adults with cerebral palsy [15–17]. The scores can also be presented in accordance with the ICF, by quantifying the scores by percentiles and applying the appropriate qualifying words. For example, minor restrictions (LIFE-H score $\geq$8), moderate (LIFE-H score 4–7) or severe restrictions (LIFE-H score $\leq$3). This provides a universally understood and clinically relevant presentation of the data [18].

Two specific elements are involved in this measure, 1) level of accomplishment of the daily activity and 2) type of assistance required (no assistance, adaptation, device or human assistance). An item score between 0 (not accomplished) to 9 (accomplished independently, without difficulty) is calculated for each life domain (scoring key is shown in Table 1). In order to account for the variable number of items within each domain of life habits and the 'non applicable' items, a scoring system has been proposed [16,19]. A weighted score was calculated by the summation of raw scores, divided by the number of applicable items [16,19]. A score may be obtained for each item, each life domain (mean of items), or for the two subscales (daily activities and social roles). We did not include the education life domain in the social roles sub-score,

Table 1. Life habits accomplishment scale.

Score	Difficulty level	Assistance type
9	No difficulty	No assistance
8	No difficulty	Assistive device (or adaptation)
7	With difficulty	No assistance
6	With difficulty	Assistive device (or adaptation)
5	No difficulty	Human assistance
4	No difficulty	Assistive device (or adaptation) and human assistance
3	With difficulty	Human assistance
2	With difficulty	Assistive device (or adaptation) and human assistance
1	Accomplished by a proxy	
0	Not accomplished	
NA	Not applicable	

Table 2. Mean LIFE-H scores by life domain categories and sub-scores (Daily activity and Social roles) and number of participants reported as experiencing severe, moderate or minor restrictions in participation.

				Participation Restrictions			
Continuous variables	**Frequency**	**Mean LIFE-H score (SD)**	**Range LIFE-H score**	**Severe n (%) (score ≤3)**	**Moderate n (%) (score 4–7)**	**Minor n (%) (Score ≥8)**	**Missing/NA n (%)**
Social Participation (LIFE-H)							
Daily activities categories							
Nutrition	166	5.91 (2.14)	0.25, 9	18 (10.8)	112 (67.5)	36 (21.7)	0
Fitness	164	7.41 (1.66)	1.25, 9	2 (1.2)	81 (48.8)	81 (48.8)	2 (1.2)
Personal care	165	6.33 (2.29)	0, 9	20(12.0)	99 (59.6)	46 (27.7)	1 (0.6)
Communication	164	5.60 (2.48)	0, 9	29 (17.5)	99 (59.6)	36 (21.7)	2 (1.2)
Housing	162	7.51 (1.69)	0.5, 9	4 (2.4)	80 (48.2)	78 (47.0)	4 (2.4)
Mobility	163	5.90 (2.11)	0.2, 9	15 (9.0)	113 (68.1)	35 (21.1)	3 (1.8)
Daily activities subscore	161	6.45 (1.65)	0.81, 8.86	8 (4.9)	126 (75.9)	27 (16.3)	5 (3.0)
Social roles categories							
Responsibility	161	3.75 (2.27)	0, 9	68 (41.0)	87 (52.4)	6 (3.6)	5 (3.0)
Employment	146	5.47 (2.83)	0, 9	34 (20.5)	76 (45.8)	36 (21.7)	20 (12.0)
Education [a]	80	4.52 (2.67)	0, 9	37 (22.2)	27 (16.3)	16 (9.6)	86 (51.8)
Relationships	159	6.66 (2.34)	0, 9	17 (10.2)	75 (45.2)	67 (40.4)	7 (4.2)
Community life	163	4.72 (2.54)	0, 9	52 (31.3)	87 (52.4)	24 (14.5)	3 (1.8)
Recreation	159	4.81 (2.38)	0, 9	44 (26.5)	93 (56.0)	22 (13.3)	7 (4.2)
Social roles subscore	141	5.17 (1.84)	0.22, 8.93	18 (10.8)	117 (70.5)	6 (3.6)	25 (15.1)

[a]Education not included in social roles subscore.

Table 3. Parent report influences of environmental factors on the accomplishment of daily activities (n = 166).

Environmental factors	Barrier n (%)	No influence n (%)	Facilitator n (%)	Does not apply n (%)	Missing/I don't know n (%)
Social environment Subscale	2 (1.2)	63 (38.0)	45 (27.1)	56 (33.7)	[a]
Social networks					
Family situation	13 (7.8)	6 (3.6)	125 (75.3)	10 (6.0)	12 (7.2)
Support from family	16 (9.6)	12 (7.2)	115 (69.3)	13 (7.8)	10 (6.0)
Support from friends	44 (26.5)	21 (12.7)	70 (42.2)	19 (11.4)	12 (7.2)
Support from neighbours	34 (20.5)	1 (0.6)	45 (27.1)	26 (15.7)	60 (36.1)
Support from colleagues	13 (7.8)	15 (9.0)	107 (64.5)	18 (10.8)	13 (7.8)
Attitudes of people around					
Families and close friends	9 (5.4)	9 (5.4)	120 (72.3)	16 (9.6)	12 (7.2)
Attitudes of friends	15 (9.0)	26 (15.7)	95 (57.2)	13 (7.8)	17 (10.2)
Attitudes of colleagues	7 (4.2)	13 (7.8)	118 (71.2)	11 (6.6)	17 (10.2)
Attitudes of superiors	8 (4.8)	12 (7.2)	121 (72.3)	8 (4.8)	17 (10.2)
Attitudes of neighbours	12 (6.1)	52 (31.3)	65 (39.2)	19 (11.4)	21 (12.7)
Attitudes of service providers	15 (7.2)	20 (10.1)	107 (64.5)	5 (3.0)	22 (13.3)
Attitudes of strangers	26 (15.7)	43 (12.0)	69 (41.6)	8 (4.8)	23 (13.9)
Attitudes of people when there in a group (class, crowd)	22 (13.3)	25 (12.6)	93 (56.0)	5 (3.0)	24 (14.5)
Religious beliefs of people in your community	7 (4.2)	60 (15.1)	53 (31.9)	22 (13.3)	24 (14.5)
Employment services					
Counseling and employment seeking services	13 (7.8)	33 (19.8)	43 (25.9)	55 (33.1)	22 (13,3)
Current availability of jobs in your community	40 (24.1)	26 (15.7)	15 (9.0)	55 (33.1)	30 (18.1)
Job criteria/tests	38 (22.9)	23 (13.9)	13 (7.8)	57 (34.3)	35 (21.1)
Currently employed only					
Their workplace	6 (3.6)	7 (4.2)	77 (46.4)	76 (45.8)	[a]
Requirements of work tasks	7 (4.2)	4 (2.4)	81 (48.8)	74 (44.6)	[a]
Their work hours	6 (3.6)	6 (3.6)	76 (45.8)	77 (46.4)	[a]
Union structures	3 (1.8)	28 (16.9)	15 (9.0)	120 (72.3)	[a]
Employee services	2 (1.2)	17 (10.2)	40 (24.1)	107 (64.5)	[a]
Financial Resources					
Personal income	23 (13.8)	24 (14.5)	93 (56.0)	7 (4.2)	22 (13.3)
Public disability programs (e.g. Disability pensions)	16 (9.6)	16 (9.6)	108 (65.1)	2 (1.2)	22 (13.3)
Private health insurance programs	16 (9.6)	35 (21.1)	68 (41.0)	28 (16.9)	22 (13.3)
Commercial services					
Availability of business (e.g. shopping centres)	12 (7.2)	29 (17.5)	88 (53.0)	18 (10.8)	22 (13.3)
Services offered by business	11 (6.6)	43 (25.9)	66 (39.8)	22 (13.3)	24 (14.5)
Other support services					
Support workers other than family	7 (4.2)	15 (9.0)	105 (63.3)	23 (13.9)	16 (9.6)
Home care services	7 (4.2)	34 (20.5)	40 (24.1)	70 (42.2)	15 (9.0)
Health services (e.g. hospital, medical clinic)	9 (5.4)	25 (15.1)	100 (60.2)	15 (9.0)	17 (10.2)
Physical and social rehabilitation services in community	7 (4.2)	39 (23.5)	38 (22.9)	62 (37.3)	20 (12.0)
Vocational services in community	11 (6.6)	40 (24.1)	30 (18.1)	60 (36.1)	25 (15.1)
Social integration support services (eg social work, residential resources)	14 (8.4)	34 (20.5)	42 (25.3)	51 (30.7)	25 (15.1)
Educational services					
Educational service in community (e.g. TAFE)	2 (1.2)	5 (3.0)	31 (18.7)	7 (4.2)	121 (72.9)
Access to student loans	1 (0.6)	36 (21.7)	5 (3.0)	1 (0.6)	123 (74.1)
Other educational services	1 (0.6)	15 (9.0)	7 (4.2)	21 (12.7)	122 (73.5)
Physical environment subscale	7 (4.2)	64 (38.6)	59 (35.5)	36 (21.7)	[a]
Public infrastructure					
Public transport	36 (21.7)	19 (11.4)	57 (34.3)	41 (24.7)	13 (7.8)

Table 3. Cont.

Environmental factors	Barrier n (%)	No influence n (%)	Facilitator n (%)	Does not apply n (%)	Missing/I don't know n (%)
Specially routed buses/trains for people with disabilities	29 (17.5)	28 (16.9)	29 (17.5)	67 (40.4)	13 (7.8)
Long distance transport (e.g. bus, plane)	19 (11.4)	45 (27.1)	33 (19.9)	51 (30.7)	21 (12.7)
Communication services (e.g. telephone, internet)	13 (7.8)	33 (19.9)	67 (40.4)	37 (22.2)	16 (9.6)
Radio media services	8 (4.8)	57 (34.3)	37 (22.2)	47 (28.3)	17 (10.2)
Television media services	8 (4.8)	0	98 (59.0)	37 (22.2)	23 (13.9)
Community organization services					
Cultural services	6 (3.6)	18 (10.8)	104 (62.7)	22 (13.3)	16 (9.6)
Religious organizations	6 (3.6)	45 (27.1)	54 (32.5)	45 (27.1)	16 (9.6)
Athletic and recreational organization services	11 (6.6)	19 (11.4)	105 (63.3)	17 (10.2)	14 (8.4)
Community organizations (e.g. craft/social groups)	11 (6.6)	33 (19.9)	68 (41.0)	37 (22.2)	17 (10.2)

[a]'Missing/I don't know' data presented with 'Does not apply' data column due being unable to distinguish between the two categories for these specific questions.

as many participants had already left school and thus this life domain was only applicable to less than half of the sample (n = 80). Parent reported level of satisfaction was scored within each life domain and was reported on a 5-point likert scale 0 (very dissatisfied) to 4 (very satisfied). The satisfaction score is reported separately and used to evaluate the individual's quality of social participation [14].

Environment: Measure of the Quality of the Environment (MQE). The MQE was designed to identify environmental factors which were facilitators or barriers to participation and has been used to measure their influence on people with stroke, cerebral palsy and spinal cord injuries [7,20–25]. The items correspond to the environmental factors described within the ICF [20] and cover six domains: social support and attitudes (14), income, labour and income security (15), government and public services (27), equal opportunities and political orientations (10), physical environment and accessibility (38) and technology (5). Generally the last two domains refer to the physical environment (40 items) while the remainder refer to the social environment (69 items) [7].

Emotional and behavioural problems: Developmental Behaviour Checklist – Adult Version (DBC-A). The DBC-A is 107-item checklist which measures emotional and behavioural problems and was developed specifically for use with adults with intellectual and/or developmental disability. Each behavioural response is scored as 0 (not true as far as you know), 1 (somewhat or sometimes true) or 2 (very true or often true). The DBC-A has been found to have acceptable test-retest and inter-rater reliability and convergent ability has been demonstrated with two measures of behavioural disturbances of adults with intellectual disability [26].

Functioning in activities of daily living: Index of Social Competence (ISC). The Index of Social Competence (ISC) [27] was used to measure domains of communication, self-care and community skills. This measure discriminates well between different levels of ability [28].

Data Analysis

Descriptive statistics including means, standard deviations and ranges, were used to describe the participation (LIFE-H) and environment (MQE) data. Univariate relationships between independent variables and the outcome, subscores of the LIFE-H, were examined using analysis of variance and chi-squared tests. Logistic regressions with binary outcomes were used in the final models allowing for adjustment for confounding variables. The outcome was binary as we combined those who reported the environment as having 'no influence' or being a 'barrier' together and compared them to those who reported the environment as a facilitator. It is useful to identify those environmental factors which are facilitators to then provide targets for intervention to make a positive impact on participation for young people with Down syndrome. Confounding variables were identified through the use of the ICF. Examining the relationship between participation and environment required accounting for confounding variables which represented the other domains of the ICF. Therefore the confounding variables which were adjusted for in the final model were age and gender (personal factors), emotional and behavioural problems (impairment of body functions and structures) and functioning in activities of daily living (activity) [1]. Unadjusted and adjusted models were reported separately. STATA 11 was used for all analyses [29].

Results

Families of 197/223 (88.3%) young people returned the 2011 Down syndrome 'NOW' questionnaire. This study will focus on the 166/197 (84.3%) families who returned the parent report questionnaires with sufficient data on the participation and environment measures. The majority (136/166, 81.9%) of the young adults lived with their parents in their family home, others lived with other family or friends (11/166, 6.6%), five lived in a group home (3.0%) and four young adults lived alone (2.4%).

Participation

Eight (4.9%) young adults were reported by their parents as experiencing severe restrictions in participation in daily activities, 126 (75.9%) moderate and 27 (16.3%) minor restrictions. Participation in social roles was reported as severely restricted in 18 young adults (10.8%), moderate for 117 (70.5%) and a minor restriction for six (3.6%)(Table 2). The domain reported with the lowest participation score was the responsibilities domain (mean 3.75 SD 2.27), which relates to recognizing the value of money, making purchases and planning budgets. Participation in education (mean 4.52, SD 2.67), community life (mean 4.72 SD 2.54) and recreation (mean 4.81, SD 2.38) also scored low participation scores (Table 2). These are all domains normally included in the

Table 4. Univariate relationship between social participation and independent variables (n = 166).

	Social Participation (LIFE-H) (0–9)					
	Daily activities sub-score			Social roles sub-score		
Independent variables	**Frequency**	**Mean (SD)**	**P-value**	**Frequency**	**Mean (SD)**	**P-value**
Personal factors						
Gender						
Male	88 (53.0)	6.37 (1.78)	0.50	77 (46.4)	5.02 (1.8)	0.28
Female	73 (44.0)	6.54 (1.49)		64 (38.6)	5.36 (1.88)	
Missing	5 (3.0)	–		25 (15.1)	–	
Age group						
16≤20 year olds	36 (21.7)	6.01 (1.79)	0.11	29 (17.5)	4.79 (1.61)	0.44
21≤25 year olds	52 (31.3)	6.38 (1.72)		46 (27.7)	5.32 (2.01)	
26≤32 year olds	73 (44.0)	6.71 (1.49)		66 (39.8)	5.24 (1.80)	
Missing	5 (3.0)	–		25 (15.1)	–	
Environmental factors						
Annual family income						
$78000 and above	72 (43.4)	6.58 (1.55)	0.47	36 (21.7)	5.22 (1.91)	0.88
Between $41600 and $77999	33 (19.9)	6.18 (1.61)		27 (16.3)	5.04 (1.41)	
Less than $41599	42(25.3)	6.33 (1.81)		65 (39.2)	5.07 (2.03)	
Missing	19 (11.4)	–		38 (22.9)		
Place of residence						
Family home	136 (81.9)	6.32 (1.67)	0.14	120 (72.3)	5.04 (1.81)	0.34
Group home/hostel	5 (3.0)	6.40 (1.46)		4 (2.4)	5.35 (2.16)	
Living alone	4 (2.4)	7.02 (0.80)		3 (1.8)	5.74 (1.71)	
Living with family/friends	11 (6.6)	7.48 (1.53)		9 (5.4)	6.14 (1.99)	
Missing	10 (6.0)	–		30 (18.1)	–	
Living Region						
Major city (Perth)	117 (70.5)	6.42 (1.65)	0.70	102 (61.4)	5.09 (1.79)	0.40
Regional/remote	44 (26.5)	6.53 (1.66)		39 (23.5)	5.38 (1.95)	
Missing	5 (3.0)	–		25 (15.1)	–	
MQE Subscales						
Social networks						
Barrier	12 (7.2)	5.46 (2.01)	0.01	10 (6.0)	4.36 (1.49)	0.14
No influence	42 (25.3)	6.13 (1.84)		34 (20.5)	4.90 (1.79)	
Facilitator	94 (56.6)	6.69 (1.35)		87 (52.4)	5.37 (1.76)	
Missing	18 (10.8)	–		35 (21.1)	–	
Attitudes of others						
Barrier	5 (3.0)	4.16 (2.08)	<0.01	5 (3.0)	4.01 (1.42)	0.24
No influence	52 (31.3)	6.33 (1.44)		43 (25.9)	5.22 (1.59)	
Facilitator	89 (53.6)	6.71 (1.50)		81 (48.8)	5.34 (1.79)	
Missing	20 (12.0)			37 (22.3)	–	
Employment services						
Barrier	19 (11.4)	6.12 ((1.93)	0.21	16 (9.6)	4.66 (1.75)	0.088
No influence	42 (25.3)	6.53 (1.51)		38 (22.9)	5.22 (1.82)	
Facilitator	59 (35.5)	6.80 (1.31)		57 (34.3)	5.67 (1.59)	
Missing	46 (27.7)	–		55 (33.1)	–	
Financial resources						
Barrier	13 (7.8)	5.09 (2.33)	<0.01	9 (5.4)	3.99 (1.56)	0.10
No influence	37 (22.3)	6.48 (1.39)		31 (18.7)	5.41 (1.61)	
Facilitator	92 (55.4)	6.55 (1.55)		85 (51.2)	5.25 (1.85)	
Missing	24 (14.5)	–		41 (24.7)	–	

Table 4. Cont.

	Social Participation (LIFE-H) (0–9)					
	Daily activities sub-score			Social roles sub-score		
Independent variables	**Frequency**	**Mean (SD)**	**P-value**	**Frequency**	**Mean (SD)**	**P-value**
Commercial services						
Barrier	11 (6.6)	5.55 (2.21)	0.057	8 (4.8)	4.73 (1.84)	0.04
No influence	37 (22.3)	6.34 (1.50)		34 (20.5)	4.69 (1.69)	
Facilitator	76 (45.8)	6.68 (1.39)		70 (42.2)	5.53 (1.59)	
Missing	42 (25.3)	–		54 (32.5)	–	
Other support services						
Barrier	5 (3.0)	4.70 (2.79)	0.04	5 (3.0)	4.08 (1.68)	0.29
No influence	55 (33.1)	6.19 (1.69)		48 (28.9)	5.05 (1.87)	
Facilitator	78 (47.0)	6.58 (1.59)		69 (41.6)	5.31 (1.77)	
Missing	28 (16.9)	–		44 (26.5)	–	
Education services						
Barrier	1 (0.6)	7.78 (0)	0.72	1 (0.6)	6.65 (0.0)	0.62
No influence	18 (10.8)	6.34 (1.47)		15 (9.0)	5.26 (1.87)	
Facilitator	25 (15.1)	6.44 (1.91)		21 (12.7)	4.94 (1.82)	
Missing	122 (73.5)	–		129 (77.7)	–	
Public infrastructure						
Barrier	17 (10.2)	5.67 (2.00)	0.05	14 (8.4)	4.85 (1.70)	0.22
No influence	49 (29.5)	6.55 (1.37)		45 (27.1)	5.12 (1.83)	
Facilitator	61 (36.7)	6.75 (1.69)		55 (33.1)	5.60 (1.66)	
Missing	39 (23.5)	–		52 (31.3)	–	
Community organization services						
Barrier	4 (2.4)	4.34 (1.97)	0.01	3 (1.8)	3.55 (1.72)	0.10
No influence	38 (22.9)	6.34 (1.44)		35 (21.1)	5.01 (1.87)	
Facilitator	98 (59.0)	6.62 (1.56)		85 (51.2)	5.42 (1.61)	
Missing	26 (15.7)	–		43 (25.9)	–	
Physical environment subscore						
Barrier	6 (3.6)	4.33 (1.54)	<0.01	5 (3.0)	3.34 (1.26)	<0.01
No influence	57 (34.3)	6.42 (1.45)		51 (30.7)	5.06 (1.77)	
Facilitator	62 (37.3)	6.90 (1.52)		56 (33.7)	5.80 (1.49)	
Missing	41 (24.7)	–		54 (32.5)	–	
Social environment subscore						
Barrier	2 (1.2)	2.76 (1.13)	<0.01	2 (1.2)	2.77 (1.36)	0.01
No influence	44 (26.5)	6.33 (1.67)		37 (22.3)	4.88 (1.68)	
Facilitator	61 (36.7)	6.76 (1.21)		59 (35.5)	5.60 (1.54)	
Missing	59 (35.5)	–		68 (41.0)	–	
Day Occupation						
Still at school	10 (6.0)	5.68 (2.14)	<0.001	7 (4.2)	4.37 (2.00)	<0.001
Open employment	35 (21.1)	7.15 (1.13)		33 (19.9)	5.99 (1.73)	
Training	20 (12.0)	6.90 (1.25)		18 (10.8)	5.56 (1.28)	
Sheltered employment	61 (36.7)	6.60 (1.47)		59 (35.5)	5.32 (1.57)	
Day recreation program	33 (19.9)	5.30 (1.90)		24 (14.5)	3.65 (2.05)	
Not working	2 (1.2)	7.39 (0.8)		0	–.	
Missing	5 (3.0)	–		25 (15.1)	–	

social roles subscore but for this study we did not include the education domain. Participation in housing and fitness domains scored the highest of the domains within the LIFE-H (mean 7.51 SD 1.69, mean 7.41 SD 1.66, respectively). The housing domain involved taking part in housekeeping tasks, entering and exiting the home and using household equipment (furniture, lighting and

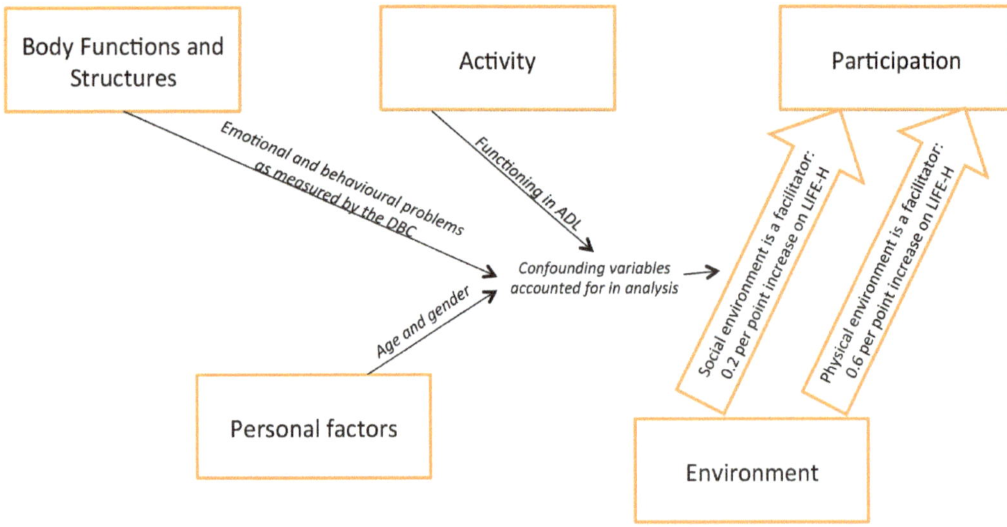

Figure 1. Relationship between social participation and the physical and social environment.

outdoor equipment). The fitness domain described participating in physical activities and relaxation activities as well as sleep and getting in and out of bed.

Environment

Parent perception of whether the environmental factor within the MQE was a major obstacle or major facilitator was scored on a 7-point Likert scale. Reponses to each item are presented in Table 3. Two continuous scores were calculated by summing the items and dividing into percentiles, one describing the physical environment and one describing the social environment. Approximately one third of the parents who provided data on the MQE reported the social environment as mainly a facilitator to participation (n = 45, 27.1%) and just over one third reported the physical environment as mainly a facilitator (n = 59, 35.5%). Just over one third reported the social and physical environment as having no influence (n = 63, 38.0%, n = 64, 38.6%, respectively) and a very small proportion reported the overall social and physical environment as a barrier to participation (n = 2, 1.2%, n = 7, 4.2%). Data for the remaining families concerning the influence of the overall social and physical environment were missing, reported as 'I don't know' or 'Does not apply' (Table 3).

Within the social environment sub-scale the most commonly reported facilitators to participation were the family situation (n = 125, 75.3%), attitudes of families and close friends (n = 120, 72.3%), colleagues (n = 118, 71.2%) and superiors (n = 121, 72.3%). The most commonly reported barriers to participation in the social environment were related to support from friends (n = 44, 26.5%) and neighbours (n = 34, 20.5%), current availability of jobs (n = 40, 24.1%) and job criteria (n = 38, 22.9%) and attitudes of strangers (n = 26, 15.7%).

Relationship between participation and physical and social environment

The two subscores of the participation measure, daily activities and social roles, and their relationship with independent variables including demographics, behavior, and environmental factors are presented in Table 4. There was no difference in participation in daily activities or social roles by gender, family income or place of residence. Attitudes of others were associated with participation in daily activities, with those parents who considered attitudes of others to be a facilitator or have no influence reporting a higher participation score (mean 6.33 SD 1.44, mean 6.71 SD 1.50, respectively) than those who considered attitudes of others to be a barrier (mean 4.16 SD 2.08). Similarly, those who considered social networks to be a barrier were more likely to report lower participation in daily activities (mean 5.46 SD 2.01) than those who considered social networks to be a facilitator or have no influence (mean 6.13 SD 1.84, mean 6.69 SD 1.35, respectively). Those who considered the influence of commercial services such as grocery stores, restaurants and shopping centres as a facilitator to participation reported higher participation in social roles (mean 5.53 SD 1.59) than those who considered them as barriers (mean 4.73 SD 1.84). This relationship was weaker for participation in daily activities (Table 4).

The unadjusted logistic regression model showed that when the physical and/or social environment was considered as a facilitator, compared to being no influence or a barrier, then participation in social roles increased (coef 0.89, 95%CI 0.28, 1.52, coef 0.83, 95%CI 0.17, 1.49, respectively)(Table 5). Confounding variables of age, gender, emotional and behavioural problems as measured by the DBC and functioning in activities of daily living (ADL) as measured by ISC were included in the adjusted regression model (Table 5). The addition of these confounding variables reduced the strength of the relationship between the facilitating effect of the social environment and increased participation in social roles (coef 0.20, 95%CI −0.47, 0.87). This was similar for the physical environment, however the effect persisted more so than for the social environment (coef 0.60, 95% CI −0.40, 1.24). These results are graphically represented in Figure 1. We considered stratifying the regression analysis by level of functioning in order to investigate if there were differences in the participation outcome. Other studies have identified that functioning in activities of daily living can be associated with different domains of participation [11,30,31]. However when we explored this interaction in this study within the regression between functioning in ADL and environment no association was found.

Table 5. Binary logistic regressions of the relationship between the physical and social environment and participation in social roles.

		Social roles subscale of LIFE-H					
		Unadjusted model*			Adjusted model (n = 93)		
	Freq	Coeff†	95% CI	p-value	Coeff†	95% CI	p-value
Physical environment subscore							
Barrier/No influence		Reference			Reference		
Facilitator	112	0.89	0.28, 1.52	0.005	0.60	−0.40, 1.24	0.06
Social environment subscore							
Barrier/No influence		Reference			Reference		
Facilitator	98	0.83	0.17, 1.49	0.015	0.20	−0.47, 0.87	0.59

Note: Adjusted model includes confounding variables age, gender, emotional and behavioural problems, functioning in ADL.
*The unadjusted models are two separate models, physical environment (n = 112) and social environment (n = 98), whereas the adjusted model is one single model.
†Per point increase on the outcome measure, Social Roles subscale of the LIFE-H.

Discussion

Young people with Down syndrome were reported to have more difficulty participating in social roles (e.g. relationships, community life, recreation etc.) than they did participating in daily activities (e.g. personal care, communication, housing etc.). The majority of young people with Down syndrome experience moderate participation restrictions in daily activities and social roles. We found that young adults' participation in social roles was considered from a parental perspective to be influenced by the physical environment (including public infrastructure and community organization services) more than by the social environment, however both were weak associations. Of concern, is the fact that the most commonly reported barriers to participation were negative attitudes of strangers, and lack of support from friends, availability of jobs and public transport. The most commonly cited facilitators to young person participation reported by parents were family and close friends, young person's current workplace (if they were employed), and attitudes of superiors and colleagues of the young person.

The main strength of this study is that it is framed within the internationally recognized disability framework, the ICF. Examining the complex situation of the environment's influence on social participation while accounting for personal (age and gender) and impairment factors (emotional and behavioural problems) can be clarified through the use of the ICF. Another strength is the quantitative description through a standardized measure of social participation and the influence of the environment of young people with Down syndrome through the use of cases ascertained from a population-based database [8]. The high response fraction enables further generalization of findings to the wider population of young people with Down syndrome across Australia and internationally and perhaps intellectual disability from other causes. However, there were some missing data in the environment (MQE) and participation (LIFE-H) measures. The cross-sectional design of this study meant we were unable to define the causal direction of the relationship between participation and environment. Another consideration is the fact that the young people may not consider barriers to participation in the same way as their parents. However, a significant strength is that there were barriers to participation identified from the parents' perspective (for example attitudes of others, availability of jobs and public transport) that have the potential to be modified through policy and intervention strategies.

The finding of a relationship between the physical environment as a facilitator and increased participation in social roles was interesting. We had hypothesized that the social environment would have had a stronger influence on participation in social roles. Elements of the physical environment included public transport, cultural and religious services and recreational and community organization. Previous research into factors that were barriers to social inclusion from the perspectives of young people with an intellectual disability highlighted four main elements, one of which related to the physical environment. This element was the location of their house, and the availability of transport to and from the house [32]. In Ireland, barriers to leisure participation for adolescents with intellectual disability were 'access to' and 'location of' leisure facilities from both young person and parent perspectives [33]. Inclusion of the variables representing the body functions and structures and activity domains of the ICF reduced the strength of the relationship, further highlighting the complex interaction between the social-psychological and biological factors that contribute to overall functioning. Emerging evidence suggests that the physical environment has the potential to have a large impact on the participation for young adults with intellectual disability and provides a new avenue for intervention.

From the parents' perspective, our study shows that the attitudes of others act as a barrier to participation for young people with Down syndrome. Previous research involving people with an intellectual disability has explored social distance and described the relative willingness of an individual to take part in relationships of varying degrees of intimacy with a person who has a stigmatized identity [34]. The authors of this research reported that older people and people with lower education levels endorsed a higher level of social distance between themselves and people with an intellectual disability [34]. Research has highlighted that public knowledge of intellectual disability and causal beliefs are particularly under-researched areas and that one of the main reasons for lay people's reluctance to interact with people with intellectual disability is due to discomfort and anxiety [35]. Clearly, public campaigns which promote education and understanding around people with intellectual disability could play a role in limiting social distance and in turn facilitate participation in social roles for people with Down syndrome.

Workplace characteristics including attitudes of superiors and colleagues and the work environment in general were cited by parents as facilitators to participation for those young people who were employed. A questionnaire study involving 643 Australian employers who had employed a person with a disability found that the person with a disability was reported as better than the 'average' employee on reliability variables (attendance and sick leave) and maintenance variables (recruitment, safety, insurance costs) [36]. Also, a Canadian study which surveyed the public on views on employment of people with intellectual disabilities found that the people surveyed believed that employing a person with a disability in a workplace would not have a negative effect on the workplace. However, the respondents did highlight lack of employment training programs for people with intellectual disability as a major obstacle to gaining their employment [37]. People with intellectual disability who participated in focus groups and were asked about their perspective on barriers to social inclusion did not cite being employed as a way to improve their inclusion [38]. However, those who were employed, often mention social inclusion as a valued outcome of participating in employment [39]. While young people with Down syndrome have been reported to find it difficult to find appropriate and suitable jobs [40,41], it is encouraging that once they were in the workplace, their environment was supportive.

This study has focused on the environmental factors that families reported as facilitators to participation in order to identify avenues for intervention. However, factors reported as barriers to participation are important to consider. Overall, there were very small proportions of families who reported the social or physical environment as a barrier, yet just over one third of families reported that the social and physical environment had 'no influence' on their sons/daughters participation. Service providers who are aiming to facilitate increased participation for young people with intellectual disabilities should consider adjusting these existing social and physical environmental factors, which act as no influence, to have a positive influence on participation.

There is a developing body of knowledge which reports the impact which negative community attitudes have on social inclusion for young people with intellectual disability [32]. Reports of increased rates of violence against people with disabilities including intellectual disability is concerning [42]. In the United States it has been reported that those people with an intellectual disability had a higher risk of violent victimization than persons with any other type of disability and those with intellectual disability experience a higher frequency of sexual assault, robbery and aggravated assault than those with a sensory disability [43]. A review involving studies from United States, Australia, England and Spain found higher prevalence of physical and sexual abuse maltreatment towards people with intellectual disability compared to those without intellectual disability [44]. There is an urgent need to address the lack of population-level data which clearly defines this issue, to then effectively guide resource allocation and service delivery [44,45].

Conclusion

Through the use of the internationally renowned framework, ICF, this study has highlighted that young people with Down syndrome experience participation restrictions in involvement in social roles. Parents reported that elements of the environment negatively influence participation including negative attitudes of strangers, and lack of support from friends, availability of jobs and public transport. This study has highlighted the important influence of the physical environment on social participation. This is an influence which may have been previously overlooked and has great potential to be modifiable.

Acknowledgments

We would like to acknowledge the valuable input from the other chief investigators of this project Professor Nick Lennox, Associate Professor Vivienne Riches and Professor Carol Bower.

Author Contributions

Conceived and designed the experiments: HL JB KF SG GL SE BT TP. Performed the experiments: HL JB KF SG. Analyzed the data: KF PJ. Contributed reagents/materials/analysis tools: KF SG HL JB PJ. Contributed to the writing of the manuscript: KF HL SG JB PJ GL SE BT TP.

References

1. World Health Organization (2001) ICF: International classification of functioning, disability and health. Geneva: World Health Organisation.
2. Schneidert J, Hurst R, Miller J, Ustan B (2003) The role of the environment in the international classification of functioning, disability and health (ICF). Disability and Rehabilitation 25: 588–595.
3. Foley K-R, Dyke P, Girdler S, Bourke J, Leonard H (2012) Young adults with intellectual disability transitioning from school to post-school: a literature review framed within the ICF. Disability and Rehabilitation 20: 1747–1764.
4. Productivity Commission (2011) Disability Care and Support. Canberra.
5. Colver A (2006) Study protocol: SPARCLE - a multi-centre European study of the relationship of environment to participation and quality of life in children with cerebral palsy. Biomed Central Public Health 6: 105–115.
6. Colver A, Dickinson H, Parkinson KN, Arnaud C, Beckung E, et al. (2010) Access of children with cerebral palsy to the physical, social and attitudinal environment they need: a cross sectional European study. Disability and Rehabilitation: 1–8.
7. Levasseur M, Desroisers J, Tribble DS (2008) Do quality of life, participation and environment of older adults differ according to level of activity? Health and Quality of Life Outcomes 6: 30–41.
8. Yoder PJ, Warren SF (2002) Effects of prelinguistic milieu teaching and parent responsivity education on dyads involving children with intellectual disabilities Journal of Speech, Language, and Hearing Research 45: 1158–1174.
9. Fougeyrollas P, Noreau L, St-Michael G, Boschen K (2008) Measure of the Quality of the Environment. Quebec, Canada: RIPPH/INDCP.
10. Noreau L, Fougeyrollas P, Vincent C (2002) The LIFE-H: Assessment of the quality of social participation. Technology and Disability 14: 113.
11. Foley K-R, Jacoby P, Girdler S, Bourke J, Pikora T, et al. (2013) Functioning and post-school transition outcomes for young people with Down syndrome. Child: Care, Health & Development 39: 789–800.

12. Bourke J, Ricciardo B, Bebbington A, Aiberti K, Jacoby P, et al. (2009) Maternal physical and mental health in children with Down syndrome. Journal of Pediatrics 153: 320–326.
13. Foley K-R, Girdler S, Downs J, Jacoby P, Bourke J, et al. (2014) Family quality of life is associated with the day occupations of young people with Down syndrome. Social Psychiatry and Psychiatric Epidemiology.
14. Fougeyrollas P (1998) Social consequences of long term impairments and disabilities: conceptual approach and assessment of handicap. International Journal of Rehabilitation Research 21: 127.
15. Noreau L, Lepage C, Boissiere L, Picard R, Fougeyrollas P, et al. (2007) Measuring participation in children with disabilities using the Assessment of Life Habits. Developmental Medicine and Child Neurology 49: 666.
16. Noreau L, Desrosiers J, Robichaud L, Fougeyrollas P, Rochettes A, et al. (2004) Measuring social participation: reliability of the LIFE-H in older adults with disabilities. Disability and Rehabilitation 26: 346.
17. Desroisers J, Noreau L, Rochette A, Carbonneau MA, Fontaine L, et al. (2007) Effect of a home leisure education program after stroke: a randomized controlled trial. Archives of Physical Medicine and Rehabilitation 88: 1095–1100.
18. Fougeyrollas P, Tremblay A, Noreau L, St-Onge M, Dumont S (2006) Subjective measurment of participation and environmental barriers and facilitators in population surveys: use of standardised tools with a sub-sample of the Quebec Activity Limitations Survey (QALS). Living in our environment: the promise of the ICF Vancouver, British Columbia.
19. Fougeyrollas P, Noreau L, St-Michael G (2001) Life habits measure - shortened version (LIFE-H 3.1). Quebec, Canada: CQCIDIH.
20. Levasseur M, Desroisers J, Noreau L (2004) Relationship between environment and quality of life of older adults with physical disabilities. Physical and Occupational Therapy in Geriatrics 22: 37–53.
21. Vik K, Nygard L, Lilja M (2007) Perceived environmental influence on participation among older adults after home-based rehabilitation. Physical and Occupational Therapy in Geriatrics 25: 1–20.
22. Fougeyrollas P, Noreau L, St-Michael G, Boschen K (1999) Measure of the quality of the environment, Version 2.0. Lac St-Charles, Quebec, Canada: International Network of the Disability Creation Process; Canadian Society for the International Classification of Impairments, Disabilities and Handicaps.
23. Rochette A, Desroisers J, Noreau L (2001) Association between personal and environmental factors and the occurence of handicap sitations following a stroke. Disability and Rehabilitation 23: 559–569.
24. Boschen K, Noreau L, Fougeyrollas P (1998) The measure of the quality of the environment: a reliability study in young adults with cerebral palsy. World Congress of Occupational Therapy. Montreal.
25. Boucher N, Dumas F, Maltais DB, Richards CL (2010) The influence of selected personal and environmental factors on leisure activities in adults with cerebral palsy. Disability and Rehabilitation 32: 1328–1338.
26. Mohr C, Tonge BJ, Einfeld SL (2005) The development of a new measure for the assessment of psychopathology in adults with intellectual disability. Journal of Intellectual Disability Research 49: 469–480.
27. McConkey R, Walsh J (1982) An index of social competence for use in determining the service needs of mentally handicapped adults. Journal of mental deficiency research 26: 47–61.
28. McEvoy J, Dagnan DJ (1993) The psychometric properties of the Index of Social Competence: A British replication. The Irish Journal of Psychology 14: 286–292.
29. Statacorp (2003) Stata Statistical Software. Release 80. College Station, Texas: Stata Corporation.
30. Rihtman T, Tekuzener E, Parush S, Tenenbaum A, Bachrach SJ, et al. (2010) Are the cognitive functions of children with Down syndrome related to their participation? Developmental Medicine and Child Neurology 52: 72–78.
31. Wuang YP, Su CY (2011) Correlations of sensory processing and visual organisation ability with participation in school aged children with Down syndrome. Research in Developmental Disabilities 32: 2398–2407.
32. May D (2001) Becoming adult: school leaving, jobs and the transition to adult life. In: May D, editor. Transition and change in the lives of people with intellectual disabilities. London: Jessica Kingsley Publishers.
33. Buttimer J, Tierney E (2005) Patterns of leisure participation among adolescents with a mild intellectual disability. Journal of Intellectual Disabilities 9: 25–42.
34. Nuehring ML, Sitlington PL (2003) Transition as a vehicle: moving from high school to an adult vocational service provider. Journal of Disability Policy Studies 14: 23–36.
35. Scior K (2011) Public awareness, attitudes and beliefs regarding intellectual disability: a systematic review. Research in Developmental Disabilities 32: 2164–2182.
36. Graffam J, Smith K, Shinkfield A, Polzin U (2002) Employer benefits and costs of employer a person with a disability. Journal of Vocational Rehabilitation 17: 251–263.
37. Burge P, Ouellette-Kuntz H, Lysaght R (2007) Public views on employment of people with intellectual disabilities. Journal of Vocational Rehabilitation 26.
38. Abbott S, McConkey R (2006) The barriers to social inclusion as perceived by people with intellectual disabilities. Journal of Intellectual Disabilities 10: 275–287.
39. Simons K (1998) Home, work and inclusion: the social policy implications of supported living and employment opportunities for people with learning disabilities. York: Joseph Rowntree Foundation.
40. Banks P, Jahoda A, Dagnan D, Kemp J, & Williams V (2010) Supported Employment for People with Intellectual Disability: The Effects of Job Breakdown on Psychological Well-Being. Journal of Applied Research in Intellectual Disabilities 23: 344–354.
41. Kober R, Eggleton IRC (2005) The effect of different types of employment on quality of life. Journal of Intellectual Disability Research 49: 756–760.
42. Hughes K, Bellis MA, Jones L, Wood S, Bates G, et al. (2012) Prevalence and risk of violence against adults with disabilities: a systematic review and meta-analysis of observational studies. The Lancet 379.
43. Rand MR, Harrell E (2009) National crime victimisation survey: crime against people with disabilities, 2007. Washington, DC: US Department of Justice. 1–12 p.
44. Horner-Johnson W, Drum CE (2006) Prevalence of maltreatment of people with intellectual disabilities: a review of recently published research. Mental Retardation and Developmental Disabilities Research Reviews 12: 57–69.
45. Soylu N, Alpaslan AH, Ayaz M, Esenyel S, Oruc M (2013) Psychiatric disorders and characteristics of abuse in sexually abused children and adolescents with and without intellectual disabilities. Research in Developmental Disabilities 34: 4334–4342.

9

Quantifying and Modeling Birth Order Effects in Autism

Tychele Turner, Vasyl Pihur, Aravinda Chakravarti*

Center for Complex Disease Genomics, McKusick-Nathans Institute of Genetic Medicine, Johns Hopkins University School of Medicine, Baltimore, Maryland, United States of America

Abstract

Autism is a complex genetic disorder with multiple etiologies whose molecular genetic basis is not fully understood. Although a number of rare mutations and dosage abnormalities are specific to autism, these explain no more than 10% of all cases. The high heritability of autism and low recurrence risk suggests multifactorial inheritance from numerous loci but other factors also intervene to modulate risk. In this study, we examine the effect of birth rank on disease risk which is not expected for purely hereditary genetic models. We analyzed the data from three publicly available autism family collections in the USA for potential birth order effects and studied the statistical properties of three tests to show that adequate power to detect these effects exist. We detect statistically significant, yet varying, patterns of birth order effects across these collections. In multiplex families, we identify V-shaped effects where middle births are at high risk; in simplex families, we demonstrate linear effects where risk increases with each additional birth. Moreover, the birth order effect is gender-dependent in the simplex collection. It is currently unknown whether these patterns arise from ascertainment biases or biological factors. Nevertheless, further investigation of parental age-dependent risks yields patterns similar to those observed and could potentially explain part of the increased risk. A search for genes considering these patterns is likely to increase statistical power and uncover novel molecular etiologies.

Editor: Andrew Whitehouse, The University of Western Australia, Australia

Funding: This research was supported by grants from the NIH (Autism Center for Excellence, MH081754) and the Simons Foundation Autism Research Initiative. The funders had no role in study design, analysis, decision to publish, or preparation of the manuscript.

Competing Interests: The authors have declared that no competing interests exist.

* E-mail: aravinda@jhmi.edu

Introduction

Autism is a genetic disorder whose molecular basis is incompletely understood. The characterized genetic component of autism, to date, accounts for only <10% of all cases [1]. The most convincing genetic etiologies arise from syndromes which display autism as one part of the phenotype, such as the Fragile(X) [2] and Rett [3], or other single genes with rare mutations in autism, such as those in SHANK3 [4,5]. Among patients with a diagnosis of autism spectrum disorder (ASD), an excess of maternal 15q11–13 duplications [6] and other chromosomal abnormalities are observed in a small subset of cases. Most patients have no identifiable molecular mutation. However, at the phenotypic level, the increased concordance in identical versus fraternal twins, as well as the increased risk of autism spectrum disorders to siblings of a proband, indicate that autism is highly heritable [7,8]. Familial patterns of autism clearly show that the disorder is "sex-dependent multifactorial" with numerous genes, likely interacting with environmental and lifestyle factors, increasing risk to family members of a proband and affecting four times as many males as females [9,10]. The genetic basis for these inherited factors remains to be discovered.

A central feature of most genetic models is that the risk of affection depends on genotype but not position within the family. The latter is rare for a Mendelian disorder with exceptions occurring where disease mutations are strongly dependent on parental age and/or the mutation is dynamic [11]. In contrast, for complex diseases, empirical risks often depend on birth rank. Indeed, for autism, there is some evidence for such a birth order effect for disease severity. In the first study, 16 multiplex families showed a birth order effect where the second affected child tended to have a lower nonverbal IQ [12]. In a follow-up study of 144 multiplex families, the authors found that there was a significant decrease of nonverbal IQ score in the second affected child [13], confirming this effect. A third study of birth order in 106 multiplex families also demonstrated various effects on autism symptom domains across birth ranks [14]. The biological causes of these findings remain unexplored and the generality of birth rank effects in autism has not been systematically investigated.

A birth order effect can arise from both biological (genetic) or demographic (social) causes. Irrespective of etiology, this risk may increase or decrease with birth rank so that the last-borns or first-borns, respectively, are more likely to be affected [15]. In addition, a V-shaped risk distribution in which the middle ranks within a family are either the most or least (inverse V-shaped) likely to be affected has been suggested as a possibility [16].

The simplest demographic cause of an apparent birth order effect is the curtailment of reproduction after the birth of a child with a serious illness. More generally, one might consider social reproduction models where the probability of future births is dependent on disease severity and the number of pre-existing affected children, thus giving rise to patterns where affected offspring are skewed towards later births. A second demographic explanation for the birth order effect can be attributed to intense disease surveillance and curtailment within particular reproductive age-groups so that almost all incident cases occur outside that age-group. For example, in Down syndrome the risk increases with maternal age but in western societies with maternal-age based screening most affected births occur to younger women.

In addition to demographic considerations, there are several well-documented biological causes for birth order effects that act through age. First, the risk of disease may depend on paternal or maternal age and thus increase with increasing birth rank [17]. For example, the risk of an aneuploid zygote, such as trisomy 21, increases significantly with maternal age [18] while some *de novo* gene mutations, such as in achondroplasia, increase with paternal age [19,20]. Other, more complicated, patterns could arise due to maternal-fetal incompatibility, that is rank- and not age-dependent, such as in Rh-disease, where earlier pregnancies increasingly sensitize the mother towards later pregnancies [21,22]. Finally, although not completely deduced at this time, epigenetic effects could be one additional factor impacting birth rank effects [23]. All these scenarios, be they demographic or biological, suggest that birth order effects either increase or decrease across birth ranks. Invoking either demographic or biological models for a V-shaped birth rank distribution is admittedly difficult but statistically feasible. Nevertheless, it is quite likely that these arise where the causes are heterogeneous with some families showing an increasing and others a decreasing birth effect trend.

To the best of our knowledge, a comprehensive formal assessment of overall birth order effect in autism, at least in the families now being extensively used for genetic investigations, has not been attempted. Consequently, in this study, we explore whether such birth rank trends exist in the three major and widely-available US autism family collections, namely, AGRE (Autism Genome Resource Exchange) [24], NIMH (National Institute of Mental Health: https://www.nimhgenetics.org/), and SSC (Simons Simplex Collection) [25]. Previous studies in autism have used a two sample paired t-test to assess autism severity differences between siblings of early and late births. In this manuscript, we propose three nonparametric statistical tests that *directly* examine deviations from the expected uniformity in the distribution of affected offspring across birth ranks. The proposed testing procedures differ in their efficiency depending on the shape of the birth order effect as shown by the results of our systematic simulation studies. Having access to large autism collections with hundreds of families allows a test for birth order effect in both simplex and multiplex families. We demonstrate that these effects are statistically significant and that different collections vary in the patterns they manifest. Consequently, these effects impact the search for autism genes.

Materials and Methods

Autism Family Collections

This study was conducted under ethics approval by the Johns Hopkins University School of Medicine Institutional Review Board (IRB) and was deemed to be exempt from full IRB review under exemption category 4. The families examined in this study were ascertained by the Autism Genome Resource Exchange (called the AGRE collection) [24], the National Institute of Mental Health (NIMH) (https://www.nimhgenetics.org/), and the Simons Foundation (Simons Simplex Collection (SSC)) [25]. All data were collected by AGRE, NIMH, and SSC under their respective IRBs. The AGRE and NIMH collections are primarily composed of multiplex families whereas the SSC is a simplex family collection. All samples were ascertained within the United States; selected features of the cases and families used in this study are summarized in Table 1. The main criterion for including families in the birth order study was choosing two-parent families with a minimum of two offspring with known birth dates. Additionally, we excluded families with discordant twins and counted concordant twins as one individual.

The two multiplex collections used in this study were the NIMH and AGRE collections. For the most part, both sets consist of families with at least two offspring affected with an autism spectrum disorder. The NIMH data comes from the NIMH distribution 6.0 pedigree files while the AGRE data was obtained from the AGRE January 2010 pedigree files. For AGRE, year of birth data was obtained from Vlad Kustanovich at AGRE (personal communication, 2010). Across all families, we counted all those with a diagnosis of autism or ASD as affected. In the AGRE collection, 346 families met these criteria and contained 744 individuals with autism (60%) among a total of 1,234 children. In the NIMH collection, 396 families met these criteria and contained 840 individuals with autism (60%) among a total of 1,393 children. These two collections have families in common so that we combined the data sources to obtain a single non-duplicated dataset of 485 families containing 1,030 individuals with autism (60%) among a total of 1,716 children. The Simons Simplex Collection (SSC) consists of simplex families with at least two offspring only one of whom had a diagnosis of ASD. We obtained the data from the SSC v.7.1 data release to identify 1,119 individuals with autism (47%) among a total of 2,392 children. The high frequency of autism in all families show the ascertainment bias induced in these collections.

Statistical Methods

We extended and generalized three different tests for the birth order effect and assessed their statistical power by computer simulations under different, but biologically relevant, types of disease risk profiles. A software package implementing these tests is freely available from the authors. A brief description of each test follows.

The rank-sum test [15] is perhaps the most intuitive non-parametric test for testing a birth order effect. In a sibship of size two or greater let r_{ij} denote the birth position of the ith child in the jth family. We compare the sum of r_{ij}'s for affected individuals with what would be expected in the absence of a birth order effect, i.e. a discrete uniform distribution on [1,N] of being affected at any

Table 1. Summary statistics of autism collections.

Family Collection	# families	# children	# affected	sibship size	# affected sibs
AGRE	346	1,234	744	3–9	2–5
NIMH	396	1,393	840	3–10	2–5
AGRE + NIMH	485	1,716	1,030	3–10	2–5
SSC	1,119	2,392	1,119	2–6	1

Table 2. Linear trend power calculations for three birth order statistical tests.

N	Test	Birth order model				
		Uniform	Linear	V-shaped	Mixed linear ($p_0=0.9$)	Mixed linear ($p_0=0.3$)
500	Rank-sum	0.05	0.74	0.06	0.55	0.14
	Inverse rank-sum	0.04	0.07	0.28	0.07	0.06
	χ^2-type	0.06	0.38	0.03	0.25	0.03
1000	Rank-sum	0.03	0.97	0.05	0.82	0.29
	Inverse rank-sum	0.01	0.06	0.45	0.07	0.02
	χ^2-type	0.01	0.68	0.10	0.43	0.10

birth position given the sibship size N>2. The test statistic is defined as:

$$S=\sum_{j=1}^{M}\sum_{i=1}^{N_j} r_{ij}a_{ij}, \tag{1}$$

where M is the number of families, N_j is the number of siblings in family j and,

$$a_{ij}=\begin{cases}1 \text{ if the i}^{th}\text{child of the j}^{th}\text{family is affected}\\ 0 \text{ otherwise}\end{cases} \tag{2}$$

To test the null hypotheses of no birth order effect, we perform a permutation test to obtain the distribution of S under the null hypothesis. To accomplish this, for the same number of families M and the same number of children in each family n_i, we randomly permute the disease status a_{ij} within each family j. This general

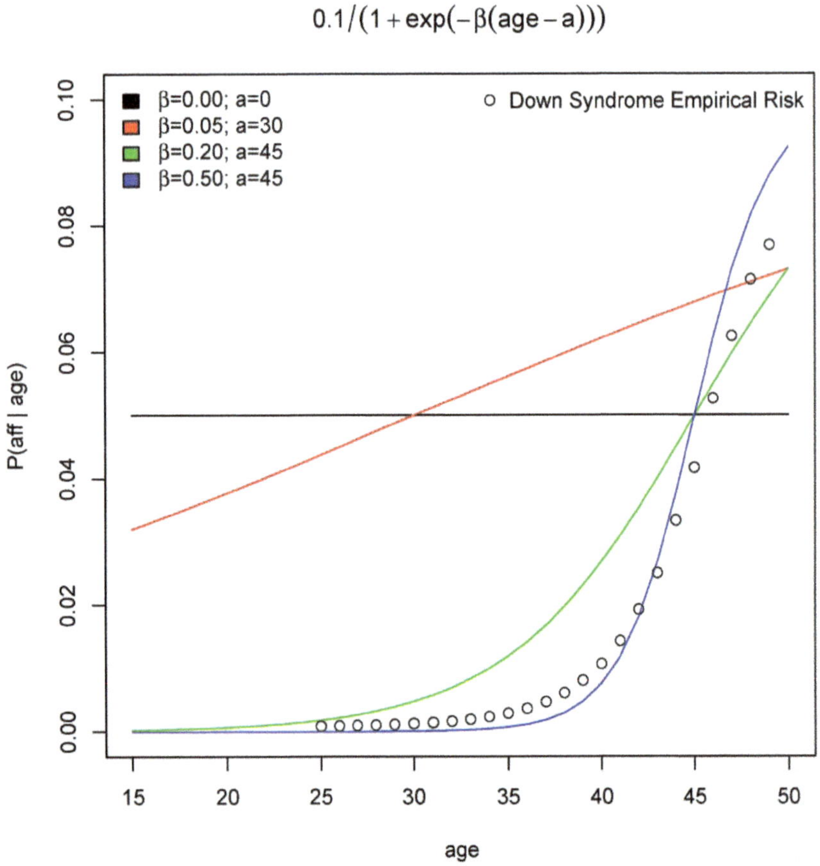

Figure 1. Logistic models for disease risk as a function of parental age; β is the rate of increase of logistic risk and a is the age in years at which risk is 50%.

scheme preserves the overall structure and dependence in our observed data, including the number of affected offspring in each family, while generating a possible realization of the data under the null hypothesis. For each permuted null outcome, we compute the test statistics $S_i^*, i=1,\ldots,K$ and the two-sided p-value as:

$$p=\frac{\#(|S_i^*-\overline{S}|>|S-\overline{S}|)}{K}, \quad (3)$$

Where $|S|$ is the absolute value of S, $\#$ denotes the number of times, $\overline{S}$ is the mean of S_i^*'s and K is the number of permutations.

Although the above test may be useful for linear changes in risk, it is inefficient whenever the risk distribution across births is V-shaped [16]. To remedy this situation, we consider an alternative ranking scheme where birth ranks are also weighted in a V-shaped manner (Table S1). The test statistics, permutation procedure and hypothesis testing are exactly the same as above (equations 1–3). The advantage of the new ranking is that it is capable of detecting complicated patterns of birth order effect, for example, when the probability of being affected is large for both early and late born offsprings. We call this the 'inverse rank-sum test.'

The third test of the birth order is a direct comparison of the observed and expected numbers of affecteds at each birth rank using a χ^2-type test [26] that uses the actual counts of affected offspring at each birth position and not the ranks (Table S2). The test statistic has the familiar form of

$$X^2=\sum_{k=1}^{\max(N_j)}\frac{(O_k-E_k)^2}{E_k}, \quad (4)$$

and yet the distribution under the null hypothesis is not a central χ^2 distribution because the observations are not independent. The observed counts for the ith birth rank are simply calculated as the total counts across appropriate sibship sizes, i.e.,

$$O_i=\sum_{z=max(i,2)}^{max(N_j)} n_{zi}. \quad (5)$$

The expected counts for the ith birth rank are computed under the assumption of uniform distribution of affected siblings within each sibship size. Thus,

$$E_i=\sum_{z=max(i,2)}^{max(N_j)}\frac{n_{z.}}{z}. \quad (6)$$

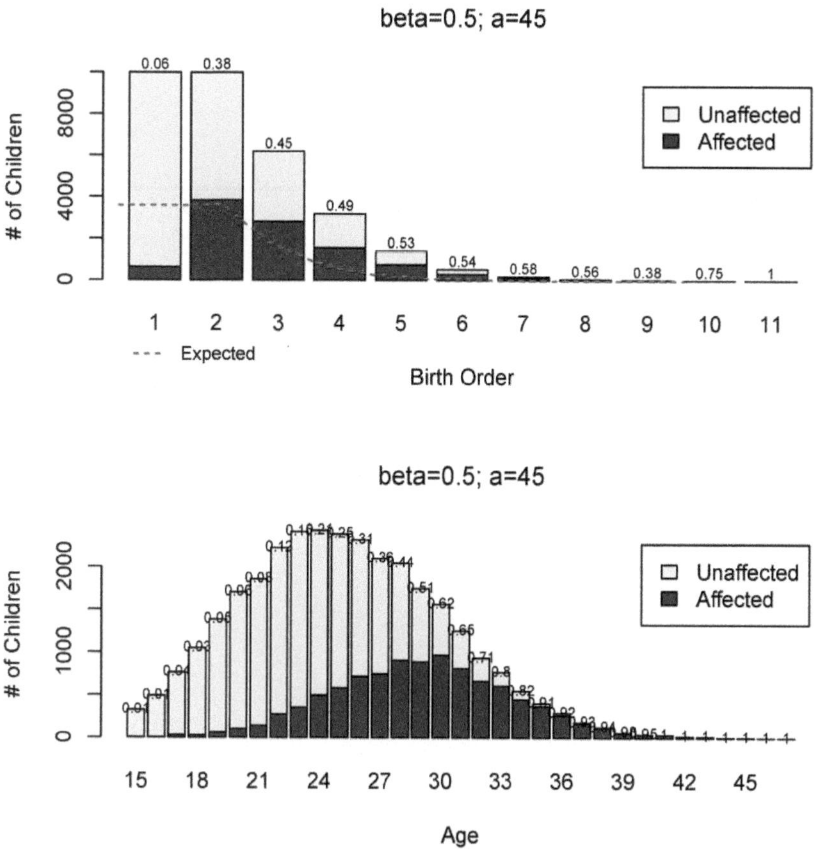

Figure 2. Example of effect of age-dependent logistic risk on birth order effect. For the most extreme age-dependent risk increase in Figure 1 ($\beta=0.5$; $a=45$) we show the distribution of offspring, both affected and unaffected, by (a) birth rank, and (b) parental age, by simulations of 10,000 nuclear families with Poisson distribution of sibship size with mean 2.39. At the top of each bar the fraction of affected offspring at that birth rank is shown.

Analogous to the first two tests, we resort to a permutation technique to assess statistical significance and to obtain a p-value.

Results

Before analysis of the real data, we first assessed statistical power and the optimal behavior of the three tests under a variety of biological models of birth order effect. We performed extensive Monte-Carlo simulations to easily accommodate a variety of risk models. In the first set of simulations, we assumed five simple models where disease risk was (a) independent of birth rank, (b) linearly dependent on birth rank (we tested only an increasing risk since the decreasing model is statistically equivalent), (c) V-shaped birth order effect; (d) and (e) were mixtures of linear but opposite birth rank trends in 9:1 (increasing/decreasing) and 3:7 proportions. To generate family structures, we used a Poisson distribution for sibship sizes with mean $\lambda = 2.39$ (the US average value). The probability of being affected at each birth rank z was computed as a linear function of birth ranks as:

$$P(aff|z) = \frac{0.4+0.05z}{\sum_{t\in[1,N]} 0.4+0.05t},$$

where N is the sibship size. Both intercept and slope were selected such that the increased risk was substantial but not exceedingly large.

We estimated statistical power for 500 and 1,000 families under the five linear models. These results are shown in Table 2. All three statistical tests are well-behaved in that the nominal Type I error is below 5% under the null hypothesis. As expected, the power increases with the number of families analyzed and can be considerable even for 500 families. Among the three tests, the rank-sum statistic has the largest power for detecting linear trends (including a mixture of linear effects), while the inverse rank-sum test is best for V-shaped effects, as expected. Interestingly, the χ^2-type test proves to be a good compromise between the two other

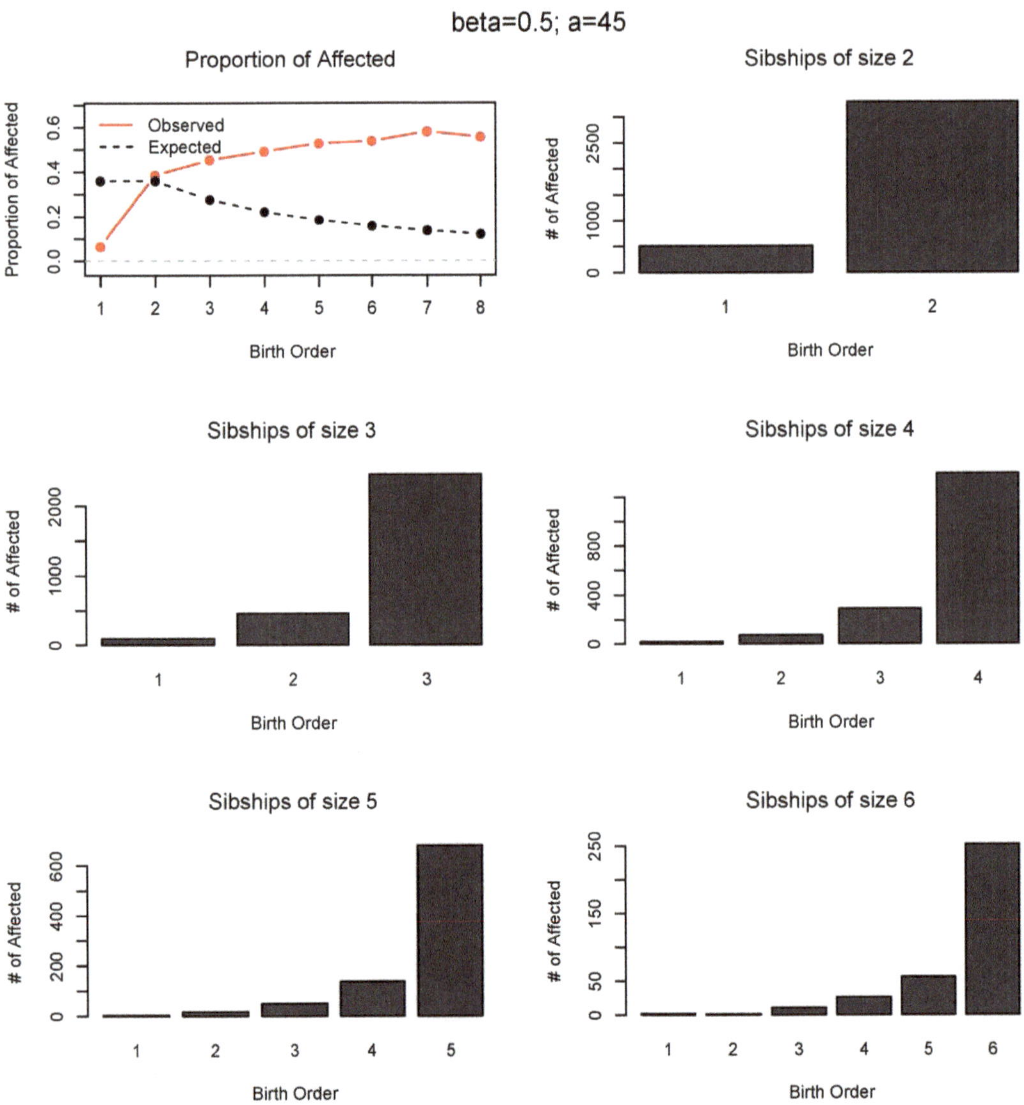

Figure 3. Statistical distribution of birth order effect of the data in Figure 2. Proportion of observed and expected numbers of affected offspring at each birth rank and the numbers of affected offspring for each sibship size and birth order is shown.

tests and is capable of detecting both types of nonuniform birth effects in the data. Its robust performance makes it the test of choice for the birth order effect, although it is less powerful than at least one of the other tests when the risk effects are either linear or V-shaped. In contrast, one has to keep in mind that both the rank-sum and inverse rank-sum test are likely to miss more complicated patterns of birth order effects.

Although the previous power calculations are encouraging, we wanted to model risk using known genetic mechanisms. In other words, we know of many genetic mechanisms that vary risk by age as opposed to birth order. Thus, we wanted to assess how age-dependent risks would manifest themselves as birth rank effects. A commonly accepted biological risk model is logistic where risk of disease is age-dependent and the precise dependence is modeled by three parameters: β (intrinsic increase/decrease rate), *b* (the maximum risk) and *a* (age-factor whereby an individual reaches half the maximum risk):

$$P(aff|age) = \frac{b}{1+e^{-\beta(age-a)}}. \quad (7)$$

We considered four sets of parameters to model three classes of risk, namely, where disease risk was (a) independent of age, (b) linearly increasing with age (we tested only an increasing risk since the decreasing model is statistically equivalent), (c) logistic increase in risk with lower and higher rates of increase at later ages. These risk profiles are shown in Figure 1 with *b* assumed to be 0.1 for all cases. Empirically observed risk rates for Down Syndrome that shows a maternal-age effect are also plotted in open circles providing a reasonable benchmark for the four models. To generate family structures, we again used a Poisson distribution for sibship sizes with mean λ = 2.39. Parameter selection for the four models was motivated by presenting reasonable yet somewhat

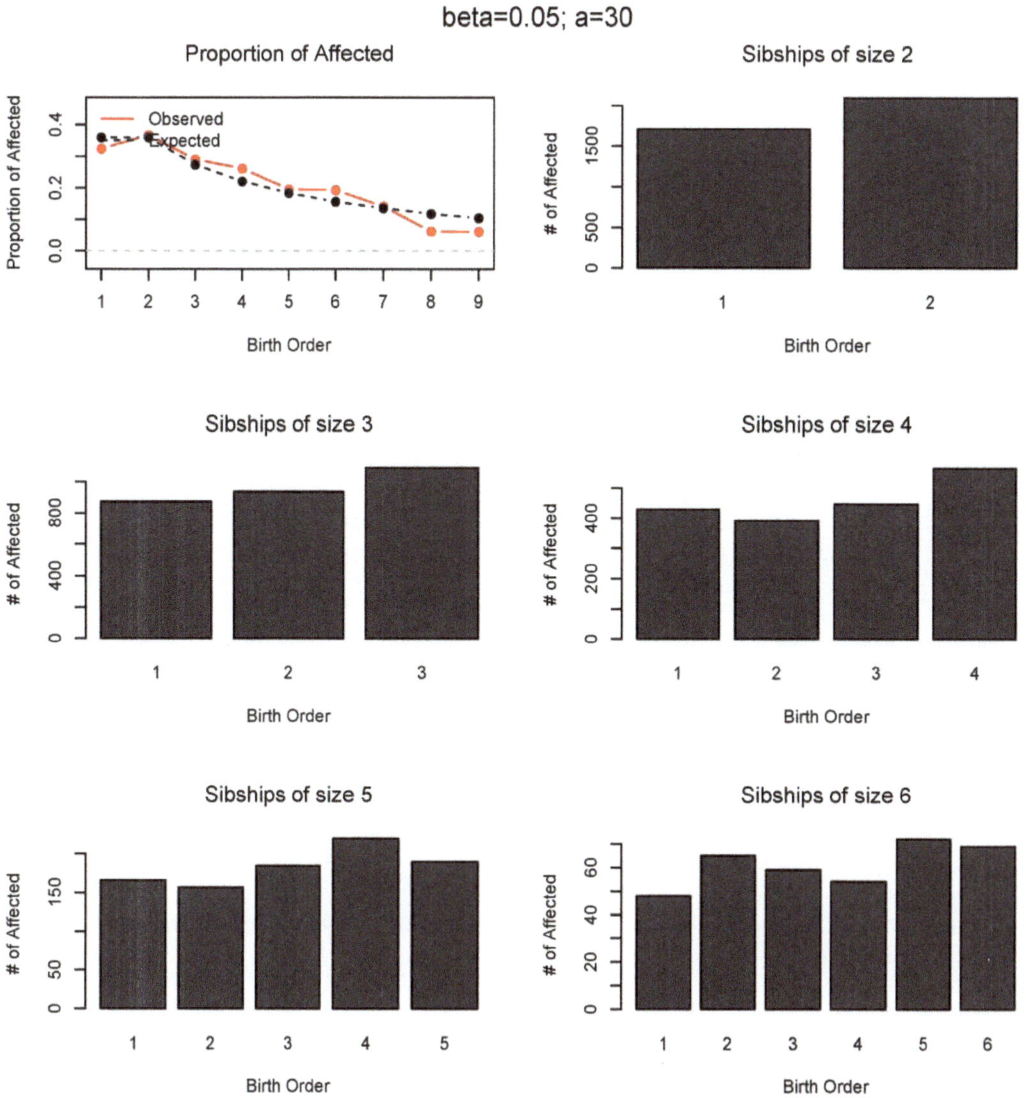

Figure 4. Statistical distribution of birth order effect for the linear model (β = 0.05; *a* = 30). Proportion of observed and expected numbers of affected offspring at each birth rank and the numbers of affected offspring for each sibship size and birth order is shown. Linear risk increase in parental age translates into an approximately linear risk increase in birth ranks.

Table 3. Logistic model power calculations for three birth order statistical tests.

N	Test	Birth order model			
		$\beta=0$; a=0	$\beta=0.05$; a=30	$\beta=0.2$; a=45	$\beta=0.5$; a=45
150	Rank-sum	0.06	0.23	1.00	1.00
	Inverse rank-sum	0.06	0.07	0.46	1.00
	χ^2-type	0.03	0.14	1.00	1.00
500	Rank-sum	0.03	0.64	1.00	1.00
	Inverse rank-sum	0.01	0.04	0.91	1.00
	χ^2-type	0.03	0.33	1.00	1.00
1000	Rank-sum	0.04	0.87	1.00	1.00
	Inverse rank-sum	0.04	0.03	1.00	1.00
	χ^2-type	0.05	0.54	1.00	1.00

different risk patterns. In the no-birth effect model both β and a are set to 0; for the linear model, $\beta=0.05$ and $a=30$, and for the two logistic curves, $a=45$ is selected as the age at which the risk reaches half of its maximum b at two different rates ($\beta=0.2$ and $\beta=0.5$). The model with $\beta=0.5$ and $a=45$ is clearly the one closest to the observed risk pattern in Down Syndrome and is of primary interest as a potential 'model' for the autism age-dependent risk profile.

To examine the nature of birth rank effects recovered we simulated 10,000 families with logistic risks and the parameters $\beta=0.5$ and $a=45$. The proportion of affected offspring by birth rank and the distributions of parental age for both affected and unaffected offspring are shown in Figure 2. The shift to the right in the two age distributions is very apparent and is also reflected in the birth ranks, especially in the deficiency of the first-born affected children. Figure 3 demonstrates the exponential increase in risk for all sibship sizes in *birth rank*, measured as proportion of affected at each rank, which directly corresponds to the underlying increase in risk by parental age. The expected and observed proportions of affected offsprings by birth rank differ substantially (top left) and the χ^2-type test is highly significant ($p<0.001$). In Figure 4, we examine a linear risk model as a function of parent's age that translates approximately into a linear risk in birth ranks. This model corresponds to $\beta=0.05$ and $a=30$ and is also plotted in red in Figure 1. The χ^2-type test for the birth order effect in these 10,000 families is also highly significant ($p<0.001$) although the departure of observed to expected proportions is not as substantial as in the previous logistic example. Nevertheless, we still observe an increase in risk at each sibship size and the overall test confirms this effect. To estimate the statistical power for these logistic models we again resort to Monte-Carlo simulations. The estimated power for sample sizes 150, 500 and 1,000 families based on 100 simulations is shown in Table 3. Clearly, the rank-sum test has the largest power in all scenarios, followed by the χ^2-type test. As expected, the inverse rank-sum test has the least power for monotonic patterns of risk increase and should not be used in such cases.

Finally, we utilized all three statistical tests and 10,000 permutations each to assess birth order effects in the multiplex AGRE and NIMH data sets and the simplex SSC data set; these results are presented in Table 4. Three trends are evident from these analyses. First, all three autism collections show statistically significant evidence of birth order effects in at least one test. Second, the χ^2-type test was significant in all three autism collections. Third, the results from the multiplex collections are more significant than those from the simplex families.

Based on the results of power analysis and assumed birth order effects, we can infer that the multiplex collections are not significant for the linear effect (rank-sum test) but very significant for the V-shaped effect (inverse rank-sum test), whereas the SSC showed an opposite pattern. In the combination dataset (AGRE + NIMH), shown in Table 5, we obtained insignificant results for the linear trend but significant results for the V-shaped effect. Thus overall, in both sets of families, the multiplex families are different in their risk profiles across births than the simplex families. Furthermore, in simplex families there is an excess of the affecteds at rank two which is the main driver for the observed birth order effect (Figure 5). On the other hand, in multiplex families the excess at rank 2 is followed by below expected counts in the following birth ranks, contributing to the inverse V-shape effect (Figure 6).

Due to large gender differences in autism prevalence, gender specific analyses in each of the collections were performed. Intriguingly, as reported in Table 5, gender specific birth order results are identified only within the SSC. For the AGRE + NIMH families both female-only and male-only families show significance for a V-shaped birth effect with a greater significance in males likely due to their larger sample size. Whether the genetic effect is larger in female-only families cannot be assessed with the sample sizes available (n = 58 affected females in 29 families). This multiplex effect shows a greater number of affecteds at the middle ranks peaking at birth rank 2 (Figure 6). On the other hand, for the SSC, affected females do not exhibit any birth order effect, whereas, affected males have a very significant linear increasing birth order effect (Figure 5, Figure S1). The effect is greater in simplex male-only affected families than it is in the overall simplex families. The absence of effect in simplex female-only affected families supports

Table 4. Results of three birth order tests in the autism collections.

Family Collection	Rank-sum test	Inverse rank-sum test	χ^2-type test
AGRE	0.786	$<10^{-4}$	$<10^{-4}$
NIMH	0.500	$<10^{-4}$	$<10^{-4}$
SSC	0.013	0.066	0.017

Table 5. Results of three birth order effect tests in the autism collections by gender.

Family Collection	# of affected	# of families	rank-sum test	inverse rank-sum test	χ^2-type test
AGRE + NIMH	1,030	485	0.382	$<10^{-4}$	$<10^{-4}$
AGRE + NIMH (affected females only)	58	29	0.354	0.0096	0.0409
AGRE + NIMH (affected males only)	658	317	0.959	$<10^{-4}$	0.014
SSC	1,119	1,119	0.013	0.066	0.017
SSC (affected females only)	150	150	0.410	0.460	0.819
SSC (affected males only)	969	969	0.004	0.076	0.005

the idea that females, who are less commonly affected, show a more characteristic genetic etiology. If birth order effects are similar to our simulated example, there is some evidence that we should have had enough detection power if it were true.

To examine both collections for parental age we also studied the parental ages for all individuals for whom this information was available. Overall, the distribution of affected children and unaffected children across parental ages did not differ (Figure

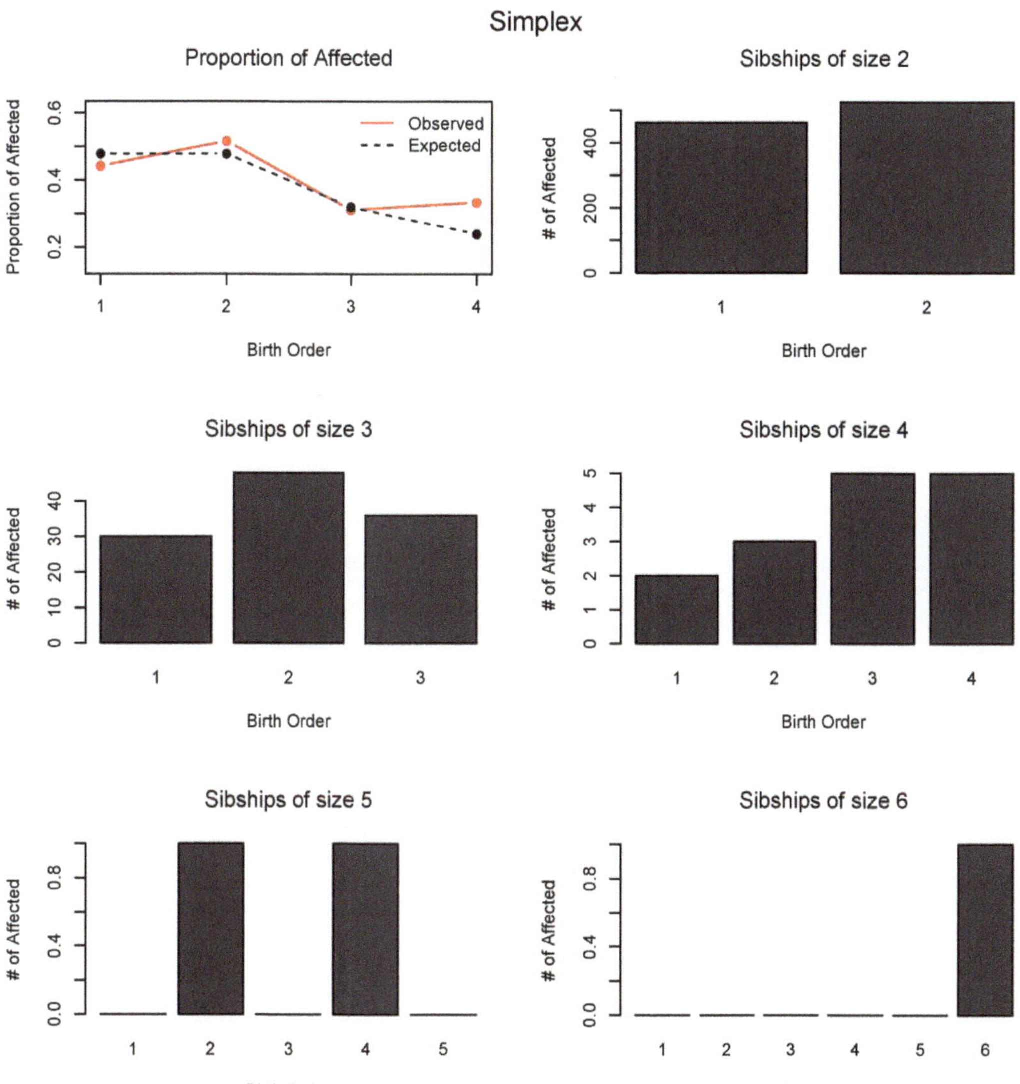

Figure 5. Proportion of observed and expected numbers of affected offspring at each birth rank for simplex families. The data for the numbers of affected offspring for each sibship size and birth order is shown.

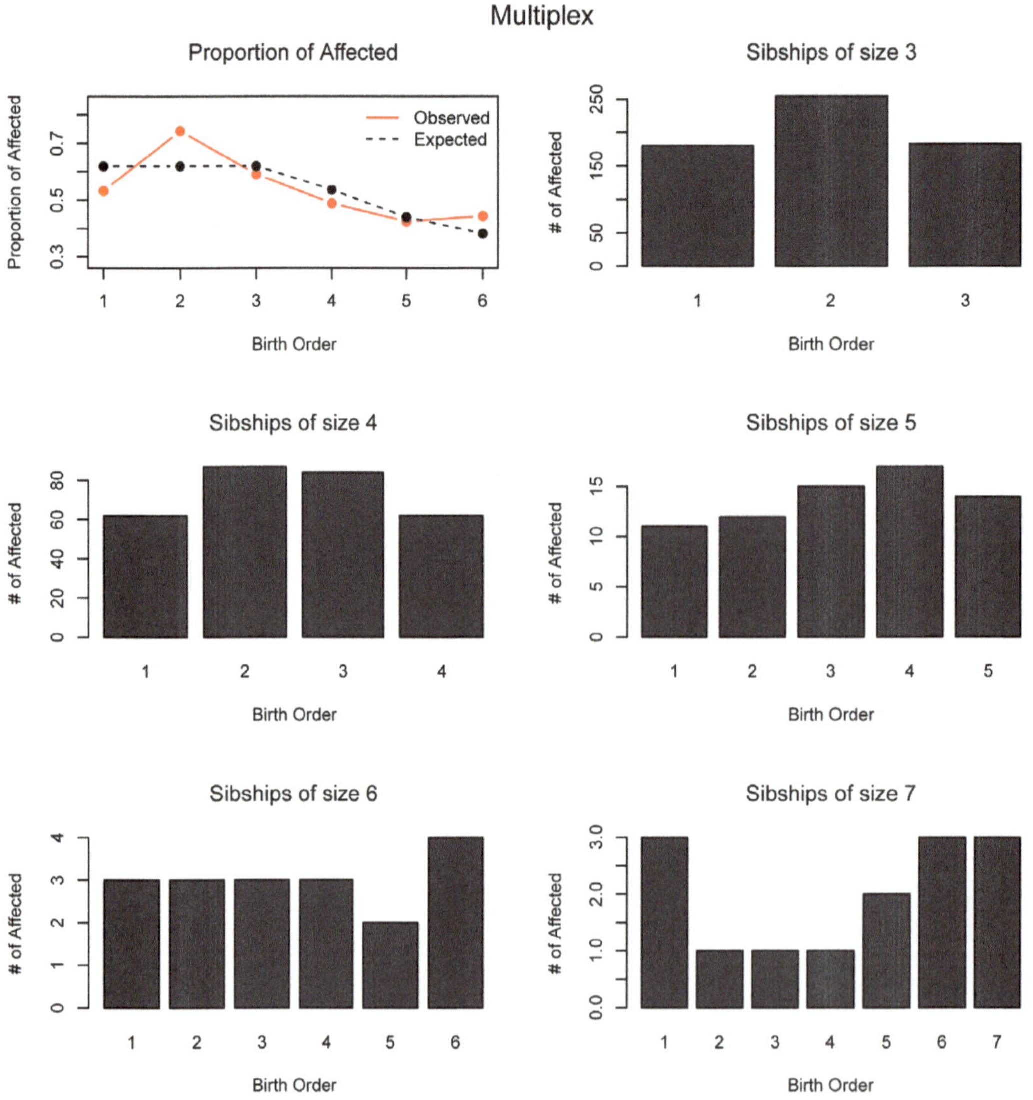

Figure 6. Proportion of observed and expected affected offspring at each birth rank for multiplex families. The data for the numbers of affected offspring for each sibship size and birth order is shown.

S2) but the proportion of affected children of all the children showed trends very similar to the birth order effects (Figure S3).

Discussion

In this study, we analyzed three autism datasets (AGRE, NIMH, SSC) for familial birth order effects in multiplex and simplex families. To accomplish this we generalized and implemented three different statistical tests for birth order effects and carried out a series of simulations studies to assess their performance under different birth order patterns. We demonstrated the proposed rank-sum, inverse rank-sum and the χ^2 -type tests to be best at detecting linear, V-shape, and general types of patterns, respectively. The χ^2 -type test proved to be the most robust test, capable of identifying arbitrary deviations from the expected distribution, although slightly less efficient when the true risk profiles are either linear or V-shaped.

Application of each test to the simplex collection identified significant linear birth order effects confirmed by both the rank-sum and the χ^2 -type tests. Looking at the results visually confirms an increasing linear effect that peaks around rank 2 (Figure 5). A demographic cause of this effect could arise from curtailment after the affected child is born. This is unlikely because a family size of 2 is common in the USA. More intriguing biological mechanisms include parental age effects, maternal-fetal incompatibility, and potential epigenetic factors. Parental age effects could arise as paternal or maternal. Well documented examples are maternal age effects in Down Syndrome from aneuploidy [18,27] and paternal age effects in Achondroplasia from recurrent male mutation [19,20]. Maternal age effects arise from non-disjunction whereas paternal age effects arise from point mutations due to increased numbers of replication in the male germline [28]. Considerations of these effects guide researchers to examine *de novo* mutations (both copy number and substitutions) in individuals with autism. Maternal-fetal incompatibility such as in Rh-disease are difficult to detect with current genomic studies: with increased risk to subsequent births this is a potential consideration for autism etiology. This type of effect should be carefully studied through the development of novel genetic methods. Lastly, epigenetic changes across pregnancies may exist but remain an enigma.

In the multiplex families, the inverse-rank sum test and the χ^2 – type test were both significant and indicated an inverse V-shape birth order effect in which the middle ranks are more commonly affected as can be seen in Figure 6. They are highest at rank two and decrease until birth rank 5 in which the number of sibships of size 5 are so small that the effect is no longer observed. This V-shaped effect is most likely a result of a heterogenous collection of families with differing birth order effects. A major factor to consider is ascertainment bias when selecting large multiplex families. This bias results because families are not chosen at random but likely with probability proportional to the number of affected children. The simplex collection was not randomly chosen either and families had to meet very stringent criteria to be added to the collection and required an unaffected sibling. Whereas the SSC commonly excluded families with other relatives who also had autism, multiplex families were collected with the purpose of having multiple affected individuals.

This study shows birth order effects do exist in autism and that some underlying biological cause may account for these effects. The *de novo* mutation associated with parental age hypothesis has been put forth in the recent past in particular for simplex families. [29] Certainly, this study adds weight to this hypothesis in that simplex family effects are linear and increasing. In addition, multiplex families do appear to be highly heterogenous and may be a result of *de novo* parental age effects in combination with genetic segregation patterns. One should not immediately discount other possibilities such as ascertainment bias or sibship curtailment. In addition, with the mysterious nature of autism causation it may be time to consider newer models and possibilities such as maternal-fetal incompatibility and/or epigenetic changes. Perhaps this can lead to specific studies of maternal genotype and fetal environment.

Supporting Information

Figure S1 The expected and observed numbers of affected males and females by birth rank in simplex and multiplex autism families.

Figure S2 Distribution of parental age at birth of affected (red) and unaffected (black) offspring in simplex and multiplex autism families.

Figure S3 Proportion of affected children of all children at each parental age.

Table S1 The inverse ranking scores used for the inverse rank-sum test. Offspring that are either early born or late born are given larger linear ranks as compared to the middle born children.

Table S2 Observed number of affected individuals for each sibship size and birth rank.

Acknowledgments

We thank all the families from the AGRE, NIMH, and SSC collections who have willingly provided information to make this study possible. We gratefully acknowledge the resources provided by the Autism Genetic Resource Exchange (AGRE) Consortium and the participating AGRE families. In particular, we thank Vlad Kustanovich for providing the year of birth data for the AGRE collection. We thank the NIMH for providing access to phenotypic information. We are grateful to all of the families at the participating SFARI Simplex Collection (SSC) sites, as well as the principal investigators (A. Beaudet, R. Bernier, J. Constantino, E. Cook, E. Fombonne, D. Geschwind, D. Grice, A. Klin, D. Ledbetter, C. Lord, C. Martin, D. Martin, R. Maxim, J. Miles, O. Ousley, B. Peterson, J. Piggot, C. Saulnier, M. State, W. Stone, J. Sutcliffe, C. Walsh, E. Wijsman). We appreciate obtaining access to phenotypic data on SFARI Base. Approved researchers can obtain the SSC population dataset described in this study (https://ordering.base.sfari.org/~browse_collection/archive[sfari_collection_v7]/ui:view) by applying at https://base.sfari.org.

Author Contributions

Conceived and designed the experiments: TT VP AC. Performed the experiments: TT VP. Analyzed the data: TT VP. Contributed reagents/materials/analysis tools: TT VP AC. Wrote the paper: TT VP AC.

References

1. Geschwind DH (2008) Autism: many genes, common pathways? Cell 135: 391–395.
2. Verkerk AJ, Pieretti M, Sutcliffe JS, Fu YH, Kuhl DP, et al. (1991) Identification of a gene (*FMR-1*) containing a CGG repeat coincident with a breakpoint cluster region exhibiting length variation in fragile X syndrome. Cell 65: 905–914.
3. Amir RE, Van den Veyver IB, Wan M, Tran CQ, Francke U, et al. (1999) Rett syndrome is caused by mutations in X-linked *MECP2*, encoding methyl-CpG-binding protein 2. Nature Genet 23: 185–188.
4. Durand CM, Betancur C, Boeckers TM, Bockmann J, Chaste P, et al. (2007) Mutations in the gene encoding the synaptic scaffolding protein *SHANK3* are associated with autism spectrum disorders. Nature Genet 39: 25–27.
5. Moessner R, Marshall CR, Sutcliffe JS, Skaug J, Pinto D, et al. (2007) Contribution of *SHANK3* mutations to autism spectrum disorder. Amer J Hum Genet 81: 1289–1297.
6. Cook EH, Jr., Lindgren V, Leventhal BL, Courchesne R, Lincoln A, et al. (1997) Autism or atypical autism in maternally but not paternally derived proximal 15q duplication. Amer J Hum Genet 60: 928–934.
7. Bailey A, Le Couteur A, Gottesman I, Bolton P, Simonoff E, et al. (1995) Autism as a strongly genetic disorder: evidence from a British twin study. Psychol Med 25: 63–77.
8. Steffenburg S, Gillberg C, Hellgren L, Andersson L, Gillberg IC, et al. (1989) A twin study of autism in Denmark, Finland, Iceland, Norway and Sweden. J Child Psychol Psychiatry 30: 405–416.
9. Fombonne E (2003) Epidemiological surveys of autism and other pervasive developmental disorders: an update. J Autism Dev Disord 33: 365–382.
10. Risch N, Spiker D, Lotspeich L, Nouri N, Hinds D, et al. (1999) A genomic screen of autism: evidence for a multilocus etiology. Am J Hum Genet. 65: 493–507.
11. Emison ES, Garcia-Barcelo M, Grice EA, Lantieri F, Amiel J, et al. (2010) Differential contributions of rare and common, coding and noncoding Ret mutations to multifactorial Hirschsprung disease liability. Am J Hum Genet. 87: 60–74.
12. Lord C (1992) Birth order effects on nonverbal IQ in families with multiple incidence of autism or pervasive developmental disorder. J Autism Dev Disord 22: 663–666.
13. Spiker D, Lotspeich LJ, Dimiceli S, Szatmari P, Myers RM, et al. (2001) Birth order effects on nonverbal IQ scores in autism multiplex families. J Autism Dev Disord 31: 449–460.
14. Reichenberg A, Smith C, Schmeidler J, Silverman JM (2007) Birth order effects on autism symptom domains. Psychiatry Res 150: 199–204.
15. Haldane JB, Smith CA (1948) A simple exact test for birth-order effect. Ann Eugen 14: 117–124.
16. Barton DE, David FN (1958) A test for birth order effect. Ann Hum Genet 22: 250–257.
17. Erickson JD (1978) Down syndrome, paternal age, maternal age and birth order. Ann Hum Genet 41: 289–298.
18. Sherman SL, Petersen MB, Freeman SB, Hersey J, Pettay D, et al. (1994) Non-disjunction of chromosome 21 in maternal meiosis I: evidence for a maternal age-dependent mechanism involving reduced recombination. Hum Mole Genet 3: 1529–1535.
19. Risch N, Reich EW, Wishnick MM, McCarthy JG (1987) Spontaneous mutation and parental age in humans. Am J Hum Genet 41: 218–248.
20. Wilkin DJ, Szabo JK, Cameron R, Henderson S, Bellus GA, et al. (1998) Mutations in fibroblast growth-factor receptor 3 in sporadic cases of achondroplasia occur exclusively on the paternally derived chromosome. Am J Hum Genet 63: 711–716.

21. Landsteiner K, Weiner AS (1941) Studies on Agglutinogen (Rh) in Human Blood Reacting with Anti-Rhesus Sera and with Human Isoantiboides. J Expt Med 74: 309–320.
22. Broman B (1950) The significance of the Rh factor in obstetrics. Acta Obstet et Gynecol Scand 30: 75–82.
23. Ogbuanu IU, Karmaus WJ, Zhang H, Sabo-Attwood T, Ewart S, et al. (2010) Birth order modifies the effect of IL13 gene polymorphisms on serum IgE at age 10 and skin prick test at ages 4, 10, and 18: a prospective birth cohort study. " Allergy Asthma Clin Immunol 6: 6.
24. Geschwind DH, Sowinski J, Lord C, Iversen P, Shestack J, et al. (2001) The autism genetic resource exchange: a resource for the study of autism and related neuropsychiatric conditions. Amer J Hum Genet 69: 463–466.
25. Fischbach GD, Lord C (2010) The Simons Simplex Collection: a resource for identification of autism genetic risk factors. Neuron. 68: 192–195.
26. Halperin M (1953) The Use of χ^2 in Testing Effect of Birth Order. Ann Eugen 18: 99–106.
27. Hassold T, Abruzzo M, Adkins K, Griffin D, Merrill M, et al. (1996) Human aneuploidy: incidence, origin, and etiology. Environ Mol Mutagen 28: 167–175.
28. Crow JF (2000) The origins, patterns and implications of human spontaneous mutation. Nat Rev Genet 1: 40–47.
29. Zhao X, Leotta A, Kustanovich V, Lajonchere C, Geschwind DH, et al. (2007) A unified genetic theory for sporadic and inherited autism. Proc Natl Acad Sci 104: 12831–12836.

10

Mitotic Spindle Defects and Chromosome Mis-Segregation Induced by LDL/Cholesterol—Implications for Niemann-Pick C1, Alzheimer's Disease, and Atherosclerosis

Antoneta Granic[1,2], Huntington Potter[1]*

1 Department of Neurology and Linda Crnic Institute for Down Syndrome, University of Colorado School of Medicine, Aurora, Colorado, United States of America, 2 Institute for Ageing and Health, Campus for Ageing and Vitality, Newcastle University, Newcastle upon Tyne, United Kingdom

Abstract

Elevated low-density lipoprotein (LDL)-cholesterol is a risk factor for both Alzheimer's disease (AD) and Atherosclerosis (CVD), suggesting a common lipid-sensitive step in their pathogenesis. Previous results show that AD and CVD also share a cell cycle defect: chromosome instability and up to 30% aneuploidy–in neurons and other cells in AD and in smooth muscle cells in atherosclerotic plaques in CVD. Indeed, specific degeneration of aneuploid neurons accounts for 90% of neuronal loss in AD brain, indicating that aneuploidy underlies AD neurodegeneration. Cell/mouse models of AD develop similar aneuploidy through amyloid-beta (Aß) inhibition of specific microtubule motors and consequent disruption of mitotic spindles. Here we tested the hypothesis that, like upregulated Aß, elevated LDL/cholesterol and altered intracellular cholesterol homeostasis also causes chromosomal instability. Specifically we found that: 1) high dietary cholesterol induces aneuploidy in mice, satisfying the hypothesis' first prediction, 2) Niemann-Pick C1 patients accumulate aneuploid fibroblasts, neurons, and glia, demonstrating a similar aneugenic effect of intracellular cholesterol accumulation in humans 3) oxidized LDL, LDL, and cholesterol, but not high-density lipoprotein (HDL), induce chromosome mis-segregation and aneuploidy in cultured cells, including neuronal precursors, indicating that LDL/cholesterol directly affects the cell cycle, 4) LDL-induced aneuploidy requires the LDL receptor, but not Aß, showing that LDL works differently than Aß, with the same end result, 5) cholesterol treatment disrupts the structure of the mitotic spindle, providing a cell biological mechanism for its aneugenic activity, and 6) ethanol or calcium chelation attenuates lipoprotein-induced chromosome mis-segregation, providing molecular insights into cholesterol's aneugenic mechanism, specifically through its rigidifying effect on the cell membrane, and potentially explaining why ethanol consumption reduces the risk of developing atherosclerosis or AD. These results suggest a novel, cell cycle mechanism by which aberrant cholesterol homeostasis promotes neurodegeneration and atherosclerosis by disrupting chromosome segregation and potentially other aspects of microtubule physiology.

Editor: Ken Arai, Massachusetts General Hospital/Harvard Medical School, United States of America

Funding: Supported by the Byrd Alzheimer's Institute, the Eric Pfeiffer Chair for Research on Alzheimer's Disease, The University of Colorado, Denver and the NIA (AG025711; AG037942). Some imaging experiments were performed in the University of Colorado Anschutz Medical Campus Advanced Light Microscopy Core supported in part by NIH/NCRR Colorado CTSI Grant Number UL1 RR025780. Contents are the authors' sole responsibility and do not necessarily represent official NIH views. The funders had no role in study design, data collection and analysis, decision to publish, or preparation of the manuscript.

Competing Interests: The authors have declared that no competing interests exist.

* E-mail: huntington.potter@ucdenver.edu

Introduction

High levels of dietary cholesterol and plasma LDL have been found to constitute a common risk factor for both atherosclerosis/cardiovascular disease and for Alzheimer's disease, but the mechanism(s) of this effect are incompletely understood [1,2]. Atherosclerosis is characterized by localized accumulations of lipids, inflammatory cells, smooth muscle cells and calcified cell debris [3], while Alzheimer's disease (AD) is characterized by aberrant oligomerization/polymerization of two misfolded proteins–extracellular amyloid-beta (Aß) assembled into amyloid deposits, and intracellular hyperphosphorylated tau assembled into neurofibrillary tangles [4–6]. We sought to determine whether there is a common pathogenic pathway by which cholesterol/LDL promotes the development of both atherosclerosis and Alzheimer's disease.

Genetic, biochemical, and transgenic mice studies of mutations that cause familial forms of AD (FAD) have identified the Aß peptide as central to AD pathogenesis, with Apolipoprotein E (ApoE), Tau, and microtubules being required for Aß to oligomerize/polymerize and induce synaptic loss, neurodegeneration, and dementia [4–7].

Cell Cycle Defects and Chromosome Mis-segregation in AD

One mechanism by which Aß evidently causes neurodegeneration is by interfering with cell cycle. For example, we proposed that AD subjects would exhibit chromosome mis-segregation and the accumulation of aneuploid, particularly trisomy 21 cells and then used primary skin fibroblasts to demonstrate such trisomy 21 mosaicism and a trend toward chromosome 18 mosaicism in both familial and sporadic AD (SAD) patients [8–11]. AD lymphocytes also showed trisomy 21 mosaicism and premature centromere division, a mechanistic precursor to chromosome mis-segregation [9,12–16]. Work from several laboratories confirmed and extended these results to buccal cells and brain neurons, with trisomy 21 constituting 10% of neurons in late stage AD brain [17–21].

We investigated the mechanism of this cell cycle defect and found that mutations in the presenilin 1 (*PS1*) and amyloid precursor protein (*APP*) genes that cause FAD directly induce chromosome mis-segregation and up to 20% aneuploidy in lymphocytes and neurons of transgenic mice and in transfected cells. Indeed the Alzheimer Aß peptide, the proteolytic product of the PS1 based γ-secretase enzyme on the APP protein and the key player in AD pathogenesis, also induces abnormal spindle structure and chromosome mis-segregation, including human trisomy 21 and mouse trisomy 16 in transgenic mice, transfected cells, and cell-free Xenopus egg extracts [22–24,25–28]. We found that his profound defect in mitosis in AD results from Aß inhibition of certain mitotic kinesin motor proteins, including kinesin5/Eg5, that are essential for the structure and function of the mitotic spindle [24].

That chromosome mis-segregation and the consequent development of aneuploidy plays an essential role in AD pathogenesis is indicated by the finding that following the development of 30% aneuploid neurons during the early stages of AD, the specific loss of these aneuploid neurons in the transition from mild cognitive impairment to late stage AD can account for 90% of the neuronal cell loss observed at autopsy [21].

The finding of trisomy 21 mosaicism in AD is particularly interesting because of the universal presence of AD-like pathology and neurodegeneration in full trisomy 21 Down syndrome (DS) patients [8,29–31], and the finding that early onset inherited AD can be caused by a single duplicated *APP* gene on one chromosome 21 [32,33]. Evidently a 50% excess of APP and its product Aß are sufficient for the development of AD. Case studies of patients with trisomy 21 mosaicism and no intellectual impairments of the DS type who developed AD by age 40 demonstrates that a small percentage of trisomy 21 cells can, over a lifetime, lead to and/or contribute to the pathogenesis of AD [8,25,34–37].

Disruption of Cholesterol Homeostasis in Neurodegenerative Diseases

Because the generation and loss of aneuploid neurons appears to underlie the majority of AD neurodegeneration, it is essential to understand the mechanism by which such aneuploidy arises during the preclinical stage of the disease. Clearly, the overproduction of the Aß peptide may be partly responsible. However, defects in cholesterol homeostasis may also play a role in AD pathogenesis [38–43]. For example AD, and cardiovascular disease (CVD) share risk factors (e.g., high plasma cholesterol and a high cholesterol and/or saturated fat diet), and the severity of atherosclerotic lesions in AD brains correlates with the extent of AD pathology [38,40]. Likewise, FAD transgenic mice fed a high cholesterol diet develop accelerated amyloid burden and steeper cognitive decline compared to animals on regular chow [39,43]. Conversely, inhibition of endogenous cholesterol synthesis with statins has been associated with a reduced risk of AD and decreased amyloid deposits in humans and animals [42]. Finally, ApoE is the major cholesterol transporter in the brain, and inheritance of the *ApoE ε4* allele is the strongest genetic risk factor for sporadic AD [44]. ApoE particularly ApoE4 directly associates with Aß and catalyzes its polymerization into neurotoxic assemblies [7].

A dysregulation of cholesterol homeostasis has also been implicated in other chronic neurodegenerative diseases, including Niemann-Pick (NPC), Huntington, and Parkinson's disease [39,43]. Specifically, a direct association between disrupted intracellular cholesterol trafficking and consequent neuronal loss, gliosis, and formation of neurofibrillary tangles (NFT) in individuals carrying a mutation in the *NPC1* or *NPC2* gene has been established. Loss-of function mutations in these genes cause sequestration of unesterified cholesterol in late endosomes/lysosomes in a number of cells and tissues, but are most deleterious for brain development and health, triggering progressive neuropathology, ataxia, dementia and premature death in early adolescence [43]. Recent studies utilizing human samples and cellular and animal models of NPC revealed interesting parallels between AD and NPC neuropathogenesis, which include endosomal/lysosomal dysfunction, glial-mediated inflammation, NFTs and Aß accumulation especially in *ApoE ε4* carriers, cholesterol dyshomeostasis, and cell cycle reactivation [27,28,39,43]. However, unlike AD [8–21], the presence of chromosomal abnormalities such as aneuploidy in peripheral and brain cells has not been reported in NPC.

These pathological correlations and our finding that Aß induces chromosome mis-segregation prompted us to investigate whether cholesterol might also induce aneuploidy in AD and possibly NPC and atherosclerosis. The latter hypothesis was reinforced by reports that each atherosclerotic plaque harbors a monoclonal proliferation of aneuploid smooth muscle cells [45–52].

To test these hypotheses, we asked whether cholesterol and lipoproteins induce chromosomal mis-segregation *in vivo* and *in vitro* and then investigated the mechanism of their observed novel aneugenic effect.

Results

To investigate whether lipoproteins and cholesterol affect chromosome segregation, we approached the project in three phases. First, metaphase chromosome analysis and fluorescence *in situ* DNA hybridization (FISH) were used to determine whether LDL/cholesterol increases the levels of total and chromosome specific aneuploidy *in vivo*: in mice fed a high cholesterol diet and in human Niemann-Pick patients with a mutation in the *NPC1* gene, which is implicated in cholesterol trafficking and atherosclerosis but has not previously been associated with a defect in chromosome segregation, although mitosis-specific epitopes have been observed in NCP1 brains [53,54] (Figure 1,2). Then, to establish that lipoproteins/cholesterol were directly responsible for the aneuploidy we observed in cholesterol-fed mice and NPC1 patients, we analyzed the chromosomes of different cells in culture after exposure to various lipids, including water solubilized cholesterol (Figures 3–4). Particular attention was paid to assessing the aneuploidy of chromosomes 7, 12, 14, 18 and 21, as mis-segregation of several of these chromosomes has been found in AD [9,11–23] and in atherosclerotic lesions [46–51]. We then investigated the mechanism by which lipoproteins/cholesterol induce chromosome mis-segregation by analyzing their effect in cells lacking the low density lipoprotein receptor (*LDLR*) or the *APP* gene or exposed to calcium chelators or ethanol to counter the intracellular signaling and the membrane rigidifying effect of cholesterol (Figures 5–8). Finally we determined whether cholesterol treatment induces DNA damage (Figure 9) or disrupts the mitotic spindle, for example leading to multiple centrosomes

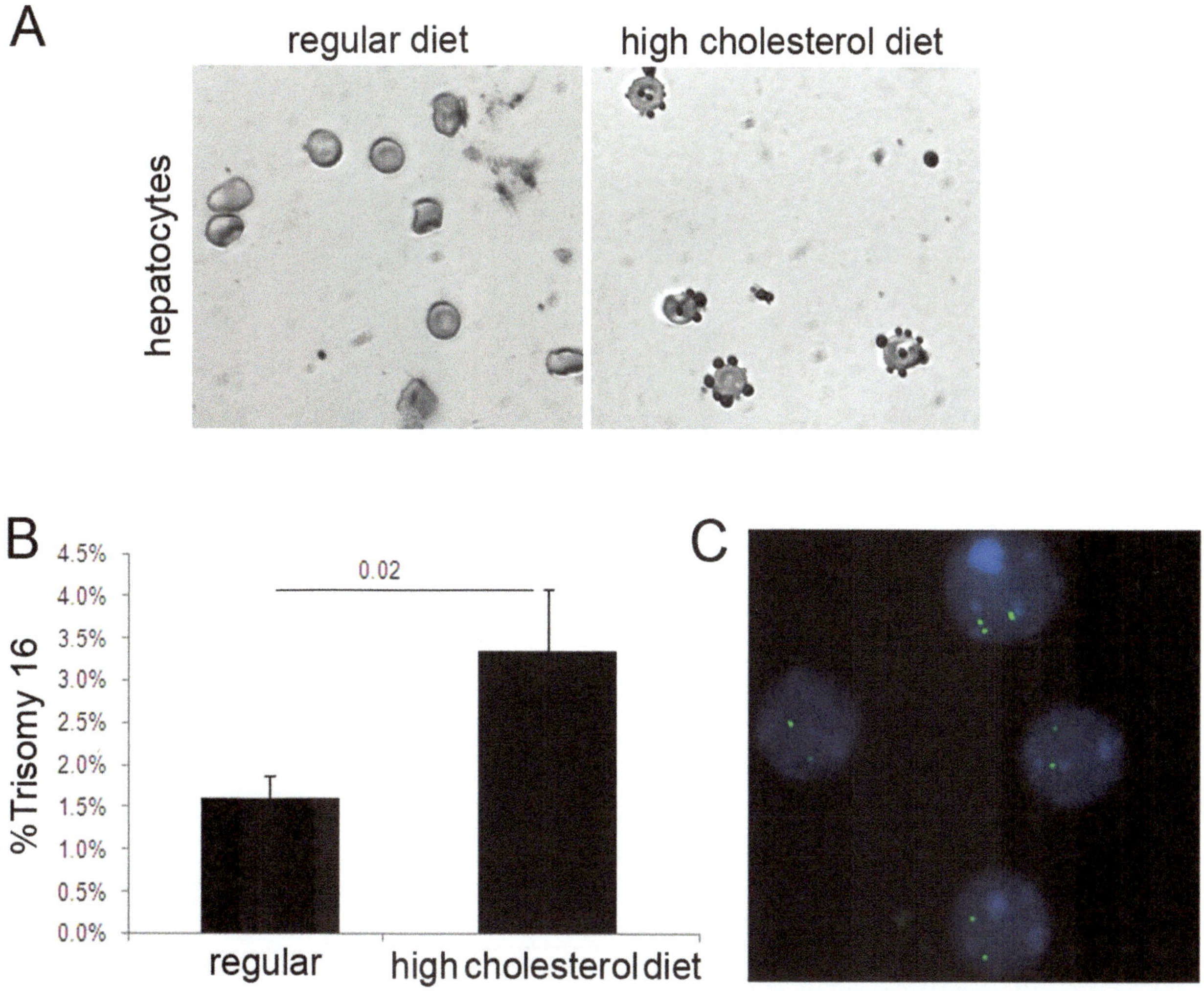

Figure 1. Increased cholesterol induces chromosome aneuploidy in vivo. (A) Mouse hepatocytes (hematoxylin blue stain; light gray in micrograph) were stained with Oil-Red-O stain (red stain, dark gray in micrograph) to detect accumulation of lipid droplets, a sign of liver steatosis and a consequence of dyslipidemia in mice fed a high cholesterol diet (right panel). (B–C) Quantitative FISH analysis for chromosome 16 showed that young wild-type mice fed a high (1.05%) cholesterol, atherogenic diet for 12 weeks developed higher levels of trisomy 16 in spleen cells compare to mice fed regular chow.

(MOCs), lagging chromosomes and mis-aligned/displaced DNA or disarrayed microtubules, all of which are known causes of chromosome mis-segregation/instability (Figure 10).

Cholesterol Dyshomeostasis Induces Aneuploidy *in vivo*

Mice fed a high cholesterol diet develop aneuploidy in splenocytes. The effect of hypercholesterolemia on chromosome-segregation in peripheral cells (T-splenocytes) and in brain cells was assessed in atherosclerosis-susceptible wild-type mice, the C57BL/6 strain [55]. One-month-old (nontransgenic) mice (4 males and 4 females) were randomly assigned to normal mouse chow (0% cholesterol) or a high cholesterol (~1.05%) diet (two mouse pairs per group) for 12 weeks. Mice fed the regular diet consumed on average 50.62±8.34 g/mouse pair/week (~172 Kcal of Digestible Energy (DE)/mouse pair/week), while mice on the high cholesterol diet consumed on average 50.83±11.14 g/mouse pair/week (~229 Kcal of DE/mouse pair/week). Because of the difference in caloric value between the diets, mice on the high cholesterol diet gained on average 2½ times more weight than mice fed regular chow ($p<0.05$). Pathological examination at sacrifice confirmed that only mice on the high cholesterol diet developed hepatic steatosis, a sign of dyslipidemia, which was confirmed with Oil-Red-O staining of isolated hepatocytes (Figure 1A).

Primary splenocyte cultures and brain cell suspensions from mice on the regular and atherogenic diets were analyzed for aneuploidy. FISH analysis of concanavalin A-stimulated spleen T-cells from mice fed the high cholesterol diet showed a significant increase in trisomy 16 compared to T-splenocytes of mice fed the regular diet (Fig. 1B,C), but there was no induction of aneuploidy in brain cells (0.76% versus 0.65%, $p=0.3$). The fact that diet-induced hypercholesterolemia has not been reported to affect brain cholesterol homeostasis in wild-type mice suggests that serum cholesterol may have induced the spleen cell aneuploidy while sparing the brain. It is also possible that 12 weeks is sufficient time to induce the development of aneuploid cells in mitotically active peripheral (lymphatic) tissues of animals fed cholesterol, but is insufficient to allow accumulation of significant aneuploidy in the brain resulting from relatively less active neurogenesis.

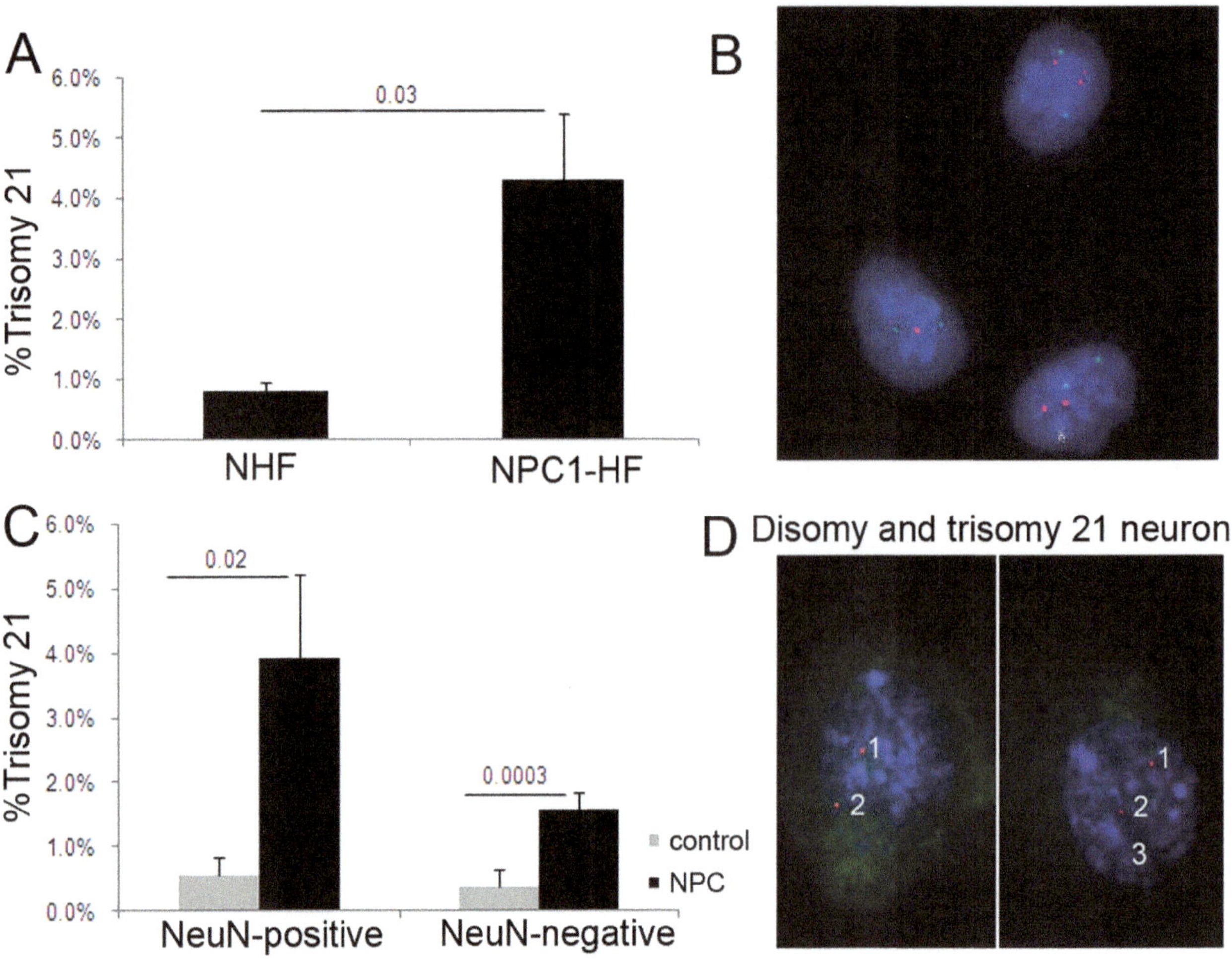

Figure 2. Increased trisomy 21 aneuploidy in fibroblasts and in glia and neurons of Niemann-Pick C1 patients. (A,B) FISH analysis with a DNA probe for chromosome 21 (red) and chromosome 12 (green) of fibroblasts derived from NPC1 patients (NPC1-HF) showed an increase in trisomy 21 cells compared to age-matched normal human fibroblasts. (C,D) Quantitative FISH analysis with a DNA probe for chromosome 21 (red) followed by staining with NeuN antibody (green) and DAPI (blue) of resuspended cells from frontal cortices of control and NPC brains revealed significantly higher levels of trisomy 21 in NPC neurons and glia compared to controls.

Niemann-Pick (*NPC1*) mutant neurons, glia, and fibroblasts accumulate elevated levels of trisomy 21. To investigate the role of disrupted peripheral and central cholesterol homeostasis in chromosome segregation in a longer-term human neurodegenerative disease model, we turned to primary cells derived from patients diagnosed with Niemann-Pick Type C (NPC) disease (Table 1). Mutations and deletions in the *NPC1* and *NPC2* genes cause impaired trafficking of unesterified cholesterol (both low density lipoprotein receptor (LDLR)-internalized and endogenously synthesized) and other lipids (e.g., glycosphingolipids), which accumulate in late endosomes and lysosomes and fail to travel to the plasma membrane and endoplasmic reticulum (ER), resulting in severe cognitive deficits [56,57]. Loss/defect in the *NPC1* gene has also been shown to promote atherosclerosis in animal models [58]. Interestingly, as was first reported in AD, mitosis-specific proteins and/or phospho-epitopes have been found to be upregulated in NPC1 brains [27,28,53,54,59–65].

To test whether cholesterol mal-distribution affects chromosome stability in NPC disease, we assessed the level of aneuploidy in primary NPC fibroblasts and brain cells hybridized with FISH probes for chromosomes 12, 21, 14 and/or 18. We observed a 4-fold increase in trisomy 21 in NPC1 fibroblasts (Figure 2A,B) compared to normal fibroblasts and an increase of aneuploidy 12 that did not reach statistical significance (2.1% versus 0.4%, $p = 0.12$). Quantitative FISH analysis of Neu-N-positive and Neu-N-negative brain cells showed 4 to 6-fold increases in trisomy 21 in both neurons and glia with the *NPC1* mutation, compared to the cells from control brains (Fig. 2C,D). However, there was no increase in aneuploidy of chromosomes 12, 14 or 18 in NPC brain cells compared to controls (0.55% vs. 0.24%, $p = 0.11$; 1.61% vs. 1.46%, $p = 0.41$; and 0.75% vs. 0.78%, $p = 0.45$, respectively).

These results are the first demonstration of a genomic instability and trisomy 21 mosaicism in Niemann-Pick disease and indicate that a cholesterol accumulation/localization defect causes chromosome mis-segregation in humans, as a high cholesterol diet did in mice.

Lipoprotein/cholesterol Induces Aneuploidy *in vitro*

hTERT-HME1 cells treated with lipoproteins develop aneuploidy. To determine whether the aneuploidy observed in NPC patients or in mice fed an atherogenic diet reflects a direct effect of lipids on mitosis, hTERT-HME1 cells were exposed to

Table 1. Characteristics of the Niemann-Pick Type C (NPC) and Control Samples.

Repository #	Age yr	Gender	Clinical Dx	Mutation of NPC assay
Control fibroblasts				
AG02101	27	female	none	N/A
AG02603	35	female	none	N/A
AG09319	24	female	none	N/A
AG09429	25	female	none	N/A
NPC1 fibroblasts				
GM18422	NK	female	NPC1	813_815delCAT & ASP874VAL
GM18390	NK	female	NPC1	ASP242HIS & SER940LEU
GM22871	4	female	NPC1	1920delG & IVS9-1009G>A
GM17912	19	female	NPC1	PRO1007ALA & THR1036MET
Control brains				
UMB754	11.5	female	asthma	N/A
UMB1864	2.5	female	streptococcus infection	N/A
UMB4725	32.2	female	hypertension	N/A
UMB55	19.6	female	auto accident injury	N/A
UMB4590	20.5	female	dilated cardiomyopathy	N/A
NPC brains				
UMB5372	11.3	female	NPC1	filipin & cholesterol esterification
UMB4214	32.3	female	NPC	confirmed NPC neuropathology
UMB4237	19.8	female	NPC	confirmed NPC neuropathology
UMBM4992M	20.1	female	NPC	NPC clinical diagnosis

yr = year; NK = not known. Human fibroblasts were purchased from Coriell and brains from NICHD Brain and Tissue Bank for Developmental Disorders. Independent T-test revealed no age difference between NPC and control brain donors (20.9±8.6 vs. 17.3±11.1, p = 0.61).

20 μg/ml oxidized LDL (OX-LDL), LDL or high density lipoprotein (HDL) for 48 hr and assessed for aneuploidy by metaphase chromosome analysis and FISH, as described. This lipid concentration was chosen to mimic the cholesterol level in human blood and to approximate tissue culture conditions. The results showed an up to 4-fold increase in abnormal chromosome complements (20% aneuploidy) in OX-LDL and LDL treated cells compared to controls and to HDL-treated cells (Figure 3A). The chromosome specific aneuploidy was further analyzed by quantitative FISH (Figure 3B–E), which revealed an induction of: 1) trisomy 21 and 12 by OX-LDL and a borderline significant induction of trisomy 21 and 12 by LDL (Figure 3B and D), and 2) induction of tetrasomy 21 and 12 by both OX-LDL and/or LDL (Figure 3C and E).

A small number of tetraploid neurons has been observed in AD brains of humans and mice and interpreted to be a consequence of aberrant cell cycle activation and DNA duplication without cell cycle completion [25,27,28,59–65]. The OX-LDL and LDL induced tetrasomy we observed in interphase hTERT-HME1 cells are most consistent with severe chromosome mis-segregation because very few tetraploid/polyploid cells were observed in the metaphase spreads (Figure 3F), which was determined by counting a total number of metaphase hyperploid/polyploid cells (having at least ≥90 chromosomes) and diploid cells (46 chromosomes [2 n]) in the portion of the slide initially analyzed for karyotype. Also, individual cells with both tetrasomy 21 and 12 occur at similar levels in treated and untreated cells (Figure 3E). Similarly in AD brain, many (10X) fewer tetraploid (4 n) neurons are observed compared to aneuploid (>2 n and <4 n) neurons [21].

LDL- induced trisomy 7 in HASM cells. To investigate the potential role of elevated lipoproteins on chromosome segregation during atherosclerosis, we tested the aneugenic effect of LDL, OX-LDL, and HDL (20 μg/ml) for 48 hr on primary human aortic smooth muscle cells (HASMC), which are prone to trisomy 7 in atherosclerotic plaques. Quantitative FISH revealed a statistically significant 3-fold increase in trisomy 7 in LDL treated cells (Figure 4).

Requirement for *LDLR* and *APP* in LDL-induced chromosome mis-segregation. 1. Lipoprotein induced aneuploidy is dependent of *LDLR*. The LDL receptor belongs to a large family of structurally and functionally related cell surface receptors that are involved in diverse cellular functions, some implicated in AD pathogenesis, including cholesterol uptake and metabolism, ApoE binding [66], and APP trafficking and processing [67,68]. More than 1000 unique *LDLR* genetic alterations have been identified that lead to Familial Hypercholesterolemia (FH), causing three to four times higher levels of blood LDL cholesterol than normal and premature CVD events, including severe atherosclerosis [69].

To investigate whether lipoprotein-induced chromosome mis-segregation requires a functional LDLR, FH primary human fibroblasts harboring mutations in both *LDLR* alleles and normal human fibroblasts were treated with 20 μg/ml of lipoproteins for 48 hr and assessed for aneuploidy. Quantitative FISH analysis revealed that LDL-treated normal human fibroblasts develop significantly higher levels of trisomy 7 compared to LDL-treated FH fibroblasts (Figure 5A).

2. Lipoprotein induced aneuploidy is independent of *APP*. Previously we found that Aß-induced aneuploidy is dependent on

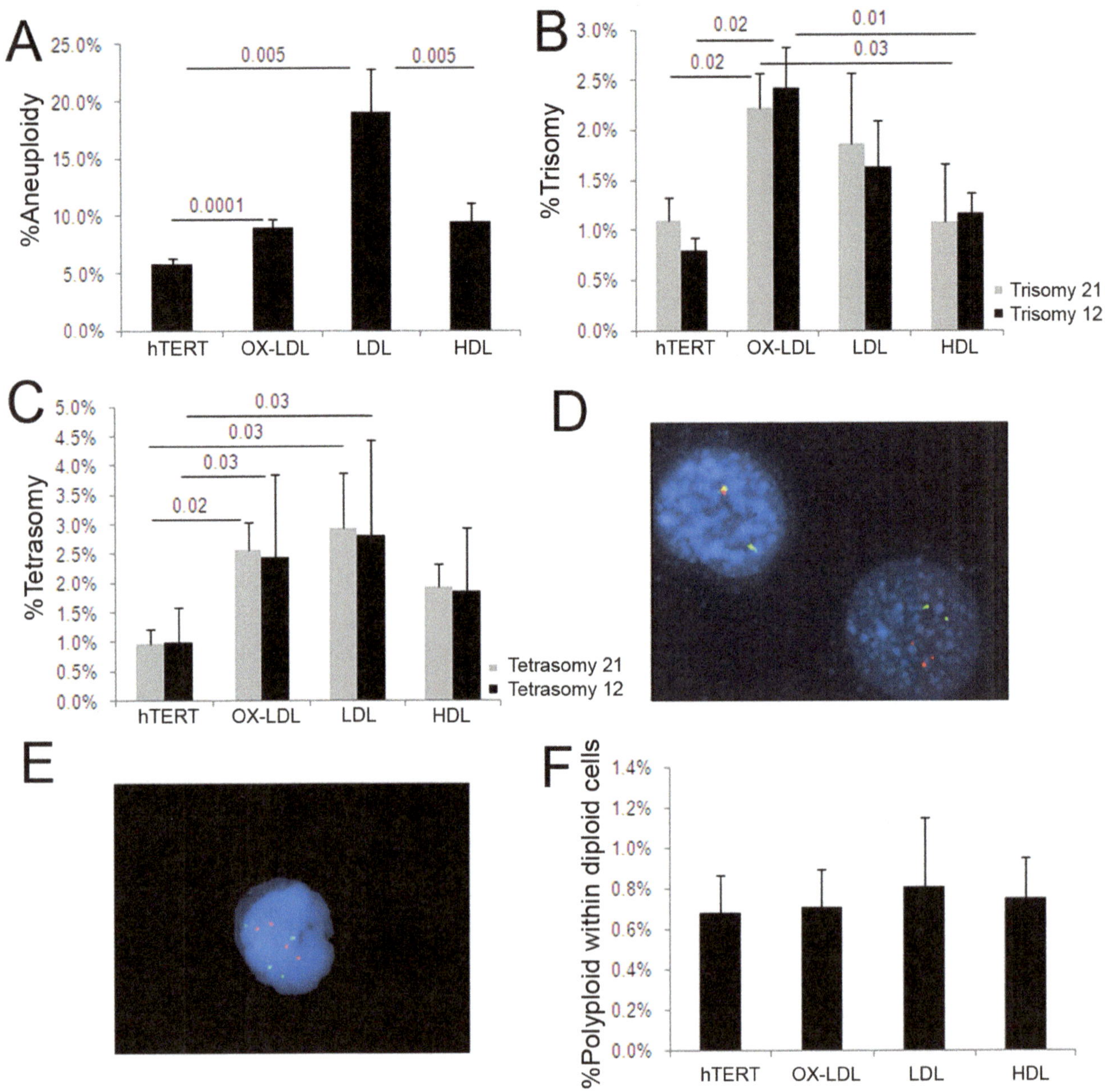

Figure 3. Lipoprotein treatment induces aneuploidy. (A) Actively growing hTERT-HME1 cells were treated with 20 μg/ml of OX-LDL, LDL or HDL for 48 hr, arrested in metaphase and Giemsa stained for karyotype analysis. All lipids induced significantly higher levels of aneuploidy compared to untreated cells, with LDL and or OX-LDL exhibiting a much stronger aneugenic effect than HDL. (B–E) FISH analysis of the same lipoprotein-treated cells showed that OX-LDL-induced trisomy 21 and trisomy 12 (B,D), and that both OX-LDL and LDL-induced tetrasomy 21 and 12 (C,E). (F) Karyotype analysis of an aliquot of the cells from the same treatment showed very few, but equal numbers of polyploid cells, indicating that the tetrasomies observed are due to chromosome mis-segregation of chromosomes 21 or 12, and not a result of chromosome duplication before cell division.

endogenous APP, possibly as a cell surface receptor to aid APP endocytosis and generation of intracellular Aß peptide or for the uptake of extracellular Aß [23,70,71].

To determine whether lipoprotein/cholesterol and Aß-induced chromosome mis-segregation are mechanistically related, we isolated primary splenocytes from *APPKO* mice and nontransgenic littermates, exposed them to lipoproteins, and scored them for chromosome 16 aneuploidy (Figure 5B). OX-LDL and LDL induced significant increases in trisomy 16 in both cell types, indicating that the aneugenic effect of lipoproteins is independent of APP expression and Aß production.

Lipids and Cholesterol-induced Aneuploidy and Spindle Defects are Mediated through Membrane Fluidity and Calcium Homeostasis

Water-Soluble Cholesterol (WsCh) induces aneuploidy *in vitro*. 1. WsCh induces aneuploidy in hTERT-HME1 cells. Cholesterol, the most abundant lipid in eukaryotic cell membranes [72], is compartmentalized into microdomains (e.g., lipid rafts),

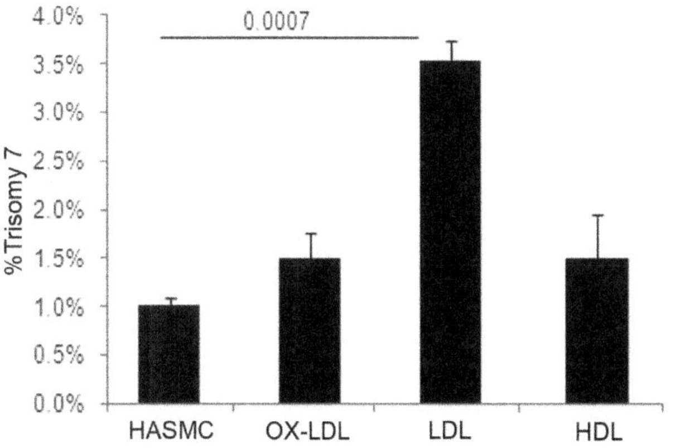

Figure 4. LDL induces trisomy 7 in human aortic smooth muscle cells. Quantitative FISH analysis of HASM cells showed an increase in trisomy 7 when incubated with 20 μg/ml of LDL, but not HDL for 48 hr.

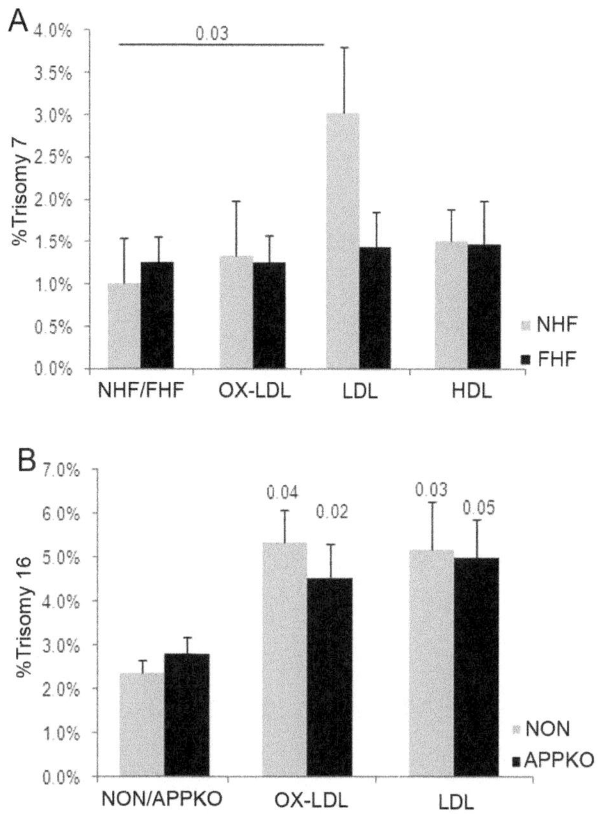

Figure 5. Lipoprotein-induced aneuploidy is dependent on LDLR and independent of APP. (A) Normal human fibroblasts (NHF) developed significantly higher levels of trisomy 7 when treated with 20 μg/ml of LDL for 48 hr compared to LDL receptor deficient human fibroblasts obtained from the patient diagnosed with familial hypercholesterolemia (FHF). (B) Quantitative FISH for chromosome 16 revealed comparable levels of trisomy 16 in primary splenocytes derived from nontransgenic (NON) and APP knockout (APPKO) mice upon incubation with 20 μg/ml of OX-LDL or LDL for 48 hr, indicating that the aneugenic activity of lipoproteins is independent of a functional APP gene and of its product Aβ.

where it is required for essential cellular functions and structure, including signal transduction and plasma membrane dynamics [73,74].

As indicated above, LDLR is used by cells to internalize external lipoproteins and is clearly required for the aneugenic effect of LDL. Methyl-β-cyclodextrin, MβCD, as cholesterol acceptor has been used to modify cellular cholesterol content, and to aid the delivery of hydrophobic cholesterol into the plasma membrane and intracellular compartments by enclosing it into its hydrophobic cavity, bypassing the need for an LDL receptor [75,76]. To directly examine the effect of cholesterol on chromosome segregation, we exposed hTERT-HME1 cells to a water-soluble MβCD:cholesterol complex (WsCh) and performed karyotype and FISH analysis. First, we conducted a set of preliminary experiments with the concentrations of 2 to 10 μg/ml of WsCh for 24 and 48 hr of incubation to determine the optimal concentration at which aneuploidy induction could be measured over the background, but no visible morphological changes or cytotoxicity could be detected. 4 μg/ml of cholesterol exposure (but not 2 μg/ml) for 48 hr induced a 2-fold increase in total aneuploidy compared to untreated cells (Figure 6A) and a significant increase in trisomy 21 and trisomy 12 (Figure 6B), without altering cell proliferation ($p = 0.25$). Taken together, these data indicate that adding cholesterol to cell membranes induces mitotic defects in the form of aneuploidy likely affecting all chromosomes.

2. WsCh induces trisomy 16 in mouse neuronal precursor cells. Induction of chromosome mis-segregation by altered membrane cholesterol in AD or NPC patients is likely to be especially detrimental during neurogenesis and/or neuro-regeneration.

To investigate the effect of cholesterol on the development of aneuploidy in neuronal precursor cells, we prepared neurospheres from prenatal brains of nontransgenic mice, treated them with WsCh, and performed FISH for chromosome 16 as described. Parallel cultures were incubated with or without WsCh for 7 days (equivalent to the two cell divisions used previously for the hTERT-HME1 cells), with fresh cholesterol-containing media being replenished every other day to allow for expansion of the spheres, a sign of neuronal precursor cell proliferation [77]. We observed >4% trisomy 16 in untreated cells (Figure 6C), as has been previously reported in developing and adult normal human and mouse brains [78–80] and a significant 2-fold increase in trisomy 16 in cholesterol treated cells (Figure 6C).

Changing membrane fluidity by ethanol attenuates lipoprotein-induced chromosome mis-segregation. The fact that the addition of cholesterol to cells induces chromosome mis-segregation is a potentially important indicator of its underlying mechanism of action. It is well established that membrane cholesterol content is directly proportional to membrane stiffness/rigidity [81], which can be increased by cholesterol enrichment or decreased by cholesterol depletion [82]. In contrast, ethanol (EtOH) increases membrane fluidity, with profound physiological effects on multiple mammalian cells, including neurons [83]. Because both lipoprotein- and MβCD-delivered cholesterol increases membrane cholesterol content and rigidity *in vitro* [81,82,84], we hypothesized that the mitotic errors induced in cells by lipoprotein/cholesterol might be caused by increased membrane rigidity, which could be counteracted by the membrane fluidizing action of ethanol.

hTERT-HME1 cells were pre-treated with 25 mM of EtOH for 24 hr and further co-incubated with lipids in EtOH-containing media. The rationales for using this concentration of EtOH were: 1) 25 mM or 0.115% corresponds to the blood alcohol levels of moderate drinkers (1–3 drinks a day, 15–45 g) which has been associated with a decrease in risk for CVD [85,86] and AD [87], 2)

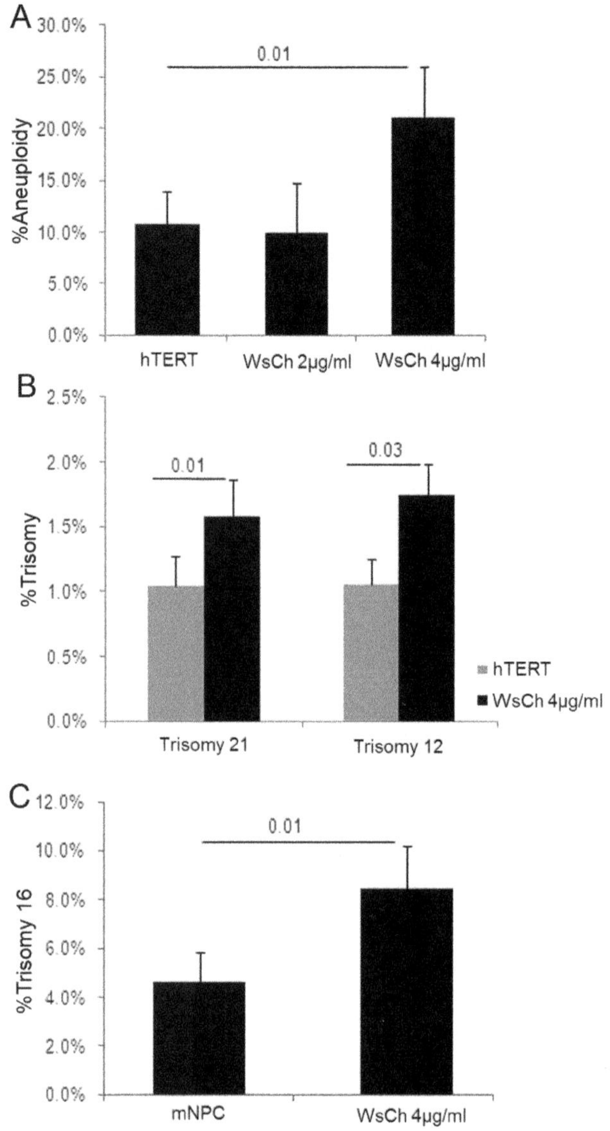

Figure 6. Increased membrane cholesterol induces aneuploidy. (A,B) Karyotype and FISH analysis showed an increase in total aneuploidy (A) and trisomy 21 and trisomy 12 (B) in hTERT cells treated for 48 hr with 4 µg/ml cholesterol made water-soluble in a methyl-β-cyclodextrin (MβCD) complex. (C) Mouse chromosome 16 DNA probe was used to measure aneuploidy levels in mouse neuronal precursor cells (mNPC) derived from prenatal brains of wild-type mice (E17–18) and incubated with and without 4 µg/ml of WsCh for 7 days. Quantitative FISH analysis showed a 2-fold increase in trisomy 16 in WsCh-treated cells compared to controls. mNPC harbored up to 4.6% endogenous aneuploidy, as reported previously in developing mouse and human brains [73].

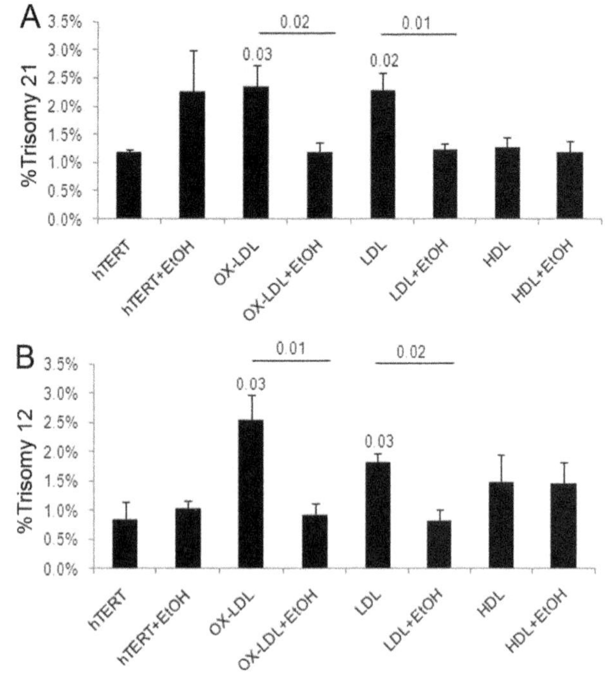

Figure 7. Ethanol attenuates lipoprotein-induced chromosome mis-segregation. (A,B) Quantitative FISH analysis of hTERT cells pre-treated with 25 mM of ethanol (EtOH) for 24 hr and co-incubated with lipoproteins and EtOH for an additional 48 hr revealed a decrease in OX-LDL and LDL-induced trisomy 21 (A) and trisomy 12 (B).

increased cholesterol efflux and cholesterol transport but unchanged cholesterol synthesis have been observed in human astrocytes *in vitro* at a concentration of 25 mM of EtOH in the presence and absence of cholesterol acceptors [88], 3) 25 mM EtOH fluidized the exofacial leaflet of the synaptic membranes [89], 4) long-term exposure of hepatic cells to 0.5% EtOH had no effect on LDLR expression or the uptake of LDL [90], and 5) our pilot experiments showed low cytotoxicity and up to ~95% cell viability after 48 hr of 25 mM EtOH exposure and only a small, non-significant induction of aneuploidy for chromosome 21 (HSA21) (Figure S1A–D).

Quantitative FISH analysis of lipoprotein/EtOH-treated cells showed a significant decrease in OX-LDL and LDL-induced trisomy 21 (Figure 7A), and trisomy 12 (Figure 7B) compared to cells exposed only to lipoproteins, indicating that fluidization of the membranes by EtOH stabilizes chromosome segregation upon lipid treatment.

Extracellular Ca++ is required for lipoprotein-induced chromosome mis-segregation. It has been postulated that perturbed calcium homeostasis plays an important role during aging and in AD pathogenesis, and calcium is essential for the function of many enzymes, for example CamKII [91]. In our recent study of Aß-induced aneuploidy, we showed that chelation of extracellular Ca++ with BAPTA prevents chromosome mis-segregation *in vitro* [23].

To elucidate whether Ca++ plays a role in lipoprotein/cholesterol-induced aneuploidy, as it does in Aß-induced aneuploidy, we conducted experiments with hTERT-HME1 cells using two different chelating reagents, EGTA and BAPTA. First, the cells were pre-treated with 1.5 mM of EGTA for three minutes before incubation with 20 µg/ml of lipoproteins for 48 hr, then analyzed by FISH. EGTA reduced by 3-fold the OX-LDL induced trisomy 21 (Figure 8A), and tetrasomy 21 and 12 (Figure 8B). The change in mitotic index between EGTA-treated cells with or without lipids (e.g. LDL) was not significant (107±29 vs. 81±42, p = 0.77, respectively).

hTERT-HME1 cells were also pre-incubated with another Ca++ chelator, BAPTA for three minutes and then co-treated with lipids for 48 hr. The results showed a statistically significant BAPTA-dependent reduction in OX-LDL-induced trisomy 21 and 12 (Figure 8C), and a borderline decrease in trisomy 21 in

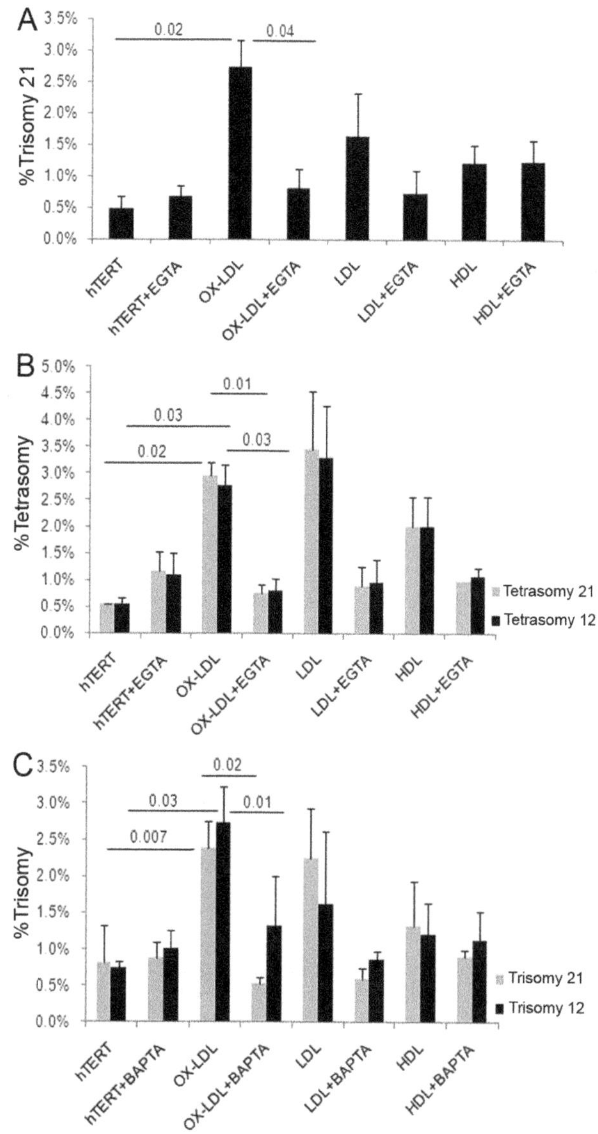

Figure 8. Role for Ca++ in lipoprotein induced chromosome mis-segregation. (A–C) Quantitative FISH analysis with a dually labeled DNA probe for chromosomes 21 and 12 showed a significant reduction in trisomy 21 (A), tetrasomy 21 and tetrasomy 12 (B) in hTERT cells pre-treated with 1.5 mM of Ca++ chelator EGTA followed by OX-LDL compared to cells treated only with OX-LDL. Cells pre-treated with 1 mM BAPTA had significantly lower levels of OX-LDL-induced trisomy 21 and trisomy 12 (C) compared to the cells grown without chelator.

LDL-treated samples ($p = 0.065$; Figure 8C). Quantification and comparison of mitotic indices in BAPTA-treated hTERT cells with or without lipids (e.g., LDL) revealed no significant difference in number of metaphases per slide (67±18 vs. 69±37, $p = 0.92$, respectively), indicating that extracellular calcium chelation does not affect the progression of the cells through the cell cycle.

Cholesterol treatment does not cause DNA damage. Aneuploidy is characteristic of transformed cells and has been hypothesized to play an essential role in carcinogenesis [92]. Radiation, DNA-damaging chemicals, or genetic mutations, for example affecting mis-match repair, can lead to double strand breaks in genomic DNA [93], which has been shown to lead to chromosome mis-segregation and aneuploidy. However, we found no increase in double strand breaks as assessed by 53 BP1 immunocytochemistry after 48 hr treatment of hTERT cells with water-soluble cholesterol (Figure 9).

Cholesterol disrupts the mitotic spindle. There are many mechanisms by which genes or agents can induce chromosome mis-segregation [94]. For example, in Aß-treated cells and Xenopus egg extracts, the mitotic spindles become shortened and bent and the DNA becomes delocalized [24]. We treated hTERT-HME1 cells with 4 µg/ml WsCh for 24 hr and analyzed the mitotic spindles after staining with α-tubulin and γ-tubulin antibodies. As shown in Figure 10, cholesterol induced a multitude (30%) of aberrant mitotic/microtubule structures with disarrayed microtubules and displaced DNA being particularly prominent in mitotic structures.

Discussion

We report a set of findings that reveal a novel cholesterol-dependent cell cycle defect that may be involved in the pathogenesis of Nieman-Pick C1 Disease, Alzheimer's Disease and cardiovascular disease/atherosclerosis. Specifically: 1) Medium-term exposure to dietary cholesterol induces chromosome mis-segregation in peripheral tissues of young wild-type mice, 2) Disturbance in intracellular cholesterol homeostasis and obstructed cholesterol trafficking to the plasma membrane in NPC-1 patients is associated with an 4 to 6-fold increase in the proportion of trisomy 21 fibroblasts, neurons and glia, 3) Atherogenic lipoproteins (i.e., LDL, OX-LDL) and cholesterol, but much less so the protective HDL, induce chromosome mis-segregation, including trisomy HSA12, HSA21, and HSA7 and MMU16 in primary human and mouse cells *in vitro*, 4) Lipoproteins apparently require a functional LDL receptor but not the presence of the *APP* gene to exert their aneugenic effect, 5) Cholesterol exposure disrupts the mitotic spindle and induces disarrayed microtubules and displaced DNA, and 6) Reduction in either plasma membrane fluidity or Ca++ homeostasis decreases lipoprotein/cholesterol-induced aneuploidy *in vitro*.

Aneugenic Effect of Lipoproteins and Cholesterol: Implications for AD and NPC

The present data complement and extend previous work showing that up 30% of AD human and mouse neurons and other cells are aneuploid due to either environmental or complex genetic influences. Although cholesterol and other aneugens, such as mutant *PS* or *APP* genes or the Aß peptide, affect all chromosomes in cultured cells, the lack of selection against trisomy 21 neurons probably accounts for their preponderance in AD and NPC-1 brain. The finding that LDL/cholesterol induces chromosome mis-segregation in the absence of *APP* indicates that the aneugenic pathways initiated by Aß and LDL are, at least in their early steps, separate and independent. While our analyses of actively dividing peripheral cells and precursor brain cells were limited to a few human and only one validated mouse chromosome probe, a comprehensive investigation of other peripheral and brain cells (i.e., neurons and glia) is warranted to fully understand the rate and type of chromosome instability in relation to changed cholesterol homeostasis.

Although there is some indication that aneuploid neurons develop normally in human brains, possibly increasing neuronal diversity [17,95], the large number of aneuploid neurons in AD and NPC must arise from mitosis, either from disease-related neurogenesis, from reactivation of the cell cycle in normally-post-mitotic neurons, or both. A number of studies reported

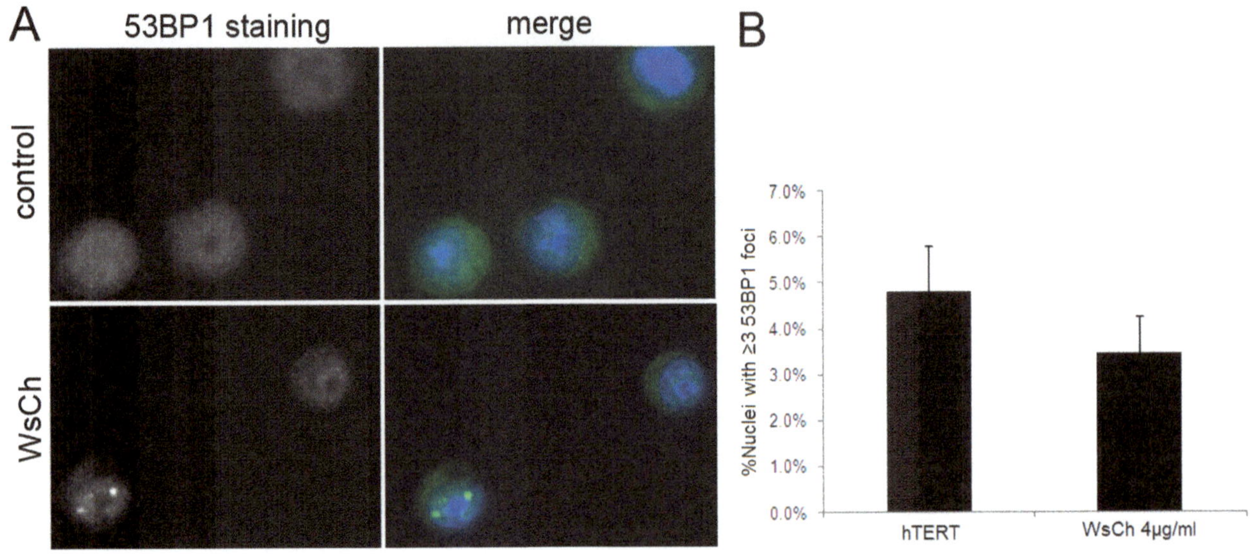

Figure 9. Cholesterol does not cause DSBs in hTERT-HM1 cells. (A) hTERT-HME1 cells were exposed to 4 μg/ml of cholesterol for 48 hr and immunostained for a double-strand breaks (DSBs) marker, the p53 binding protein 53 BP1. Immunofluorescent 53 BP1 (green) foci in nuclei (DAPI, blue) of control and cholesterol-treated cells were counted. (B) There was no statistically significant ($p = 0.06$) increase in DSBs events (≥3 foci per nucleus) in cholesterol-treated compared to untreated cells. The nuclei containing ≥4 foci were extremely rare.

neuronal aneuploidy and tetraploidy of several chromosomes in the human brains diagnosed with AD [17,18,20,21]. Here we did not observe a cholesterol-dependent increase in tetraploid cells (i.e., cells that had duplicated every chromosome, but failed to divide, or had not yet divided), but mitosis specific epitopes have been observed in a small number of neurons in AD and NPC brain or in mouse models of AD, and have been interpreted as indicative of such reactivation of the cell cycle and the consequent development of aneuploid neurons [25,27,28,53–64]. However, the frequency of such tetraploid (4 n) neurons in AD is certainly less than 10% of the frequency of aneuploidy cells (with DNA content between 2 n and 4 n) [21], and some researchers report that the number of tetraploid cells is actually the same in brains from AD and control individuals and are exclusively non-neuronal [96]. Nevertheless, if neurons are induced to re-enter the cell cycle in response to neurodegenerative disease, the resulting mitosis and cell division might well be abnormal and result in the observed increase in aneuploidy, rather than tetraploid neurons.

While we failed to observe a change in ploidy in the brains of mice fed a high cholesterol diet, possibly due to the 1) length of dietary exposure, 2) reduced neurogenesis, 3) young age of the mice, and 4) low or nonexistent exchange of cholesterol and its metabolites across the intact blood-brain barrier (BBB), a peripheral induction of trisomy 16 in mitotically active tissues may be an initiating event that precedes the induction of brain aneuploidy once the extracerebral damage reaches a critical point and the BBB is compromised.

In conclusion, AD and NPC1 exhibit cell cycle abnormalities, to which excess lipoproteins, particularly LDL, can contribute and lead to the chromosome mis-segregation, aneuploidy and neurodegeneration observed in these diseases. Furthermore, the fact that aneuploid neurons also characterize other cognitive brain diseases, such as Frontotemporal Dementia [97] (also Granic et al., unpublished), Down syndrome and Ataxia-Telangiectasia [20], suggests that chromosome mis-segregation and the development of aneuploidy neurons may be a general feature of neurodegeneration.

Chromosome Instability in Atherosclerosis: Implications for AD

Several studies have reported the hyperproliferation of aneuploid smooth muscle cells within atherosclerotic plaques [45–52], which our data suggest may be induced by elevated LDL-cholesterol. Specifically, during the initiation of atherosclerosis, a single smooth muscle cell that, as a consequence of aneuploidy, suffers altered gene regulation may lose checkpoint control or become more responsive to autocrine or paracrine growth factors (for example by becoming trisomy for chromosome 7, which encodes the PDGF receptor) and then hyper-proliferating to generate the observed thickening of the vascular wall. The fact that aneuploid cells are prone to apoptosis fits this model well, for apoptosis of smooth muscle cells is thought to be an essential contributor to the formation of atherosclerotic plaques [98]. Cholesterol induced aneuploidy would also be expected to initiate atherosclerosis in the brain, which can lead to the reduced blood flow and the development of 'vascular dementia' often seen AD patients [40–43,99,100].

Furthermore, the fact that inheritance of the *ApoE ε4* allele is the strongest known risk factor for developing sporadic AD other than age [101] (i.e., ApoE being the major cholesterol carrier protein in the brain [102]), also strengthens the potential significance of lipoprotein/cholesterol-induced aneuploidy for the pathogenesis of AD. LDL and ApoE4 also promote atherosclerosis [103], which is characterized by hyperproliferation of aneuploid cells, as discussed above [45–52], extending the connection between lipid-induced aneuploidy and both CVD and AD. Finally, the fact that Aß causes chromosome mis-segregation and aneuploidy [23] and that atherosclerosis arises in the AD brain and in mouse models of AD [40,104] suggests that Aß itself may trigger the mis-segregation event that initiates the atherogenic process in AD.

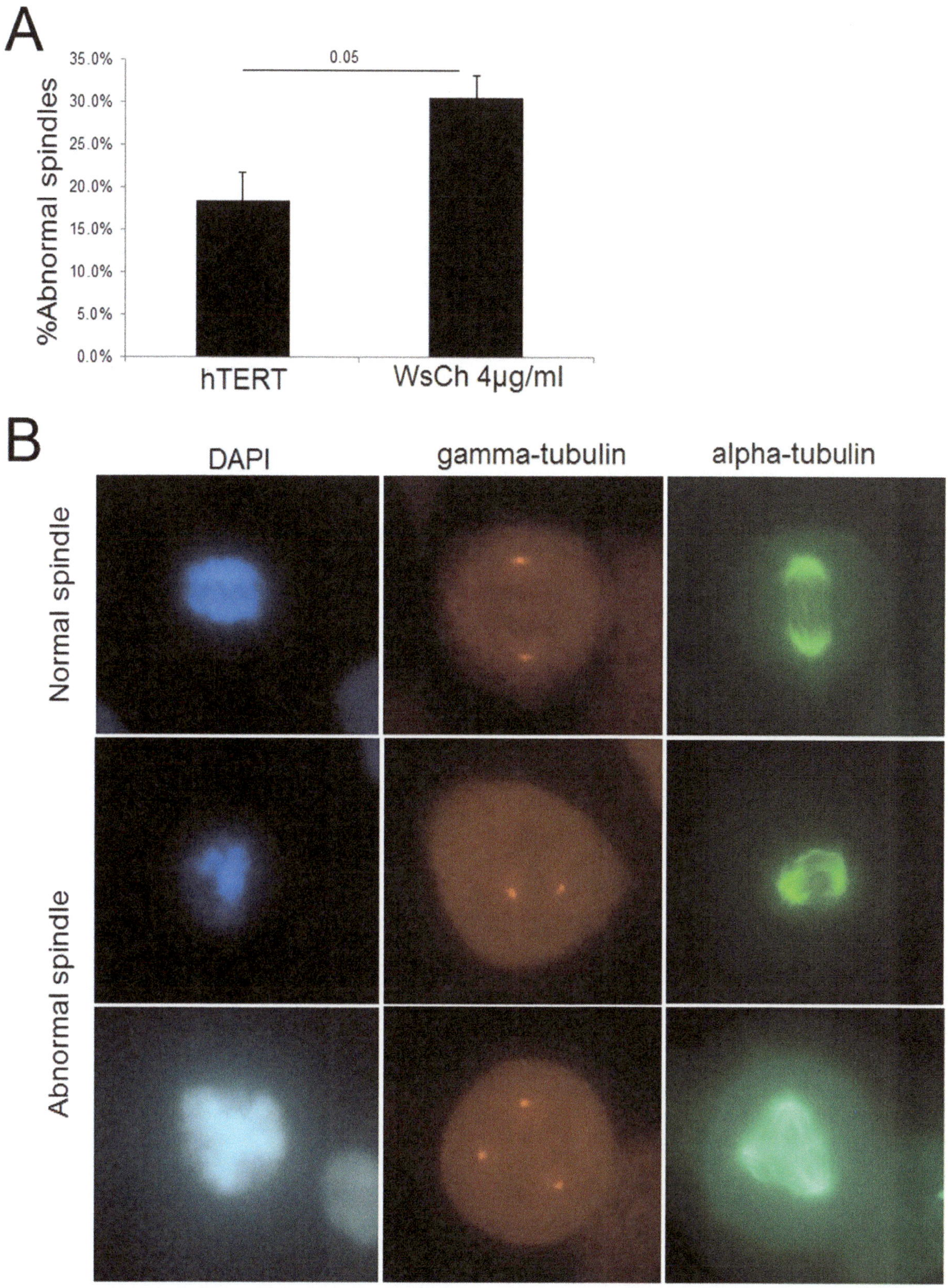

Figure 10. Mitotic spindle structure disrupted by cholesterol. (A) hTERT cells were treated for 24 hr with 4 μg/ml WsCh and the structure of the mitotic spindles observed and analyzed for abnormal DNA localization, lagging chromosomes, super-numerary centrosomes, and dis-arrayed microtubules. There was a significant increase in abnormal mitotic spindle structure induce by cholesterol exposure, with dis-arrayed microtubules and mis-localized DNA being the most prominent defects. (B) Examples of normal spindles in untreated cells and abnormal spindles in cholesterol-treated cells.

Mechanisms by which Aneuploidy may Contribute to Neurodegeneration in AD

There are several ways in which cholesterol (or Aß)-induced aneuploidy may contribute to cognitive decline in AD and related disorders. The most straightforward mechanism would be that aneuploid cells, with their altered genetic complements and thus altered gene expression are inherently prone to apoptosis/degeneration, as has been shown in many experimental systems [21,105–107]. Indeed, as discussed above, the specific loss of (especially of non-trisomy 21) aneuploid neurons accounts for 90% of neurodegeneration in AD [9–23]. When the aneuploid neuronal progenitors and neurons harbor trisomy 21 or 16 and accumulate in the brains of AD patients and FAD transgenic mice respectively, overexpression of *APP* and other chromosome 21/16 genes will occur. That such imbalance may further contribute to disease onset and progression is evident in individuals harboring trisomy 21 mosaicism [25,34–37] or an *APP* gene duplication [32,33]. Similarly, the reduced neurogenesis and reduced neuronal number in Down syndrome [108], may result from the constitutive over expression of *APP* and production of Aß and the consequent induction of the cell cycle defect of chromosome mis-segregation.

Another possibility supported by the data, is that, like Aß, cholesterol disrupts chromosome segregation through inhibition of normal MT function. In addition to inducing defective neurogenesis as we demonstrate above, MT dysfunction could also affect neuronal plasticity. For example, we have found that Aß causes chromosome mis-segregation directly by binding to and inhibiting certain MT-dependent kinesin family motor proteins that are essential for mitotic spindle function [24]. These enzymes are also present in neurons, where they direct plasma neurotransmitter and neutrophin receptor localization and function at the plasma membrane [Ari et al. unpublished data]. As altered cholesterol homeostasis also disrupts microtubule structure and function, it could similarly affect receptor localization.

Finally, the counteracting effect of ethanol on lipid-induced chromosomal instability *in vitro* supports the hypothesis that the chromosome mis-segregation induced by lipoproteins is attributable to the increased membrane rigidity induced by cholesterol. We hypothesize that membrane stiffness upon cholesterol exposure may be restored by the fluidizing action of ethanol, making the cell less prone to mitotic errors. The fluidizing effect of ethanol on cell membranes is well established [83,88,89] and was proposed here as a possible mechanism for the reduction in aneuploidy in the cells co-incubated with cholesterol and alcohol, although no measurements of membrane fluidity were employed. Significantly, Aß peptide also increases membrane rigidity [109]. In the light of these data and the finding of aneuploid cells in AD brain and atherosclerotic plaques discussed above, it is interesting that moderate ethanol consumption has been linked to reduced risk of both CVD and AD [85–87,110]. Prospective studies of microtubule stabilizers and/or ethanol or other modifiers of membrane fluidity may open new approaches to the prevention of neurodegenerative and cardiovascular disease.

Conclusion

In this study we have presented *in vitro* and *in vivo* evidence that cholesterol dyshomeostasis, a common risk factor for NPC-1 and two age-related diseases (i.e., AD and atherosclerosis) may exert its pathogenic effect in part through disruption of the cell cycle. Specifically lipoprotein/cholesterol-induced chromosome instability/mis-segregation may be an underlying cytogenetic trait and part of the pathogenic pathway of multiple disorders, which opens new avenues for research and therapy.

Materials and Methods

Cell Line

hTERT-HME1 cells. The hTERT-HME1 cell line (Clontech) is a primary human mammary epithelial cell line that permanently expresses the telomerase reverse transcriptase and can thus divide indefinitely while retaining normal function, phenotype, and karyotype [111,112]. The cell line was cultured in supplemented Mammary Epithelium Basal Medium (MEBM, Lonza) as described elsewhere [23].

Primary Cells

HASMC. Human Primary Aortic Smooth Muscle Cells (HASMC) were isolated from healthy human aorta and cryopreserved as secondary culture at the density $>5\times10^5$ cells per vial (ScienCell Research Laboratories). The cells were maintained in the Smooth Muscle Cell Medium according to manufacturer's specifications (SMCM; ScienCell Research Laboratories). Cells are subcultured when they were 90% confluent in 2 µg/ml poly-L-lysine (Sigma)-coated cell culture dishes.

Human fibroblasts. LDL receptor-negative human skin fibroblasts harboring two mutations, *C240-F* and *Y160-ter*, which cause a severe form of familial hypercholesterolemia (FH), fibroblasts with functional LDL receptor, four different human fibroblasts harboring *NPC1* mutations and four age-matched controls were obtained from Coriell Cell Repositories and cultured according to their recommended protocol.

Generation and maintenance of mNPCs. Mouse neurosphere cultures and derived neuronal precursor cells were established from non-transgenic prenatal brains (E17–E18) following a modified protocol by [77] and maintained according to [113].

Mouse splenocytes and brain cells. Mouse spleens and brains were harvested and processed to yield a cell suspension and prepared for karyotype and FISH analysis according to procedures previously described [22,23].

Human brain cells. Frozen samples of frontal cortices from patients with the Niemann-Pick type C1 disease (age 20.88±8.64) and age, gender and race matched control brain tissues (age 17.26±11.07) were obtained from the NICHD Brain and Tissue Bank for Developmental Disorders at the University of Maryland (Baltimore, MD). Cell suspensions were prepared as previously described for mouse brains [23] and processed for FISH. Filipin and NeuN co-immunolabeling revealed significantly more cholesterol staining in the intracellular compartment in NPC neurons compared to controls.

Mice, Feeding and Diets

Housing of and procedures involving all animals, including the time-pregnant C57BL/6 mice were approved by the USF Institutional Animal Care and Use Committee.

Wild-type mice. Eight one-month-old nontransgenic C57BL/6 mice (4 males and 4 females) (Jackson Lab) were caged in standard housing in pairs, and were fed *ad libitum* for 12 weeks with either regular chow, or high cholesterol diet (Harlan Laboratories) with free excess to fresh water. Food intake and weight gain were monitored and recorded weekly. The mice were anesthetized with i.p. injection of sodium pentobarbital (50 mg/kg weight), and the tissues harvested and inspected for pathological changes. Mice from dietary intervention were transcardially perfused with 0.9% saline before internal organs of interest were removed.

Diets. Regular mouse chow (2018 Tekland Global 18% Protein Rodent Diet, Harlan Laboratories) contains 5% crude plant-based oil (fat), 0% cholesterol, and supplies 3.3 Kcal/g of Digestible Energy (DE). Custom-made high cholesterol diet (TD.95286, Harlan) consists of 21% milk fat (fat and 0.05% cholesterol), 1% of cholesterol, and provides 4.5 Kcal/g of DE.

APPKO mice. Mice lacking an *APP* gene and their non-transgenic littermates were 3–4 months of age (Jackson Labs) and had C57BL/6 background strain. The spleens were used for primary cell cultures and lipoprotein/cholesterol treatments.

Reagents and Kits

Lipoproteins. Human oxidized LDL (protein concentration 2 mg/ml), human LDL (protein concentration 5 mg/ml) and human HDL (protein concentration 10 mg/ml) were purchased from Biomedical Technologies Inc. Water-Soluble Cholesterol (WsCh) (Sigma; 31.8 mg of pure cholesterol in 0.6 g total weight of solid, balanced in methyl-beta-cyclodextrin) was resuspended in sterile water.

Other reagents, kits and DNA probes. EGTA (Sigma) and BAPTA (Calbiochem) were used as Ca++ buffering reagent at 1.5 mM and 1 mM, respectively. hTERT-HM1 cells are cultured in medium that has 2.65 mM calcium. Absolute (without benzene) ethyl alcohol (Sigma-Aldrich) was prepared as a sterile aqueous 1 M solution and aliquoted. Filipin complex (Sigma) was dissolved in DMSO (Sigma) and stored at −20°C in small aliquots and protected from light. Giemsa stain (Gibco/Invitrogen) was diluted freshly in 1X GURR buffer (GibcoBRL Life Technologies) to stain metaphase chromosomes. Mouse anti-neuronal nuclei (NeuN) AlexaFluor® antibody (Millipore) and VectaShield with DAPI (Vector Laboratories) was used to label neurons and nuclei, respectively. Anti-53BP1 rabbit polyclonal (Abcam) and Alexa-Fluor 488 goat-anti-rabbit antibody (Invitrogen, Molecular Probes) were used to detect DNA double-strand breaks (DSBs) foci, anti-α-tubulin (clone B-5-1-2, Sigma) and AlexaFluor 488 goat-anti-mouse antibodies (Invitrogen) were used to stain mitotic spindles, and anti-γ-tubulin (Sigma) and AlexaFluor 594 goat-anti-rabbit antibodies (Invitrogen) were utilized to detect centrosomes. Nick Translation Kit (Roche) and Spectrum Green or Spectrum Orange dUTPs (Vysis) were used to generate the chromosome 16 BAC probe as previously described [22]. Ethanol Assay Kits (BioVision) and BioTek Synergy HT micro-plate reader (BioTek Instruments) for colorimetric assay (O.D. 570 nm), and Gen5™ (BioTek Instruments) data analysis software were used to measure ethanol concentration in the media at baseline, after 24 and 48 hr of exposure following manufacturer's instructions. Oil-Red-O staining kit (American MasterTech) was used to stain for neutral lipids accumulation in mouse hepatocytes. Fluorescently labeled DNA probes detecting human chromosome 21, 12, and, 18, 14 and 7 (LSI® TEL/AML1 ES Dual Color Translocation Probe, LSI® IGH (14q32)/MALT1(18q21) Dual Color Dual Fusion Probe and LSI® D7S522 (7q31) SpectrumOrange ™/CEP® 7 SpectrumGreen™, respectively) were purchased from Abbott, Vysis.

In Vitro Incubation with Lipoproteins/Cholesterol

Two days prior to treatment/incubation, freshly passaged hTERT cells ($1–3\times10^5$ cells/2 ml) were plated in 100 mm tissue culture dishes in MEBM to assure 60%–70% confluency on the day of the treatment. The cells were then incubated for 48 hr at the concentration of 20 μg/ml of lipoproteins or 2 and 4 μg/ml of WsCh.

Seven parallel experiments were used to assess the effect of lipoproteins on chromosome segregation (i.e., karyotype analysis and chromosome specific aneuploidy) and six separate experiments to test the aneugenic effect of cholesterol. The same cell passages were used for the set of parallel experiments involving Ca++ chelating reagents, BAPTA or EGTA performed as in [23].

Similarly, two days before lipid treatment, freshly passaged HASMC, human fibroblasts with and without a functional LDL receptor or hTERT-HME1 cells were seeded onto pre-coated (2 μg/ml of poly-L-lysine, Sigma) single glass chamber slides (8.6 cm^2 growth surface/well) (BD Bioscience) at the density of 100,000 and 200,000 cells per slide respectively. After 24 or 48 hr of lipid/cholesterol incubation, the cells were rinsed twice with 1X PBS without Ca and Mg (Cellgro), immediately fixed with either cold 3:1 anhydrous methanol and acetic acid fixative or methanol, and incubated at −20°C for 30 min.

Mouse non-transgenic and *APPKO* spleen cells were similarly incubated with lipoproteins for 48 hr, harvested and fixed for FISH analysis as described [22,23].

In Vitro Ethanol and Lipoprotein/Cholesterol Incubation

To assure an exact and consistent ethanol (EtOH) concentration in treated cells, we used a modified closed chamber system protocol by Adickes et al. [114]. Prior to ethanol and lipoproteins co-treatments, several pilot experiments were conducted to examine the viability of hTERT-HME1 cells in the closed chamber, and to establish cytotoxicity of 25 mM and 50 mM of EtOH for 6, 12 and 24 hr on cell morphology, proliferation and survival (Trypan Blue dye exclusion). Based on these results, triplicate experiments were conducted with 25 mM EtOH for 24 hr followed the next day by lipoproteins (20 μg/ml) and WsCh (4 μg/ml) and EtOH co-incubation for 48 hr. A small aliquot of EtOH containing media from two samples was collected at the baseline, 24 and 48 hr to measure alcohol concentration using colorimetric assay (Ethanol Assay Kit, BioVision). Lastly, the cells were harvested and fixed for FISH analysis.

Metaphase Chromosome Analysis

After colcemid treatment, hTERT-HME1 cells were harvested and the metaphase chromosomes counted as described [22,23]. Genus 2.81® software was used for chromosome analysis (Applied Imaging). At least 40–45 metaphases were analyzed per each sample.

Fluorescence in situ Hybridization (FISH)

Prior to hybridization, all slides were aged at room temperature followed by hybridization procedures recommended by Abbott, Vysis and by protocols and mouse and human probes described above and previously [22,23]. Hybridizations were done according to manufacturer's instructions (Abbott, Vysis) for the selected probes in a HyBrite hybridization chamber (Vysis) followed by DAPI II (Abbott, Vysis) or Vectashield with DAPI (Vector Laboratories) counterstain.

FISH Followed by Immunocytochemistry of NPC1 Brain Cells

To assess neuronal versus glial cell aneuploidy in NPC1 and control brains, we used a combination of FISH and immunocytochemistry [23]. Briefly, immediately after FISH, brain cells were incubated in 1XPBS for 10 min, blocked in 10% goat serum/0.1% Triton X-100 PBS solution for 1 hr followed by overnight incubation in conjugated Ms X Neuronal Nuclei AlexaFluor 488 (Millipore) 1:100 antibody prepared in 1% BSA/0.1% Triton X-

100 1XPBS. After final washes in 1XPBS, the cells were stained with DAPI II counterstain.

Immunocytochemical Quantification of Double Strand Breaks

Double strand breaks, an indication of DNA damage were identified in cholesterol-treated hTERT-HME1 cells by immunostaining for 53 BP1-containing foci. First, cell pellets were fixed in 70% cold ethanol, dropped onto Frosted slides (Fisher Scientific) and air-dried. Second, immediately after fixation in 4% paraformaldehyde for 10 min, and three 1XPBS washes, the cells were permeabilized in 0.2% Triton X-100 1XPBS solution for 10 min, blocked in 5% BSA 1XPBS/0.1% Tween-20 for 30 min, and incubated in 1% BSA 1XPBS/0.1% Tween-20 solution containing anti-53 BP1 rabbit polyclonal antibody (Abcam), 1:400 for 1 hr followed by AlexaFluor 488 goat-anti-rabbit antibody (Invitrogen), 1:300 incubation for the same time period. After several 1XPBS washes, the cells were stained with DAPI II (Vector).

Immunocytochemistry for Spindle Analysis

Upon fixation in methanol, cholesterol treated hTERT-HME1 cells were co-immunostained for mitotic spindles and centrosomes with anti-α-tubulin (Sigma) and anti-γ-tubulin antibodies (Sigma) 1:1000, followed by AlexaFluor 488 goat-anti-mouse and AlexaFluor 594 goat-anti-rabbit secondary antibodies (Invitrogen, Molecular Probes), 1:2000 incubation, respectively and Vectashield mounting medium with DAPI staining (Vector) as described [23].

Oil-Red-O Staining

Cell suspension of snap-frozen livers (2 from mice fed a regular and 2 from mice fed a high cholesterol diet) were made in 1XPBS, dropped onto pre-wetted slides, and stained with the Oil-Red-O staining kit following manufacturer's procedures for frozen tissues with slight modifications (American MasterTech). Hematoxylin stained single cells and cell aggregates (blue) were evaluated under phase microscopy (Zeiss Imager M1) for the presence of lipid droplets (red).

Image Acquisition and Analysis

FISH hybridization signals were analyzed according to Abbott/Vysis guidelines as described in [22,23] using a Nikon Eclipse E1000 fluorescence microscope with a 4912 CCIR high performance COHU CCD Camera and Genus 2.81® software (Applied Imaging) or a Zeiss Imager M1 microscope with a CV-M4+CL high resolution camera and Axiovision4.6 software (Zeiss) or a Zeiss Axiovert 135 with AxioCam HRc (Zeiss). The frequencies of nuclei containing 0, 1, 2 or 3 53 BP1 signals were recorded in treated and control cells, and mitotic spindle phenotypes were analyzed as described [22]. On average, between 700 and 1,000 interphases per each sample/treatment were scored for aneuploidy, and 400 NeuN positive and NeuN negative NPC1 brain cells were analyzed for DNA hybridization signals. More than 450–600 cells for each of three samples of both WsCh-treated and control were assessed for 53 BP1 foci, and more than 45–80 spindles from each of four samples of both treated and control cells were analyzed for spindle abnormalities.

Hematoxylin and Oil-Red-O stained mouse hepatocytes and cell aggregates from mice fed a regular and high cholesterol diet were compared and contrasted for amount of red staining under phase microscopy (Zeiss).

Statistical Analysis

Paired Student's T-test was used to compare the aneuploidy induced by various lipoproteins with or without Ca++ chelating reagents and ethanol in different cell lines across multiple experiments and in spleen and brain cells of mice fed different diets, and to compare the percentages of nuclei containing 1 to 3 DSBs foci and the levels of abnormal spindle events between treated and untreated cells. Independent T-test was used to compare the aneuploidy between NPC1 fibroblasts and NPC1 brain cells and appropriate controls. Three to 7 treatments with lipids/cholesterol for each cell line, and triplicate experiments with chelators and ethanol were conducted and scored for aneuploidy. Four to 5 primary NPC1 cells sources and controls and at least 6–12 mice were analyzed for each graph.

Ethics statement. All experiments were carried out in accord with the University of South Florida guidelines for examination of human tissue and the ethical treatment of animals. Because the only human tissues were cell lines and autopsy brain tissue obtained from biorepositories, and we were not provided any identifying information, the experiments are exempt. The animal work was carried out under the USF IACUC oversight and approval (M3785; Promoters and Inhibitors of Alzheimer's Disease Pathology, Colony and R3138 and R3786 (different times); Promoters and Inhibitors of Alzheimer's Disease Pathology, Research).

Supporting Information

Figure S1 25 mM of Ethanol (EtOH) does not induce aneuploidy within 48 hr. hTERT-HME1 cells were treated with 25 mM EtOH for 24 and 48 hr in a closed chamber system. (A) No induction of trisomy 21 (or trisomy 12) was observed, but there was an increase in tetrasomy 21 (presumably cells in G2), within 24 hr (B). After further incubation in EtOH-containing media, levels of such tetrasomy 21 cells returned to background (C–D).

Acknowledgments

The chromosome 16 BAC is a kind gift from Dr. Bruce Lamb. Human tissue was obtained from the NICHD Brain and Tissue Bank for Developmental Disorders at the University of Maryland, Baltimore, MD. The authors thank Dr. Susan Lee for early experiments, Dr. Jaya Padmanabhan for scientific discussions and Michelle Norden for the mice genotyping and assistance with the surgical procedures and mouse dietary study.

Author Contributions

Conceived and designed the experiments: AG HP. Performed the experiments: AG. Analyzed the data: AG HP. Wrote the paper: AG HP.

References

1. Anstey KJ, Lipnicki DM, Low LF (2008) Cholesterol as a risk factor for dementia and cognitive decline: A systematic review of prospective studies with meta-analysis. Am J Geriatr Psychiatry 16: 343–354.
2. Dolan H, Crain B, Troncoso J, Resnik SM, Zonderman AB, et al (2010) Atherosclerosis, dementia, and Alzheimer's disease in the Baltimore Longitudinal Study of Aging Cohort. Ann Neurol 68: 231–240.
3. Steinberg D (2002) Atherogenesis in perspective: Hypercholesterolemia and inflammation as partners in crime. Nat Med 8: 1211–1217.

4. Querfurth HW, LaFerla HW (2010) Alzheimer's disease. N Engl J Med 362: 329–344.
5. Hardy J (2006) Alzheimer's disease: the amyloid cascade hypothesis: an update and reappraisal. J Alzheimers Dis 9: 151–153.
6. Lee VM, Trojanowski JQ (2006) Progress from Alzheimer's tangles to pathological tau points towards more effective therapies now. J Alzheimers Dis 9: 257–262.
7. Potter H, Wisniewski T (2012) Apolipoprotein E: Essential catalyst of the Alzheimer amyloid cascade. Int J Alz Dis 2012 article ID 489428doi:10.1155/2012/489428.
8. Potter H (1991) Review and hypothesis: Alzheimer disease and Down syndrome–chromosome 21nondisjunction may underlie both disorders. Am J Hum Genet 48: 1192–1200.
9. Potter H, Ma J, Das S, Geller LN, Benjamin M, et al. (1995) Beyond ß-protein: New steps in the pathogenic pathway to Alzheimer's disease. In: Iqbal K, J.A. Mortimer JA, Winblad B, Wisniewski HM, editors. Research advances in Alzheimer's disease and related disorders. Hoboken: John Wiley and Sons Ltd. 643–654.
10. Li J, Xu M, Zhou H, Ma J, Potter H (1997) Alzheimer presenilins in the nuclear membrane, interphase kinetochores, and centrosomes suggest a role in chromosome segregation. Cell 90: 917–927.
11. Geller LN, Potter H (1999) Chromosome missegregation and trisomy 21 mosaicism in Alzheimer's disease. Neurobiol Dis 6: 167–179.
12. Migliore L, Testa A, Scarpato R, Pavese N, Petrozzi L, et al. (1997) Spontaneous and induced aneuploidy in peripheral blood lymphocytes of patients with Alzheimer's disease. Hum Genet 101: 299–305.
13. Migliore L, Botto N, Scarpato R, Petrozzi L, Cipriani G, et al. (1999) Preferential occurrence of chromosome 21 malsegregation in peripheral blood lymphocytes of Alzheimer disease patients. Cytogenet Cell Genet 87: 41–46.
14. Trippi F, Botto N, Scarpato R, Petrozzi L, Bonuccelli U, et al. (2001) Spontaneous and induced chromosomal damage in somatic cells of sporadic and familial Alzheimer's disease patients. Mutagenesis 16: 321–327.
15. Migliore L, Boni G, Bernardini R, Trippi F, Colognato R, et al. (2006) Susceptibility to chromosome malsegregation in lymphocytes of women who had a Down syndrome child in young age. Neurobiol Aging 27: 710–716.
16. Živković L, Spremo-Potparević, Djelić N, Bajić V (2006) Analysis of premature centromere division (PCD) of the chromosome18 in peripheral blood lymphocytes in Alzheimer disease patients. Mech Ageing Dev 127: 892–896.
17. Kingsbury MA, Yung YC, Peterson SE, Westra JW, Chun J (2006) Aneuploidy in the normal and diseased brain. Cell Mol Life Sci 63: 2626–2641.
18. Mosch B, Morawski M, Mittag A, Lenz D, Tarnok A, et al. (2007) Aneuploidy and DNA replication in the normal human brain and Alzheimer's disease. J Neurosci 27: 6859–6867.
19. Thomas P, Fenech M (2008) Chromosome 17 and 21 aneuploidy in buccal cells is increased with ageing and in Alzheimer's disease. Mutagenesis 23: 57–65.
20. Iourov IY, Vorsanova SG, Liehr T, Yurov YB (2009) Aneuploidy in the normal, Alzheimer's disease and ataxia-telangiectasia brain: differential expression and pathological meaning. Neurobiol Dis 34: 212–220.
21. Arendt T, Brückner MK, Mosch B, Lösche A (2010) Selective cell death of hyperploids neurons in Alzheimer's disease. Am J Path 177: 15–20.
22. Boeras DI, Granic A, Crespo NC, Rojiani AM, Potter H (2008) Alzheimer's presenilin 1 causes chromosome missegregation and aneuploidy. Neurobiol Aging 29: 3119–3128.
23. Granic A, Padmanabhan J, Norden M, Potter H (2010) Alzheimer Abeta peptide induces chromosome mis-segregation and aneuploidy, including trisomy 21: requirement for tau and APP. Mol Biol Cell 21: 511–520.
24. Borysov SI, Granic A, Padmanabhan J, Walczak CE, Potter H (2011) Alzheimer Aβ disrupts the mitotic spindle and directly inhibits mitotic microtubule motors. Cell Cycle 10: 1–14.
25. Granic A, Potter H (2011) Down syndrome model of Alzheimer's disease: beyond trisomy 21 nondisjunction. In: Dey S, editor. Genetics and etiology of Down syndrome. Rijeka: InTech. 159–176.
26. Migliore L, Coppede F, Fenech M, Thomas P (2011) Association of micronucleus frequency with neurodegenerative diseases. Mutagenesis 26: 85–92.
27. Yurov YB, Vorsanova SG, Iourov IY (2011) The DNA replication stress hypothesis of Alzheimer's disease. Scientific World Journal 11: 2602–2612.
28. Arendt T (2012) Cell cycle activation and aneuploid neurons in Alzheimer's disease. Mol Neurobiol 46: 125–35.
29. Epstein CJ (1990) The consequences of chromosome imbalance. Am J Med Genet Suppl. 7: 31–37.
30. Glenner GG, Wong CW (1984) Alzheimer's disease and Down's syndrome: sharing of a unique cerebrovascular amyloid fibril protein. Biochem Biophys Res Commun 122: 1131–1135.
31. Wisniewski KE, Wisniewski HM, Wen GY (1985) Occurrence of neuropathological changes and dementia of Alzheimer's disease in Down's syndrome. Ann Neurol 17: 278–282.
32. Sleegers K, Brouwers N, Gijselinck I, Theuns J, Goossens D, et al. (2006) APP duplication is sufficient to cause early onset Alzheimer's dementia with cerebral amyloid angiopathy. Brain 129: 2977–2983.
33. Rovelet-Lecrux A, Hannequin D, Raux G, Le Meur N, Laquerrière A, et al (2006) APP locus duplication causes autosomal dominant early-onset Alzheimer disease with cerebral amyloid angiopathy. Nat Genet 38: 11–12.
34. Rowe IF, Ridler MAC, Gibberd FB (1989) Presenile dementia associated with mosaic trisomy 21 in a patient with a Down syndrome child. Lancet 2: 229.
35. Schapiro MB, Kumar A, White B, Grady CL, Friedland RP, et al. (1989) Alzheimer's disease (AD) in mosaic/translocation Down's syndrome (DS) without mental retardation. Neurology 39: 169.
36. Hardy J, Goate A, Owen M, Rossor M (1989) Presenile dementia associated with mosaic trisomy 21 in a patient with a Down syndrome child. Lancet 2: 743.
37. Ringman JM, Rao PN, Lu PH, Cederbaum S (2008) Mosaicism for trisomy 21 in a patient with young-onset dementia: a case report and brief literature review. Arch Neurol 65: 412–415.
38. Sparks DL (1997) Coronary artery disease, hypertension, ApoE, and cholesterol: a link to Alzheimer's disease. Ann N Y Acad Sci 826: 128–146.
39. Burns M, Duff K (2002) Cholesterol in Alzheimer's disease and tauopathy. Ann N Y Acad Sci 977: 367–375.
40. Beach TG, Wilson JR, Sue LI, Newell A, Poston M, et al. (2007). Circle of Willis atherosclerosis: association with Alzheimer's disease, neuritic plaques and neurofibrillary tangles. Acta Neuropathol 113: 13–21.
41. Jones L, Holmans PA, Hamshere ML, Harold D, Moskvina D, et al. (2010) Genetic evidence implicates the immune system and cholesterol metabolism in the aetiology of Alzheimer's disease. PLoS ONE 5: e13950.
42. Wolozin B (2004) Cholesterol and the biology of Alzheimer's disease. Neuron 41: 7–10.
43. Vance J (2012) Dysregulation of cholesterol balance in the brain: contribution to neurodegenerative disease. Dis Model Mech 5: 746–755.
44. Kim J, Basak JM, Holtzman DM (2009) The role of apolipoprotein E in Alzheimer's disease. Neuron 63: 287–303.
45. Benditt EP, Benditt JM (1975) Evidence for a monoclonal origin of human atherosclerotic plaques. Proc Natl Acad Sci U S A 70: 1753–1756.
46. Casalone R, Granata P, Minelli E, Portentoso P, Giudici A, et al. (1991) Cytogenetic analysis reveals clonal proliferation of smooth muscle cells in atherosclerotic plaques. Hum Genet 87: 139–143.
47. Vanni R, Licheri S (1991) Clonal cytogenetic changes in atherosclerotic plaques including trisomy 20. Dis Markers 9: 81–85.
48. Matturri L, Cazzullo A, Turconi P, Lavezzi AM (1997) Cytogenetic aspects of cell proliferation in atherosclerotic plaques. Cardiologia 42: 833–836.
49. Matturri L, Cazzullo A, Turconi P, Lavezzi AM, Vandone PR, et al (2001) Chromosomal alterations in atherosclerotic plaques. Atherosclerosis 154: 755–761.
50. Murry CE, Gipaya CT, Bartosek T, Benditt EP, Schwartz SM (1997) Monoclonality of smooth muscle cells in human atherosclerosis. Am J Pathol 151: 697–705.
51. Andreassi MG, Botto N, Colombo MG, Biagini A, Clerico A (2000) Genetic instability and atherosclerosis: can somatic mutations account for the development of cardiovascular diseases? Environ Mol Mutagen 35: 265–269.
52. Miniati P, Sourvinos G, Michalodimitrakis M, Spandidos DA (2001) Loss of heterozygosity on chromosomes 1, 2, 8, 9 and 17 in cerebral atherosclerotic plaques. Int J Biol Markers16: 167–171.
53. Zhang M, Li J, Chakrabarty P, Bu B, Vincent I (2004) Cyclin-dependent kinase inhibitors attenuate protein hyperphosphorylation, cytoskeletal lesion formation, and motor defects in Niemann-Pick Type C mice. Am J Pathol165: 843–53.
54. Zhang M, Wang X, Jiang F, Wang W, Vincent I, et al. (2010) Mitotic epitopes are incorporated into age-dependent neurofibrillary tangles in Niemann-Pick disease type C. Brain Pathol 20: 367–377.
55. Paigen B, Ishida BY, Verstuyft J, Winters RB, Albee D (1990) Atherosclerosis susceptibility differences among progenitors of recombinant inbred strains of mice. Arteriosclerosis 10: 316–332.
56. Mukherjee S, Maxfield FR (2004) Lipid and cholesterol trafficking in NPC. Bioch Biophys Acta 1685: 28–37.
57. Peake KB, Vance JE (2010) Defective cholesterol trafficking in Niemann-Pick C-deficient cells. FEBS Letters 584: 2731–2739.
58. Zhang JR, Coleman T, Langmade SJ, Scherrer DE, Lane L, et al. (2008) Niemann-Pick C1 protects against atherosclerosis in mice via regulation of macrophage intracellular cholesterol trafficking. J Clin Invest 118: 2281–2290.
59. Vincent I, Rosado M, Davies P (1996) Mitotic mechanisms in Alzheimer's Disease? J Cell Biol 132: 423–425.
60. Arendt T, Rödel L, Gärtner U, Holzer M (1996) Expression of the cyclin-dependent kinase inhibitor p16 in Alzheimer's disease. Neuroreport 7: 3047–3049.
61. Smith TW, Lippa CF (1995) TI Ki-67 immunoreactivity in Alzheimer's disease and other neurodegenerative disorders. J Neuropathol Exp Neurol 54: 297–303.
62. Nagy Z, Esiri MM, Cato AM, Smith AD (1997) Cell cycle markers in the hippocampus in Alzheimer's disease. Acta Neuropathol 94: 6–15.
63. Yang Y, Varvel NH, Lamb BT, Herrup K (2006) Ectopic cell cycle events link human Alzheimer's disease and amyloid precursor protein transgenic mouse models. J Neurosci 26: 775–784.
64. Lopes JP, Blurton-Jones M, Yamasaki TR, Agostinho P, LaFerla FM (2009) Activation of cell cycle proteins in transgenic mice in response to neuronal loss but not amyloid-beta and tau pathology. J Alzheimers Dis16: 541–549.
65. Varvel NH, Bhaskar K, Patil AR, Pimplikar SW, Herrup K, et al. (2008) Abeta oligomers induce neuronal cell cycle events in Alzheimer's disease. J Neurosci 28: 10786–10793.

66. Herz J, Bock HH (2002) Lipoprotein receptors in the nervous system. Annu Rev Biochem 71: 405–434.
67. Marzolo MP, Bu G (2009) Lipoprotein receptors and cholesterol in APP trafficking and proteolytic processing, implications for Alzheimer's disease. Semin. Cell Dev Biol 20: 191–200.
68. Abisambra JF, Fiorelli T, Padmanabhan J, Neame P, Wefes I, et al. (2010) LDLR expression and localization are altered in mouse and human cell culture models of Alzheimer's disease. PLoS ONE 5: e8556.
69. Leigh SE, Foster AH, Whittall RA, Hubbart CS, Humphries SE (2008) Update and analysis of the University College London low density lipoprotein receptor familial hypercholesterolemia database. Ann Hum Genet 72: 485–498.
70. Lorenzo A, Yuan M, Zhang Z, Paganetti PA, Sturchler-Pierrat C, et al. (2000) Amyloid beta interacts with the amyloid precursor protein: a potential toxic mechanism in Alzheimer's disease. Nat Neurosci 3: 460–464.
71. Shaked GM, Kummer MP, Lu DC, Galvan V, Bredesen DE, et al. (2006) Abeta induces cell death by direct interaction with its cognate extracellular domain on APP (APP 597–624). FASEB J 20: 1254–1256.
72. Bloch K (1991) Cholesterol: evolution of structure and function. In: Vance DE, Vance JE, editors. Biochemistry of lipids, lipoproteins and membranes. Amsterdam: Elsevier. 363–381.
73. Brown DA, London E (2000) Structure and function of sphingolipid and cholesterol-rich membrane rafts. J Biol Chem 275: 17221–17224.
74. Simons K, Toomre D (2000) Lipid rafts and signal transduction. Nat Rev Mol Cell Biol 1: 31–39.
75. Christian AE, Haynes MP, Phillips MC, Rothblat GH (1997) Use of cyclodextrins for manipulating cellular cholesterol content. J Lipid Res 38: 2264–2272.
76. Härtel S, Diehl HA, Ojeda F (1998) Methyl-beta-cyclodextrins and liposomes as water-soluble carriers for cholesterol incorporation into membranes and its evaluation by a microenzymatic fluorescence assay and membrane fluidity-sensitive dyes. Annal Biochem 258: 277–284.
77. Pacey L, Stead S, Gleave JA, Tomczyk K, Doering L (2006) Neural stem cell culture: neurosphere generation, microscopical analysis and cryopreservation. Protocol Exchange doi:10.1038/nprot.2006.215. Available: http://www.nature.com/protocolexchange/protocols/77. Accessed 8 October 2010.
78. Yang AH, Kausal D, Rehen SK, Kriedt K, Kingsbury MA, et al (2003) Chromosome segregation defects contribute to aneuploidy in normal neural progenitor cells. J Neurosci 23: 10454–10462.
79. Yurov YB, Iourov IY, Vorsanova SG, Liehr T, Kolotii AD, et al (2007) Aneuploidy and confined chromosomal mosaicism in the developing human brain. PloS ONE 2: e558.
80. Peterson SE, Westra JW, Paczkowski CM, Chun J (2008) Chromosomal mosaicism in neural stem cells. Methods Mol Biol 438: 197–204.
81. Demel RA, De Kruyff B (1976) The function of sterols in membranes. Biochim Biophys Acta 457: 109–132.
82. Abramov AY, Ionov M, Pavlov E, Duchen MR (2011) Membrane cholesterol content plays a key role in the neurotoxicity of β-amyloid: implications for Alzheimer's disease. Aging Cell 10: 595–603.
83. Bae MK, Jeong DK, Park NS, Lee CH, Cho BH, et al. (2005) The effect of ethanol on physical properties of neuronal membranes. Mol Cell 19: 356–364.
84. Badea MG, Sima A, Jinga VV, Hörer O (1989) The interaction between human low density lipoproteins and bovine aortic endothelial cells. Measurements of membrane fluidity. Physiologie 26: 95–100.
85. Rimm EB, Williams P, Fosher K, Criqui M, Stampfer MJ (1999) Moderate alcohol intake and lower risk of coronary heart disease: meta-analysis of effects on lipids and haemostatic factors. BMJ 319: 1523–1528.
86. Di Castelnuovo A, Costanzo S, Donati MB, Iacoviello L, de Gaetano G (2010) Prevention of cardiovascular risk by moderate alcohol consumption: epidemiologic evidence and plausible mechanisms. Intern Emerg Med 5: 291–297.
87. Luchsinger JA, Tang MX, Siddiqui M, Shea S, Mayeux R (2004) Alcohol intake and risk of dementia. J Am Geriatr Soc 52: 540–546.
88. Guizzetti M, Chen J, Oram JF, Tsuji R, Dao K, et al. (2007) Ethanol induces cholesterol efflux and up-regulates ATP-binding cassette cholesterol transporters in fetal astrocytes. J Biol Chem 282: 18740–18749.
89. Schroeder F, Morrison WJ, Gorka C, Wood WG (1988) Transbilayer effects of ethanol on fluidity of brain membrane leaflets. Biochim Biophys Acta 946: 85–94.
90. Dashti N, Franklin FA, Abrahamson DR (1996) Effect of ethanol on the synthesis and secretion of apoA-I and apoB-containing lipoproteins in HepG2 cells. J Lipid Res 37: 810–824.
91. Woods NK, Padmanabhan J (2012) Neuronal calcium signaling and Alzheimer's disease. In: Islam S, editor. Calcium signaling Adv Exp Med Biol. New York: SpringerLink. 1193–1217.
92. Duesberg P, Li R (2003) Multistep carcinogenesis: a chain reaction of aneuploidization. Cell Cycle 2: 202–210.
93. Horn S, Barnard S, Rothkamm K (2011) Gamma-H2AX-based dose estimation for whole and partial body radiation exposure. PLoS ONE 6: e25113.
94. King RW. (2008) When 2+2 = 5: the origins and fates of aneuploid and tetraploid cells. Biochim Biophys Acta 1786: 4–14.
95. Rehen SK, McConnell MJ, Kaushal D, Kingsbury MA, Yang AH, et al. (2001) Chromosomal variation in neurons of the developing and adult mammalian nervous system. Proc Natl Acad Sci U S A 98: 13361–13366.
96. Westra JW, Barral S, Chun J (2009) A reevaluation of tetraploidy in the Alzheimer's disease brain. Neurodegener Dis 6: 221–229.
97. Rossi G, Dalprà L, Crosti F, Lissoni S, Sciacca FL, et al (2008) A new function of microtubule-associated protein tau: involvement in chromosome stability. Cell Cycle 15: 1788–1794.
98. Clarke MC, Littlewood TD, Figg N, Maguire JJ, Davenport AP, et al. (2008) Chronic apoptosis of vascular smooth muscle cells accelerates atherosclerosis and promotes calcification and medial degeneration. Circ Res 102: 1529–1538.
99. Honig LS, Kukull W, Mayeux T (2005) Atherosclerosis and AD: analysis of data from the US National Alzheimer's Coordinating Center. Neurology 64: 494–500.
100. Solomon A, Kivipelto M, Wolozin B, Zhou J, Whitmer RA (2008) Midlife serum cholesterol and increased risk of Alzheimer's and vascular dementia three decades later. Dement. Geriatr Cogn Disord 28: 75–80.
101. Roses AD (1996) Apolipoprotein E alleles as risk factor in Alzheimer's disease. Annu Rev Med 47: 387–400.
102. Mahley RW (1988) Apolipoprotein E: Cholesterol transport protein with expending role in cell biology. Science 240: 622–630.
103. Bennet AM, Di Angelantonio E, Ye Z, Wensley F, Dahlin A, et al (2007) Association of apolipoprotein E genotypes with lipid levels and coronary risk. JAMA 298: 1300–1311.
104. Li L, Cao D, Garber DW, Kim H, Fukuchi K (2003) Association of aortic atherosclerosis with cerebral beta-amyloidosis and learning deficits in a mouse model of Alzheimer's disease. Am J Pathol 163: 2155–2164.
105. Busciglio J, Yankner BA (1997) Apoptosis and increased generation of reactive oxygen species in Down's syndrome neurons in vitro. Nature 378: 776–779.
106. McConnell MJ, Kaushal D, Yang AH, Kingsbury MA, Rehen SK, et al (2004) Failed clearance of aneuploid embryonic neural progenitor cells leads to excess aneuploidy in the Atm-deficient but not the Trp53-deficient adult cerebral cortex. J Neurosci 24: 8090–8096.
107. Kai Y, Wang CC, Kishigami S, Kazuki Y, Abe S, et al (2009) Enhanced apoptosis during early neuronal differentiation in mouse ES cells with autosomal imbalance. Cell Res 19: 247–258.
108. Guidi S, Bonasoni P, Ceccarelli C, Santini D, Gualtieri F, et al. (2008) Neurogenesis impairment and increased cell death reduce total neuron number in the hippocampal region of fetuses with Down syndrome. Brain Pathol 18: 180–197.
109. Eckert GP, Wood WG, Mullere WE (2005) Membrane disordering effects of beta-amyloid peptides. Subcell Biochem 38: 319–337.
110. Brust JC (2010) Ethanol and cognition: indirect effects, neurotoxicity and neuroprotection: a review. Int. J. Environ. Res. Public Health 7: 1540–1557.
111. Jiang XR, Jimenez G, Chang E, Frolkis M, Kusler B, et al. (1999) Telomere expression in human somatic cells does not induce change associated with transformend phenotype. Nat Genet 21: 111–114.
112. Morales CP, Holt SE, Quellette M, Kaur KJ, et al. (1999) Absence of cancer-associated changes in human fibroblasts immortalized with telomerase. Nat Genet 21: 115–118.
113. Marchenko S, Flanagan L (2007) Passing human neuronal stem cells. J Vis Exp7: e263, doi:10.3791/263. Available: http://www.jove.com/video/263/passaging-human-neural-stem-cells. Accessed 12 October 2010.
114. Adickes ED, Mollner TJ, Lockwood SK (1988) Closed chamber system for delivery of ethanol to cell culture. Alcohol 23: 377–381.

An Examination of the Relationship between Hotspots and Recombination Associated with Chromosome 21 Nondisjunction

Tiffany Renee Oliver[1,2*⁹], Candace D. Middlebrooks[1⁹], Stuart W. Tinker[1], Emily Graves Allen[1], Lora J. H. Bean[1], Ferdouse Begum[3], Eleanor Feingold[3,4], Reshmi Chowdhury[4], Vivian Cheung[5,6], Stephanie L. Sherman[1]

1 Department of Human Genetics, Emory University School of Medicine, Atlanta, Georgia, United States of America, 2 Department of Biology, Spelman College, Atlanta, Georgia, United States of America, 3 Department of Biostatistics, Graduate School of Public Health, University of Pittsburgh, Pittsburgh, Pennsylvania, United States of America, 4 Department of Human Genetics, Graduate School of Public Health University of Pittsburgh, Pittsburgh, Pennsylvania, United States of America, 5 Howard Hughes Medical Institute, University of Michigan, Ann Arbor, Michigan, United States of America, 6 Department of Human Genetics, University of Michigan, Ann Arbor, Michigan, United States of America

Abstract

Trisomy 21, resulting in Down Syndrome (DS), is the most common autosomal trisomy among live-born infants and is caused mainly by nondisjunction of chromosome 21 within oocytes. Risk factors for nondisjunction depend on the parental origin and type of meiotic error. For errors in the oocyte, increased maternal age and altered patterns of recombination are highly associated with nondisjunction. Studies of normal meiotic events in humans have shown that recombination clusters in regions referred to as hotspots. In addition, GC content, CpG fraction, Poly(A)/Poly(T) fraction and gene density have been found to be significant predictors of the placement of sex-averaged recombination in the human genome. These observations led us to ask whether the altered patterns of recombination associated with maternal nondisjunction of chromosome 21 could be explained by differences in the relationship between recombination placement and recombination-related genomic features (i.e., GC content, CpG fraction, Poly(A)/Poly(T) fraction or gene density) on 21q or differential hot-spot usage along the nondisjoined chromosome 21. We found several significant associations between our genomic features of interest and recombination, interestingly, these results were not consistent among recombination types (single and double proximal or distal events). We also found statistically significant relationships between the frequency of hotspots and the distribution of recombination along nondisjoined chromosomes. Collectively, these findings suggest that factors that affect the accessibility of a specific chromosome region to recombination may be altered in at least a proportion of oocytes with MI and MII errors.

Editor: Beth A. Sullivan, Duke University, United States of America

Funding: This work was supported by R01 HD38979, R01 HL083300 and UL1TR000454. The funders had no role in study design, data collection and analysis, decision to publish, or preparation of the manuscript.

Competing Interests: The authors have declared that no competing interests exist.

* E-mail: Toliver4@spelman.edu

⁹ These authors contributed equally to this work.

Introduction

Trisomy 21, leading to Down Syndrome (DS), is the most common autosomal trisomy among live-born infants, occurring in approximately 1 in 700 live-births, and is caused mainly by the failure of chromosome 21 to properly segregate during oogenesis [1]. Increased maternal age and altered number and location of recombination events have been found to be associated with maternal meiotic errors involving chromosome 21 [2,3]. Specifically, the absence of recombination [4] or the presence of a single recombinant event near the telomere of 21q [2] are associated with maternal meiosis I (MI) errors and these associations appear to be independent of the age of the oocyte (i.e., maternal age at the time of birth of the infant with trisomy 21) [5]. Meiosis II (MII) errors appear to be driven by different age and recombination traits: MII errors are associated with the placement of a recombinant event near the centromere of 21q [2] and this association increases with increasing age of the oocyte [5].

Studies of normal meiotic events in humans show that the placement of recombination is not a random event. Rather, both cis and trans-acting factors have been found to be associated with the placement of recombination. Specifically, GC content, CpG fraction and Poly(A)/Poly(T) fraction have each been found to be significant predictors of placement of sex-averaged recombination events in the human genome [6]. In addition, sequence variation in the zinc-finger domain of the gene *Proline Rich Domain Containing 9* (PRDM9) has a major impact on the location of recombination in humans [7,8,9,10]. Specifically, allelic differences in the zinc finger binding domain of *PRDM9* explain approximately 80% of the heritable variation in "hotspot usage" " (i.e. the frequency in which recombination occurs within linkage disequilibrium (LD) or "historically"-defined hotspots) [8,11,12]. The observation that both cis and trans-acting factors are associated with the placement of recombination led us to question whether the altered patterns of recombination associated with nondisjunction of chromosome 21 could be explained by differences in the relationship between recombination and genomic features (i.e., GC content, CpG fraction, Poly(A)/Poly(T) fraction or gene density) on 21q or differential hot-spot usage. This paper presents the first analyses of the relationship between recombination rate and the quantity of genomic features or LD-defined hotspots specifically along chromosome 21 in oocytes with a normal meiotic outcome, a MI nondisjunction error or a MII nondisjunction error.

Materials and Methods

Ethics Statement

The work presented in this publication was approved by the Emory Univeristy Institutional Review Board. All participants in provided written consent which indicated that the individual (1) agreed for study personnel to proceed with the interview and (2) consented for biological specimens to be obtained from them and their child. All information obtained during participant interviews and related to sample collection were catalogued electronically and de-identified.

Trisomic Population

Families with an infant with full trisomy 21 were recruited through a multisite study of risk factors associated with chromosome mal-segregation [2,13,14]. Parents and the infant donated a biological sample (either blood or buccal) from which DNA was extracted. Only families in which DNA was available from both biological parents and the child with trisomy 21 were included, leading to a total of 297 maternal MI and 277 maternal MII cases of trisomy 21 (Table 1).

Trisomic Population Genotyping and Quality Control

Samples were genotyped at 1536 SNP loci on 21q by the Center for Inherited Disease Research using the Illumina Golden Gate Assay. The most centromeric SNP was rs2259403 (13,615,252 bp) and the most telomeric was rs7116 (46,909,248 bp). The average number of SNPs per 500 kb bin was 25.56 with a standard deviation of 25.91 with over 70% of cases exhibiting a recombinant having recombination breakpoints smaller than 1 Mb. Mendelian inconsistencies and sample mix-ups were identified using RelCheck among the trios. In addition, parental genotyping data were used to identify poorly performing SNPs.

Table 1. Population Sample Sizes.

Meiotic Outcome Group and Recombination Type	Number of samples
MI Single	222
MI Proximal	75
MI Distal	75
MII Single	202
MII Proximal	75
MII Distal	75
Normal Single	1272
Normal Proximal	342
Normal Distal	342

SNPs that met the following criteria were excluded from our analyses: minor allele frequency (MAF) <0.01, deviation from Hardy Weinberg Equilibrium (HWE) ($p<0.01$), heterozygosity > 0.60 or > 10% missingness. We also excluded SNPs on a family-by-family basis if >50% of the genotype data for a proband had low intensity levels. As it relates to our exclusion of SNPs with a heterozygosity rate of >0.60, while we understand that is a very conservative/stringent cutoff, we did indeed examine the distribution of cases by stage and origin upon changing the heterozygosity rate and we did not see any significant changes in stage (data not shown). In addition, for a significant majority of our cases, stage and origin had been previously determined using STR data and compared to what was identified with our SNP only data.

Determining Stage and Origin of Meiotic Chromosome Mal-Segregation

Individuals with trisomy 21 have three copies of chromosome 21 and thus display three alleles for each SNP genotyped on chromosome 21. In instances where trisomy 21 is caused by a maternal meiotic error, for each SNP examined, one of these alleles is inherited from dad, while the other two are inherited from mom. Maternal meiotic errors were confirmed upon determining that trisomic offspring inherited two alleles from mom and one from dad for SNPs genotyped on chromosome 21. Only cases of maternal origin were included in our analyses. Once the maternal origin of the meiotic error was established, markers located in the pericentromeric region (13,615,252 bp – 16,784,299 bp) of 21q were used to infer the stage of the meiotic error, MI or MII. If maternal heterozygosity was retained in the trisomic offspring, we concluded a MI error. If maternal heterozygosity was reduced to homozygosity, we concluded a MII error. In this assay, we cannot distinguish between the different types of underlying errors that might lead to an MII error. For example, sister chromatids that fail to separate during anaphase of MII or an error that is initiated in MI and not resolved properly in MII both lead to the contribution of sister chromatids to the gamete. Also, if sister chromatids prematurely separate in MI, some configurations will lead to both sister chromatids segregating to the same pole in MII. Lastly, when all informative markers in the parent of origin were reduced to homozygosity, the origin of nondisjunction was inferred to be a post-zygotic, mitotic error and excluded from the study.

Identifying the Location of Recombination – Trisomic Samples

After genotyping quality control measures were implemented and SNP data were combined with STR data from our previous studies [3], we defined the location of recombinant events. The breakpoints of a single recombinant event were defined by a minimum of either one STR or eight consecutive, informative SNPs flanking the recombination breakpoint. An exception to this rule occurred when the most proximal or most distal informative markers on 21q indicated the presence of recombinant event. In these instances, a minimum of either one STR or four consecutive, informative SNPs were required to define the breakpoints of recombination. The presence of a double recombinant event was defined by a minimum of either one STR or 8 consecutive, informative SNPs flanking the recombination breakpoint on each side for both events.

Euploid Population

SNP genotyping data for normally segregating chromosomes 21 were taken from families recruited for 1) the Autism Genetic Research Exchange (AGRE) (N = 743) [15], 2) the Framingham

Heart Study (FHS) (N = 764) [16] and 3) the GENEVA Dental Caries Study (N = 107) [17] (Table 1). All families were two-generation families with a minimum of three children. This was necessary to define specific recombination profiles for each parent child transmission.

Euploid Population Genotyping and Quality Control

The AGRE samples were genotyped for SNPs genome-wide using the Infinium(R) HumanHap550-Duo BeadChip. The AGRE data included genotypes at 520,017 markers genome-wide, however 11,473 markers were excluded from the analysis due to deviation HWE ($p<10^{-7}$). After quality control measures were completed, there was genotype information for 7,810 SNPs on 21q for the AGRE dataset. The FHS samples were genotyped for SNPs genome-wide using the Genome-Wide Human SNP Array 5.0. The FHS data included genotypes at 500,568 markers. However, 22,000 markers were excluded from the analysis due to deviation from HWE ($p<10^{-7}$). After quality control measures were completed, there was genotype information for 6,705 SNPs on 21q for the FHS dataset. The GENEVA samples were genotyped using the Illumina 610-Quad Array. The GENEVA dataset included genotypes at 620,901 SNPs. 58,610 markers were excluded from the analysis due to deviation from HWE ($p<10^{-5}$), a MAF < 0.02. After quality control measures were completed, there was genotype information for 8,189 SNPs on 21q from the GENEVA population. All SNP locations were based on human NCBI Build 36 (hg18).

Identifying the Location of Recombination – Euploid Samples

For the AGRE, FHS and GENEVA datasets, genotype data from members of two-generation families with three or more children were used to infer the location of recombination along the maternal chromosome 21. Our approach and software are described in Chowdhury et al. [18]. Briefly, parental genotypes were used to identify informative markers. Then, using these markers, genotypes of the children were compared to identify alleles inherited identical-by-descent from the mothers and fathers. Between two sibs, a switch from sharing the same maternal allele to not sharing was scored as a maternal recombination event.

Examining the Relationship Between Genomic Features and Recombination

We used linear regression models to assess the relationship between the quantity of recombination and the quantity of each variable of interest found within regions across 21q. We divided 21q into 500 kb bins and calculated the quantity of each variable within a bin. We chose this bin size based on our level of refinement of recombination break-points. For the genomic features, we quantified the amount of each bin occupied by each genomic feature of interest, GC content, CpG content, Poly(A)/Poly(T) content were calculated as the proportion of each bin occupied by each feature however the number of genes per bin was calculated for gene density. Data on genomic features were based on the hg18 build of the human genome and retrieved from the following tables within the USCS Genome Browser: gc5Base, CpGIslandExt and rmsk (repeat master), UniGene_3 and RefGene. As for hotspots, we used the number of LD-defined hotspots, as defined by Myers et. al.[19] per bin as the predictor variable (Figure S1). The outcome variable was defined as the proportion of all chromosome 21 single or double recombinant events that occurred within the bin. As it is well known that single recombination events cluster in the telomeric and centromeric regions of 21q for the MI and MII error groups (Fig. 1), respectively, we included bin location as a variable in our models as it may be a confounding variable. We stratified analyses by chromosomes with single and double recombinant events (Figs. 2 and 3, Table 1) as mechanisms of chromosome 21 nondisjunction may differ based on the number of recombinant events on 21q[2,3,5,14]. Univariate linear regression was then used to determine whether there was significant correlation between the quantity of each predictor variable and the proportion of recombination within a bin ($p\leq0.05$).

General linear regression models were used to test for differences in the slopes of the regression models between comparison groups (MI or MII versus Controls) for each predictor. That is, to compare MI error to normal meiotic outcomes, we included the interaction term of comparison group by genomic feature within a bin. This type of model was also used to compare MII errors with controls. Once again, we included bin location as a covariate for the reason stated above.

Results

Association between genomic features along chromosome 21q and the proportion of recombination events

We first examined meiotic events with one detectable recombinant event on 21q (Table 2). In regression models that included both the specific genomic feature (i.e., GC content, CpG fraction, Poly(A)/Poly(T) fraction or gene density) and the location of the bin along 21q, only location, was found to be a significant predictor of the amount of recombination for the vast majority of features. This is consistent with previous work that has established altered placement of recombination as a significant risk factor for chromosome 21 nondisjunction [2,3]. There was one exception to this pattern: among the MII errors with a single recombinant, both location and GC content were significant predictors of the amount of recombination. This suggests that among MII single recombinant events, where the increased risk is associated with a pericentromeric recombinant, there may be a preference for recombination to occur in regions with elevated GC content and close to the centromere.

We then looked at meiotic events with two detectable recombinants and separated the analyses by the proximal and distal event. For proximal recombinant events (Table 3), GC and CpG content as well as bin location were found to be positively correlated with recombination among MI and MII errors; no association for these features was found among normal meiotic control recombinant events of this type (Table 3). Poly(A)/Poly(T) fraction was found to be inversely correlated with the amount of recombination among MI and MII errors and normal outcomes. Collectively these observations suggest that MI and MII proximal recombinant events occur in GC rich regions more often than statistically expected if there was no relationship between the

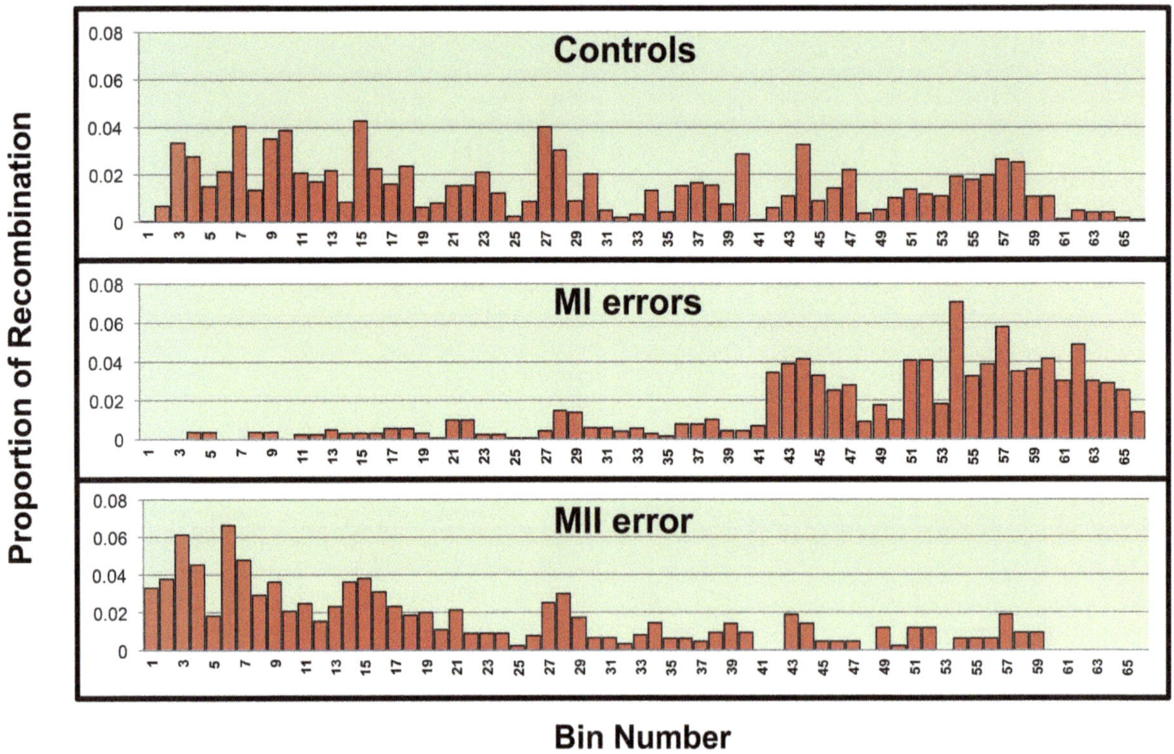

Figure 1. The distribution of single recombination events across the long arm of 21q by population. 21q was divided into 66 500 kb bins and the proportion of recombination in each bin from chromosomes with only one recombinant event is depicted above.

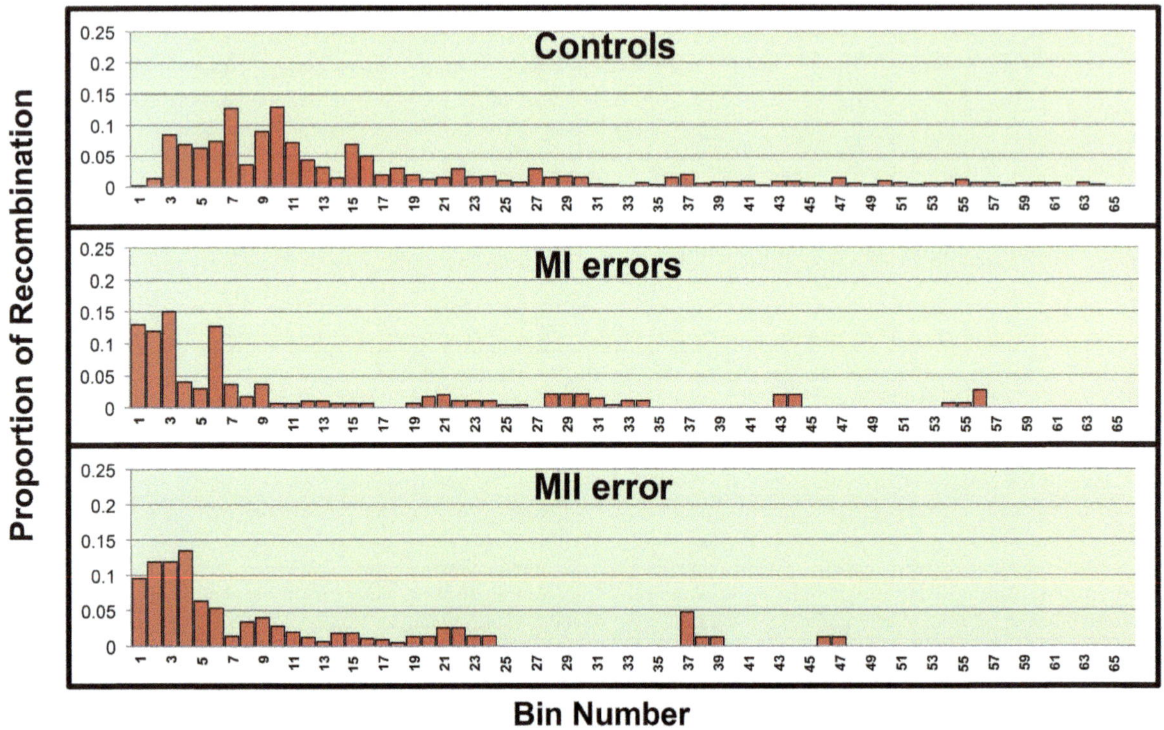

Figure 2. The distribution of the proximal recombinant of a double recombinant event across the long arm of 21q by population. 21q was divided into 66 500 kb bins and the distribution of recombination in each bin from the proximal recombinant event of chromosomes displaying two recombinant events is depicted above.

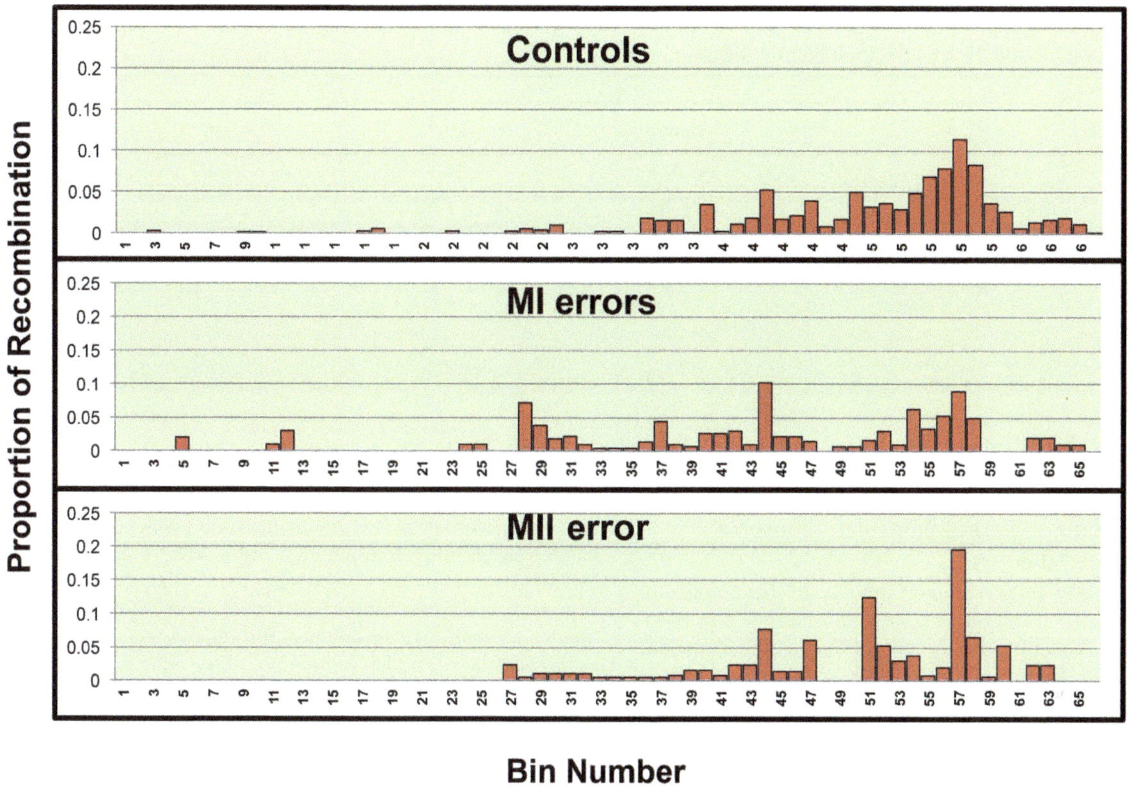

Figure 3. The distribution of the distal recombinant of a double recombinant event across the long arm of 21q by population. 21q was divided into 66 500 kb bins and the distribution of recombination in each bin from the distal recombinant event of chromosomes displaying two recombinant events is depicted above.

amount of recombination and GC (or CpG) content. We did not find any associations between genomic features and recombination among our MI and MII distal recombination events (Table 4).

Hotspot usage among normally disjoined chromosome 21 events

We examined LD-defined hotspots first among normally disjoining chromosomes (controls). We looked separately at those with one recombinant event and those with two recombinant events. Among those with one detectable event, we found a significant positive association between the number of hotspots per bin and the proportion of recombination per bin ($p<.0001$) (Table 5). Similarly, among those with two detectable events, we found that the proportion of proximal and distal recombinant events within a bin was significantly associated with LD-defined hotspots density ($p=0.001$ and $<.0001$, respectively, Table 5). Thus, as expected, the amount of recombination per bin is positively correlated with historical hotspot density suggesting that historical hotspots are used for recombination along normally segregating chromosomes 21.

Table 2. Values of slopes/beta coefficients for GC, CpG, PolyAT and gene denisty for single recombinants stratified by meiotic outcome group.

Predictor Variable	Controls	MI	MII
GC	−0.0108	0.0377	**0.0856***
21q location	−0.0002	0.0006*	−0.0008*
CpG	−0.145	−0.3102	0.161
21q location	−0.0002	0.0008*	−0.0006*
Poly(A)/Poly(T)	−0.0354	−0.1311	−0.4959
21q location	−0.0002*	0.0006*	−0.0007*
Gene Density	−0.0005	−0.0041	0.0044
21q location	−0.0002*	0.0007*	−0.0006*

Beta values for each genomic feature adjusted for bin variable. Beta coefficients/slopes that are significantly different from zero are marked with an asterisk ($p<0.05$)*.

Table 3. Values of slopes/beta coefficients for GC, CpG, PolyAT and gene density for the proximal recombinant of a double recombinant event stratified by meiotic outcome group.

Predictor Variable	Controls	MI	MII
GC	0.167	0.366*	0.477*
21q location	−0.001*	−0.002*	−0.002*
CpG	0.36	0.891*	1.099*
21q location	−0.001	−0.001*	−0.001*
Poly(A)/Poly(T)	−1.739*	−3.237*	−3.612*
21q location	−0.001*	−0.001*	−0.002*
adjusted Gene Density	0.0137	0.019	0.005
21q location	−0.001*	−0.001*	−0.001*

Beta values for each genomic feature adjusted by bin variable. Beta coefficients/slopes that are significantly different from zero are marked with an asterisk ($p<0.05$)*.

Hotspot usage among nondisjoined chromosome 21events due to MI errors

We first examined single recombinants along 21q. Similar to normally segregating chromosomes, we found hotspot density to be a positively correlated with the proportion of recombination within a bin ($p=0.0006$, Table 5). In order to determine whether the strength of the relationship between recombination and hotspot density differed between control and MI single recombinant events, we next tested whether the strength of the association between the proportion of recombination and hotspot density among MI errors significantly differed from that of controls and found no evidence for different patterns (Fig. 4A, $p=0.43$).

Among nondisjoining chromosomes with two detectable recombinants we separated analyses by the proximal and distal event. We did not detect a significant relationship between hotspot density and the proportion of recombination per bin for proximal recombinants (fig. 5A, table 5). For distal recombinant events, we found that recombination was significantly associated with LD-defined hotspot density (Table 5, $p=0.02$), however for the patterns of association did not differ between MI and controls (Fig. 6A, $p=0.21$).

Hotspot usage among nondisjoined chromosome 21events due to MII errors

As for MII, we detected a significant positive correlation between hotspot density and the proportion of recombination across 21q for single recombinants. The association patterns differed significantly from that of controls (Fig. 4B, $p=0.01$), with MII single recombinant events being less correlated with hotspot density than controls. Among MII errors with two recombinant events, as with MI errors, we did not detect a significant correlation between the proportion of recombination per bin and the density of LD-defined hotspots in the proximal region (fig 5B, table 5). For MII distal events, there was a significant positive association between LD-defined hotspot density and the proportion of recombination per bin (Table 5, $p=0.02$). The association patterns did not differ significantly between MII versus control events (Fig. 6B, $p=0.69$).

Discussion

Association between genomic features along chromosome 21 and the proportion of recombination events along 21q

In our analysis of the relationships between our genomic features of interest and the proportion of recombination per bin, we found several genomic features to be associated with recombination, although these results were not consistent among recombination types (single, double proximal or distal event). Based on the lack of patterns, we were unable to draw any significant conclusions. We do note that our large sample of normal maternal meiotic events ($n=1,272$) for 21q did not show many of the relationships found in the study of Kong et al.[20].

Table 4. Values of slopes/beta coefficients for GC, CpG, Poly(A)/Poly(T) and gene density for the distal recombinant of a double recombinant event stratified by meiotic outcome group.

Predictor Variable	Controls	MI	MII
GC	−0.039	−0.098	0.037
21q location	0.001*	0.001*	0.001*
CpG	−0.705*	−0.573	−0.558
21q location	0.001*	0.001*	0.001*
Poly(A)/Poly(T)	−0.215	0.195	−0.794
21q location	0.001*	0.0004*	0.001*
Gene Density	0.002	0.001	−0.008
21q location	0.001*	0.0004*	0.001*

Beta values for each genomic feature adjusted by bin variable. Beta coefficients/slopes that are significantly different from zero are marked with an asterisk*.

Table 5. Beta coefficient/slope values for hotspots variable adjusted by bin variable and stratified by meiotic outcome group and number of recombinants on chr21.

Recombination Type	Predictor Variable	Controls	MI	MII
Single Recombination	Hotspot count	0.002*	0.002*	0.001*
	Bin location	−0.0002*	0.0007*	−0.0006*
Double Recombination -Proximal	Hotspot count	0.003*	−0.0005	0.0002
	Bin location	−0.001*	−0.0009	−0.001
Double Recombination - Distal	Hotspot count	0.0034*	0.002*	0.0028*
	Bin location	0.0007*	0.0004*	0.0007*

Beta coefficients/slopes that are significantly different from zero are marked with an asterisk*.

We attribute this to a difference in the study design, not to the sample size, as both studies had comparable numbers of meiotic events. First, we restricted our analysis to 21q, whereas the original associations were found through the analysis of the entire genome. Second, the Kong et al. study the sex-averaged associations based on 628 paternal and 629 maternal meiotic outcomes; we only examined maternal recombination events. Taken together, a study of sex-specific, chromosome-specific associations of genomic features and recombination may provide further insights into the control of recombination.

Hotspot usage among nondisjoined chromosome 21 events

Our findings with regard to LD-defined historical hotspots differ between our meiotic outcomes groups and provide some insight into recombination-associated nondisjunction. First, we gain confidence that our analyses are able to identify associations with hotspot usage, as our findings from normally disjoining chromosomes 21 are consistent with expectation. That is, using our sample of normal meiotic events, our statistical analysis showed the expected pattern of increased recombination in the LD-defined hotspots for single events and double recombinant events on 21q. As it relates to MI errors, our analysis of single recombinants indicated an association of recombination with the distribution of LD-defined hotspots along 21q, similar to controls, suggesting that these events occur preferentially near or within LD-defined hotspots. This is interesting as our previous studies have shown that the average location of MI single recombinant events is approximately 10 Mb closer to the telomere of 21q than normal single recombinant events [21]. As a result, it does not appear that the altered patterns of recombination associated with MI errors can be explained by differential hotspot usage.

We found different patterns of association for MII single recombinant events compared with those for MI-single recombinants events and controls. Specifically, we found that the proportion of single recombinants across 21q per bin is significantly correlated with LD-defined hotspots; however, this association is not as strong as it is in controls. From our most

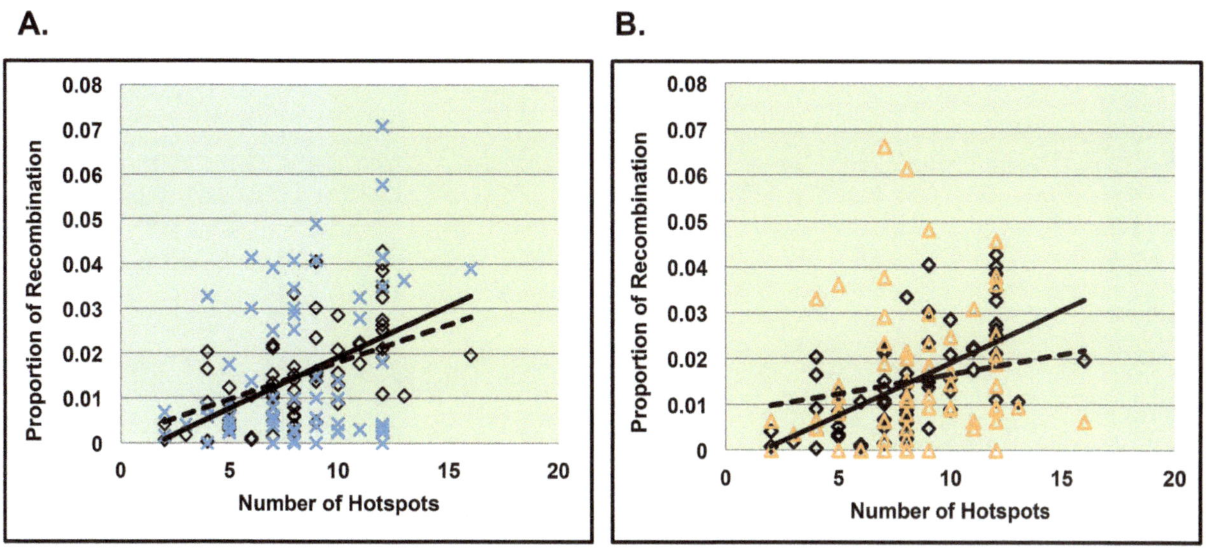

Figure 4. Comparison of the relationship between hotspot usage between MI and MII cases and Controls. Figure 4A and 4B represent MI and MII cases respectively with only one recombinant event on 21q. The solid line represents the relationship between the number of hotspots per bin and the proportion of recombination per bin along normally segregating chromosomes 21. The dotted line represents the relationship between the number of hotspots per bin and the proportion of recombination per bin along chromosomes 21 from MI errors (figure 4A) and MII errors (figure 4B).

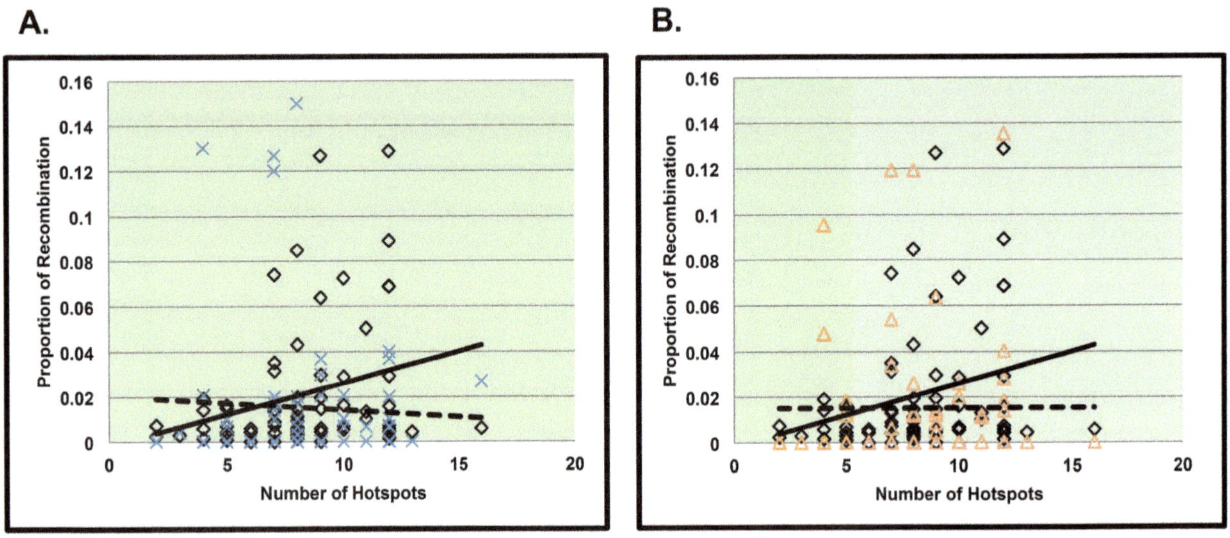

Figure 5. Comparison of slopes between MI or MII errors and controls for the proximal recombinant of double recombinant events. Figures 5A and 5B represent data from the proximal recombinant event of chromosomes displaying two recombinant events on 21q. The solid line represents the relationship between the number of hotspots per bin and the proportion of recombination per bin along normally segregating chromosomes 21. The dotted line represents the relationship between the number of hotspots per bin and the proportion of recombination per bin along chromosomes 21 from MI errors (figure 5A) and MII errors (figure 5B).

recent work, recombination along 21q among MII errors is more proximally located: average location 22.60 Mb on 21q compared with 27.53 Mb on 21q among normal events [21]. Potentially factors characteristic of pericentromeric DNA such as chromatin structure or epigenetic modifications may affect the accessibility of a specific chromosome region to recombination in at least a proportion of oocytes with meiotic errors.

In our analysis of double recombinants events, we found similar results with respect LD-defined hotspots among MI and MII errors. We detected a significant relationship between LD-defined hotspots for the distal recombinant events among doubles, but not the proximal events. Furthermore, the lack of evidence for an association in the proximal region differed from that in controls where an association was detected (i.e., significant interaction). Oliver et al. [21]. found that the unusual pericentromeric proximal

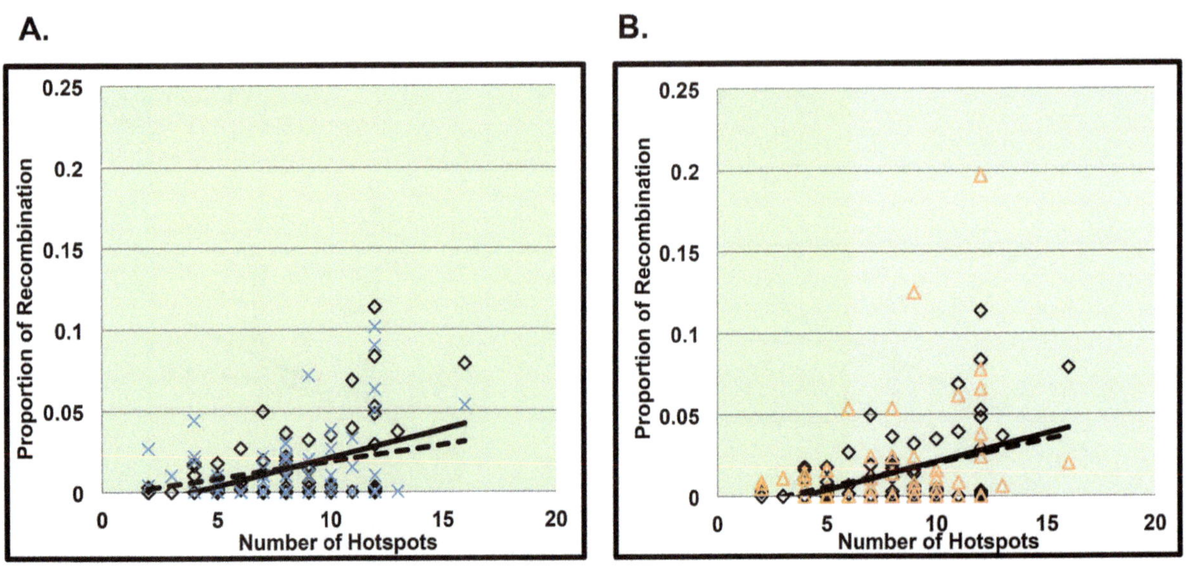

Figure 6. Comparison of slopes between MI or MII errors and controls for the distal recombinant of double recombinant events. Figures 6A and 6B represent data from the distal recombinant event of chromosomes displaying two recombinant events on 21q. The solid line represents the relationship between the number of hotspots per bin and the proportion of recombination per bin along normally segregating chromosomes 21. The dotted line represents the relationship between the number of hotspots per bin and the proportion of recombination per bin along chromosomes 21 from MI errors (figure 6A) and MII errors (figure 6B).

events imposed a risk for MII nondisjunction and were associated with increased maternal age, but this pattern was not found among MI errors. Further work is needed to synthesize these results with those based on location of the events along nondisjoined chromosomes 21.

We do not provide consistent evidence that genomic features present at the site of recombination or differential hotspot usage are implicated in the nondisjunction of chromosome 21. However, altered patterns of recombination on 21q have long-been identified to be associated with an increased risk for chromosome 21 nondisjunction. Thus we believe that either the absence or altered physical placement of recombination may be more important as it relates to the risk for chromosome 21 nondisjunction. Moving forward we plan to take a genome-wide approach in efforts to identify genetic factors implicated in the altered patterns of recombination associated with chromosome 21 nondisjunction.

Supporting Information

Figure S1 Distribution of Hotspots along 21q. Hotspot counts for each of the 66 bins across 21q.

Acknowledgments

We would like to thank our lab personnel, recruiters and the families that participated in this study. We would also like to thank Dr. Mary Marazita [M.M] for contributing data on the location of recombination along properly segregating chromosomes. This data was derived from the GENEVA dental caries study.

Author Contributions

Conceived and designed the experiments: TO SS CM EF LB. Performed the experiments: TO CM. Analyzed the data: TO CM SS EF LB EGA ST. Contributed reagents/materials/analysis tools: VC FB RC SS. Wrote the paper: TO CM EF SS VC.

References

1. Sherman SL, Allen EG, Bean LH, Freeman SB (2007) Epidemiology of Down syndrome. Ment Retard Dev Disabil Res Rev 13: 221–227.
2. Lamb NE, Feingold E, Savage A, Avramopoulos D, Freeman S, et al. (1997) Characterization of susceptible chiasma configurations that increase the risk for maternal nondisjunction of chromosome 21. Hum Mol Genet 6: 1391–1399.
3. Oliver TR, Feingold E, Yu K, Cheung V, Tinker S, et al. (2008) New insights into human nondisjunction of chromosome 21 in oocytes. PLoS Genet 4: e1000033.
4. Warren AC, Chakravarti A, Wong C, Slaugenhaupt SA, Halloran SL, et al. (1987) Evidence for reduced recombination on the nondisjoined chromosomes 21 in Down syndrome. Science 237: 652–654.
5. Oliver TR, Tinker SW, Allen EG, Hollis N, Locke AE, et al. (2011) Altered patterns of multiple recombinant events are associated with nondisjunction of chromosome 21. Hum Genet.
6. Holmquist GP, Ashley T (2006) Chromosome organization and chromatin modification: influence on genome function and evolution. Cytogenet Genome Res 114: 96–125.
7. Berg IL, Neumann R, Lam KW, Sarbajna S, Odenthal-Hesse L, et al. (2010) PRDM9 variation strongly influences recombination hot-spot activity and meiotic instability in humans. Nat Genet.
8. Hinch AG, Tandon A, Patterson N, Song Y, Rohland N, et al. (2011) The landscape of recombination in African Americans. Nature 476: 170–175.
9. Berg IL, Neumann R, Sarbajna S, Odenthal-Hesse L, Butler NJ, et al. (2011) Variants of the protein PRDM9 differentially regulate a set of human meiotic recombination hotspots highly active in African populations. Proc Natl Acad Sci U S A 108: 12378–12383.
10. Kong A, Thorleifsson G, Gudbjartsson DF, Masson G, Sigurdsson A, et al. (2010) Fine-scale recombination rate differences between sexes, populations and individuals. Nature 467: 1099–1103.
11. Baudat F, Buard J, Grey C, Fledel-Alon A, Ober C, et al. (2010) PRDM9 is a major determinant of meiotic recombination hotspots in humans and mice. Science 327: 836-840.
12. Fledel-Alon A, Leffler EM, Guan Y, Stephens M, Coop G, et al. (2011) Variation in human recombination rates and its genetic determinants. PLoS One 6: e20321.
13. Freeman SB, Allen EG, Oxford-Wright CL, Tinker SW, Druschel C, et al. (2007) The National Down Syndrome Project: design and implementation. Public Health Rep 122: 62–72.
14. Lamb NE, Freeman SB, Savage-Austin A, Pettay D, Taft L, et al. (1996) Susceptible chiasmate configurations of chromosome 21 predispose to non-disjunction in both maternal meiosis I and meiosis II. Nat Genet 14: 400–405.
15. Weiss LA, Shen Y, Korn JM, Arking DE, Miller DT, et al. (2008) Association between microdeletion and microduplication at 16p11.2 and autism. N Engl J Med 358: 667–675.
16. Dawber TR, Meadors GF, Moore FE Jr (1951) Epidemiological approaches to heart disease: the Framingham Study. Am J Public Health Nations Health 41: 279–281.
17. Polk DE, Weyant RJ, Crout RJ, McNeil DW, Tarter RE, et al. (2008) Study protocol of the Center for Oral Health Research in Appalachia (COHRA) etiology study. BMC Oral Health 8: 18.
18. Chowdhury R, Bois PR, Feingold E, Sherman SL, Cheung VG (2009) Genetic analysis of variation in human meiotic recombination. PLoS Genet 5: e1000648.
19. Myers S, Bottolo L, Freeman C, McVean G, Donnelly P (2005) A fine-scale map of recombination rates and hotspots across the human genome. Science 310: 321–324.
20. Kong A, Gudbjartsson DF, Sainz J, Jonsdottir GM, Gudjonsson SA, et al. (2002) A high-resolution recombination map of the human genome. Nat Genet 31: 241–247.
21. Oliver TR, Tinker SW, Allen EG, Hollis N, Locke AE, et al. Altered patterns of multiple recombinant events are associated with nondisjunction of chromosome 21. Hum Genet.

12

Non-Invasive Epigenetic Detection of Fetal Trisomy 21 in First Trimester Maternal Plasma

Ji Hyae Lim[1], Shin Young Kim[1], So Yeon Park[1], Shin Yeong Lee[1], Mi Jin Kim[1], You Jung Han[2], Si Won Lee[2], Jin Hoon Chung[2], Moon Young Kim[2], Jae Hyug Yang[2], Hyun Mee Ryu[1,2]*

1 Laboratory of Medical Genetics, Medical Research Institute, Cheil General Hospital and Women's Healthcare Center, Seoul, Korea, **2** Department of Obstetrics and Gynecology, Cheil General Hospital and Women's Healthcare Center, KwanDong University college of Medicine, Seoul, Korea

Abstract

Background: Down syndrome (DS) is the most common known aneuploidy, caused by an extra copy of all or part of chromosome 21. Fetal-specific epigenetic markers have been investigated for non-invasive prenatal detection of fetal DS. The phosphodiesterases gene, *PDE9A*, located on chromosome 21q22.3, is completely methylated in blood (*M-PDE9A*) and unmethylated in the placenta (*U-PDE9A*). Therefore, we estimated the accuracy of non-invasive fetal DS detection during the first trimester of pregnancy using this tissue-specific epigenetic characteristic of *PDE9A*.

Methodology/Principal Findings: A nested, case-control study was conducted using maternal plasma samples collected from 108 pregnant women carrying 18 DS and 90 normal fetuses (each case was matched with 5 controls according to gestational weeks at blood sampling). All pregnancies were singletons at or before 12 weeks of gestation between October 2008 and May 2009. The maternal plasma levels of *M-PDE9A* and *U-PDE9A* were measured by quantitative methylation-specific polymerase chain reaction. *M-PDE9A* and *U-PDE9A* levels were obtained in all samples and did not differ between male and female fetuses. *M-PDE9A* levels did not differ between the DS cases and controls (1854.3 *vs* 2004.5 copies/mL; $P = 0.928$). *U-PDE9A* levels were significantly elevated in women with DS fetuses compared with controls (356.8 *vs* 194.7 copies/mL, $P < 0.001$). The sensitivities of *U-PDE9A* level and the unmethylation index of *PDE9A* for non-invasive fetal DS detection were 77.8% and 83.3%, respectively, with a 5% false-positive rate. In the risk assessment for fetal DS, the adjusted odds ratios of *U-PDE9A* level and UI were 46.2 [95% confidence interval: 7.8–151.6] and 63.7 [95% confidence interval: 23.2–206.7], respectively.

Conclusions: Our findings suggest that *U-PDE9A* level and the unmethylation index of *PDE9A* may be useful biomarkers for non-invasive fetal DS detection during the first trimester of pregnancy, regardless of fetal gender.

Editor: Qamaruddin Nizami, Aga Khan University, Pakistan

Funding: This study was supported by a research grant from the Life Insurance Philanthropy Foundation. The funders had no role in study design, data collection and analysis, decision to publish, or preparation of the manuscript.

Competing Interests: The authors have declared that no competing interests exist.

* E-mail: hmryu@yahoo.com

Introduction

Prenatal testing is an integral component of obstetric practice. Detection of chromosomal aneuploidy has been considered the most common and important aspect of prenatal testing. Aneuploidy refers to changes in the numbers of chromosomes present inside a cell, and phenotypic effects are caused by an increased or decreased gene dosage as a result of gaining or losing a particular chromosome. The most common aneuploidy is trisomy 21, refered to as Down syndrome (DS), which occurs in 1 in 800 live births worldwide and is caused by an extra copy of all or part of chromosome 21 [1]. DS is associated with intellectual impairment, severe learning difficulties, and mortality caused by long-term health problems such as heart disease [1]. The incidence of fetal DS increases in a maternal age-dependent manner [1,2].

Worldwide, millions of pregnant women undergo prenatal testing including screening tests and invasive diagnostic procedures for fetal DS detection every year. The current screening protocol for fetal DS involves a blood test for maternal protein biomarkers associated with DS (maternal serum alpha fetoprotein, unconjugated estriol, human chorionic gonadotrophin, and inhibin-A) as well as fetal ultrasound evaluations of nuchal translucency. However, the detection rate for each factor ranges from 25% to 68% with false-positive rate of 5% [3,4]. Therefore, multiple screening tests are usually performed to increase the detection rate for fetal DS at 11–12 weeks and 16–18 weeks of gestation. However, such integrated tests have disadvantages such as increased cost due to the use of multiple biomarkers and psychological burden on the patient as they wait to obtain results in the second trimester (16–18 weeks of gestation). Moreover, 5% of normal pregnant women with false-positive results undergo unnecessary invasive diagnostic processes such as amniocentesis or chorionic villus sampling (CVS) for fetal DS detection. Such invasive diagnostic tests are expensive, require expert technicians, and carry a risk of miscarriage of approximately 1% [5,6]. Therefore, non-invasive prenatal test that allow for the direct analysis of fetal genetic material in maternal blood have been investigated as alternative methods to reduce the need for invasive procedures and to improve the efficacy of current screening tests for fetal DS.

Cyclic nucleotide phosphodiesterases (PDEs) catalyze the hydrolysis of cyclic adenosine 30,50-monophosphate (cAMP) and/or cyclic guanosine 30,50-monophosphate (cGMP) [7]. The human *PDE9A* gene, located on chromosome 21q22.3, encodes a cGMP-specific PDE that is expressed in most tissues, but not in blood [8,9]. Due to its location and contribution to the regulation of the steady-state cellular concentrations of cyclic nucleotides, *PDE9A* is a possible candidate gene for diseases such as bipolar affective disorder [9], and Guipponi *et al.* suggested that its overexpression might be involved in DS [9]. Recently, Chim *et al.* performed a systematic search for fetal-specific epigenetic markers on chromosome 21 [10], during which they found that the *PED9A* region is completely methylated in the maternal blood (*M-PED9A*) and unmethylated in fetal (placental) tissues (*U-PED9A*). Therefore, they reported that this marker was independent of fetal gender and genotype, and hence could be applied to all fetal-maternal pairs for non-invasive detection of fetal sequences on chromosome 21. However, the usefulness of *PED9A* in the non-invasive prenatal detection of fetal DS has not yet been clinically validated.

The aim of this study was to estimate the accuracy of non-invasive fetal DS detection using tissue specific-methylation in *PDE9A* and to evaluate the potential of *PDE9A* as a new biomarker for the first trimester detection of fetal DS.

Materials and Methods

Ethics statement

This study was conducted according to the principles expressed in the Declaration of Helsinki. Appropriate institutional review board approval was obtained from the Ethics Committee at Cheil General Hospital for this study (#CGH-IRB-2008-43). Written informed consent was obtained from each participant before blood draws for the collection of samples and subsequent analysis.

Study participants and samples

We performed a nested case-control study of women who enrolled in the Cheil General Hospital Non-invasive Prenatal Diagnosis Study (CNPD). Participants in the CNPD were recruited from 2008 for non-invasive prenatal diagnosis of rare and incurable fetal diseases. Participants were women who received prenatal care at Cheil General Hospital. For the current study, 108 women were selected from a larger sample of 793 women enrolled in the CNPD according to criteria described below. All pregnancies were singletons at or before 12 weeks of gestation between October 2008 and May 2009.

The case group consisted of 18 women who were subsequently detected to be carrying a DS fetus by amniocentesis or CVS for fetal karyotyping. Each case was paired with five controls that were matched according to gestational week at blood sampling (Table S1). The control group ($n = 90$) included women who delivered healthy normal neonates at term (37 weeks of gestation or more) without medical or obstetric complications, such as hypertension, diabetes, renal insufficiency, congenital anomalies, or fetal demise. Before maternal blood sampling, ultrasonography was recommended to establish the viability of each singleton pregnancy and to confirm gestational age calculated from the time of last menstruation. Maternal, fetal, and infant records were collected prospectively and maintained in an electronic database. None of the participants had histories of preexisting hypertension, diabetes mellitus, liver disease, or chronic kidney disease.

Isolation of Plasma and DNA

Ten milliliters of peripheral blood were collected from each participant into ethylenediaminetetraacetic acid (EDTA) tubes. Immediately after sampling, maternal peripheral blood samples were centrifuged at 1,600 g for 10 minutes at 4°C and the plasma portion was recentrifuged at 16,000 g for 10 minutes to minimize any additional release of maternal DNA. Circulating fetal DNA was extracted from 1.5 mL of maternal plasma using the QIAamp DSP Virus Kit (Qiagen, Hilden, Germany), according to the manufacturer's recommendations. Each DNA sample was eluted into 50 μL of sterile, DNase-free water. The samples were coded for subsequent blinded analysis.

Quantitative methylation-specific polymerase chain reaction (qMSP)

Differences in methylation of *PDE9A* in maternal blood cells and placenta were confirmed by bisulphite genomic sequencing (Fig. 1, Methods S1). Levels of *M-PDE9A* and *U-PDE9A* in maternal plasma were measured by qMSP assays as previously described [10,11].

DNA extracted from plasma was bisulphite-converted using the EZ DNA Methylation Kit (Zymo Research, Orange, CA, USA) and then eluted into 30 μL. For the validation of bisulphite conversion, a synthetic DNA oligonucleotide for the *U-PDE9A* region and genomic DNA extracted from peripheral blood cells were used as positive and negative controls, respectively. The PCR reaction solution contained 12.5 μL iQ Supermix (Bio-Rad, Hercules, CA, USA), 200 nM hydrolysis probe (Applied Biosystems, Foster City, CA, USA), 400 nM primers (Applied Biosystems, Foster City, CA, USA), and 5 μL converted DNA per 25 μL total reaction volume. The primers and hydrolysis probes used for qMSP assay were as follows; for *M-PDE9A*, forward primer: 5′-CGG TGA GTG CGC GTC GC-3′, reverse primer: 5′-CCA ACC ATC CCG AAA AAG CG-3′, and probe: 5′-TTC GGT GAC GTT ACG CGG T-3′, for *U-PDE9A*, forward primer: 5′- GGT TTG TTT TGG TGA GTG TGT GTC GT-3′, reverse primer: 5′- CCC AAC CAT CCC AAA AAA GCA-3′, and probe: 5′-TTT GTT TGG TGA TGT TAT GTG GTT T-3′. The probes for *M-PDE9A* and *U-PDE9A* were dual-labeled with 6-carboxyfluorescein (FAM) and minor groove-binding non-fluorescent quencher (MGBNFQ). The thermal profile consisted of an initial denaturation step of 95°C for 10 minutes followed by 50 cycles of 95°C for 15 seconds, 60°C for 30 seconds, and 72°C for 30 seconds. Calibration curves were prepared for each assay by serial dilutions of single-stranded synthetic DNA oligonucleotides specific to the *M-PDE9A* and *U-PDE9A* amplicons. The sequences of the synthetic DNA were as follows; for *M-PDE9A*: 5′-CGG TGA GTG CGC GTT GCG GGT TTT GTT CGG TGA CGT TAC GCG GTT TTT TCG TTT TTT CGG GAT GGT TGG-3′, for *U-PDE9A*: 5′-GGT TTG TTT TGG TGA GTG TGT GTT GTG GGT TTT GTT TGG TGA TGT TAT GTG GTT TTT TTG TTT TTT TGG GAT GGT TGG G-3′.

Levels were calculated as copies/mL as previously described [12]. Strict precautions were taken to prevent contamination, and multiple negative-control water blanks were included in every analysis. To reduce inter-experimental variation, each extraction was repeated in triplicate. The final data reflect the means of the results (Table S2 and S3). All samples were analyzed blindly.

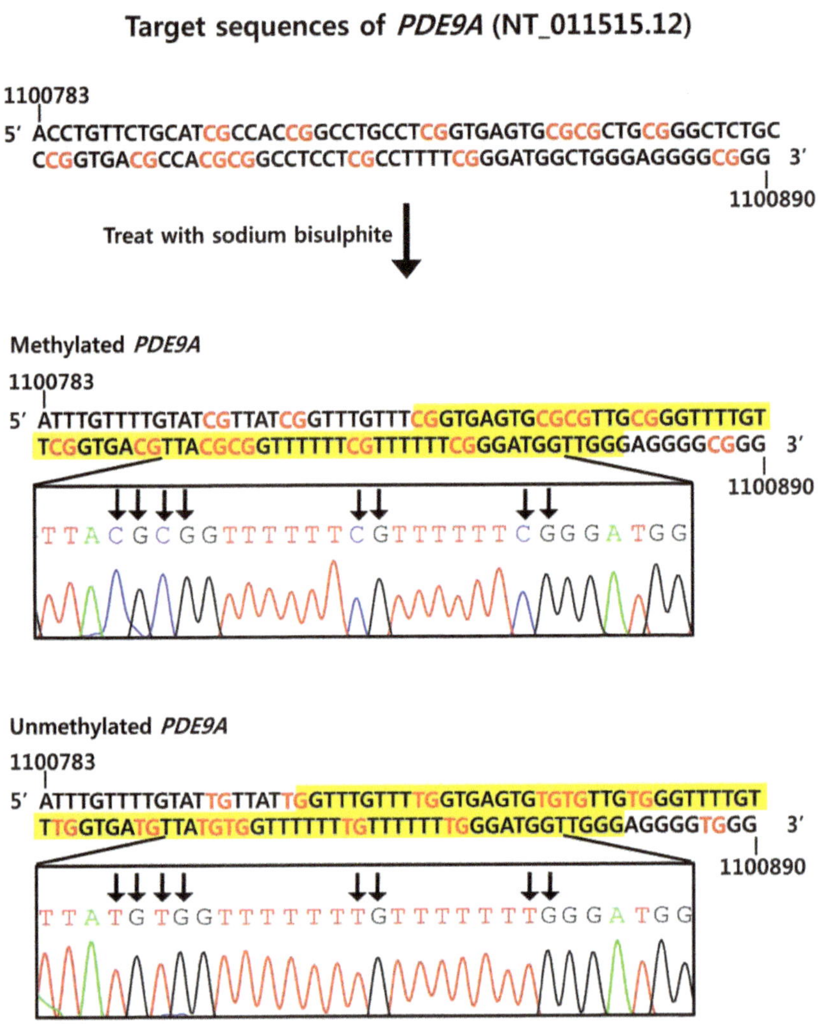

Figure 1. Bisulfite genomic sequencing of *PDE9A*. The red characters in the sequences indicate methylation CpG sites of the *PDE9A* gene. Methylated CpG sites of *PDE9A* were detected in maternal blood cells and placental tissues. Unmethylated CpG sites of *PDE9A* were detected only in placental tissues. Yellow boxes indicate the regions that were amplified by the methylation-specific polymerase chain reaction.

Statistical Analysis

The clinical characteristics of the study population were compared between cases and controls using the Mann-Whitney U test and the χ^2 test. The accuracy for detecting fetal DS was analyzed with factors such as *U-PDE9A* level and unmethylation index (UI). The UI is calculated as {*U-PDE9A* level/(*M-PDE9A* level+*U-PDE9A* level)}X100. The accuracy of fetal DS detection was determined with the fetal karyotyping results. Receiver operating characteristics (ROC) curve analysis was performed to assess the optimal cutoff value as described in our previous study [13]. The optimal cutoff was set at a 5% false-positive rate for comparisons with the accuracy of current screening test for fetal DS. The sensitivity, positive predictive value (PPV), negative predictive value (NPV), and odds ratio (OR) were calculated with 95% confidence intervals (CIs) using the EpiMax Table Calculator (http://www.healthstrategy.com/epiperl/epiperl.htm). Overall accuracy was estimated according to the area under the ROC curve (AUC). Multiple logistic regression analysis was used to estimate the values of *U-PDE9A* levels and UI as risk factors for fetal DS, controlling for potential confounding factors. Potential confounding factors included maternal age, body mass index, and nulliparity at the time of blood sampling. Adjusted ORs (adjORs) and their 95% CIs were calculated. In all tests, thresholds of $P<0.05$ were set for statistical significance. Statistical analyses were performed using the Statistical Package for Social Sciences 12.0 (SPSS Inc., Chicago, IL, USA).

Results

The clinical characteristics are given in Table 1. At blood sampling, maternal age, gravidity, and body mass index did not significantly differ between the cases and controls ($P>0.05$ for all). The median gestational age was 7.5 weeks in both case and control groups. Forty-four percent of participants in the case group and 41% of participants in the control group were nulliparous; this difference between cases and controls was not significant ($P=0.799$). Fetal gender-ratio and tobacco use also were not different between the two groups ($P>0.05$ for both).

In the analysis of *M-PDE9A* and *U-PDE9A* levels according to fetal gender, median levels of *M-PDE9A* were 1956.0 (interquartile range: 1592.5–2411.2) and 2023.1 (interquartile range: 1650.0–2310.3) copies/mL in male and female fetus-bearing participants,

Table 1. Clinical characteristics in cases and controls.

Characteristics	Case (N = 18)	Control (N = 90)	*P* value
At blood sampling			
Maternal age (years)	36.1 (31.3–38.0)	31.1 (29.1–34.8)	0.059 [a]
Gestational age (weeks)	7.5 (6.0–9.0)	7.5 (6.0–9.0)	0.999 [a]
Body mass index (kg/m^2)	22.2 (20.6–24.0)	21.4 (19.3–23.3)	0.180 [a]
Nulliparity	8 (44.4)	37 (41.1)	0.799 [b]
Gravidity	2.0 (1.0–3.3)	2.0 (2.0–3.0)	0.331 [a]
Gender-ratio of fetus (male:female)	7:11	44:46	0.606 [b]
Tobacco use	1 (5.6)	6 (6.7)	0.999 [b]

Values are median (interquartile range) or number (%).
a: Mann-Whitney U test, b: χ^2 test.

respectively. Levels of *U-PDE9A* were 213.6 (interquartile range: 155.1–308.4) and 209.6 (interquartile range: 156.3–283.5) copies/mL in male and female fetus-bearing participants, respectively. Levels of *M-PDE9A* and *U-PDE9A* were not significantly different between fetal genders (P>0.05 for all, Fig. 2). In the analysis of *M-PDE9A* and *U-PDE9A* levels according to fetal karyotype, levels of *M-PDE9A* were not different between the DS cases and controls [1854.3 (interquartile range: 1653.3–2446.3) *vs* 2004.5 (interquartile range: 1605.2–2316.9)copies/mL, P= 0.928, Fig. 3]. However, levels of *U-PDE9A* were significantly higher in the cases compared to controls [356.8 (interquartile range: 314.8–437.4) *vs* 194.7 (interquartile range: 143.0–263.6) copies/mL, P<0.001, Fig. 3].

The accuracies of *U-PDE9A* level and UI for the detection of fetal DS are shown in Table 2. The cutoff value for each factor was set at the 5% false-positive rate by ROC analysis. Sensitivity, PPV, and NPV were compared at an equivalent false-positive rate. The ROC curves of *U-PDE9A* level and UI are presented in Fig. 4. The *U-PDE9A* cutoff level of 320 copies/mL had a sensitivity of 77.8%, PPV of 73.7%, and NPV of 95.5% in differentiating women carrying a DS fetus from women carrying a normal fetus, and the AUC was 0.907 (95% CI: 0.833–0.981) with a standard error (SE) of 0.038 (P<0.001). The UI cutoff value of 14 had a sensitivity of 83.3%, PPV of 75.0%, NPV of 96.6%, and the AUC was 0.927 (95% CI: 0.851–1.003) with an SE of 0.039 (P<0.001). These findings were confirmed using sample karyotypes (Table S1).

We analyzed the accuracy of *U-PDE9A* levels and UI for detecting fetal DS based on gestational weeks at blood sampling (Table 3). The sensitivity of *U-PDE9A* level was higher at 9–12 weeks of gestation than at 5–8 weeks of gestation, whereas the sensitivity of UI was higher at 5–8 weeks of gestation than at 9–12 weeks of gestation. The specificities of both tests were higher at 9–12 weeks of gestation than at 5–8 weeks of gestation. All cases showing false-positive and false-negative results were observed at or before a gestational age of 10 weeks (Table 4).

We analyzed the associations between each factor and the risk of DS. As listed in Table 5, the risk of DS was significantly increased in women with values greater than the cutoff values compared with women whose values were less than the cutoff values for *U-PDE9A* level or UI (OR [95% CI]: 59.5 [12.1–340.7] for *U-PDE9A* level, 85.0 [15.5–564.2] for UI). After adjusting for potential confounding factors such as maternal age, body mass index, and nulliparity at blood sampling, the adjORs of *U-PDE9A* level and UI were 46.2 (95% CI: 7.8–151.6) and 63.7 (95% CI: 23.2–206.7), respectively. Women with *U-PDE9A* levels and UI greater than the cutoff values were at dramatically higher risk of fetal DS in both unadjusted and adjusted analyses, compared with women with values less than the cutoff values.

Discussion

Our findings demonstrate that *U-PDE9A* and UI are effective biomarkers for the non-invasive detection of fetal DS during the

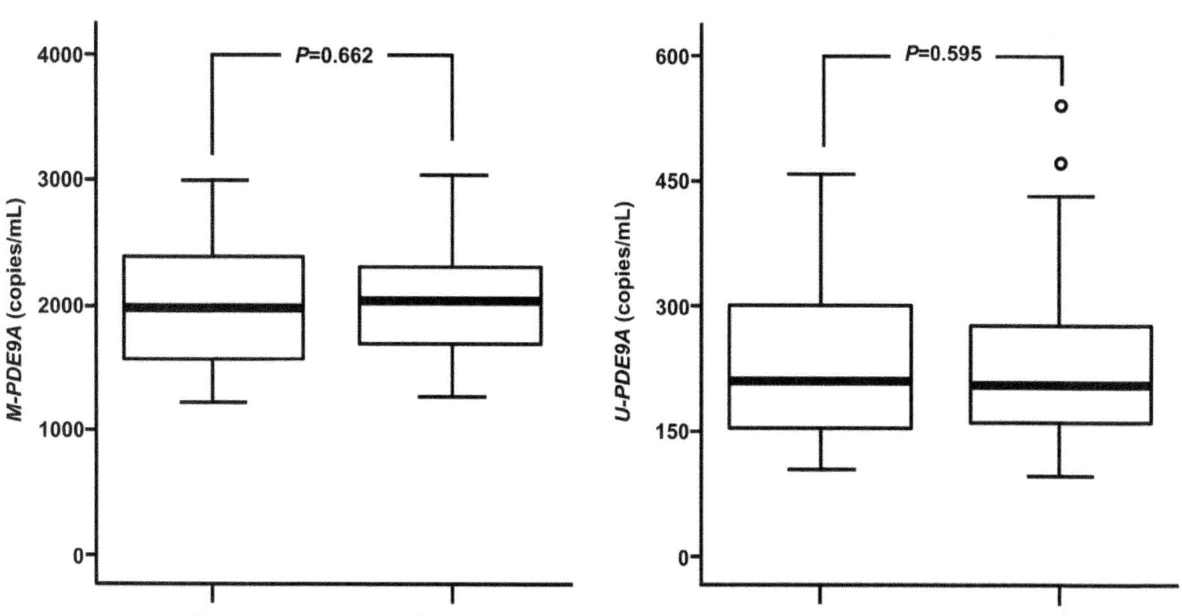

Figure 2. Levels of *M-PDE9A* and *U-PDE9A* in maternal plasma according to fetal gender. The upper and lower limits of the boxes and the lines across the boxes indicate the 75th/25th percentiles and the medians, respectively. The upper and lower error bars indicate the 90th and 10th percentiles, respectively. The circles indicate outliers. Levels were analyzed by the Mann-Whitney U-test.

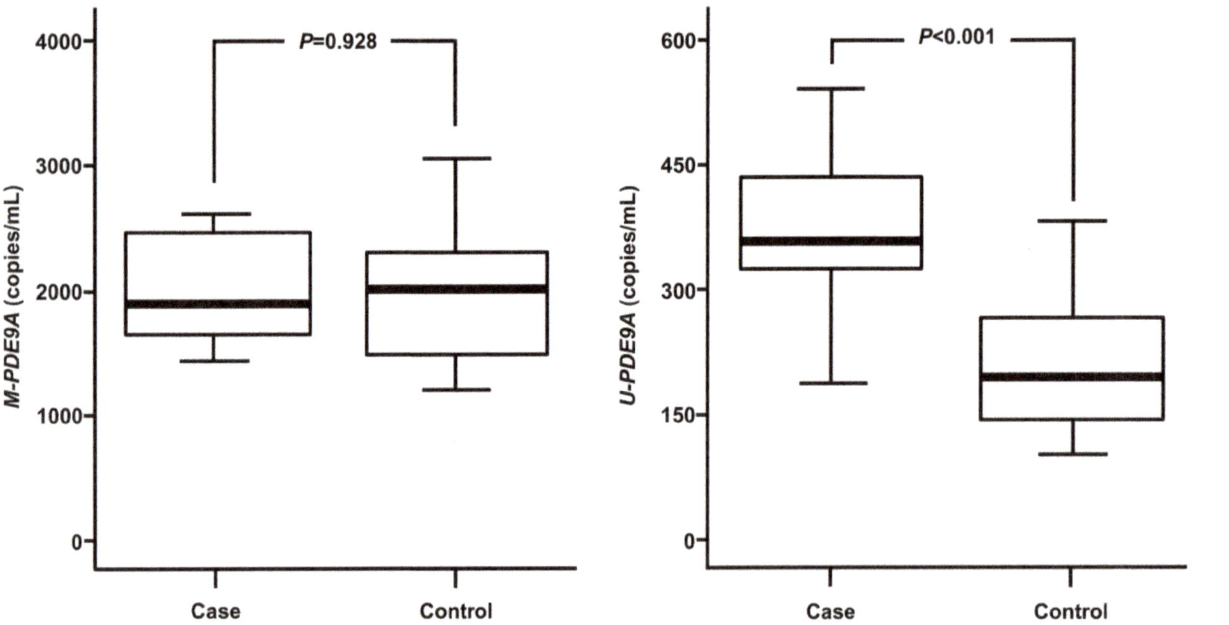

Figure 3. Levels of *M-PDE9A* and *U-PDE9A* in maternal plasma according to fetal karyotype. The upper and lower limits of the boxes and the lines across the boxes indicate the 75th/25th percentiles and the medians, respectively. The upper and lower error bars indicate the 90th and 10th percentiles, respectively. Levels were analyzed by the Mann-Whitney U-test.

first trimester of pregnancy. We determined that *U-PDE9A* levels and UI were significantly elevated in pregnant women carrying DS fetuses compared to women carrying normal fetuses in the first trimester, regardless of fetal gender. Moreover, pregnant women with high values for *U-PDE9A* and UI were at an increased risk of carrying a DS fetus. Therefore, we suggest that *U-PDE9A* and UI may be useful biomarkers for non-invasive fetal DS detection using circulating fetal DNA from maternal plasma, regardless of fetal gender.

Current screening tests for fetal DS detection increases detection rate by integration of multiple methods, such as measurement of nuchal translucency and blood tests for numerous maternal serum markers, including alpha fetoprotein, unconjugated estriol, human chorionic gonadotrophin, and inhibin-A, but at a higher screen-positive rate (approximately 16–22%) [3,4]. Moreover, diagnostic test currently requires obtaining samples of fetal cells directly from the uterus for genetic analysis, either through CVS between 11 and 14 weeks gestation or amniocentesis after 15 weeks. However, these invasive procedures present a small but significant risk of miscarriage in normal pregnancies [5,6]. Therefore, the development of non-invasive prenatal tests for DS detection using circulating fetal DNA in maternal plasma has been considered as a potential alternative to improve current screening tests and to reduce the need for invasive procedures, such as amniocentesis or CVS.

Epigenetics is the study of molecular phenomena that affect gene expression, but which do not involve alterations in DNA sequences. The best-studied epigenetic phenomenon is the process of DNA methylation, which suppresses gene expression and

Table 2. The utility of measurements for detection of fetal Down syndrome.

	Cutoff	Sensitivity	PPV	NPV
U-PDE9A level (copies/mL)	320	0.778 (0.557–0.891)	0.737 (0.537–0.863)	0.955 (0.912–0.982)
Unmethylation index	14	0.833 (0.635–0.940)	0.750 (0.563–0.855)	0.966 (0.923–0.990)

The cutoff was set at 5% false positive rate by ROC curve analysis. To compare detection accuracies of factors, sensitivity, positive predictive value (PPV), and negative predictive value (NPV) were calculated at equivalent false positive rate. The number in parentheses indicates the 95% confidence interval.

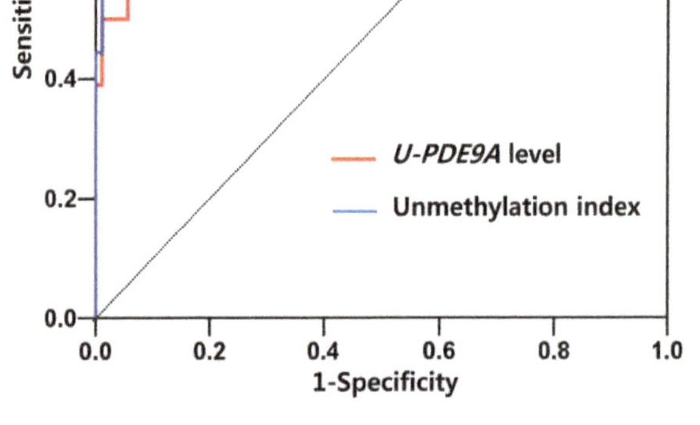

Figure 4. The ROC curves of *U-PDE9A* level and unmethylation index. The ROC curves of unmethylation index and *U-PDE9A* level are represented by blue and red lines, respectively.

Table 3. Detection accuracy according to gestational weeks.

	Gestational weeks	Case (correct N/total N)	Control (correct N/total N)	Sensitivity	Specificity	PPV	NPV
U-PDE9A Level	5–8	10/13	61/65	0.769 (0.509–0.925)	0.938 (0.886–0.970)	0.714 (0.472–0.859)	0.953 (0.900–0.985)
	9–12	4/5	24/25	0.800 (0.347–0.982)	0.960 (0.869–0.996)	0.800 (0.347–0.982)	0.960 (0.869–0.996)
Unmethylation index	5–8	11/13	61/65	0.846 (0.588–0.970)	0.938 (0.887–0.963)	0.733 (0.510–0.841)	0.968 (0.915–0.994)
	9–12	4/5	24/25	0.800 (0.347–0.982)	0.960 (0.869–0.996)	0.800 (0.347–0.982)	0.960 (0.869–0.996)

PPV, positive predictive value; NPV, negative predictive value.
The number in parentheses indicates the 95% confidence interval.

exhibits tissue-specific patterns [14]. In a prior study, Poon *et al.* demonstrated that it was possible to develop fetal DNA markers based on differential DNA methylation patterns between maternal and fetal tissues [15]. This strategy has led to the recognition that the *SERPINB5* gene on chromosome 18, which codes for maspin, is hypomethylated in the placenta, but hypermethylated in maternal blood cells [15]. Therefore, it has been suggested that the measurement of the ratio of single nucleotide polymorphisms (SNP) in the hypomethylated version of the *SERPINB5* gene might allow the detection of fetal trisomy 18 [16].

Similar studies have been performed for non-invasive prenatal detection of fetal DS using circulating fetal DNA. Recently, Papageorgiou *et al.* reported that the application of fetal-specific methylation ratio led to correct diagnosis of fetal DS [17] and Tong *et al.* reported that epigenetic-genetic chromosome dosage using hypermethylated *HLCS* and a paternally inherited fetal SNP allele could be applied for the prenatal diagnosis of trisomy 21 for both male and female fetuses [18]. However, these studies were performed with maternal blood samples that were taken during the late-first or second trimesters (11.1–14.4 weeks of gestation in Papageorgiou *et al.* [17]; 12–21 weeks of gestation in Tong *et al.* [18]) and the samples ware small (14 cases and 26 controls in a blinded analysis by Papageorgiou *et al.* [17]; 14 cases and 33 controls in Tong *et al.* [18]). Moreover, these studies did not control for gestational weeks at blood sampling, which can affect the concentrations of circulating fetal DNA [17,18]. Despite these limitations, previous studies suggest that diagnostic strategies using fetal-specific epigenetic markers may be advantageous compared to current biochemical screening methods for fetal DS. Therefore, searches for fetal-specific epigenetic markers on chromosome 21

Table 4. Cases showing false-positive and false-negative results.

Factors	Condition	Value	Gestational weeks	Karyotype
U-PDE9A level (cutoff: 320 copies/mL)	False-negative (N = 4)	228.4	6	47,XX,+21
		280.6	6	47,XX,+21
		186.6	7	47,XY,+21
		255.9	9	47,XX,+21
	False-positive (N = 5)	361.6	6	46,XX
		381.1	7	46,XY
		345.9	7	46,XX
		351.8	8	46,XX
		366.5	10	46,XY
Unmethylation index (cutoff: 14)	False-negative (N = 3)	9.5	6	47,XX,+21
		8.7	7	47,XY,+21
		12.9	9	47,XX,+21
	False-positive (N = 5)	16.5	6	46,XY
		15.8	7	46,XX
		14.9	8	46,XY
		14.4	8	46,XX
		15.3	10	46,XY

Table 5. Odds ratios for fetal Down syndrome.

	Case (N = 18)	Control (N = 90)	Unadjusted OR (95%CI)	Adjusted OR (95% CI)*
U-PDE9A level (copies/mL)				
Lower than 320	4	85	1.0	1.0
320 or higher	14	5	59.5 (12.1–340.7)	46.2 (7.8–151.6)
Unmethylation index				
Lower than 14	3	85	1.0	1.0
14 or higher	15	5	85.0 (15.5–564.2)	63.7 (23.2–206.7)

OR, odds ratio; CI, confidence interval.
*Adjusted for maternal age, body mass index, and nullipara at blood sampling.

are important for non-invasive prenatal detection of fetal DS. Recently, Chim *et al.* performed a systematic search for such markers on chromosome 21 [10] and reported that 22 of the 114 studied genomic regions were differentially methylated between maternal and fetal (placental) tissues. On the basis of this tissue-specific methylation, they proposed the use of fetal-DNA markers, such as *U-PDE9A*, which are completely methylated in maternal blood cells but unmethylated in the placenta for non-invasive prenatal detection of fetal sequences on chromosome 21. However, the usefulness of such markers in non-invasive prenatal test for fetal DS has not yet been confirmed.

In the present study, we investigated the utility and accuracy of *U-PDE9A* levels and UI for use in non-invasive prenatal detection of DS using circulating fetal DNA from the first trimester. We conducted a nested case-control study controlling for gestational weeks at blood sampling; each case was matched carefully with 5 controls according to gestational weeks at blood sampling (Table S1). Furthermore, all samples were obtained during the first trimester (12 weeks of gestation or less) and the sample number was larger than those of prior studies [17,18]. In this study, *U-PDE9A* levels and UI were significantly elevated during the first trimester in pregnant women carrying DS fetuses, regardless of fetal gender. The fetal DS detection rates of the two factors were higher than those of serum screening markers and nuchal translucency measurements, which are generally performed in the first trimester [3,4]. Moreover, the detection rates of *U-PDE9A* and UI for fetal DS were far superior to those of Y chromosome-specific markers, such as *DYS14* or *SRY*, in maternal serum [19]. Furthermore, Y chromosome-specific markers are limited to use for male fetuses. Therefore, we suggest that *U-PDE9A* levels and UI are effective markers for use in non-invasive prenatal detection of DS during the first trimester regardless of fetal gender, and in fact, these markers may detect fetal DS more effectively than current screening tests for fetal DS. However, the sensitivities of *U-PDE9A* level and the UI were lower or similar (77.8% for *U-PDE9A* levels and 83.3% for UI) than those of second trimester quadruple screening tests (81%). Moreover, false-positive and false-negative results were observed at or before 10 weeks of gestational age. Accordingly, non-invasive fetal DS detection using these markers may have limited clinical applications prior to 10 weeks of gestation. Therefore, improvements in detection rate by applications of other detection methods such as digital PCR or direct comparisons with fetal-specific DNA markers on reference chromosomes may facilitate the clinical use of these markers.

In non-invasive prenatal testing, the analysis of fetal genetic loci in maternal plasma is still problematic because circulating fetal DNA is present in small amounts. To solve this problem, many researchers have suggested methods such as size fractionation [20,21]. Prior studies have demonstrated that more than 99% of circulating fetal DNA is less than 313 bp in length, whereas circulating maternal DNA is significantly longer [20,21]. This discovery enables the possibility of circulating fetal DNA enrichment by size fractionation using a number of methods. Most simply, gel electrophoresis of DNA extracted from maternal plasma has been used to select for low molecular weight DNA. Other methods include the use of kits and columns that rely either on the inability of large molecular weight DNA to pass through, or by the retention of low molecular weight DNA [22,23]. In recent studies, Clausen *et al.* reported that using the DSP Virus Kit resulted in a higher yield of circulating fetal DNA compared with total circulating DNA from maternal plasma [22]. Legler *et al.* suggested that the DSP Virus Kit is an optimal method for extracting high yields of circulating fetal DNA from total plasma [23]. In this study, we used the DSP Virus Kit to extract circulating fetal DNA from maternal plasma. Therefore, we were able to detect fetal DNA identifiers, such as *U-PDE9A*, at as early as five weeks of gestation.

To our knowledge, this is the first study to estimate the accuracy of non-invasive fetal DS detection using *U-PDE9A* analysis in circulating fetal DNA from first trimester maternal plasma. Our data indicate that *U-PDE9A* and UI may be useful markers for non-invasive prenatal detection for fetal DS in all fetal-maternal pairs, regardless of fetal gender. Additionally, high *U-PDE9A* levels and UI may be suitable biomarkers for identifying pregnant women carrying fetuses with DS. Accordingly, these markers may be useful in the development of effective and reliable tests for non-invasive detection of fetal DS. However, the use of this method may create ethical and social issues because the results may impact decisions to terminate or continue the pregnancy. Therefore, the use of this method should be carefully considered in clinical situation and should not be used in the present clinical settings unless more research is done. Furthermore, this method needs to be further refined to achieve higher sensitivity and specificity. Additionally, this study is limited by its small sample size and inclusion of only Korean patients. Therefore, a larger-scale study within different ethnic populations will need to be performed to assist the introduction of the diagnostic strategy used in this study.

Supporting Information

Methods S1 There are included sample processing and DNA extraction for bisulfite genomic sequencing of *PDE9A*, bisulfite genomic sequencing of *PDE9A*, and

limit of detection for quantitative methylation-specific polymerase chain reaction.

Table S1 DNA samples from participants in this study.

Table S2 Unmethylated *PDE9A* levels obtained from 108 samples.

Table S3 Methylated *PDE9A* levels obtained from 108 samples.

Acknowledgments

We thank the following physicians and their associated staff who took the time and effort to participate in this study: Joung Yeol Han, MD, PhD, Jun Seek Choi, MD, PhD, Hyun Kyong Ahn, MD, PhD, Jin Hoon Chung, MD, PhD, Min Hyoung Kim, MD, PhD, You Jung Han, MD, Da Eun Lee, PhD, Jin Woo Kim, MS, Bom Yi Lee, MS, Do Jin Kim, MS, Ju Yeon Park, BS, Eun Young Choi, BS, Yeon Woo Lee, BS, Ah Rum Oh, BS, and So Min Seo, BS. We thank Daehun Peah, MD, PhD and In Soo Kang, MD, PhD for statistical analysis of the data.

Author Contributions

Conceived and designed the experiments: JHL HMR. Performed the experiments: SYK SYL MJK. Analyzed the data: JHL SYP SWL. Contributed reagents/materials/analysis tools: YJH SWL JHC MYK JHY. Wrote the paper: JHL SWL HMR.

References

1. Driscoll DA, Gross S (2009) Clinical practice. Prenatal screening for aneuploidy. N Engl J Med 360: 2556–2562.
2. Hook EB, Cross PK, Schreinemachers DM (1983) Chromosomal abnormality rates at amniocentesis and in live-born infants. JAMA 249: 2034–2038.
3. Malone FD, Canick JA, Ball RH, Nyberg DA, Comstock CH, et al. (2005) First-trimester or second-trimester screening, or both, for Down's syndrome. N Engl J Med 353: 2001–2011.
4. Wapner R, Thom E, Simpson JL, Pergament E, Silver R, et al. (2003) First-trimester screening for trisomies 21 and 18. N Engl J Med 349: 1405–1413.
5. Mujezinovic F, Alfirevic Z (2007) Procedure-related complications of amniocentesis and chorionic villous sampling: a systematic review. Obstet Gynecol 110: 687–694.
6. Reddy UM, Mennuti MT (2006) Incorporating first-trimester Down syndrome studies into prenatal screening: executive summary of the national institute of child health and human development workshop. Obstet Gynecol 107: 167–173.
7. Soderling SH, Beavo JA (2000) Regulation of cAMP and cGMP signalling: new phosphodiesterases and new functions. Curr Opin Cell Biol 12: 174–179.
8. Fisher DA, Smith JF, Pillar JS, St Denis SH, Cheng JB (1998) Isolation and characterisation of PDE9A, a novel human cGMPspecific phosphodiesterase. J Biol Chem 273: 15559–15564.
9. Guipponi M, Scott HS, Kudoh J, Kawasaki K, Shibuya K, et al. (1998) Identification and characterisation of a novel cyclic nucleotide phosphodiesterase gene (PDE9A) that maps to 21q22.3: alternative splicing of mRNA transcripts, genomic structure and sequence. Hum Genet 103: 386–392.
10. Chim SS, Jin S, Lee TY, Lun FM, Lee WS, et al. (2008) Systematic search for placental DNAmethylation markers on chromosome 21: toward a maternal plasma-based epigenetic test for fetal trisomy 21. Clin Chem 54: 500–511.
11. Lim JH, Park SY, Kim SY, Kim DJ, Choi JE, et al. (2011) Effective detection of fetal sex using circulating fetal DNA in first-trimester maternal plasma. FASEB J doi: 10.1096/fj.11-191429.
12. Lo YM, Tein MS, Lau TK, Haines CJ, Leung TN, et al. (1998) Quantitative analysis of fetal DNA in maternal plasma and serum: implications for non-invasive prenatal diagnosis. Am J Hum Genet 62: 768–775.
13. Lim JH, Kim SY, Park SY, Yang JH, Kim MY, et al. (2008) Effective prediction of preeclampsia by a combined ratio of angiogenesis-related factors. Obstet Gynecol 111: 1403–1409.
14. Rakyan VK, Down TA, Thorne NP, Flicek P, Kulesha E, et al. (2008) An integrated resource for genome-wide identification and analysis of human tissue-specific differentially methylated regions (tDMRs). Genome Res 18: 1518–1529.
15. Poon LL, Leung TN, Lau TK, Chow KC, Lo YM (2002) Differential DNA methylation between fetus and mother as a strategy for detecting fetal DNA in maternal plasma. Clin Chem 48: 35–41.
16. Chim SS, Tong YK, Chiu RW, Lau TK, Leung TN, et al. (2005) Detection of the placental epigenetic signature of the maspin gene in maternal plasma. Proc Natl Acad Sci U S A 102: 14753–14758.
17. Papageorgiou EA, Karagrigoriou A, Tsaliki E, Velissariou V, Carter NP, et al. (2011) Fetal-specific DNA methylation ratio permits noninvasive prenatal diagnosis of trisomy 21. Nat Med 17: 510–513.
18. Tong YK, Chiu RW, Akolekar R, Leung TY, Lau TK, et al. (2010) Epigenetic-genetic chromosome dosage approach for fetal trisomy 21 detection using an autosomal genetic reference marker. PLoS One 5: e15244.
19. Farina A, LeShane ES, Lambert-Messerlian GM, Canick JA, Lee T, et al. (2003) Evaluation of cell-free fetal DNA as a second-trimester maternal serum marker of Down syndrome pregnancy. Clin Chem 49: 239–242.
20. Chan KC, Zhang J, Hui AB, Wong N, Lau TK, et al. (2004) Size distributions of maternal and fetal DNA in maternal plasma. Clin Chem 50: 88–92.
21. Li Y, Zimmermann B, Rusterholz C, Kang A, Holzgreve W, et al. (2004) Size separation of circulatory DNA in maternal plasma permits ready detection of fetal DNApolymorphisms. Clin Chem 50: 1002–1011.
22. Clausen FB, Krog GR, Rieneck K, Dziegiel MH (2007) Improvement in fetal DNA extraction from maternal plasma. Evaluation of the NucliSens Magnetic Extraction system and the QIAamp DSP Virus Kit in comparison with the QIAamp DNA Blood Mini Kit. Prenat Diagn 27: 6–10.
23. Legler TJ, Liu Z, Mavrou A, Finning K, Hromadnikova I, et al. (2007) Workshop report on the extraction of foetal DNA from maternal plasma. Prenat Diagn 27: 824–829.

13

Investigating and Correcting Plasma DNA Sequencing Coverage Bias to Enhance Aneuploidy Discovery

Dineika Chandrananda[1,2]*, Natalie P. Thorne[1,2], Devika Ganesamoorthy[3,4], Damien L. Bruno[3], Yuval Benjamini[5], Terence P. Speed[1,5], Howard R. Slater[3,4], Melanie Bahlo[1,6]

1 Bioinformatics Division, The Walter and Eliza Hall Institute of Medical Research, Melbourne, Australia, **2** Department of Medical Biology, University of Melbourne, Melbourne, Australia, **3** Victorian Clinical Genetics Services Cytogenetics Laboratory, Murdoch Childrens Research Institute, Melbourne, Australia, **4** Department of Paediatrics, University of Melbourne, Melbourne, Australia, **5** Department of Statistics, University of California, Berkeley, California, United States of America, **6** Department of Mathematics and Statistics, University of Melbourne, Melbourne, Australia

Abstract

Pregnant women carry a mixture of cell-free DNA fragments from self and fetus (non-self) in their circulation. In recent years multiple independent studies have demonstrated the ability to detect fetal trisomies such as trisomy 21, the cause of Down syndrome, by Next-Generation Sequencing of maternal plasma. The current clinical tests based on this approach show very high sensitivity and specificity, although as yet they have not become the standard diagnostic test. Here we describe improvements to the analysis of the sequencing data by reducing GC bias and better handling of the genomic repeats. We show substantial improvements in the sensitivity of the standard trisomy 21 statistical tests, which we measure by artificially reducing read coverage. We also explore the bias stemming from the natural cleavage of plasma DNA by examining DNA motifs and position specific base distributions. We propose a model to correct this fragmentation bias and observe that incorporating this bias does not lead to any further improvements in the detection of fetal trisomy. The improved bias corrections that we demonstrate in this work can be readily adopted into existing fetal trisomy detection protocols and should also lead to improvements in sub-chromosomal copy number variation detection.

Editor: Fengfeng Zhou, Shenzhen Institutes of Advanced Technology, China

Funding: This work was supported by the Victorian State Government Operational Infrastructure Support and Australian Government NHMRC IRIISS. Additional support provided by Australian Postgraduate Awards (to DC and DG); The John and Patricia Farrant Scholarship (to DC); National Science Foundation VIGRE Graduate Fellowship (to YB); National Health and Medical Research Council Australia Fellowship (grant number 575503 to TPS); National Institutes of Health (grant number 5R01 GM083084-03 to TPS.) and an Australian Research Council Future Fellowship (grant number FT100100764 to MB). The funders had no role in study design, data collection and analysis, decision to publish, or preparation of the manuscript.

Competing Interests: The authors have declared that no competing interests exist.

* E-mail: chandrananda@wehi.edu.au

Introduction

Detection of trisomy 21, also known as Down syndrome, has long been considered the driving force for prenatal diagnosis. This disorder, which causes severe intellectual and developmental disability, is the most common fetal chromosomal defect with a prevalence of 1 in 700 newborns [1]. Other aneuploidy conditions such as trisomy 13 (Patau Syndrome) and trisomy 18 (Edwards Syndrome) are more lethal in infants but are much less frequent [2,3]. Efforts to develop non-invasive prenatal tests (NIPT) for detection of these chromosome abnormalities have been spurred on by the increasing maternal age in developed countries and the associated increase in the risk of fetal aneuploidy [4,5].

The 1997 discovery of the existence of cell-free fetal DNA in maternal plasma [6] provided a new avenue for non-invasive prenatal testing. A decade and a half of concentrated research efforts coupled with the recent rapid advances of Next-Generation Sequencing (NGS), have now allowed sequencing based aneuploidy tests to be clinically translated in several countries including USA and China. Since the initial proof-of-principle studies in 2008 [7,8], the NGS platform type, sequencing scope and depth used in NIPT have been rapidly changing, in the quest for greater sensitivity of trisomy detection and the need to investigate sub-chromosomal copy number changes in the fetus in the most cost-effective manner [9,10].

Characteristics and biology of cell-free fetal DNA

Nucleic acids can be found in cell-free form in human plasma and serum [11]. This DNA has recently been demonstrated to be predominately of hematopoietic origin [12] and apoptosis has consistently been shown as a major source of this cell-free DNA (cfDNA) [13–15]. However, other biological sources have also been implicated and there remains uncertainty in the field as to the involvement of various processes such as the active secretion of cfDNA by cells and the role of membrane proteins in protecting cfDNA in circulation [16,17].

In early pregnancy, 3–20% of the DNA in maternal plasma comes from the developing fetus [18–20] and this proportion is shown to increase with gestational age [21,22]. An inverse relationship has been described between the fetal proportion and maternal weight, indicating a possible dilution effect [23,24]. Fetal cfDNA is detectable from the 7th week of gestation and the most likely source is thought to be apoptosis of placental (i.e. extra-embryonic) cells [25,26].

Paired-end sequencing of plasma DNA has revealed that the fragments are generally around 166 bp in size with a small proportion exhibiting a length close to 340 bp [27]. The major peak in the size distribution is very similar to the length of DNA that is wrapped around a nucleosomal core unit (approximately 146 bp plus a linker fragment of DNA between 20–90 base pairs [28]). The 340 bp signal corresponds to a di-nucleosomal structure. The same study showed that fetal fragments were generally shorter than 150 bp.

NGS-based Down syndrome detection

While a few clinically available tests use targeted sequencing to select DNA fragments from specific chromosomes [29,30], the majority currently utilize a genome-wide sequencing protocol that has been shown to be reproducible in multiple studies [24,31–33]. The largest clinical validation studies that use whole-genome sequencing have all used variations of the "molecular-counting" approach.

This approach attempts to identify an increase in DNA fragments originating from the aneuploidy chromosome in the fetus without distinguishing between maternal and fetal DNA, using either lab-based or bioinformatics methods. The tests calculate the relative amounts of plasma DNA fragments originating from the different chromosomes and determine if there is an increase beyond what is expected for a euploid pregnancy assuming that this increase stems from a copy number change in the fetus. In a pregnancy with fetal trisomy 21, there would be a slight increase in the amount of DNA derived from chromosome 21 in maternal plasma compared with the DNA from other chromosomes. The extent of this increase is dependent on the fetal DNA proportion, in that, if fetal DNA constitute 10% of the ccfDNA in a pregnancy with fetal trisomy 21, we would anticipate a 5% increase in the copy number of chromosome 21 fragments in maternal plasma. This can be assessed by comparing the chromosome 21 read counts for an unspecified pregnancy to that of a set of controls (euploid pregnancies).

Biases in sequencing data

Since the tests attempt to detect small increases in the chromosomal representation, they incorporate steps in their analysis that adjust for the bias inherent in NGS data which lead to inter- and intra-chromosomal read count variability.

Table 1. Clinical details and sequencing data statistics of recruited samples.

Sample Index	Sample ID	Fetal Karyotype	Total Sequence Reads Generated (HiSeq 2000)	Reads Uniquely Aligned (Novoalign)	Reads Uniquely Aligned (BWA)
1	NIPD-03_TM	47, XX, +21	31,081,981	26,236,069	25,199,455
2	NIPD-03_TMR*	47, XX, +21	32,282,282	28,346,871	27,521,416
3	NIPD-04_TM	47, XY, +21	40,278,804	35,421,320	34,594,910
4	NIPD-04_TMR*	47, XY, +21	38,031,790	33,324,563	32,436,346
5	NIPD-05_TM	46, XX	33,885,622	29,897,378	29,186,676
6	NIPD-05_TMR*	46, XX	31,936,055	28,391,920	27,739,819
7	NIPD-07_TM	47, XY, +21	24,767,047	20,878,567	20,050,937
8	NIPD-07_TMR*	47, XY, +21	24,955,598	21,922,674	21,287,065
9	NIPD-09_TM	46, XY	26,987,293	23,723,020	23,164,487
10	NIPD-09_TMR*	46, XY	31,019,583	27,134,946	26,400,672
11	NIPD-13_TM	46, XY	28,932,490	25,534,678	24,925,205
12	NIPD-13_TMR*	46, XY	32,691,501	29,063,410	28,394,889
13	NIPD-48_TM	46, XY	31,048,049	27,414,008	26,758,810
14	NIPD-51_TM	46, XY	31,303,893	27,363,033	26,587,761
15	NIPD-54_TM	46, XX	32,519,963	28,835,431	28,135,842
16	NIPD-56_TM	46, XY	32,568,205	28,658,808	27,943,150
17	NIPD-58_TM	46, XY	28,960,279	25,087,238	24,309,884
18	NIPD-60_TM	47, XY, +21	32,137,330	28,409,821	27,687,323
19	NIPD-50_TM	47, XY, +21	33,458,803	29,815,550	29,158,995
20	NIPD-52_TM	46, XY	30,801,889	27,449,087	26,835,869
21	NIPD-53_TM	46, XX	33,135,305	29,454,208	28,740,525
22	NIPD-59_TM	46, XX	33,321,758	29,621,383	28,948,308
23	NIPD-61_TM	46, XX	38,287,043	34,235,072	33,502,284
24	NIPD-62_TM	46, XY	33,183,117	29,674,630	29,047,689
25	NIPD-23_TM	46, XX	29,852,910	26,152,316	25,492,998
26	NIPD-30_TM	46, XX	32,038,077	28,463,745	27,840,119
27	NIPD-63_TM	46, XX	32,085,733	28,679,366	28,097,170
28	NIPD-65_TM	46, XY	35,094,568	31,339,712	30,653,822
29	NIPD-66_TM	47, XY, +21	35,411,652	31,237,019	30,450,668

*Sample IDs with the suffix TMR belong to the re-amplified libraries.

Table 2. Genome-wide coverage at each sampling proportion for the 29 datasets after Novoalign mapping and subsequent read filtering.

Proportion of reads sampled	Average number of reads	Range	Mean fold coverage
original	26,174,727	18,832,054–32,733,023	0.42X
0.75	19,719,795	14,172,672–24,677,526	0.31X
0.5	13,206,439	9,483,101–16,539,568	0.21X
0.25	6,635,982	4,761,496–8,317,675	0.11X
0.125	3,328,165	2,387,989–4,173,351	0.053X
0.0625	1,667,889	1,196,946–2,091,602	0.026X
0.0312	854,222	613,083–1,071,927	0.014X

One such bias is the Guanine-Cytosine content (GC) bias which is uni-modal in nature as the read coverage is maximized for genomic regions with 40–50% GC with coverage decreasing at the extreme values. The current tests predominantly incorporate a locally weighted scatterplot smoothing (LOESS) correction step as described by Alkan et al. [34] to correct for GC. This involves binning the read counts into non-overlapping windows and calculating the GC content of these windows (a 50 Kb bin size is in wide use). A LOESS curve is fitted to the plot of bin counts vs. bin GC to obtain predicted values that are used to correct the raw counts.

A second source of bias stemming from the alignment of short read data is the inability of sequence reads to map unambiguously or uniquely to highly repetitive regions of the genome. This mappability bias is generally dealt with by removal of such regions (annotated in the RepeatMasker database [35]) rather than quantifying the mappability and correcting for it.

Statistical test for trisomy

Different research groups use different algorithms to test for aneuploidy in the bias corrected data. Since they generally have access to large sample sizes of both normal and aneuploid pregnancies they are able to make use of these samples to perform an empirical bias adjustment, per chromosome, in their statistical analysis [31,36].

Motivation

In this work, we present a post-sequencing protocol that utilizes a more sensitive GC correction (based on the work of Benjamini and Speed [37]) as well as a correction for mappability. We also show an additional source of bias due to fragmentation that is inflated in plasma cfDNA when compared to genomic DNA. The fragmentation effect is the position-specific pattern of nucleotides around DNA fragment ends. Plasma DNA shows different and stronger patterns than genomic DNA due to the fragments originating from a biological process and possible nuclease activity rather than a random shearing during the DNA fragmentation step of library preparation. This bias is investigated in depth to illustrate its relationship with the GC bias. We then extend the improved GC correction to incorporate the fragmentation bias.

The motivation of our work is to compare between different bias correction protocols in order to recommend an optimal correction procedure. Since optimization of the test statistic can be considered a separate research area, we use the simple Z-score method described by Chiu et al. in 2008 and 2011 [7,19], to benchmark the results of our correction methods. Furthermore, the Z-score method has been the basis of many of the subsequent tests so we used this test statistic for our comparisons. We find that considerable improvements in trisomy detection are achieved using our recommended pipeline.

Materials and Methods

Ethics Statement

This study was approved by the Royal Children's Hospital (RCH) Human Research Ethics Committee (HREC). All participants gave written informed consent to the protocol approved by the RCH HREC (reference number 31080A).

Subject recruitment and clinical information

Pregnant women in their first and second trimester of pregnancy were recruited through the Victoria Clinical Genetics Service (VCGS) after providing informed written consent. All

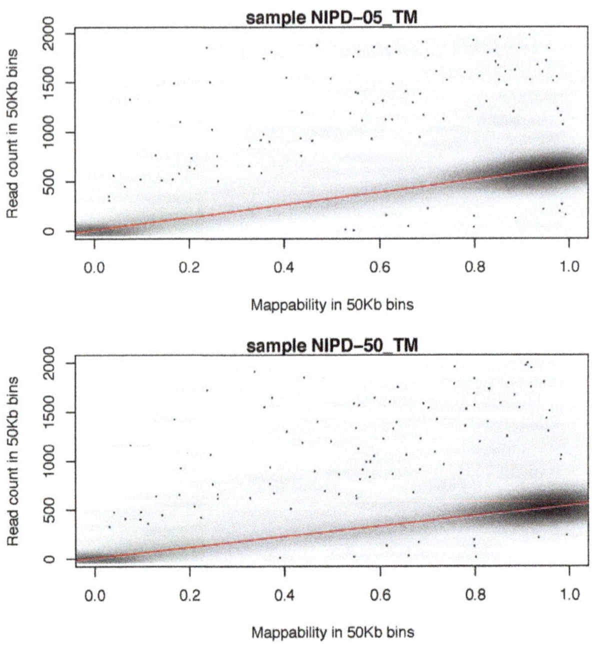

Figure 1. Mappability bias. The smoothed scatter plot of the mappability (as calculated by mapping the fragmented hg19 reference to itself using Novoalign) against the read count in 50 Kb genomic windows shows a linear relationship. Extreme bin counts have been removed for plotting.

participants donated 10 mL of peripheral blood. Samples used in this study were collected prior to any invasive testing and all were from singleton pregnancies.

Two patient groups were included: The first were women who had received a post-test low-risk score by Combined First Trimester Screening. Samples from these women were assumed as euploid and used as 'normal' controls; pregnancy outcomes were consistent with categorizing these as 'likely' euploid. The second were women with a diagnosis of fetal trisomy 21, which was made by chromosome analysis of amniocentesis or chorionic villus samples.

Processing of blood samples

The collected blood samples were stored in tubes containing Ethylene Diamine Tetraacetic Acid (EDTA) and were processed within 4 hours after phlebotomy by a double-centrifugation protocol. In brief, blood was transferred into 15 mL falcon tubes and centrifuged at 1600 g for 10 minutes at 4°C to separate the blood cells and plasma. Next, plasma was transferred into 1.5 mL micro-centrifuge tubes and centrifuged at 16000 g for 10 minutes at 4°C to remove residual cells. Plasma was transferred into new microcentrifuge tubes and stored at −80°C until further processing. The blood cell fraction was stored at −20°C until further processing.

DNA library preparation and sequencing

DNA library preparation was carried out at the Murdoch Childrens Research Institute where the samples were de-identified and assigned anonymous IDs for the purposes of this study.

Cell-free DNA was isolated from plasma using the QIAamp Circulating Nucleic Acid Kit (Qiagen, Melbourne, Australia) according to the manufacturer's guidelines, with slight modifications in reagent volumes.

DNA libraries were prepared according to a modified protocol from Illumina (http://www.illumina.com/). After end-repairing, A-base tailing and adaptor ligation, standard multiplex primers were introduced by PCR with 5 mL of PCR Primer Cocktail and 25 mL of PCR Master Mix. The PCR protocol consisted of a denaturation step at 98°C for 30 seconds and 10 cycles of 98°C for 10 seconds, 60°C for 30 seconds and 72°C for 30 seconds and final extension at 72°C for 5 minutes and held at 10°C.

The size distribution of the libraries was analyzed using an Agilent Bioanalyzer and quantified with real-time PCR. The fragmentation and size selection steps in the library preparations

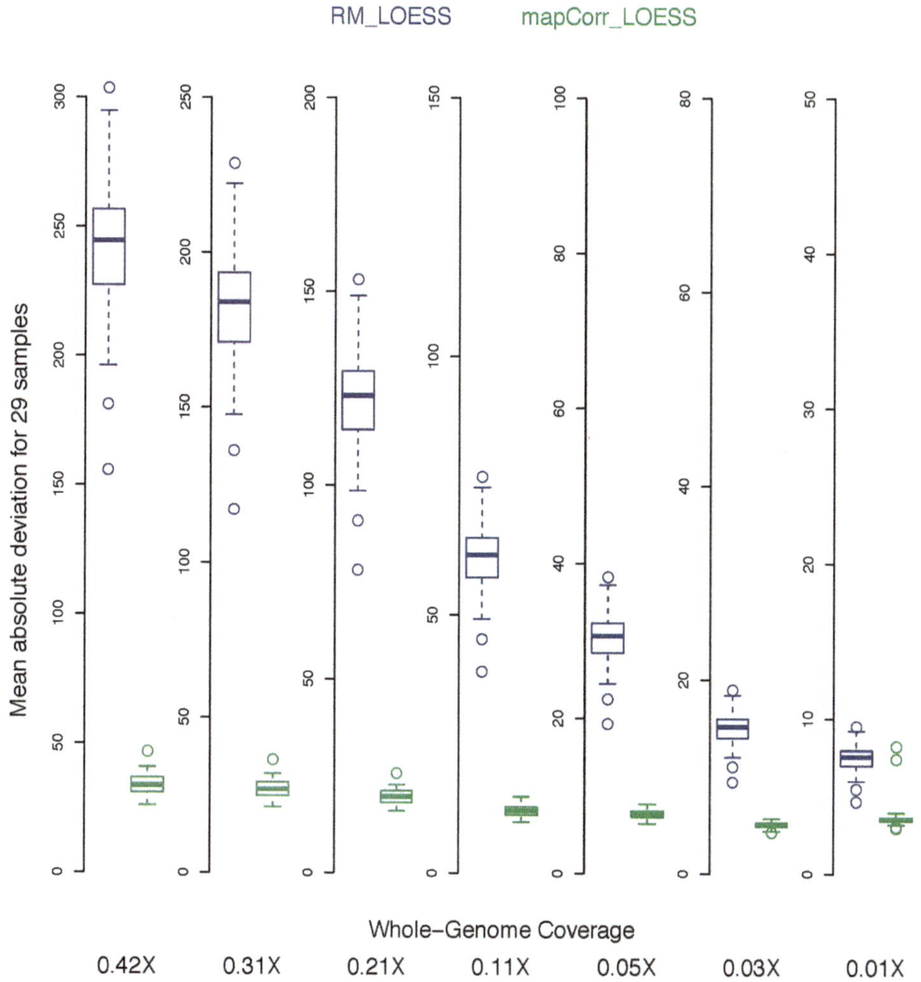

Figure 2. Comparison of the repeat handling methods. The prediction error (mean absolute deviation around the predicted rates) in the two repeat handling methods for 29 samples at different depths of coverage. RM_LOESS (blue) is the protocol where RepeatMasker regions are filtered and mapCorr_LOESS (green) is where mappability is quantified and read counts are corrected.

were omitted, as the plasma DNA molecules are naturally cleaved and exist as short fragments [27].

All samples were sequenced at the Australian Genome Research Facility on the Illumina HiSeq 2000 platform. Barcoded libraries were equally pooled in batches of 6 in one lane and sequenced with a 50-cycle single-end multiplex strategy. Thirty libraries were sequenced in total using the 6-plex format in five batches. The batches were run at different times and using different flow-cells.

Sequenced samples

Initially, blood samples from 24 pregnant women were used to make 24 DNA libraries. All samples, except one, had clinical information available on the Combined First Trimester Screening test. The single sample that was missing this information was removed from further analyses leaving 23 samples.

Six of the remaining libraries were re-amplified using either 3 or 5 cycles of PCR based on the library yield, in order to act as technical replicates in the study. Hence, twenty-nine 50 bp single-end read datasets were utilized in the subsequent analysis. Of these, 9 were from trisomy 21 cases and 20 were normals. All 29 read datasets are accessible through the Short Read Archive (http://www.ncbi.nlm.nih.gov/Traces/sra/) under the accession number SRA097799.

Sequencing data processing

Following sequencing, reads were stripped of their adapters and demultiplexed according to their barcodes. The reads for the 29 samples were then aligned to the human genome, build 37 (hg19) using Novoalign V2.08.03 (www.novocraft.com). An ambiguous human reference was used that has known SNPs encoded as IUPAC ambiguous codes. Reads that mapped to multiple-locations, those that were designated as PCR duplicates as well as reads that aligned with more than two mismatches were discarded from each dataset using a combination of Samtools V0.1.18 [38] and Picard software V1.65 (http://picard.sourceforge.net/).

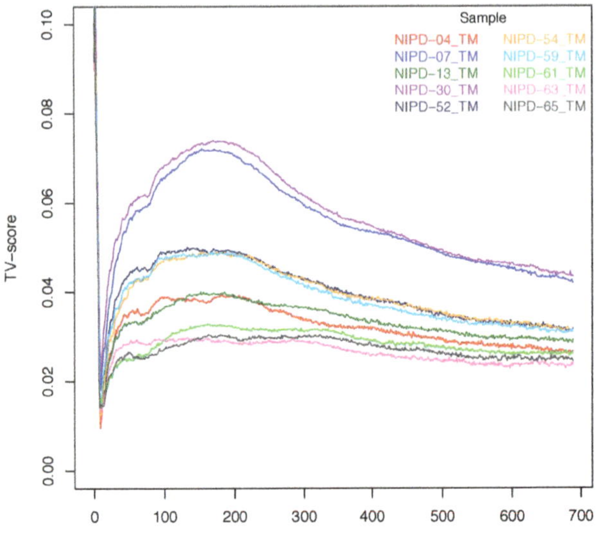

Figure 3. Estimating the optimal window size for GC content. The truncated plot of the scaled TV scores for 10 representative samples as the GC window size is varied. The TV score indicates the suitability of the window length used to calculate GC content. The peak at windows less than 10 bp demonstrates a strong GC dependent fragmentation effect. The high values in the range of 150–250 bp stems from the wide distribution of fragment lengths in plasma. The TV score is truncated for the fragmentation peak (the range for this peak for the 29 samples is between 0.11 and 0.15).

Each sample, consisting of a set of reads from an individual, had the following four bias correction protocols applied to allow comparisons in their performance. All the following analyses were performed in R [39].

1) RM_LOESS: reads that fall into repeatMasker regions (http://www.repeatmasker.org) are removed and a LOESS correction performed for GC bias (using the 'loess' R package).
2) mapCorr_LOESS: read counts are corrected according to the mappability [40] of the regions and a LOESS correction performed for GC bias.
3) mapCorr_singlePos: GC bias was estimated and corrected via the single position model [37] after correcting read counts according to the mappability of regions.
4) mapCorr_singlePos_Frag: As in 3) but corrections carried out after stratifying reads into classes based on their fragmentation signature.

Method 1 is a commonly used bias correction approach in the NIPT field, whilst methods 2)-4) represent new protocols.

In order to assess the robustness of the bias corrections, the read alignment of the 29 sequencing datasets was repeated with a different aligner, BWA (V 0.7.2-r351) [38], which uses an algorithm different to that of Novoalign. BWA is freeware and is commonly used by other researchers to align NGS data. Its algorithm is unable to utilize the ambiguous reference; hence the sequencing reads were mapped to the human genome with unmasked SNPs.

LOESS GC bias correction

The LOESS correction performed was similar to the one described by Alkan et al. 2009 [34]. The genome was segmented into non-overlapping bins of 50 Kb length and the chromosomal read coverage as well as GC content of each bin was calculated (chrY was excluded from this analysis). Bin counts are the total number of reads with the 5′ end inside the bin. GC content is the proportion of guanine and cytosine bases in the bin as per the reference genome. After filtering regions with no counts, the average read count for windows with GC content in intervals of 1% were calculated. A LOESS regression curve was fitted to this data with a span of 0.3, to determine a predicted count for each bin along the genome based on its GC content using the loess function in R. The read count of each bin was normalized by the predicted bin count to obtain the corrected value.

Fifty kb bins were used in the analyses as it is the most widely used bin size in the NIPT literature. The choice for this bin size was stated to be arbitrary in an early proof of principle publication [41].

Usage of Repeat Masker

Reads that were mapped to repeat-masker annotated sites (Repeat Library 20120124; http://www.repeatmasker.org) were discarded prior to GC correction.

Mappability correction

Short sequence reads were simulated by fragmenting the human reference genome (hg19) into overlapping fragments at one base-pair resolution. The length of the simulated reads was set to 50 bp, as this was the read length in the sequencing data. The reads were

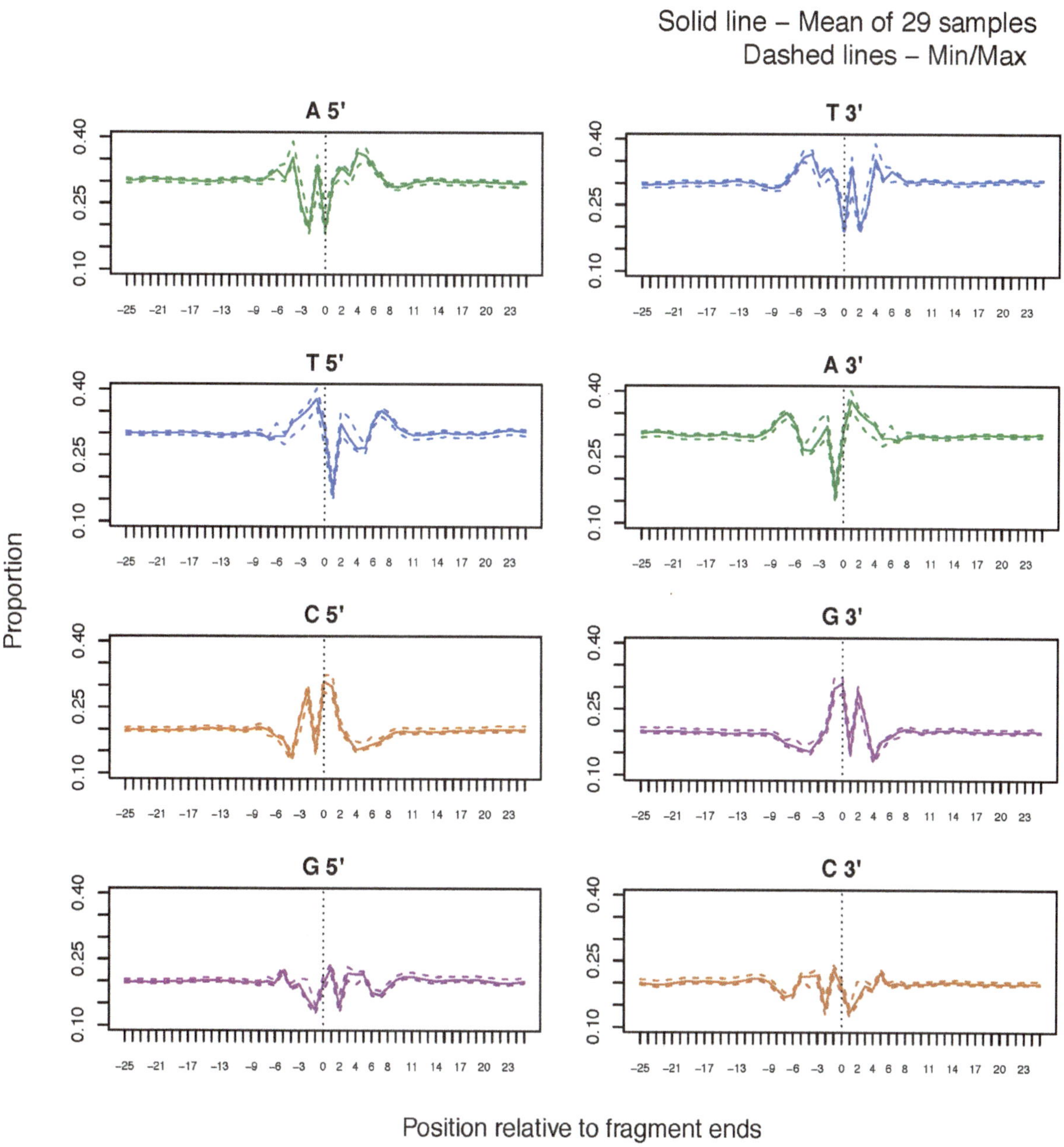

Figure 4. Investigating the fragmentation effect. The y-axis denotes the proportion of each nucleotide at fixed positions relative to the fragment 5′ and 3′ ends. The vertical line at 0 denotes the start of the read on each strand. The mean, minimum and maximum proportions of 29 samples have been plotted on the same graph and show that the variability between the samples is nearly negligible.

aligned back to the reference genome using Novoalign, and all base positions of uniquely mapping reads were identified. The proportion of 'unique' sites in the window then gives its mappability value.

The read counts in a given window were multiplied by the reciprocal of its mappability value in order to correct for this mapping bias in the sequencing data. Fifty Kb windows with less than 50% unique sites were filtered out to prevent over-correction. Data aligned using BWA were corrected with mappability annotation created using BWA.

Single-position GC bias estimation with mappability correction

Benjamini and Speed described a single-position GC bias correction model [37] and showed that it removed more bias than the commonly used LOESS method that is based on modeling read counts and GC content in non-overlapping genomic windows. The single-position model stratifies uniquely mappable positions along the genome by the GC content of the DNA fragment of fixed length beginning at the position. It then estimates a mean fragment rate for all positions with the same GC. The following steps summarize how this model was utilized in this study. All steps were carried out using the GCcorrect R package. (http://www.stat.berkeley.edu/~yuvalb/YuvalWeb/Software.html).

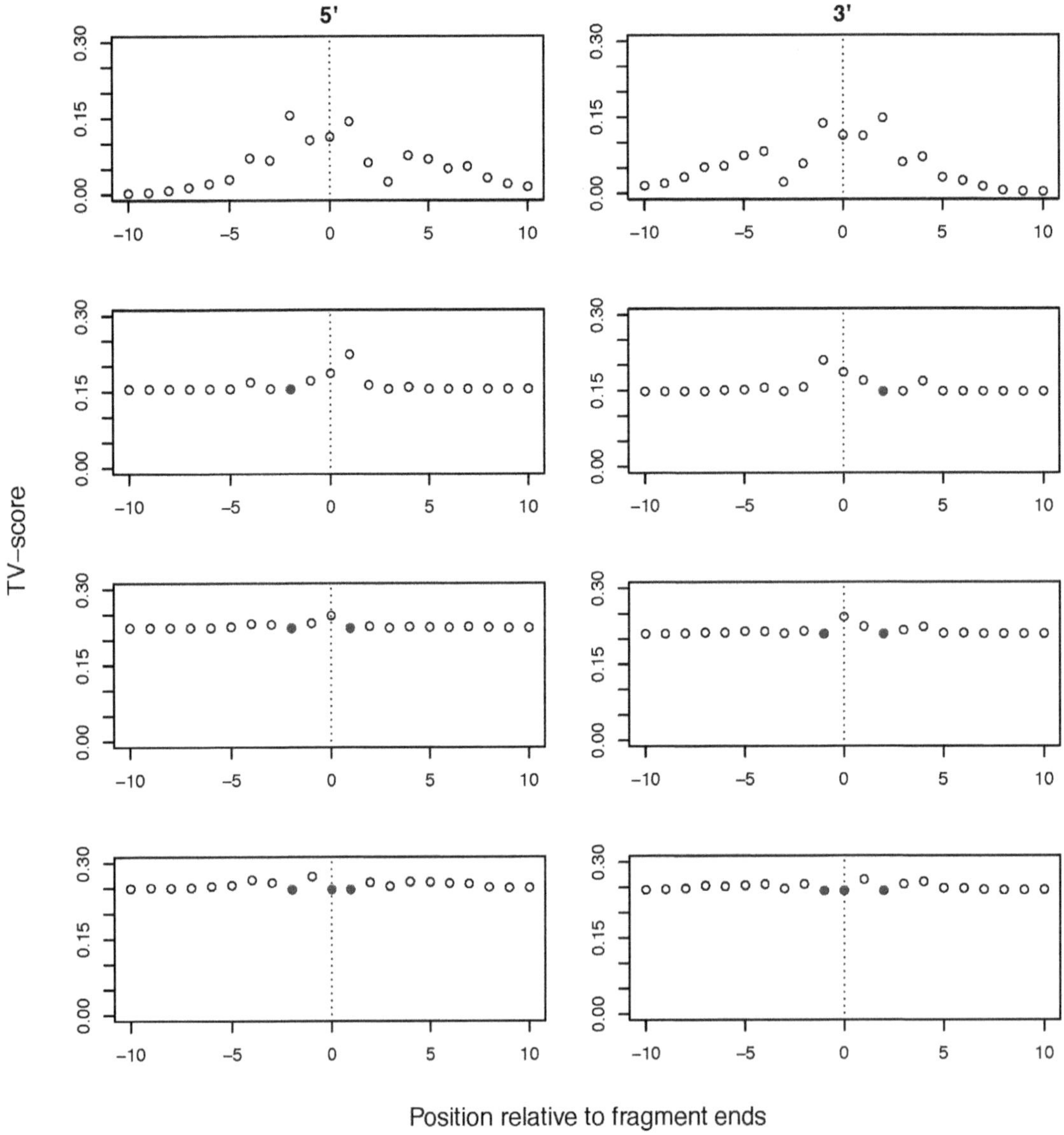

Figure 5. Defining a model for the fragmentation effect. The TV-score of one representative sample, conditioning on individual positions at breakpoints on the 5′ (right) and 3′ (left) strands sequentially, starting with −2 bp position (2nd row), then adding the 1st bp position (3rd row) and finally the 0th bp position (4th row). After each level of conditioning, the position that shows the highest TV score (in blue) is aggregated into the k-mer used to stratify the reads to set up the next conditioning step and the TV score is recalculated. Bias is no longer visibly location-specific after incorporating the 3-mer at positions −2,0,1. Hence, these positions can be used in a simplified model for the fragmentation bias.

(i) Uniquely mappable positions along the genome (denoted by x) were randomly sampled. Each position was assigned a value corresponding to the number of GC bases in a window of length l starting at position x. This was done in a strand-specific manner.

(ii) Positions of similar GC value were classed into different GC strata. The total number of positions that fall into a certain stratum gc was denoted by N_{gc}.

(iii) The number of DNA fragments F_x in each position x were counted so that the total number of fragments in each GC stratum F_{gc} could be calculated.

(iv) Mean fragment rates $\hat{\lambda}_{gc}$ were estimated for each GC stratum by taking the ratio between fragment count F_{gc} and positions N_{gc}. The plot of mean rates against GC was smoothed to obtain the predictions $\hat{\mu}_{gc}$ for each stratum.

(v) Since the GC stratum of each position x was known, the prediction per position $\hat{\mu}_x$ could be found using $\hat{\mu}_{gc}$ $\cdot\hat{\mu}_x$ was equal to 0 if the position x was not uniquely mappable.

(vi) The read counts and predictions were aggregated separately into non-overlapping genomic windows of 50 Kb after the predictions per position were calculated in order to compare with the LOESS correction protocol. The counts were normalized by the aggregated predictions per window and multiplied by the reciprocal of the mappability value of the window as described before.

Estimating the best GC window size

Benjamini and Speed found that the GC window size that captures the most variation was comparable to the length of the DNA fragments in the library. They recommended the use of the median fragment length of a sample. However, paired-end information was not available in the libraries used in this study so the fragment sizes could not be determined directly. Hence, the Total Variation from Independence score (TV-score) described by Benjamini and Speed was employed to find the optimal GC window.

The TV-score is a measure of how much of the variation in read depth is explained by conditioning on GC. Since it was known that the majority of plasma DNA fragments are shorter than 500 bp, the TV-score was calculated for GC-window sizes from one bp up to 700 bp. For each sample, the GC window that gave a high TV score and was comparable to fragment lengths of plasma DNA was used in the single position model.

Investigating the fragmentation bias in plasma DNA

In their work, Benjamini and Speed examined the fragmentation bias present in genomic DNA and investigated the effect of this bias on the coverage. They concluded that in the genomic data the bias due to fragmentation was not significant, whilst GC content of the fragments was an important factor in determining coverage. We investigated fragmentation effects in this study due to the possibility that fragmentation bias plays a more important role in cell-free DNA given its exposure to non-random, biological processes such as apoptosis, which could result in fragmentation bias effects.

The following investigations were carried out in all 29 samples using stringently mapped reads (mapping quality greater than 60) that aligned to the 5′ and 3′ strands separately. The proportions of each nucleotide (A, T, C, G) in an interval surrounding read starts were calculated to examine any perturbations in the nucleotide proportions at the sites of DNA fragmentation.

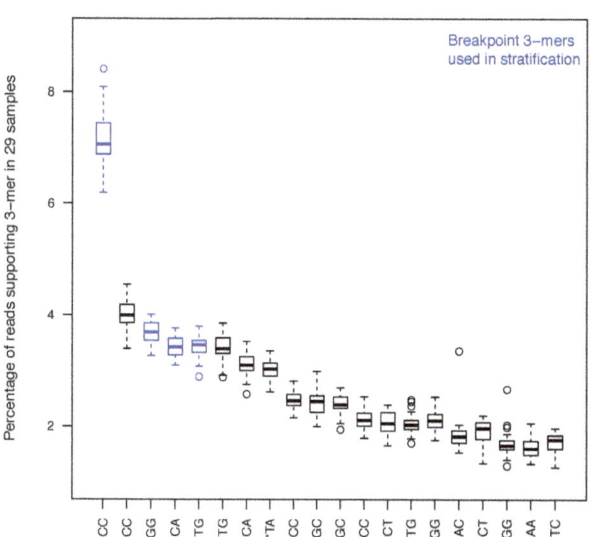

Figure 6. Investigating DNA motifs at the fragment breakpoints. The percentage of reads for the top twenty 3-mers at the 5′ breakpoint across all samples. Four high frequency motifs (shown in color) were grouped into one class and used in the stratification of reads. This grouping presented the divergent GC profiles shown in Figure 7.

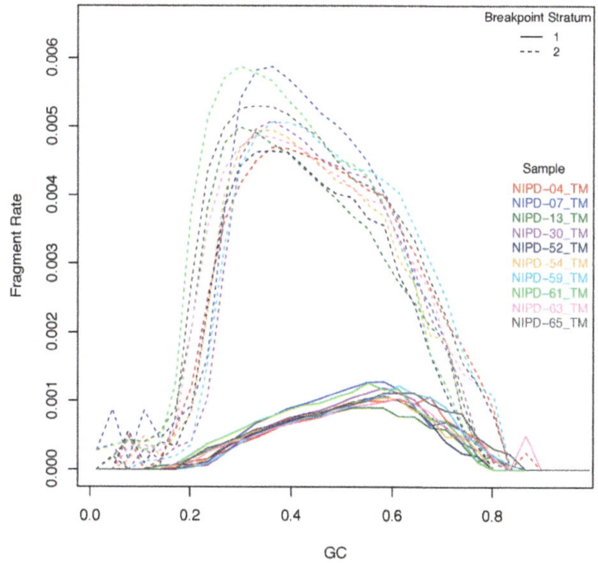

Figure 7. The GC bias profiles of the fragmentation motif classes. The GC profile of reads belonging to stratum 1 (reads with motifs C*CC, C*GG, C*CA and C*TG inferred from the positions −2, 0, 1 of the mapped reads) and stratum 2 (not any of these 4 motifs). Within each sample, the GC bias show different peak locations for the two sets of DNA fragments, indicating the need for separate corrections.

Subsequently, the TV-score statistic was used to find which positions at the cleavage site were most influential in the fragmentation bias in order to reduce the fragmentation signature involving more than 18 positions. It should be noted that the TV-score is not specific to quantifying how much of the variation in read coverage is explained by the GC content of a window hence could also be used for this purpose. Reads were stratified according to the type of base at different positions surrounding the read starts and the fragment rates in these strata were used to calculate TV scores. The TV score in this setting measures how much variation in the read coverage is explained by conditioning on the base at each position. The positions that gave a high value relative to the others were determined visually and were aggregated. Thus, reads were stratified according to the k-mer at two or more positions instead of at a single position. This process was repeated until there was no visible increase in the TV-score and resulted in a simplified model for the bias by describing a motif consisting of the second base before the fragment starts as well as the first two bases into the fragment (positions -2,0,1), other bases did not impact the TV score once these bases were included in the model. The motif of nucleotides at these positions for a given read will henceforth be referred to as its breakpoint 3-mer. For example, C*CC is the breakpoint 3-mer corresponding to C at the −2,0 and 1 positions around the breakpoint with any of the four bases allowed at the −1 position.

Four nucleotides at three positions about the breakpoint result in a possible 64 combinations (4^3) of breakpoint 3-mers. The proportions of all 3-mers were assessed for the 29 samples to detect any motifs that were consistently over-represented.

For both strands the frequency of reads for the common top twenty 3-mers was calculated and the rest were aggregated into a single class. In order to assess any strand specific fragmentation signature, a chi-square test for homogeneity was carried out to compare the proportions of the two multinomial distributions.

Incorporating fragmentation effect into the single-position model

The fragmentation bias can be corrected by applying read stratification by motif. Reads were stratified according to the breakpoint 3-mer and the single-position GC correction was carried out within each separate stratum. Stratifying reads from low-coverage datasets into 64 classes creates too many strata with low counts of fragments; hence the strata were pooled into two classes that were determined by examining the GC profiles of fragments in the strata as well as the marginal frequency distributions.

With this stratification, the single-position model produces two predicted counts for every 50 Kb genomic bin. To correct the count in a bin, its observed counts for each stratum were normalized by their respective stratum predictions. The corrected stratum bin counts were aggregated within a bin using the proportion of reads belonging to the two strata as weights.

Test for trisomy

Bias corrected sequence counts in genomic windows were used to calculate a standard Z-test of proportions as described by Chiu et al. [19]. The chromosome 21 proportion metric $\hat{p}_j$ was computed for each sample, as the total bin count for chromosome 21 divided by the sum of the bin counts for all chromosomes except for the Y chromosome. The Z-score was defined as,

$$Z_j = \frac{\hat{p}_j - p_0}{\sqrt{\frac{p_0(1-p_0)}{n}}}$$

where $\hat{p}_j$ is the chromosome 21 proportion for sample j and p_0 is the mean of the chromosome 21 proportions for the 20 non-trisomy samples (reference set, $n = 20$). A Z-score value of greater than 3 was chosen as a threshold to determine rejection of diploidy. This represents a chromosome 21 proportion greater than that of the 99.9th percentile of the reference set under the assumption of diploidy for a one-tailed Normal distribution.

Evaluation of the bias correction algorithms

The performance of the different bias correction protocols was assessed by evaluating their ability to detect the known trisomy samples as the depth of sequencing was artificially reduced. For this purpose, aligned reads in each of the 29 datasets were separately sampled without replacement to generate different proportions to simulate data of lower coverage. The proportions used were 0.75, 0.5, 0.25, 0.125, 0.0625 and 0.0312. For each sample, the sub-sampled reads were processed as described previously and the sequence data at the 7 different coverage

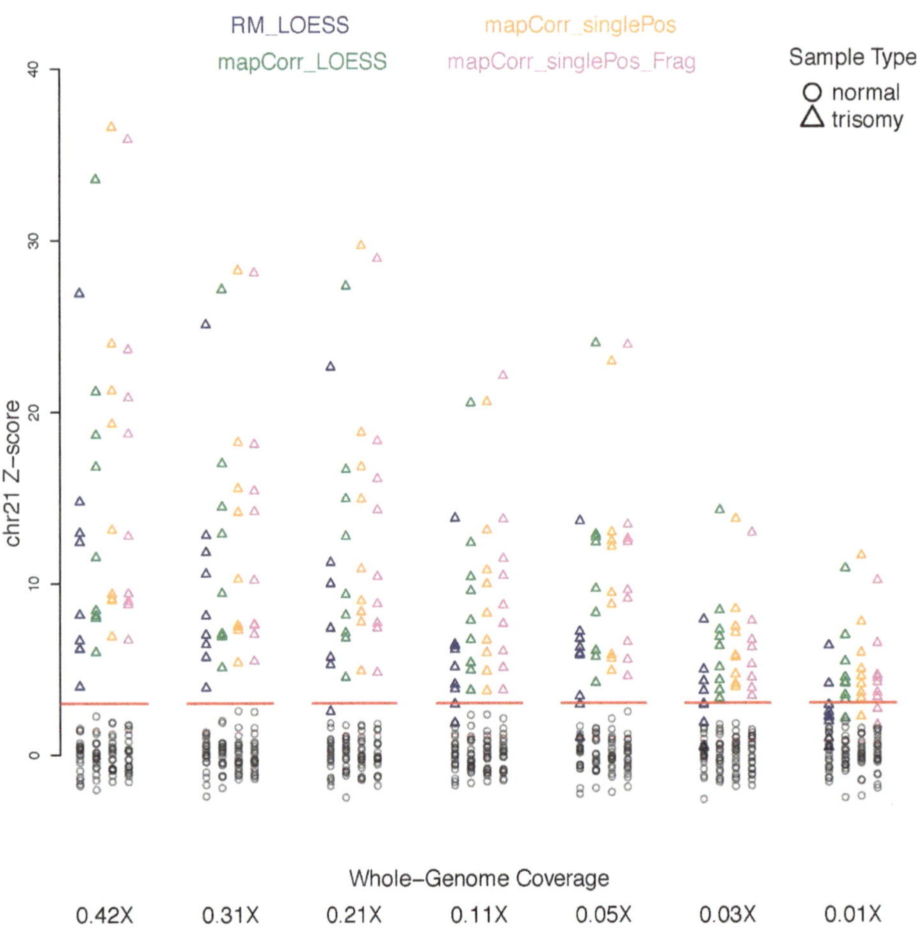

Figure 8. Performance of the bias correction algorithms. Chromosome 21 Z-scores for the four different methods as coverage is reduced. (Blue: RM_LOESS, Green: mapCorr_LOESS, Orange: mapCorr_singlePos, Violet: mapCorr_singlePos_ Frag). The red line denotes the diagnostic threshold of +3 for trisomy 21 detection.

levels (original coverage as well as the 6 lower coverage levels) were run through the four different bias correction protocols.

Firstly, the data processed using the algorithms RM_LOESS and mapCorr_LOESS was used to compare the effect of the two methods for handling repeat regions in the genome. A LOESS smoother is separately fit to the data after each repeat handling protocol was carried out. The performance of the two methods is assessed by calculating the mean of the absolute difference between the observed fragment count and the LOESS prediction in each 50 Kb genomic bin. This estimate is known as the Mean Absolute Deviation (MAD). The MAD allows the comparison of the prediction error of the two LOESS models.

Secondly, the Z-score test was performed and the accuracy of trisomy detection between all four protocols was assessed. The difference between the 95th percentile of the normal chromosome 21 Z-scores and the 5th percentile of trisomy Z-scores (known as the discriminatory distance in NIPT literature) was calculated at each coverage level, as an additional method for comparison of the protocols.

Once the most sensitive bias correction algorithm was identified, an investigation was carried out to determine if this protocol could detect trisomy in a reference free setting to mimic the situation where no reference pool was available and to investigate the necessity of using the Z-score. This was done using methodology similar to the work of Fan and Quake [41], where the corrected bin counts of each chromosome were compared to all other chromosomes within the sample in order to detect over-representation. The details of this analysis are provided in Text S1.

Results

Clinical details and sequence read statistics for the plasma DNA samples from 29 women are specified in Table 1. The gestational age of the pregnancies at the time of phlebotomy ranged from 9 to 16 weeks. Six-plex format, 50 bp single-end sequencing on the Illumina HiSeq 2000 platform generated a total number of reads ranging from 24.8 million to 40.3 million (an average of 32.1 million reads per sample). Novoalign was able to align an average of 88% of the total reads to the ambiguous reference while BWA mapped 86% to the non-ambiguous reference.

Table 2 provides coverage statistics for the 29 samples after the raw reads were processed (aligned, filtered for multi-mapping, duplicates and mismatches). At the original sequencing depth, the samples exhibited average genome wide fold coverage of 0.42X (26 million reads) using Novoalign. The coverage was gradually reduced, through subsampling of the aligned data based on the Novoalign alignment, until the number of reads was comparable to the amount generated on an Illumina MiSeq sequencer with read lengths of 50 bp (proportions 0.125–0.0312 leading to coverage of 0.053X – 0.014X). The complementary statistics for the data aligned by BWA is given in Table S1.

Assessment of mappability bias

The effect of mappability on the read coverage is shown in Figure 1 using two representative samples. The mapping bias in the plasma samples show no difference to the bias reported for genomic DNA in that the mappability effect was linear and therefore a reciprocal correction was suitable.

Repeat handling

Figure 2 presents the Mean Absolute Deviation (MAD) or prediction error in data processed using the algorithms RM_LOESS and mapCorr_LOESS. MAD estimates are presented for the 29 samples at all seven coverage levels. The protocol that made use of the mappability correction (mapCorr_LOESS) consistently gave a lower error than that which made use of the method based on removing reads identified as repetitive by RepeatMasker (RM_LOESS). For coverages between 0.42X to 0.21X, mapCorr_LOESS (green) reduces error by 80% in comparison to RM_LOESS (blue) whilst for the lower sequencing depth the reduction in error is approximately 30%.

Estimating the best GC window size for the single-position model

Figure 3 shows the TV score as the GC window length is incrementally increased from one to 700 bp for 10 representative samples. All samples showed a spike for window sizes less than 10 bp, at the start of the read fragments. This is evidence for an abundance of GC dependent motifs at the fragment breakpoints. Disregarding the fragmentation effect, high TV-scores can also be seen in the range of 150–250 bp, but the function is very flat, making it difficult to determine a maximum. Similar plots for genomic/nuclear DNA derived NGS data show clear peaks at the median fragment lengths of the DNA library [37]. In contrast, plasma data indicates a range of values that is consistent with the nucleosomal lengths associated with plasma DNA fragments and the fact that DNA was not size selected in the library preparation step. When the TV scores for a sample did not indicate a clear maximum, the window size of 180 bp was chosen, which is similar to the average length of DNA wrapped around a nucleosome. The optimal GC window size selected for each sample is provided in Table S2.

Fragmentation Effect

The investigation of base composition around the read starts presented a strong fragmentation effect. Figure 4 shows the

Table 3. Discriminatory distances for the different corrections at the 7 coverage levels.

Coverage	RM_LOESS	mapCorr_LOESS	mapCorr_singlePos	mapCorr_singlePos_Frag
0.42X	2.55	4.60	7.43	4.97
0.31X	2.67	3.20	5.04	3.88
0.21X	0.94	3.46	4.54	3.29
0.11X	0.27	2.05	2.95	2.23
0.053X	−0.19	2.69	3.40	3.36
0.026X	−1.07	1.78	2.54	2.13
0.014X	−1.07	0.52	0.94	0.28

Table 4. Accuracy estimates for the different corrections at the 7 coverage levels.

Coverage	RM_LOESS	mapCorr_LOESS	mapCorr_singlePos	mapCorr_singlePos_Frag
0.42X	100%	100%	100%	100%
0.31X	100%	100%	100%	100%
0.21X	96.6%	100%	100%	100%
0.11X	93.1%	100%	100%	100%
0.053X	93.1%	100%	100%	100%
0.026X	82.8%	100%	100%	100%
0.014X	75.9%	96.6%	96.6%	93.1%

relative abundance of nucleotides at positions up to 25 bp on either side of the fragment breakpoint (represented as the average across all 29 samples). The nucleotides show a position-specific pattern between the bases beginning 8–9 positions before the fragment and ending 8–10 positions inside the read fragment. Guanine (G) and Cytosine (C) bases are preferentially observed at the breakpoint as indicated previously by the TV score plot. There is no evidence for a strand specific fragmentation signature since the 3′ ends of the fragments show the reverse complement of the 5′ pattern. Although the pattern extends over ~18 positions, the position specific TV-score plots (Figure 5) show that the most influential bases can be found at positions −2, 0 and 1, with 0 indicating the start of reads. Hence, these positions can be used to simplify the motif structure for analysis purposes.

This fragmentation pattern was also represented in plasma DNA prepared using the beta ChIP-Seq library protocol optimized for low input DNA with no actual chromatin immunoprecipitation (data not shown). Furthermore, this fragmentation signature is highly replicable across technical replicates and independent samples with very little variability indicating that it is likely to be reflecting the existence of biological signal in the observed circulating cfDNA fragments.

A preference for specific motifs was apparent when reads were classed into the 64 possible 3-mers using the positions at −2,0,1 relative to the breakpoints. Figure 6 shows the proportions across the 29 samples using reads mapping to the 5′ strand. The C*CC motif was over-represented above all others with a median percentage of 7%. The motifs of T*CC, C*GG, C*CA, C*TG and T*TG were also given a higher preference (3–4.5%). The plot shows that the proportions have minimal variation between samples and the chi-square test for homogeneity using the motif proportions between the two DNA strands showed no evidence of originating from different distributions (p-values for the 29 samples ranged between 0.095 and 0.971).

Examination of GC bias profiles stratified for membership of each of the eight highest frequency motifs in Figure 6 showed that only four of these (C*CC, C*GG, C*CA and C*TG) influenced the differences in TVscore. Reads were stratified according to whether they had any one of these motifs (stratum 1), or not (stratum 2), with stratum 1 constituting around 16% of data in each sample. Figure 7 shows the GC bias (mean fragment rates vs. GC content) when the single-position model was run on the stratified reads. The GC-bias curve in stratum 1 shows a shift towards higher GC content compared to stratum 2.

Looking across all 29 samples, stratum 1 has the maximum number of reads observed for 60% GC on average (standard deviation = 0.04) while stratum 2 has the maximum number of reads observed at 37% GC (standard deviation = 0.08). The obvious shift in the GC peaks between the fragments of the two strata was the motivation for correcting the reads of the 2 strata separately.

Evaluation of the bias correction algorithms

Figure 8 shows the chromosome 21 Z-scores for each coverage level and bias correction protocol. Table 3 provides the discriminatory distance between the trisomy and normal Z-scores as a summary of Figure 8. Negative values of this statistic occur when the distributions of trisomy and normal Z-scores overlap eachother.

The RM_LOESS bias correction method loses sensitivity more rapidly than all the other methods as the coverage is reduced, beginning to gain false negatives at 0.2X coverage. mapCorr_-LOESS performs better than RM_LOESS at all depths. The single position GC correction performs better than a LOESS correction as it increases the separation between the trisomy and normal samples. It should be noted that the discriminatory distance of the single position protocol at 0.056X is larger than that of the RM_LOESS method at the original coverage of 0.42X. The improvement of this new protocol over the RM_LOESS method is replicated in trend in the data aligned using BWA as an alternative aligner to Novoalign (Figure S1). Stratifying by breakpoint motif does not show an improvement over the original single position model, despite showing a difference in GC profiles for reads of the two strata. These observations are further corroborated in the accuracy estimates provided in Table 4.

Figure S3 shows that the order of the trisomy samples (based on the Z-score) stays relatively constant as the coverage is reduced.

Despite the clear improvement seen in the mapCorr_singlePos model, we also see that not all intra-chromosomal variation is removed and that it is necessary to use reference samples via the Z-score to remove remaining bias, which cannot currently be modeled (Figure S2).

Discussion

In the past few years there have been major advances in the area of sequencing-based non-invasive prenatal testing (NIPT). To date, a number of large-scale clinical validation studies have shown that whole-genome sequencing of circulating cell-free DNA (ccfDNA) in maternal plasma can be used to detect fetal aneuploidy with high accuracy. Published tests including those in commercial use, utilize variations of the molecular counting approach where following the mapping of sequence reads to the human reference genome, the relative numbers of fragments per chromosomes are counted to detect deviations due to the extra genetic material in the fetus.

We have demonstrated that using a more refined method for GC correction and improvements in the handling of repetitive genomic regions can lead to substantial improvements in the sensitivity of the standard statistical test for trisomy 21 detection. We would suggest that with the rapid progression of the field and a focus on the roll out of large-scale studies some of the assumptions and practices made early on in the work should no longer be perpetuated but be replaced with improved analysis techniques such as those that we have demonstrated.

The first proof-of-principle NIPT studies dealt with the 'hard-to-map' repeat regions of the genome by aligning the sequencing reads to the repeat masked human reference. Since 50% of the genome [35] is designated as some type of repeat, it was determined that the speed, quality and quantity of mapping was lowered when aligning directly to the masked reference and that it also lead to increased false-positives in trisomy detection [42]. Later NIPT studies opted to remove any reads in the annotated regions post-alignment (using the RepeatMasker database). Even as the sequencing-based NIPT was clinically translated and the sequencing depth was dramatically reduced for cost-efficiency the practice of using RepeatMasker persisted.

This study demonstrates the application of an alternative method for repeat handling, where the mappability of regions is calculated and read counts are corrected by these values instead of using the RepeatMasker method. Our work shows that by using this 'soft' approach rather than hard filtering, one can avoid unnecessarily reducing the read coverage and increasing the variation of bin counts due to uneven removal of reads. In line with our findings, a large-scale NIPT study recently reported that filtering RepeatMasker regions in moderation rather than the current severe practice, also increases the performance of NIPT [43].

To correct the GC bias we opted to use the protocol introduced by Benjamini and Speed in 2012. In their work, using genomic DNA, it was shown that a correction based on the single position model eliminates more GC bias than a LOESS correction. Since LOESS is the method of choice in whole genome NIPT, we employed the single position GC model to investigate its performance in the setting of trisomy detection using plasma DNA. This is the first instance of the application of this model in the NIPT setting.

The result of our work shows that the single-position GC correction coupled with the aforementioned mappability correction shows a significant improvement over the LOESS method with RepeatMasker by maintaining 100% sensitivity of trisomy detection over a range of decreasing depths of coverage. In particular, the latest NGS based NIPT studies, use approximately 0.2X coverage while we demonstrate 100% sensitivity down to 0.03X or $1/7^{th}$ the data. The discriminatory distance between trisomy and normal samples is also much higher with the new bias correction. We also show that these improvements are not aligner specific by replicating the results using a different alignment algorithm.

The performance of the methods we have demonstrated would improve further if a larger pool of reference samples were available or by using reference samples that show better matching to reduce technical variation between sequencing runs [24,32,44]. Another approach made possible with larger groups of reference samples, adopted by some NIPT analysis protocols, involves matching chromosomes of interest to reference chromosomes that have similar coverage variation across sequencing runs. This is one method whereby the expected read counts are adjusted to correct remaining bias after standard intra-sample adjustments for GC and repeats [31,36]. This method is based on ad-hoc criteria and it would be desirable to identify and remove further sources of bias using justifiable approaches. Our study is carried out with a limited number of samples; hence the above methods are not applicable. By improving intra-sample bias correction strategies, we can reduce the reliance on reference samples, but as yet it is not possible to forego these entirely as we have also demonstrated.

In addition to the improvement in bias reduction, the single position model estimates corrections at the single base pair level, rather than at a binned level so it has clear advantages in terms of resolution when detecting sub-chromosomal copy number changes in the fetus. However, in an effort to benchmark our improvements against existing protocols we have not taken full advantage of these improvements. For example we bin our single base pair predictions into 50 Kb bins, using the standard protocol currently favored by researchers. We have evidence (data not shown) that further gains are possible if the size of the window for binning was reduced, analogously to Benjamini and Speed [37]. If paired-end information is available the model can also be extended to incorporate different fragment lengths as the bias stems from the GC content of the full DNA fragment. This would lead to an even more sensitive correction as plasma DNA shows a multi-modal size distribution with fetal and maternal fragments differing in lengths. We were not able to investigate the further possible gains this would make in trisomy 21 detection, as we did not have paired-end data.

We also investigated the effects due to the natural cleavage of plasma DNA using moderate coverage sequencing data, which has not been explored in depth using next generation sequencing. When using genomic DNA the input genetic material is fragmented artificially via sonication or nebulization protocols, which creates a wide array of fragment lengths. These are then size-selected depending on research specifications. In contrast, plasma DNA is fragmented by natural nuclease action and the fragments are not size selected in the library preparation for NGS.

We have shown that there are several high frequency motifs in the nucleotide frequencies spanning 8–10 positions on either side of the DNA cleavage site and that the positions on which fragment rates depend the most are the second base before the breakpoint as well as the first two bases into the fragment. We note that the cytosine rich motif that we observe at these positions has also been reported by others using cloned ccfDNA [45]. However, in an in-vitro study of the apoptotic digestion of lymphocyte chromatin, an AT-rich motif was uncovered [46], indicating that the enriched motifs we observe in our data are likely to result from a combination of biological processes.

When sequence fragments were stratified by over-represented motifs, a shift in the GC bias curve between strata was revealed, which was an indication that these fragments should be corrected separately, in two groups. However, there was no improvement over the results of the single position GC model with the mappability correction using the un-stratified data, and the stratified method performed marginally worse. This could be due to the presence of only a small subset of the reads (16%) that fall into the stratum with the enriched motifs and estimating the bias with a small number of reads at a low sequencing depth generates too much variability at the gain of little bias improvement.

The fragmentation effect seen in plasma DNA is different to that seen in genomic NGS data [37,47]. Since these observations are highly replicable across multiple samples and across different library preparation protocols we have reason to believe that these enriched motifs reflect the existence of real biological signals. Since the enzymatic action related to plasma DNA cleavage is not fully understood, the DNA fragments may stem from multiple sources, including different nucleases with differing cleavage sites and trimming of exposed fragment ends. These various processes could dilute the fragmentation motifs and result in a highly complex mixture that we only indirectly incorporate into the proposed model. We cannot rule out the possibility that there may be some motif signal arising from technical aspects of the library preparation for ccfDNA (e.g. end-repair), but this can only be teased apart by carefully designed, deep sequencing experiments.

Whilst we have employed a better correction for GC bias in plasma DNA sequencing samples, there exist further sources of bias, which are as yet unknown, and cannot currently be corrected for within samples. The removal of these sources of bias necessitates the use of reference samples. These sources of variation need to be investigated further through deeper sequencing and analysis of plasma derived DNA. Such an analysis will also extend our biological understanding of the plasma DNA cleavage process.

Supporting Information

Figure S1 Chromosome 21 Z-scores for the two main bias correction protocols as coverage is reduced in read data aligned by BWA. Blue: RM_LOESS, Orange: mapCorr_singlePos. The red line denotes the diagnostic threshold of +3 for trisomy 21 detection.

Figure S2 Reference free, intra-sample trisomy detection with the single position GC model with mappability correction. The plot of the minimum t-statistic for each chromosome in all 29 samples, calculated from pair-wise Welsh t-tests. The dashed line corresponds to the statistic associated with $\alpha<0.001/(22\times21$ comparisons).

Figure S3 Tracking samples across the different methods and coverage levels. Chromosome 21 Z-scores for the four different methods as coverage is reduced. Different symbols are used to track the trisomy samples across the different coverage levels in each bias correction protocol. (Blue: RM_LOESS, Green: mapCorr_LOESS, Orange: mapCorr_singlePos, Violet: mapCorr_singlePos_ Frag). The red line denotes the diagnostic threshold of +3 for trisomy 21 detection.

Table S1 Genome-wide coverage at each sampling proportion for the 29 datasets after BWA mapping and subsequent read filtering.

Table S2 GC window sizes for the 29 samples estimated using the TV score.

Text S1 Reference-free intra-sample trisomy detection.

Acknowledgments

The authors are grateful to the pregnant women who participated in this study. We would like to thank Keith Satterley for his help with technical issues in data storage, Dr. Ingrid Lönnstedt for discussions on the single position model and The Australian Genomic Research Facility (AGRF) staff, Dr. Sue Forrest, Dr. Matthew Stevens and Matthew Tinning, for valuable discussions about the DNA sequencing aspects of this study.

Author Contributions

Conceived and designed the experiments: MB NPT HRS DLB TPS. Performed the experiments: DG. Analyzed the data: DC. Contributed reagents/materials/analysis tools: DG DLB HRS YB. Wrote the paper: DC MB NPT DG DLB HRS YB TPS. Designed the software used in analysis: YB TPS.

References

1. Acog Practice Bulletine No 88 (2007) Invasive prenatal testing for aneuploidy. Obstetrics and Gynecology 110: 1459–1467.
2. Driscoll DA, Gross S (2009) Prenatal screening for aneuploidy. New England Journal of Medicine 360: 2556–2562–2502.
3. Wellesley D, Dolk H, Boyd PA, Greenlees R, Haeusler M, et al. (2012) Rare chromosome abnormalities, prevalence and prenatal diagnosis rates from population-based congenital anomaly registers in Europe. European Journal of Human Genetics.
4. Morris JK, Alberman E (2009) Trends in Down's syndrome live births and antenatal diagnoses in England and Wales from 1989 to 2008: analysis of data from the National Down Syndrome Cytogenetic Register. BMJ (Clinical research ed) 339.
5. Ferguson-Smith MA, Bianchi DW (2010) Prenatal Diagnosis: Past, present, and future. Prenatal Diagnosis 30: 601–604.
6. Lo YMD, Corbetta N, Chamberlain PF, Rai V, Sargent IL, et al. (1997) Presence of fetal DNA in maternal plasma and serum. Lancet 350: 485–487.
7. Chiu RWK, Chan KCA, Gao Y, Lau VYM, Zheng W, et al. (2008) Noninvasive prenatal diagnosis of fetal chromosomal aneuploidy by massively parallel genomic sequencing of DNA in maternal plasma. Proceedings of the National Academy of Sciences of the United States of America 105: 20458–20463.
8. Fan HC, Blumenfeld YJ, Chitkara U, Hudgins L, Quake SR (2008) Noninvasive diagnosis of fetal aneuploidy by shotgun sequencing DNA from maternal blood. Proceedings of the National Academy of Sciences of the United States of America 105: 16266–16271.
9. Chitty LS, Bianchi DW (2013) Noninvasive prenatal testing: the paradigm is shifting rapidly. Prenatal Diagnosis 33: 511–513.
10. Boon EMJ, Faas BHW (2013) Benefits and limitations of whole genome versus targeted approaches for noninvasive prenatal testing for fetal aneuploidies. Prenatal Diagnosis 33: 563–568.
11. Mandel P, Metais P (1948) Les acides nucléiques du plasma sanguin chez l'homme. CR Acad Sci Paris 142: 241–243.
12. Lui YYN, Chik K-W, Chiu RWK, Ho C-Y, Lam CWK, et al. (2002) Predominant hematopoietic origin of cell-free DNA in plasma and serum after sex-mismatched bone marrow transplantation. Clinical Chemistry 48: 421–427.
13. Stroun M, Lyautey J, Lederrey C, Olson-Sand A, Anker P (2001) About the possible origin and mechanism of circulating DNA: Apoptosis and active DNA release. Proceedings of the Chinese Congress of Clinical Chemistry and Laboratory Medicine 2000 313: 139–142.
14. Jahr S, Hentze H, Englisch S, Hardt D, Fackelmayer FO, et al. (2001) DNA fragments in the blood plasma of cancer patients: quantitations and evidence for their origin from apoptotic and necrotic cells. Cancer research 61: 1659–1665.
15. van der Vaart M, Pretorius PJ (2007) The origin of circulating free DNA. Clinical Chemistry 53: 2215.
16. Stroun M, Anker P (2005) Circulating DNA in higher organisms cancer detection brings back to life an ignored phenomenon. Cellular and molecular biology (Noisy-le-Grand, France) 51: 767–774.
17. Peters DL, Pretorius PJ (2011) Origin, translocation and destination of extracellular occurring DNA – a new paradigm in genetic behaviour. Clinica chimica acta; international journal of clinical chemistry 412: 806–811.
18. Lun FMF, Chiu RWK, Allen Chan KC, Yeung Leung T, Kin Lau T, et al. (2008) Microfluidics digital PCR reveals a higher than expected fraction of fetal DNA in maternal plasma. Clinical Chemistry 54: 1664–1672.
19. Chiu RWK, Akolekar R, Zheng YWL, Leung TY, Sun H, et al. (2011) Noninvasive prenatal assessment of trisomy 21 by multiplexed maternal plasma DNA sequencing: Large scale validity study. BMJ 342: 217.
20. Lo YMD, Tein MSC, Lau TK, Haines CJ, Leung TN, et al. (1998) Quantitative analysis of fetal DNA in maternal plasma and serum: Implications for noninvasive prenatal diagnosis. American Journal of Human Genetics 62: 768–775.
21. Liao GJW, Lun FMF, Zheng YWL, Chan KCA, Leung TY, et al. (2011) Targeted massively parallel sequencing of maternal plasma DNA permits efficient and unbiased detection of fetal alleles. Clinical Chemistry 57: 92–101.
22. Ariga H, Ohto H, Busch MP, Imamura S, Watson R, et al. (2001) Kinetics of fetal cellular and cell-free DNA in the maternal circulation during and after pregnancy: implications for noninvasive prenatal diagnosis. Transfusion 41: 1524–1530.
23. Ashoor G, Poon L, Syngelaki A, Mosimann B, Nicolaides KH (2012) Fetal fraction in maternal plasma cell-free DNA at 11–13 weeks' gestation: Effect of maternal and fetal factors. Fetal Diagnosis and Therapy 31: 237–243.

24. Palomaki GE, Kloza EM, Lambert-Messerlian GM, Haddow JE, Neveux LM, et al. (2011) DNA sequencing of maternal plasma to detect Down syndrome: An international clinical validation study. Genetics in Medicine 13: 913–920.
25. Wataganara T, Metzenbauer M, Peter I, Johnson KL, Bianchi DW (2005) Placental volume, as measured by 3-dimensional sonography and levels of maternal plasma cell-free fetal DNA. American Journal of Obstetrics and Gynecology 193: 496–500.
26. Alberry M, Maddocks D, Jones M, Abdel Hadi M, Abdel-Fattah S, et al. (2007) Free fetal DNA in maternal plasma in anembryonic pregnancies: Confirmation that the origin is the trophoblast. Prenatal Diagnosis 27: 415–418.
27. Fan HC, Blumenfeld YJ, Chitkara U, Hudgins L, Quake SR (2010) Analysis of the size distributions of fetal and maternal cell-free DNA by paired-end sequencing. Clinical Chemistry 56: 1279–1286.
28. Szerlong HJ, Hansen JC (2011) Nucleosome distribution and linker DNA: connecting nuclear function to dynamic chromatin structure. Biochemistry and cell biology Biochimie et biologie cellulaire 89: 24–34.
29. Norton ME, Brar H, Weiss J, Karimi A, Laurent LC, et al. (2012) Non-Invasive Chromosomal Evaluation (NICE) Study: results of a multicenter prospective cohort study for detection of fetal trisomy 21 and trisomy 18. American Journal of Obstetrics and Gynecology 207.
30. Zimmermann B, Hill M, Gemelos G, Demko Z, Banjevic M, et al. (2012) Noninvasive prenatal aneuploidy testing of chromosomes 13, 18, 21, X, and Y, using targeted sequencing of polymorphic loci. Prenatal Diagnosis 32: 1233–1241.
31. Bianchi DW, Platt LD, Goldberg JD, Abuhamad AZ, Sehnert AJ, et al. (2012) Genome-wide fetal aneuploidy detection by maternal plasma DNA sequencing. Obstetrics and Gynecology 119: 890–901.
32. Palomaki GE, Deciu C, Kloza EM, Lambert-Messerlian GM, Haddow JE, et al. (2012) DNA sequencing of maternal plasma reliably identifies trisomy 18 and trisomy 13 as well as Down syndrome: an international collaborative study. Genetics in medicine: official journal of the American College of Medical Genetics 14: 296–305.
33. Dan S, Wang W, Ren J, Li Y, Hu H, et al. (2012) Clinical application of massively parallel sequencing-based prenatal noninvasive fetal trisomy test for trisomies 21 and 18 in 11 105 pregnancies with mixed risk factors. Prenatal Diagnosis: 1–8.
34. Alkan C, Kidd JM, Marques-Bonet T, Aksay G, Antonacci F, et al. (2009) Personalized copy number and segmental duplication maps using next-generation sequencing. Nature Genetics 41: 1061–1067.
35. Smit AFA, Hubley R, Green P (1996) RepeatMasker Open-3.0. RepeatMasker Open-30.
36. Sehnert AJ, Rhees B, Comstock D, De Feo E, Heilek G, et al. (2011) Optimal detection of fetal chromosomal abnormalities by massively parallel DNA sequencing of cell-free fetal DNA from maternal blood. Clinical Chemistry 57: 1042–1049.
37. Benjamini Y, Speed TP (2012) Summarizing and correcting the GC content bias in high-throughput sequencing. Nucleic Acids Research 40: e72.
38. Li H, Handsaker B, Wysoker A, Fennell T, Ruan J, et al. (2009) The Sequence Alignment/Map format and SAMtools. Bioinformatics 25: 2078–2079.
39. R Development CoreTeam (2010) R: A language and environment for statistical computing. R Foundation for Statistical Computing Vienna, Austria.
40. Derrien T, Estellé J, Marco Sola S, Knowles DG, Raineri E, et al. (2012) Fast computation and applications of genome mappability. PLoS ONE 7: e30377.
41. Fan H, Quake S (2010) Sensitivity of noninvasive prenatal detection of fetal aneuploidy from maternal plasma using shotgun sequencing is limited only by counting statistics. PLoS ONE 5.
42. Chen EZ, Chiu RWK, Sun H, Akolekar R, Chan KCA, et al. (2011) Noninvasive prenatal diagnosis of fetal trisomy 18 and trisomy 13 by maternal plasma dna sequencing. PLoS ONE 6.
43. Jensen TJ, Zwiefelhofer T, Tim RC, Dzakula Z, Kim SK, et al. (2013) High-throughput massively parallel sequencing for fetal aneuploidy detection from maternal plasma. PLoS ONE 8: e57381.
44. Ehrich M, Deciu C, Zwiefelhofer T, Tynan JA, Cagasan L, et al. (2011) Noninvasive detection of fetal trisomy 21 by sequencing of DNA in maternal blood: a study in a clinical setting. American Journal of Obstetrics and Gynecology 204: 205.e201–205.e211.
45. Suzuki N, Kamataki A, Yamaki J, Homma Y (2008) Characterization of circulating DNA in healthy human plasma. Clinica Chimica Acta 387: 55–58.
46. Bettecken T, Frenkel ZM, Altmüller J, Nürnberg P, Trifonov EN (2012) Apoptotic cleavage of DNA in human lymphocyte chromatin shows high sequence specificity. Journal of biomolecular structure & dynamics 30: 211–216.
47. Hansen KD, Brenner SE, Dudoit S (2010) Biases in Illumina transcriptome sequencing caused by random hexamer priming. Nucleic Acids Research 38: e131.

A Role for Thrombospondin-1 Deficits in Astrocyte-Mediated Spine and Synaptic Pathology in Down's Syndrome

Octavio Garcia, Maria Torres, Pablo Helguera, Pinar Coskun, Jorge Busciglio*

Department of Neurobiology and Behavior, Institute for Memory Impairments and Neurological Disorders (iMIND), Center for the Neurobiology of Learning and Memory (CNLM), University of California Irvine, Irvine, California, United States of America

Abstract

Background: Down's syndrome (DS) is the most common genetic cause of mental retardation. Reduced number and aberrant architecture of dendritic spines are common features of DS neuropathology. However, the mechanisms involved in DS spine alterations are not known. In addition to a relevant role in synapse formation and maintenance, astrocytes can regulate spine dynamics by releasing soluble factors or by physical contact with neurons. We have previously shown impaired mitochondrial function in DS astrocytes leading to metabolic alterations in protein processing and secretion. In this study, we investigated whether deficits in astrocyte function contribute to DS spine pathology.

Methodology/Principal Findings: Using a human astrocyte/rat hippocampal neuron coculture, we found that DS astrocytes are directly involved in the development of spine malformations and reduced synaptic density. We also show that thrombospondin 1 (TSP-1), an astrocyte-secreted protein, possesses a potent modulatory effect on spine number and morphology, and that both DS brains and DS astrocytes exhibit marked deficits in TSP-1 protein expression. Depletion of TSP-1 from normal astrocytes resulted in dramatic changes in spine morphology, while restoration of TSP-1 levels prevented DS astrocyte-mediated spine and synaptic alterations. Astrocyte cultures derived from TSP-1 KO mice exhibited similar deficits to support spine formation and structure than DS astrocytes.

Conclusions/Significance: These results indicate that human astrocytes promote spine and synapse formation, identify astrocyte dysfunction as a significant factor of spine and synaptic pathology in the DS brain, and provide a mechanistic rationale for the exploration of TSP-1-based therapies to treat spine and synaptic pathology in DS and other neurological conditions.

Editor: Mel B. Feany, Brigham and Women's Hospital, Harvard Medical School, United States of America

Funding: This work was supported by grants from The Larry L. Hillblom Foundation and the National Institutes of Health (grant no. HD38466, and Alzheimers Disease Research Center grant no. AG16573). The funders had no role in study design, data collection and analysis, decision to publish, or preparation of the manuscript.

Competing Interests: The authors have declared that no competing interests exist.

* E-mail: jbuscigl@uci.edu

Introduction

Down's syndrome (DS) or the triplication of chromosome 21 (trisomy 21) is the most common genetic cause of mental retardation. The cognitive deficits in patients with DS have been associated with structural changes in the architecture and alterations in the number of dendritic spines [1]. Morphological abnormalities such as unusually long spines, shorter spines, and reduced number of spines have been documented in the cortex of DS fetuses and newborns [2,3]. Similar alterations were observed in the hippocampal formation, and additional reductions in spine number in adult DS patients have been linked to the development of Alzheimer's disease (AD) pathology [4,5]. Spine pathology is also present in the Ts65Dn mouse model of DS, which shows decreased spine and synaptic density, and aberrant spine morphology including enlarged spines, irregular spine heads, and globular spine shapes [6–8]. Since dendritic spines are the primary sites of excitatory synapses, defects in spine structure and function can result in synaptic and circuit alterations leading to cognitive impairment and the progression of AD pathology in DS patients [9]. Unfortunately, there is little information available on the cellular and molecular mechanisms involved in DS spine malformation.

In recent years, a number of studies indicate that astrocytes regulate the stability, dynamics and maturation of dendritic spines [10–13]. In addition, astrocytes participate in the regulation of synaptic plasticity and synaptic transmission [14–18]. Astrocytes modulate the establishment and maintenance of synaptic contacts through the release of soluble factors such as cholesterol [19] or thrombospondins [20], or by direct physical interaction with neuronal cells [10–13,21]. Our previous research indicates the presence of mitochondrial dysfunction and energy deficits in DS astrocytes leading to abnormal amyloid precursor protein (APP) processing and secretion, and to intracellular accumulation of amyloid β (Aβ) [22]. To investigate the role of astrocytes in DS spine pathology, we established a coculture system in which rat hippocampal neurons were plated on top of normal (NL) or DS astrocyte monolayers. Using this experimental paradigm, we found abnormal spine development and reduced synaptic density and activity in neurons growing on top of DS astrocytes, and identified thrombospondin 1 (TSP-1) as a critical astrocyte-secreted factor that modulates spine number and morphology. TSP-1 levels were markedly reduced in DS astrocytes and brain homogenates, and restoration of TSP-1 levels prevented spine and synaptic alterations. These results underscore the potential therapeutic use of TSP-1 to treat spine and synaptic pathology in DS and other neurodevelopmental or neurodegenerative conditions.

Results

Rat hippocampal neurons growing on top of human astrocytes develop extensive processes and dendritic spines

Previous reports have established the critical role of astrocytes in synapse formation [16,17,19–21] and regulation of dendritic spines [10–13]. However the role of astrocytes in DS spine pathology has not been investigated. Our previous results indicate the presence of mitochondrial dysfunction in DS astrocytes leading to alterations in protein secretion and intracellular Aβ accumulation [22]. To establish whether deficits in DS astrocyte function could be involved in spine pathology, rat hippocampal neurons were cultured on top of NL or DS astrocyte monolayers (Figure 1A). Under these conditions, rat hippocampal neurons survived well for extended periods of time and developed fast-growing axons and dendrites (Figure 1A). No differences in neuronal survival were observed between regular rat hippocampal cultures and rat hippocampal/human astrocyte cocultures (Figure S1). After 21 DIV, neurons developed numerous spines (Figure 1B) exhibiting characteristic shapes including stubby-, mushroom-, thin- and filopodium-like spines [23]. Stubby spines were especially abundant (Figure 1B). In contrast, human cortical neurons exhibited poor spine development in culture (data not shown), precluding their use for this study. Thus, to assess the capacity of DS astrocytes to sustain spine and synapse formation we utilized human cortical astrocyte/rat hippocampal neuron cocultures.

Altered spine number and morphology in hippocampal neurons growing on top of DS astrocytes

We used immunofluorescence to analyze spine formation in the cocultures at 21 DIV. For simplicity, we assessed both stubby- and mushroom-like spines as "stubby", and both thin- and filopodium-like spines as "filopodium" spines. We found a significant reduction in the total number of spines in neurons growing on top of DS astrocytes compared to neurons growing on top of NL astrocytes (NL: 9.1±0.5 per 50 μm of dendrite; DS: 7.1±0.6 per 50 μm of dendrite)(Figure 2A and B), indicating that DS astrocytes are less efficient than normal astrocytes in supporting dendritic spine formation. The reduction in spine density affected specifically stubby spines (NL: 4.6±0.5 stubby spines per 50 μm dendrite; DS: 2.1±0.3 stubby spines per 50 μm dendrite) (Figure 2C). Conversely, in DS astrocyte/hippocampal neuron cocultures we observed a significant increase in the number and

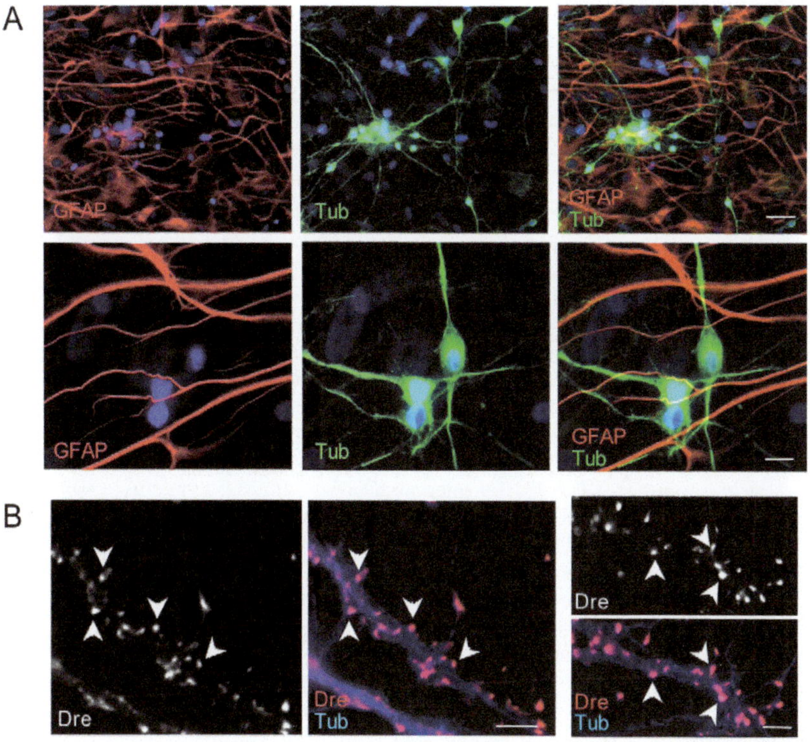

Figure 1. Human astrocyte/rat hippocampal neuron cocultures. Cocultures were prepared as described in the Methods section. **A**) After 21 DIV, the cells were fixed and immunostained with anti-GFAP (1:1000, red) to visualize astrocytes, and anti-β tubulin class III (1:1000, green) to visualize neurons. Nuclei were counterstained with Hoechst (blue). Note the significant development of neuronal processes in the cocultures. **B**) Spines (arrows) present in a typical dendritic segment visualized with anti-drebrin (1:250, red), and anti-β tubulin class III (blue). Scale bars: A: 20 μm upper panel; 10 μm lower panel. B: 5 μm.

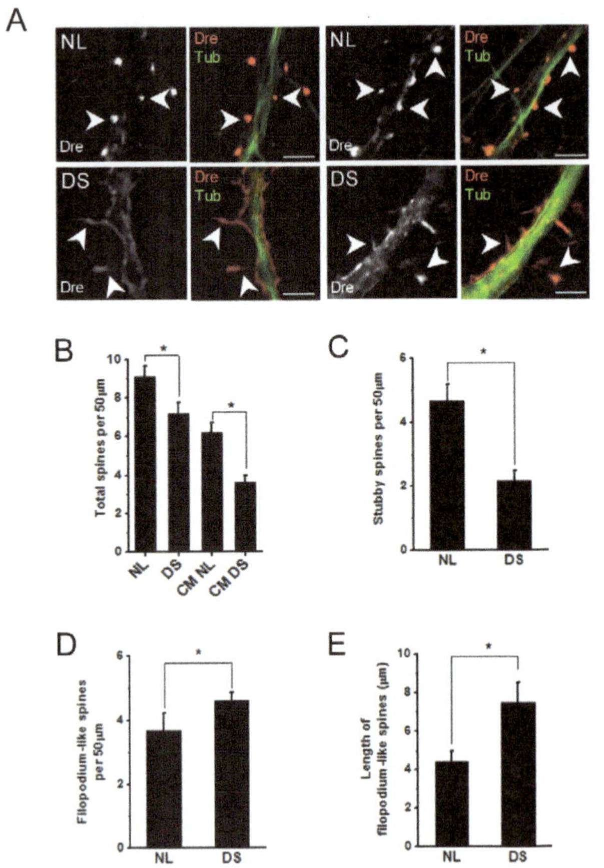

Figure 2. Spine number and morphology are altered in hippocampal neurons grown on top of DS astrocytes. A) Double immunofluorescence with anti-drebrin (red) and anti- β tubulin class III (green) illustrates typical spine morphologies (arrows) found in cocultures of neurons with NL and DS astrocytes respectively. The frequency of filopodium spines is significantly increased in DS cocultures. Scale bar: 5 µm. **B)** Image analysis indicates a significant reduction in the total number of spines in neurons grown on top of DS astrocytes or maintained in DS CM. In particular, this reduction affects stubby spines (**C**). Assessment of spine morphology in DS astrocyte cocultures shows a significant increase in the number (**D**) (NL 3.7±0.5; DS 4.6±0.2 SEM), and length (**E**) (NL 4.4±0.5; DS 7.5±1 SEM) of filopodium spines. Spine number represents the average number of spines scored in a 50 µm dendritic segment. Data were analyzed by one-way analysis of variance (ANOVA) followed by Fisher's test. All data are expressed as mean ± SEM. *$p<0.05$.

length of filopodium spines (Figure 2A, D and E), which previous studies have characterized as immature spines in hippocampal neurons [24]. Similar alterations in spine number and structure are present in DS brains [2,3,25], suggesting that astrocyte dysfunction contributes to spine pathology in DS.

Soluble factors released by astrocytes such as cholesterol or thrombospondins have been shown to modulate spine formation and the establishment and maintenance of synaptic contacts [19,20]. We assessed the effect of astrocyte-released factors on spine formation. Pure hippocampal cultures grown on polylysine and maintained with astrocyte conditioned medium (CM) exhibited somewhat lower spine density than their counterparts grown on top of astrocyte monolayers, indicating that physical contact with astrocytes is also relevant for spine formation (Figure 2B). Hippocampal neurons maintained in DS astrocyte CM showed a marked reduction in the number of spines compared to neurons maintained in NL astrocyte CM (NL CM: 6.2±0.5 spines per 50 µm of dendrite; DS CM: 3.6±0.3 spines per 50 µm of dendrite)(Figure 2B). Thus, soluble factors are critically involved in DS astrocyte-mediated spine alterations.

Reduced TSP-1 levels in DS astrocytes and DS brains

TSP-1 is an extracellular matrix protein synthesized and released by astrocytes [26], which is highly expressed during development of the nervous system [27]. It promotes neurite outgrowth and survival [28–30], neuronal migration [31,32] and synaptogenesis [20]. Recently, it has been demonstrated that TSP-1 is necessary for synaptic and motor recovery after stroke [33], suggesting that TSP-1 also participates in neuronal plasticity. Given that TSP-1 is one of the most abundant proteins secreted by human astrocytes (data not shown), and that there are marked deficits in protein secretion in DS astrocytes [22], we next analyzed TSP-1 expression and secretion in DS astrocyte cultures and brain homogenates. We found high TSP-1 expression in human astrocytes and prominent surface localization (Figure 3A-D). TSP-1 subcellular localization and staining pattern was similar in normal and DS astrocytes. Quantification of TSP-1 protein levels by ELISA demonstrated significant reductions in both DS astrocyte cell lysates and CM (Figure 3E), suggesting that reduced TSP-1 expression leads to decreased TSP-1 in DS CM. TSP-1 expression was considerably higher in fetal than in adult brain homogenates (data not shown), consistent with a significant role of TSP-1 during development [27]. A comparison of TSP-1 protein expression in fetal brain lysates showed an average reduction of 57.9% in TSP-1 levels in DS brains despite the average age of DS brain samples being almost 4 weeks younger than the average age of NL brain samples (Figure 3F). qPCR analysis of mRNA expression indicated similar mRNA levels in DS brains than in NL brains for all thrombospondin isoforms (TSP-1, -2, -3 and -4)(Figure S2), suggesting that a post transcriptional mechanism underlies the changes observed in TSP-1 in DS brains and astrocyte cultures.

TSP-1 regulates spine morphology and prevents spine alterations in neurons grown on top of DS astrocytes

We assessed the effect of TSP-1 on spine development in pure hippocampal cultures. Recombinant TSP-1 was added to the culture medium at day 7, and fresh TSP-1 was replenished every 3 days for 14 days. We used a TSP-1 dose of 250 ng/ml because it is in the range of the difference in the level of TSP-1 in CM between NL and DS astrocyte cultures (Figure 3E). TSP-1 increased significantly the number of spines compared to vehicle-treated cultures (control: 6.5±0.7 spines per 50 µm dendrite; TSP-1: 9.0±0.7 spines per 50 µm dendrite)(Figure 4A and B). The effect of TSP-1 on spine number was similar to the effect of BDNF, a well known inducer of spine development in hippocampal neurons [34,35]. Combined treatment of BDNF+TSP-1 had an additive effect on spine development, suggesting that the two factors act through non-overlapping, complementary signaling pathways (Figure 4A and B). A dose-response assay indicated that concentrations of TSP-1 between 250 ng/ml to 1250 ng/ml produced a gradual and marked increase in the number of dendritic spines in pure neuronal cultures (Figure 4C). Thus, TSP-1 is a strong promoter of spine development.

To determine whether depletion of TSP-1 is sufficient to alter spine number and morphology, NL astrocyte/hippocampal neuron cocultures were treated with anti-TSP-1 antibody to neutralize the endogenous TSP-1 secreted by NL human astrocytes. At day 7, anti-TSP-1 was added to the cultures and replenished every 3 days during 14 days. Hippocampal neurons

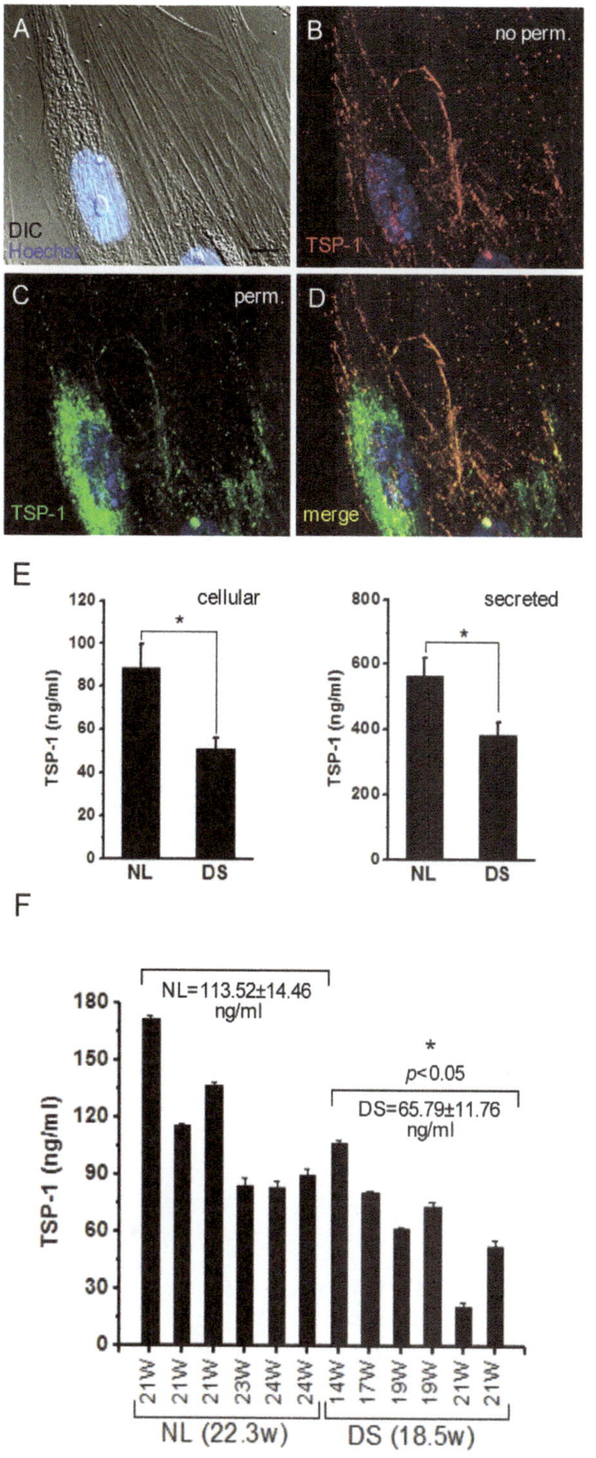

Figure 3. Reduced TSP-1 levels in DS astrocytes and DS fetal brain tissue. Human astrocytes in culture express abundant TSP-1. **A**) Differential interference contrast microscopy (DIC) image of the field shown in B-D. **B**) Cell surface TSP-1 IF prior to permeabilization of the cells (red fluorescence). **C**) After permeabilization, the preparation was incubated again with anti-TSP-1 (green fluorescence). Note the strong perinuclear staining. **D**) Merged image of the fields shown in B and C. Nuclei were counterstained with Hoechst (blue). Scale bar: 10 μm. **E**) Measurement of TSP-1 levels in homogenates (cellular) and CM (secreted) indicates significant reductions in DS astrocytes. Homogenates: NL 88.4±11.1 ng/ml, DS 51.51±4.7 ng/ml; CM: NL 564.0±54.2 ng/ml, DS 381.9±42.0 ng/ml. **F**) TSP-1 levels were measured in NL (n = 6) and DS (n = 6) fetal cortical brain samples as described in the Methods section. Average gestational ages of NL and DS samples were 22.3 weeks and 18.5 weeks respectively. The concentration of TSP-1 was markedly reduced in DS brain samples (average values above of the bars). Data were analyzed by ANOVA followed by Fisher's test. Error bars indicate the mean ± SEM. *$p<0.05$.

treated with anti-TSP-1 exhibited dramatic changes in spine morphology, including a marked reduction in the density of stubby spines, and a major increase in the frequency and length of filopodium spines (Figure 5 and Figure S3). Anti-TSP-1 previously neutralized with excess TSP-1 and non-immune IgG had no effect on spine morphology (data not shown). Conversely, addition of recombinant TSP-1 to hippocampal neurons growing on top of DS astrocytes exhibited a significant reduction of filopodium spines (Figure 6A), and a marked increase in the number of stubby spines (Figure 6B). A similar effect on spines, although of slightly smaller magnitude, was observed after the addition of BDNF to the cocultures (data not shown). Heat-inactivated TSP-1 did not have any effect on spine morphology or number (Figure 6A and B). These results demonstrate that soluble TSP-1 modulates spine morphology and that reduced expression of TSP-1 in DS astrocytes leads to abnormal spine development.

Altered spine morphology in neurons growing on top of TSP-1 KO astrocytes

To directly address the role of TSP-1 on the regulation of spine formation, rat hippocampal neurons were grown on top of astrocyte monolayers derived from wild type (WT) or TSP-1 KO mice [36]. There were no significant differences in general morphology, viability, between both cocultures (Figure 7A). However, neurons growing on top of TSP-1 KO astrocytes exhibited a striking increase in the number of filopodium spines and a marked reduction in the number of stubby spines (Figure 7B and C). Treatment of TSP-1 KO cocultures with recombinant TSP-1 for 4 days reduced significantly the number of filopodium spines and increased the number of stubby to similar levels than WT cocultures (Figure 7C). The effect of TSP-1 was more pronounced after 7 days of treatment (Figure 7C). The spine phenotype in TSP-1 KO cocultures is reminiscent to the alterations observed in DS cocultures, providing direct evidence for a role of TSP-1 on spine formation.

Synaptic density and the number of functional synapses are reduced in neurons grown on top of DS astrocytes

We investigated the effect of spine alterations and TSP-1 deficits on synapse formation and activity in DS cocultures. Synaptic density was assessed as the frequency of colocalization of the pre- and post-synaptic markers synaptophysin and PSD95 at 21 DIV [37–39]. Consistent with the alterations in spine morphology and density, we found a significant reduction in the number of synaptic contacts (NL: 12.1±1.1 synaptophysin/PSD95 colocalized puncta per 50 μm of dendrite; DS: 5.0±0.5% synaptophysin/PSD95 colocalized puncta per 50 μm of dendrite)(Figure 8A and B). To determine the number of synapses specifically localized in spines (Figure 8C), we measured the frequency of colocalization of synaptophysin, PSD95 and drebrin, (Figure 8D and Figure S4). Of the total number of synapses in the culture, represented by synaptophysin/PSD95 colocalization (Figure 8A and B), more than 50% were localized at dendritic spines, represented by synaptophysin/PSD95/drebrin colocalization (Figure 8C and D), indicating that spines are principal sites of synaptic formation in the cocultures. The number of synapses localized at spines was also

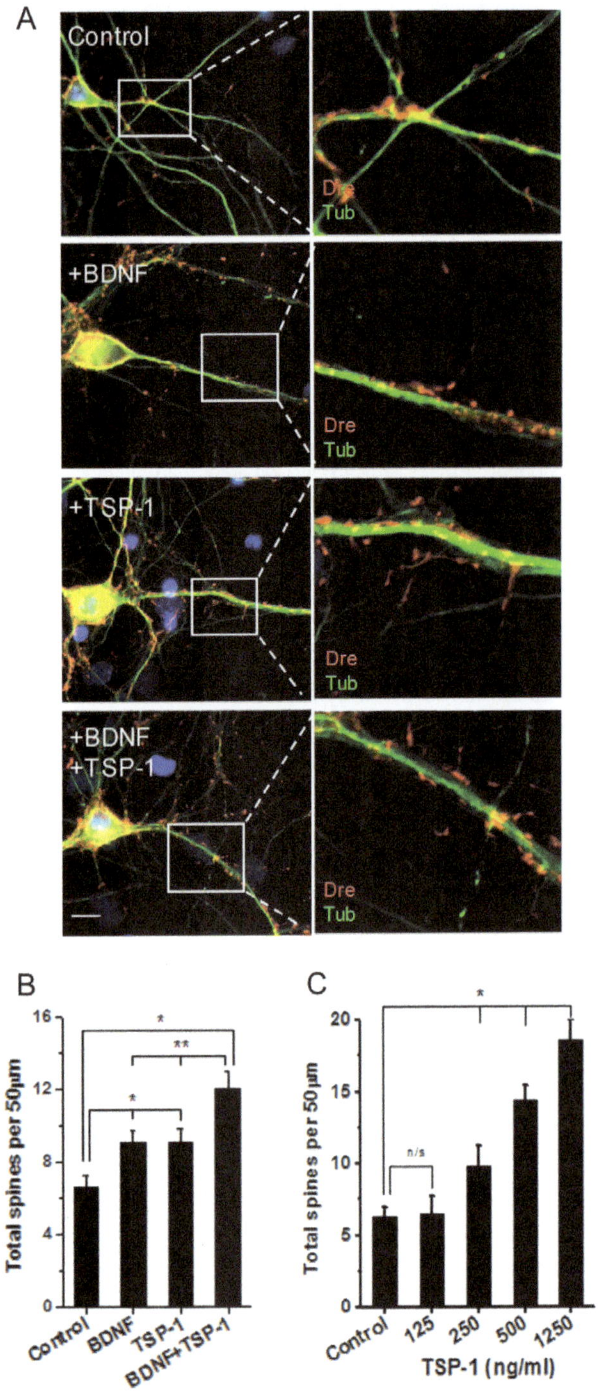

Figure 4. TSP-1 modulates spine development. A) Pure rat hippocampal cultures were incubated with BDNF (10 ng/ml), recombinant TSP-1 (250 ng/ml), or TSP-1+BDNF as described in the Methods section. Double immunofluorescence shows anti-Drebrin (red) and anti-β tubulin class III (green) immunostaining. Note abundant spine development with the treatments. Nuclei were counterstained with Hoechst (blue). Scale bar: 10 µm. **B**) TSP-1 and BDNF significantly enhance total spine number to similar levels. Coincubation with TSP-1+ BDNF produces a higher increase in spine number than either individual factor. Error bars indicate the mean ± SEM. *$p<0.05$ *vs* Control, **$p<0.05$ *vs* TSP-1 or BDNF. **C**) Increasing concentrations of TSP-1 induces a gradual increase in spine density in hippocampal neurons. Error bars indicate the mean ± SEM. *$p<0.05$.

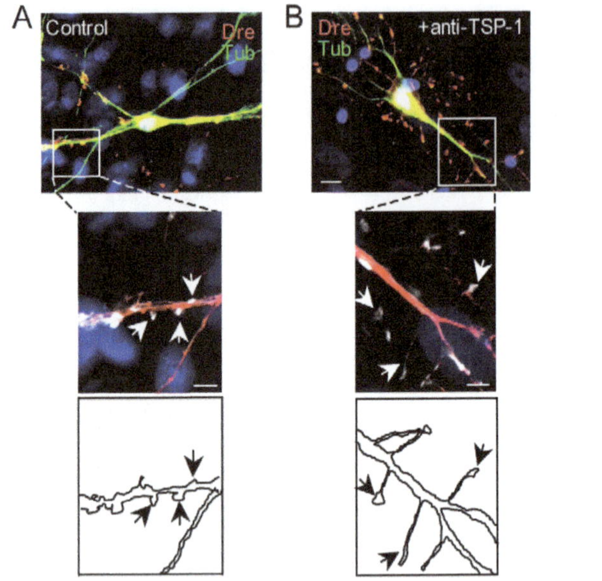

Figure 5. Depletion of TSP-1 markedly alters spine morphology. Cocultures of rat hippocampal neurons and NL astrocytes were incubated with a control IgG (**A**) or anti- TSP-1 (**B**). The region outlined by rectangles is shown at higher magnification in the panels below. Cocultures immunodepleted of TSP-1 exhibit dramatic changes in spine morphology including a marked increase in long filopodium-like spines (arrows) compared to control cultures, in which stubby spines predominate (arrows). Cocultures were fixed and immunofluorescence was performed with anti-drebrin (red) and anti- β tubulin class III (green) antibodies. The panels at higher magnification have been pseudocolored in red (tubulin) and white (drebrin) to facilitate the visualization of spine morphologies. Nuclei were counterstained with Hoechst (blue). Scale bars: 10 µm (upper panel), 5 µm (lower panel).

markedly reduced in DS cocultures (Figure 7D). To study the presence of functional synapses, we assessed vesicular uptake using the fluorescent cationic styryl fixable dye AM4-64. Depolarization induced by 20 mM KCl causes rapid vesicular uptake of A4-64,

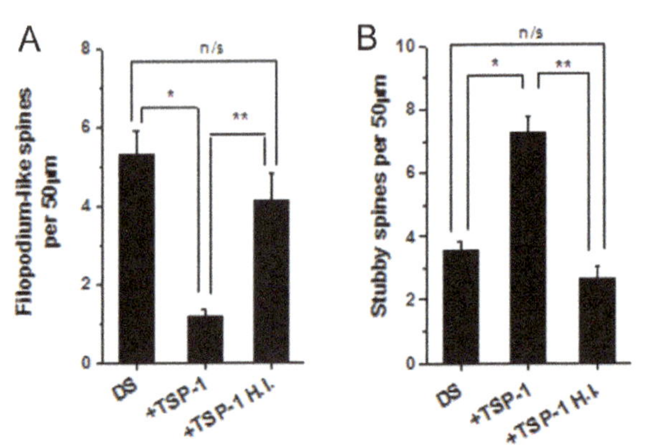

Figure 6. TSP-1 prevents spine alterations in neurons grown on top of DS astrocytes. Recombinant TSP-1 (250 ng/ml) was added to DS astrocyte/hippocampal neuron cocultures. TSP-1 induced a significant reduction in the number of filopodium-like spines (DS: 5.3±0.5; DS+TSP-1: 1.2±0.1)(**A**), and a marked increase in the number of stubby spines (DS: 3.5±0.3; DS+TSP-1: 7.2±0.5)(**B**). Heat-inactivated (H.I.) TSP-1 did not have any effect on spines. Data were analyzed by ANOVA followed by Fisher's test. Error bars indicate the mean ± SEM. *$p<0.05$, **$p<0.05$.

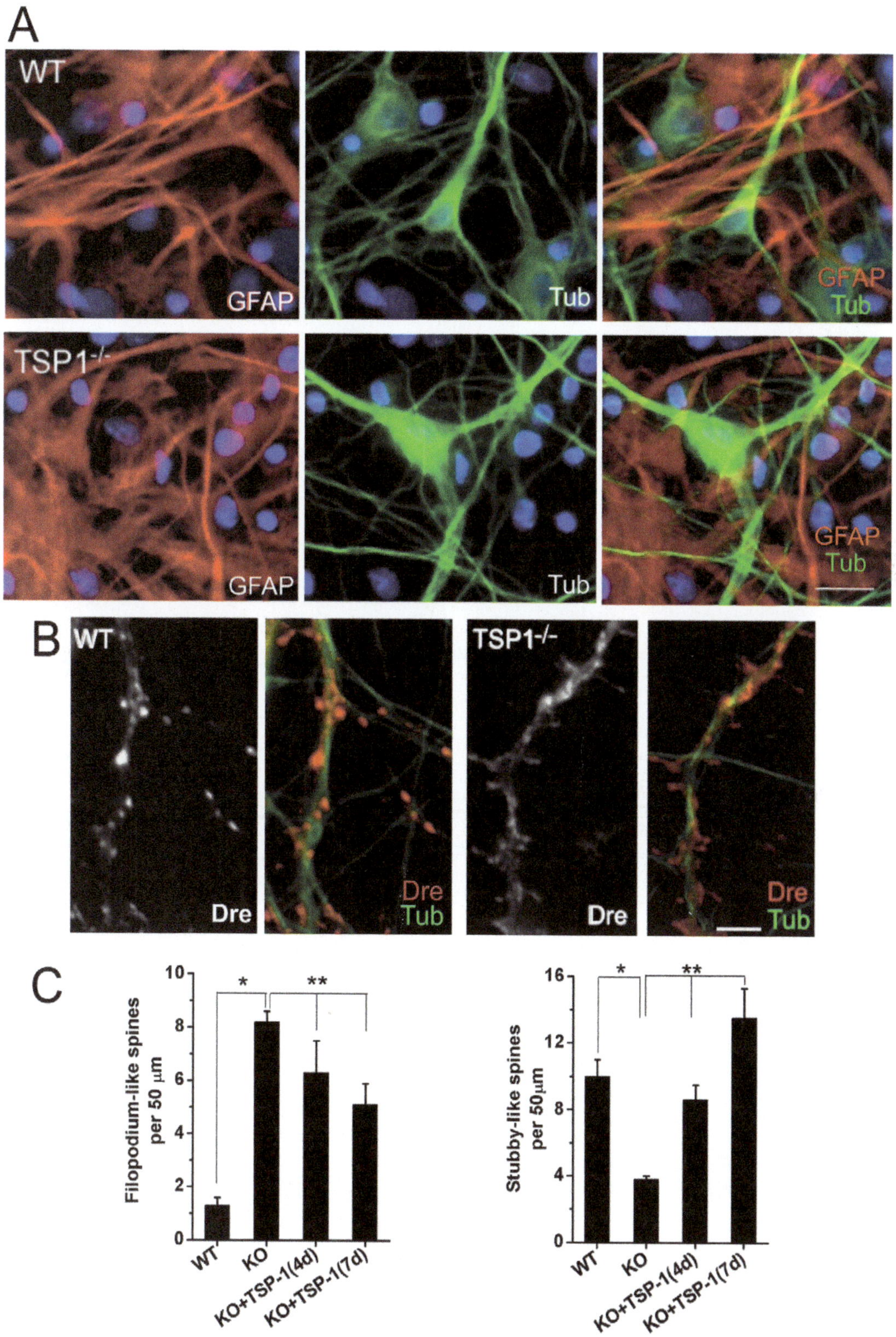

Figure 7. Altered spine morphology in neurons growing on top of TSP-1 KO astrocytes. Rat hippocampal neuron/mouse astrocyte cocultures were prepared as described in the Methods section. (**A**) After 21 DIV, the cultures were fixed and immunostained with anti-GFAP (1:1000, red), an astrocytic marker, and anti-β tubulin class III (1:1000, green), a neuronal marker. Hoechst was used for nuclear staining (blue). Similar neuronal viability and growth was observed in WT and TSP-1 KO (TSP-1$^{-/-}$) cocultures. Scale bar: 20 μm. (**B**) Double immunofluorescence with anti-drebrin (red) and anti- β tubulin class III (green) illustrates the differences in spine morphology in neurons growing on top of WT or TSP-1 astrocytes. Note the presence of numerous filopodium spines in TSP-1 KO cocultures. Scale bar: 5 μm. (**C**) Assessment of spine morphology indicates a significant increase in filopodium spines in TSP-1 KO cocultures (KO) compared to WT cocultures. Conversely, the number of stubby spines is reduced more than 50% in

TSP-1 KO cocultures. Continuous treatment with recombinant TSP-1 (250 ng/ml) during 4 days (4D) or 7 days (7D) prior to fixation at day 21 averted the spine alterations in TSP-1 KO cocultures. Spine number represents the average number of spines scored in a 50 μm dendritic segment. Data were analyzed by ANOVA followed by Fisher's test. All data are expressed as mean ± SEM. *$p<0.05$.

allowing the visualization of recycled vesicles [37], which in this case was used as an indicator of active synapses. Depolarization induced massive vesicle recycling in both NL and DS cocultures, indicating the presence of a high number of functional synapses in the cocultures (Figure 8E). However, there was a significantly lower density of A4-64-positive vesicles in DS cocultures after stimulation with KCl (Figure 8F). These findings demonstrate that the total number of synapses, the number of synapses at spines, and the number of active synapses are all reduced in DS cocultures.

TSP-1 increases synaptic density and activity in neurons grown on top of DS astrocytes

The ability of TSP-1 to modulate spine formation (Figure 4), to rescue spine defects associated with DS and TSP-1 KO cocultures (Figure 6 and 7), and its capacity to stimulate synaptogenesis [20], prompted us to examine the effect of TSP-1 treatment on synapse formation in neurons growing on top of DS astrocytes. Addition of 250 ng/ml TSP-1 resulted in a major increase in both total synaptic density (Figure 8B) and in the number of synapses localized at spines (Figure 8D). Restoration of TSP-1 levels also increased synaptic activity in DS cocultures as measured by A4-64 uptake (Figure 8E and F).

Antioxidants and mitochondrial cofactors have no effect on TSP-1 expression and secretory deficits in DS astrocytes

Protein synthesis and secretory function are highly dependent on mitochondrial energy production and are particularly vulnerable to the effects of intracellular oxidative damage. For example, APP secretory deficits in DS astrocytes are directly linked to impaired mitochondrial metabolism and abnormal secretory function [22], and increased apoptosis of DS neurons can be prevented by antioxidants [40]. To establish whether reduced expression of TSP-1 in DS astrocytes was associated with oxidative stress and/or energy deficits in DS cells, we analyzed the effect of free radical scavengers, antioxidants, and energy substrates on TSP-1 expression. DS astrocytes were treated with sPBN (100 μM), trolox (100 μM), resveratrol (100 μM), nicotinamide (15 mM), nicotinamide adenine dinucleotide (β-NAD, 15 mM), creatine (5 mM) or glucose (5 mM), and TSP-1 levels were quantified 24 hr later. None of the compounds tested were able to modify TSP-1 levels inside the cells or in the CM, suggesting that neither mitochondrial dysfunction nor oxidative stress are primary factors mediating TSP-1 deficits in DS astrocytes (Figure S5).

Discussion

Dendritic spine abnormalities have long been recognized as structural correlates of mental retardation in DS [1,9,41]. However, the origin and mechanisms involved in DS spine alterations are not known. Here, we show that: 1) DS astrocytes play a significant role in spine pathology and reduced synaptic density; 2) both DS brains and DS astrocytes show deficits in TSP-1 levels and secretion; 3) TSP-1 modulates dendritic spine development and morphology; and 4) TSP-1 addition reverts DS astrocyte-mediated spine and synaptic alterations.

Astrocytes are important modulators of neuronal development, metabolism, and synaptic activity [15,18,42,43]. Astrocyte alterations have been linked to diverse neurological conditions such as epilepsy [44–46], AD [47,48], ischemic injury [49], amyotrophic lateral sclerosis [50,51], and neurodevelopmental disorders such as Rett's syndrome [52,53] and fragile X syndrome [54]. However, the role of astrocytes in DS has received less attention. Astrocytes from DS fetal brain tissue and DS mouse models show increased concentration of intracellular calcium [55,56], altered sensitivity to oxidative stress [57], deficits in mitochondrial energy metabolism [22,58] and abnormal APP transport and secretion [22]. In addition, there is increased S100 and interleukin-1 expression in astrocytes in DS brain cortex [59,60]. Together, these results indicate the presence of metabolic alterations in DS astrocytes that can directly affect neuronal survival and development. Supporting this notion, Nelson and colleagues demonstrated that NL neurons co-cultured with TS16 mouse astrocytes exhibit reduced cholinergic function, while TS16 neurons co-cultured with WT mouse astrocytes display normal cholinergic activity [61]. Our data indicate that neurons growing on top of DS astrocytes exhibit abnormal changes in spine morphology and density, and a marked reduction in synaptic density. Hippocampal neurons cocultured on top of DS astrocytes display a high number and longer filopodium spines, and a significant reduction in the number of stubby spines (Figure 2), reminiscent of the spine pathology described in DS infant brains [2,3,62]. Filopodium spines are expressed early during hippocampal [63–65] and cortical development [66,67]. Although the function of filopodium spines is unclear, some studies suggest that they are associated with early stages of synaptic formation including spinogenesis, synaptogenesis and regulation of dendritic braching [24,64,68]. At maturity, filopodia disappear in many neurons and are replaced by stubby spines [69,70]. Astrocytes control the maturation and dynamics of dendritic spines by physical contact with neurons [10–13], and can influence synapse formation through secreted factors such as cholesterol [19], thrombospondins [20] and TNF-α [71]. Thus, functional or metabolic alterations in DS astrocytes may affect normal spine development and plasticity, ultimately leading to abnormal synapse and circuit formation.

Secretory function is integral for astrocytes neuromodulatory role. Astrocytes secrete growth factors, extracellular matrix proteins, proteases, modulators of protease activity, etc [72–74], which regulate neuronal development and survival [75], neuritogenesis [76] and synaptogenesis [19,20,77]. Human astrocytes synthesize and secrete TSP-1, an extracellular matrix component involved in cell-cell and cell-matrix communication [26,78], which is widely expressed in the developing nervous system [27]. In vitro, human astrocytes expressed high levels of TPS-1, which was detected intracellularly and at the cell surface (Figure 3A-D). TSP-1 levels were reduced in both DS astrocyte homogenates and CM, as well as in DS fetal brains, raising the possibility that in DS, TSP-1 deficits could affect critical stages of neuronal development such as neurite outgrowth [28–30,79], neuronal migration [32], or synaptogenesis [20,80]. Indeed, reduced TSP-1 activity in cocultures of NL astrocytes is sufficient to dramatically alter spine morphology (Figure 5) and synapse formation (data not shown) in hippocampal neurons. Moreover, neurons growing on top of TSP-1 KO astrocytes developed abnormal spines reminiscent to the spines in DS astrocyte cocultures. Conversely, addition of TSP-1 prevented the alterations in spine morphology and the reductions

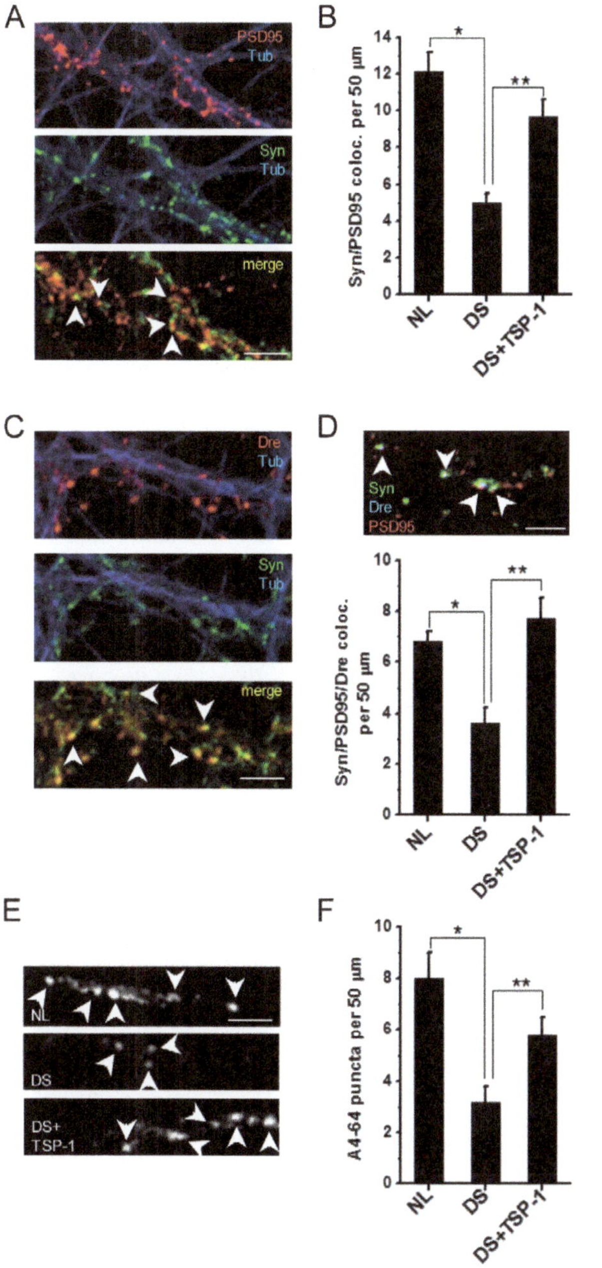

Figure 8. Reduced synaptic density in hippocampal neurons grown on top of DS astrocytes can be reversed by treatment with TSP-1. A) Colocalization of post-synaptic marker PSD-95 (1:250, red) and pre-synaptic marker synaptophysin (1:250, green)(arrows) was utilized to define synaptic contacts and to assess synaptic density. Neuronal processes were stained with tubulin class III (blue). **B**) Synaptic density was expressed as the number of colocalized puncta per 50 µm of dendrite in NL, DS and DS treated with 250 ng/ml TSP-1 cocultures. Error bars indicate the mean ± SEM. *$p<0.05$ vs cocultures of NL astrocytes, **$p<0.05$ vs cocultures of DS astrocytes. **C**) The colocalization of synaptophysin, drebrin and tubulin class III denotes the presence of synapses at spines (arrows). **D**) The number of synapses localized at spines was assessed by quantifying the triple colocalization of synaptophysin, PSD95 and drebrin (arrows). Error bars indicate the mean ± SEM. *$p<0.05$. **E**) The fluorescent cationic styryl fixable dye AM4-64, which is taken up during vesicle recycling, was used to study synaptic activity in the cocultures. AM4-64 fluorescence is shown in living NL cultures after depolarization induced by treatment with KCl (upper panel). DS cocultures present a marked decrease in AM4-64-positive vesicles after stimulation with KCl (middle panel). Treatment with TSP-1 increases synaptic activity in DS cocultures (lower panel). **F**) Quantification of AM4-64-positive puncta shows a significant reduction in DS compared to NL cocultures, which can be reverted by TSP-1 treatment. Data were analyzed by ANOVA followed by Fisher's test. All data are expressed as mean ± SEM. *$p<0.05$. Scale bars: 5 µm.

in both synaptic density and activity in neurons growing on top of DS and TSP-1 KO astrocytes. Interestingly, thrombospondin-deficient mice exhibit deficits in recovery of motor function after stroke [33], and reduced proliferation and differentiation of neuronal progenitors [81]. Thrombospondins are expressed in forebrain of human but not nonhuman primates [82], further suggesting a role for thrombospondins in synaptic plasticity and human cognition. Lastly, the loss of thrombospondins also leads to craniofacial dysmorphism [83], which is a common feature of DS subjects and DS mouse models [84,85], raising the possibility that reduced TSP-1 levels may be associated with a number of developmental anomalies present in DS.

The stimulatory effect of TSP-1 on spine formation was of similar magnitude to that of BDNF (Figure 4), pointing to a role for TSP-1 not only in synaptogenesis [20,80], but also in spine formation. Together, TSP-1 and BDNF potentiated their effect, suggesting the presence of non-redundant, complementary pathways for TSP-1 and BDNF action on spines. In this respect, thrombospondins have been shown to act at multiple levels in different signaling pathways [86]. TSP-1 can bind and activate integrin receptors to mediate neurite outgrowth [28], and some studies suggest that TSP-1 can reorganize the actin cytoskeleton through stimulation of phosphoinositide 3-kinase (PI3-K) [87]. TSP-1 can also induce changes in cell morphology through activation of the Src family of kinases, ERK 1/2 or Rac-1 [88]. In addition, many effects of TSP-1 as inhibitor of angiogenesis and tumor growth are mediated by nitric oxide [89], p38 MAPK [90], PI3-K, FAK [91] and the CD36 receptor [92]. Recent studies show that TSP-1 can interact with the α2δ-1 gabapentin receptor [93], and with neuroligin 1 during synaptogenesis [80]. Ongoing experiments are directed to establish which signaling pathway(s) engaged by TSP-1 mediates spine formation and morphology.

Mitochondrial dysfunction and oxidative stress are major factors contributing to DS altered cellular function and survival [22,40,94-96]. In DS astrocytes, energy depletion leads to abnormal APP metabolism and altered APP secretion, both of which can be prevented by treatment with antioxidants [22]. However, antioxidants or mitochondrial cofactors did not revert TSP-1 deficits in DS astrocytes (Figure S5). One possibility is that mechanism(s) regulating TSP-1 expression such as activation of purinergic receptors [97], muscarinic receptors [74], or nitric oxide-mediated signaling [89,98] could be altered in DS astrocytes. Alternatively, TSP-1 reduced levels in DS may be linked to the capacity of gamma interferon (IFN-γ) to inhibit both the production and secretion of thrombospondins without changing mRNA levels [99]. IFN-γ levels are elevated in both DS [100,101] and trisomy 16 mice [102,103]. DS individuals are hypersensitive to IFN-γ [104–107] and exhibit pronounced dysregulation in the levels of IFN-γ and other cytokines [108,109]. These actions of INF-γ in DS are likely to be related to the presence of several IFN receptor genes in chromosome 21 including IFNGR2, which is one of the subunits of the IFN-γ receptor [110]. Thus, upregulated IFN-γ signaling in DS astrocytes may lead to a downregulation of TSP-1 protein levels. Furthermore, interferons also inhibit protein glycosylation [111], which is required for TSP-1 secretion. Experiments in progress are directed to understand the role of IFN-γ signaling in the post-transcriptional regulation of TSP-1 in DS.

In summary, we found metabolic alterations in DS astrocytes that cause spine pathology and reduced synaptic density in cocultured neurons. Spine and synaptic alterations were associated with reduced expression of TSP-1, which was also significantly reduced in DS brains. Finally, the identification of a novel role for TSP-1 as a strong modulator of dendritic spine development and morphology supports the exploration of TSP-1 and downstream signaling partners as therapeutic targets to treat spine pathology and cognitive impairment in DS and other neurological conditions.

Methods

Ethics Statement

This study is part of an ongoing research protocol approved by the Health and Hospital Corporation of the City of New York, the Albert Einstein College of Medicine Committee on Clinical Investigation and the Internal Review Board of the University of California-Irvine. The protocols for obtaining post-mortem fetal brain tissue comply with all federal and institutional guidelines with special respect for the confidentiality of the donor's identity. Written informed consent was obtained from all tissue donors.

All procedures for the generation of rat hippocampal neuronal suspensions were reviewed and approved by the Institutional Care and Use Committee (IACUC) at the University of California Irvine, protocol number 2008-2779.

Cell Culture

Astrocyte cultures were established from postmortem NL and DS human fetal brain tissue samples as described [22]. Normal and DS fetal human brain samples are procured at the Human Fetal Tissue Repository, Albert Einstein School of Medicine (AECOM), NY, and received and processed in the Busciglio laboratory at UCI. Cortical tissue samples were dissociated into a single-cell suspension by incubation with 0.25% trypsin/40 µg/ml DNAse (Sigma, St Louis, MO) in PBS at 37°C for 30 min, and mechanically dissociated with a fire-polished glass Pasteur pipette. Cells were plated on the bottom of tissue culture dishes or on glass coverslips, and maintained in DMEM (Invitrogen, Grand Island, NY) supplemented with 10% fetal bovine serum (HyClone, Road Logan, UT). After growing to confluence, cells were subjected to two passages to generate pure astrocytic cultures. The identity and purity of the astrocyte cultures was confirmed by immunocytochemistry with anti-GFAP and anti-S100 antibodies. To generate the cocultures, hippocampi were dissected from rat newborn pups, incubated with trypsin, and triturated through a glass Pasteur pipette as described by Kaech and Banker [112]. The neurons were plated on top of NL or DS astrocyte monolayers at 100,000 cells/mm^2. Two hr after neuronal plating, the medium was changed to Neurobasal plus N2 and B27 supplements (Invitrogen, Grand Island, NY). Partial medium changes were performed every 5 days. Cultures were maintained for 21 days to allow for the development and maturation of dendritic spines. Under these conditions, there is minimal growth of rat astrocytes in the coculture (Figure S6). Pure hippocampal cultures were maintained in NL or DS astrocyte conditioned medium (CM) obtained from astrocyte cultures. For pure hippocampal cultures, the neurons were plated on coverslips pretreated with 1 mg/ml poly-L-lysine immediately after dissociation (Sigma, St Louis, MO). Two hr after plating, the medium was switched to NL or DS CM. Partial medium changes with fresh CM were performed every 3 days. For some experiments, astrocyte monloayers were generated from the cortex of WT and TSP-1 KO [36] newborn pups following the procedures described above.

Immunofluorescence and image analysis

Cultures were fixed with 4% paraformaldehyde/0.12 M sucrose/PBS for 15 min at 37°C, permeabilized 15 min with 0.2% Triton X-100/PBS, and blocked for 30 min in 5% bovine serum albumin/PBS. Then, the cultures were incubated with one or more of the following primary antibodies: mouse anti-drebrin, a marker of dendritic spines (1:250, Stressegen, Ann Arbor, MI), GFAP (1:1000, Sigma, St Louis, MO), anti-β-tubulin isotype III (1:1000, Sigma, St Louis, MO), mouse anti-thrombospondin-1 (1:250 Calbiochem, La Jolla, CA), anti-synaptophysin (1:250, Calbiochem, Gibbstown, NJ), anti-PSD95 (1:250, Abcam, Cambridge, MA), and anti S-100β (1:500, R&D systems, Minneapolis, MN), for 1 hr at RT, followed by a 30 min incubation in fluorescent-conjugated secondary antibody (1:500, Alexa 350, Alexa 488 and Alexa 594, Invitrogen, Eugene, OR). An Axiovert 200 inverted microscope (Zeiss, Jena, Germany) was used for examination, imaging and quantification of various parameters of spine morphology. Images were captured with a digital camera and processed using AxioVision software (Zeiss). When required, Z-stacks were captured at 500 nm intervals, processed and rendered using the Apotome imaging system (Zeiss). Spine-like protrusions were classified according to Hering and Sheng [23]. For spine assessment, dendritic spines were defined as protrusions from the surface of dendritic processes exhibiting a high concentration of drebrin [113,114]. Morphologically, we identified 2 populations of spines: stubby-/mushroom-like spines, short, small and rounded spines with or without a short neck, and filopodium-like spines, which are typically longer, thin and lack a head. For quantification, 10 neurons per culture were selected from 3–6 separate cultures. Density and morphology of spines were scored in dendritic segments approximately 50 µm away from the cell body. Spine length was measured using the measurement tool of AxioVision. Spine length was defined as the distance from the base of the neck to the tip of the spine. To assess synaptic density, the colocalization of pre- and post-synaptic markers was performed as described [37–39].

TSP-1 measurements

TSP-1 levels were determined in astrocyte cultures and fetal brain homogenates. Astrocytes were plated in 24-well plates. Cultures were washed in ice-cold PBS and collected in Eppendorf tubes in 0.1 M NaOH. The lysates were centrifuged at 14,000 rpm in an Eppendorf microcentrifuge for 30 min at 4°C, and the supernatants were used to determine the intracellular concentration of TSP-1. Aliquots of CM from the same cultures were processed to determine the level of secreted TSP-1. Samples of fetal cortex were homogenized in RIPA buffer plus protease inhibitors (Complete, Roche, Mannheim, Germany) with a Turrax homogenizer (Ika Works, Wilmington, NC), and centrifuged at 14,000 rpm for 30 min at 4°C. TSP-1 levels in the supernatant fraction were determined using a commercial ELISA kit following the vendor's instructions (R&D systems, Minneapolis, MN). For some experiments, the following compounds (purchased from Sigma, St Louis, MO) were added to pure astrocyte cultures, and TSP-1 levels were determined after 24 hr: s-PBN (100 mM), Trolox (100 µM), resveratrol (100 mM), nicotinamide (15 mM), nicotinamide adenine dinucleotide (β-NAD, 15 mM), creatine (5 mM) and glucose (5 mM).

TSP-1 treatments

Cocultures were plated in 24-well plates and human recombinant TSP-1 (R&D system Minneapolis, MN) was added every 3 days at the indicated concentrations. Control cultures were incubated with heat-inactivated TSP-1 (100°C for 5 min).

Cocultures were fixed at 21 DIV and analysis of spines was performed as described above. For some experiments, pure hippocampal cultures were treated with TSP-1 (250 ng/ml), BDNF (10 ng/ml, PeproTech Inc, Rocky Hill, NJ) or with TSP-1+BDNF.

Depletion of TSP-1

Cocultures were plated in 24-well plates. Starting at day 7, anti-TSP-1 (1:1000 Calbiochem, Gibbstown, NJ) was added to the cultures, and fresh anti-TSP-1 was replenished with partial medium changes every 3 days. Control cultures were treated with anti-TSP-1 previously neutralized with an excess of recombinant human TSP-1 or with non-immune rabbit serum. Cocultures were fixed at 21 DIV to assess spine density and morphology.

Assessment of vesicle recycling

To assess activity-dependent vesicle recycling, the cultures were incubated with the fixable fluorescent probe AM4-64 (Biotium Inc, Hayward, CA) for 5 min with or without 20 mM KCl [37]. AM4-64 fluorescent density was quantified using Axiovision.

Statistical analysis

All experiments were repeated three to six times using cultures derived from different brain specimens. Each individual experiment was performed at least in in triplicate samples. Data were analyzed by one-way analysis of variance (ANOVA) followed by Fisher's test. Results were expressed as the mean ± SEM. Significance was assessed at $p<0.05$. All results shown correspond to individual representative experiments.

Supporting Information

Figure S1 Similar viability in neurons growing on top of normal or DS astrocytes and pure rat hippocampal cultures. Hippocampi from rat newborn pups were processed as described (Kaech and Banker, 2006). Rat hippocampal cultures were plated on coverslips precoated with poly-L-lysine. To generate cocultures, the neurons were plated on top of NL or DS astrocyte monolayers. All cultures were fixed after 21 days. Cell viability was evaluated by direct examination of neuronal morphology by a blinded operator. Neurons were visualized after immunofluorescence with anti-beta tubulin class III. Nuclei were counterstained with Hoechst. Neurons with round or oval nuclei showing light blue fluorescence and intact neuronal morphology were considered viable. Cells exhibiting condensed or fragmented nuclei and/or disrupted neuronal processes were considered dead. Fluorescent images were captured at 630X final magnification. Five fields per coverslip from 3-6 independent experiments were randomly selected for scoring of live or dead neurons. Error bars indicate the mean ± SEM. *p<0.05.

Figure S2 Similar TSP-1, -2, -3 and -4 mRNA levels in normal and DS fetal brains. TSP-1, -2, -3 and -4 mRNA levels were quantified in four 18-23 week old DS fetal brains and five age-matched controls. Quantitative real-time PCR was performed with a LightCycler 480 Real-Time PCR System utilizing Light-Cycler 480 SYBR Green I Master from Roche Applied Biosciences. The expression levels were normalized using 3 housekeeping genes (HKGs), Glucose 6 Phospahate Dehydrogenase (G6DH), β-Actin (Actβ), and TATA binding protein (TBP). None of the housekeeping genes were found differentially expressed between control and DS fetal brains. The graph summarizes the fold differences of each thrombospondin isoform in DS brains compared to normal brains. Each sample was run in triplicates. The primer pairs for each gene from 5- to 3-primus end are as follows: TSP1: GCTGCACTGAGTGTCACTGTC and TCAGGAACTGTGGCATTGG; TSP2: GTGCAGGAGCGT-CAGATGT, and GGGTTGGATAAACAGCCATC; TSP3: AA-TCTCCAGTATCGATGCAATG, and GTGGCCTCC TCC TCA CAC; TSP4: CTACCGCTGTTCCTACAGC, and GAG-CCTTCATAAAATCGTACCC; G6DH: GAGCCAGATGCA-CTTCGTG and GGGCTTCTCCAGCTCAATC; Actβ: CAA-CCGCGAGAAGATGAC and GTCCATCACGATGCCAGT; TBP: TGAATCTTGGTTGTAAACTTGACC and CTCAT-GATTACCGCAGCAAA. The thermal cycle protocol consisted of an initial heat denaturation at 95°C for 5 min, followed by 45 cycles each of denaturation at 95°C for 10 sec, annealing at 60°C for 10 sec, and an extension at 72°C for 10 sec for all primer sets. The bars represent SD.

Figure S3 Increased number of filopodium spines after TSP-1 immunodepletion in neurons grown on top of normal astrocytes. The histogram shows the number of filopodium spines per 50 μm of dendrite in control cocultures and cocultures treated with anti-TSP-1 antibody. At day 7, anti-TSP-1 was added to the culture medium and replenished every 3 days during 14 days. The cultures were fixed at day 21, and the number and type of spines was quantified as described in the Methods section. Hippocampal neurons treated with anti-TSP-1 exhibited a significant increase in the frequency and length of filopodium spines. Data were analyzed by ANOVA followed by Fisher's test. Results are expressed as the mean ± SEM. *p<0.05. The experiment was repeated using 3 different cocultures in triplicate or cuadruplicate samples. The graph corresponds to an individual representative experiment.

Figure S4 Colocalization of synaptic and spine markers. Single channel images of triple immunofluorescence showing drebrin (spine marker), PSD95 (post-synaptic marker) and synapthophysin (pre-synaptic marker). The merged image is shown in Figure 7D.

Figure S5 Antioxidants and mitochondrial cofactors have no effect on TSP-1 expression and secretion in DS astrocytes. Astrocyte cultures were treated with the designated compounds as described in the Methods section. TSP-1 levels were quantified by ELISA in soluble fractions and cellular homogenates. Sodium 4-[(tert-butylimino) methyl]benzene-3-sulfonate N-oxide (s-PBN, 100 mM); trolox (100 μM); resveratrol (Resv, 100 mM); nicotinamide (Nico, 15 mM); nicotinamide adenine dinucleotide (NAD, 15 mM); creatine (cre, 5 mM); glucose (Gluco, 5 mM). Data were analyzed by ANOVA followed by Fisher's test. The results are expressed as the mean ± SEM. Values represent the mean from 6 independent experiments. *p<0.05 vs cocultures of NL astrocytes.

Figure S6 Quantification of rat astrocytes in rat hippocampal neuron/human astrocyte cocultures. Hippocampal cell suspensions were incubated for 1 hr with fluorescent microspheres (PS-Speck, Invitrogen, Carlsbad, CA), which are rapidly taken up by viable cells. The microspheres remain in the cytoplasm and do not affect cell function or survival. Then, hippocampal suspensions were plated on top of human astrocyte monolayers, cultured for 21 days, fixed, counterstained with Hoechst, and processed for image analysis. A) DIC and fluorescence image of a microscopic field in which fluorescent microspheres are apparent in one cell (arrow, putative rat astrocyte) and absent in the other three cells in the field (putative human astrocytes). Nuclei were stained with

Hoechst. Scale bar: 10 µm. B) Total number of astrocytes in the culture was assessed by scoring astrocyte nuclei, which are easily distinguishable because of their size (3 to 5 times larger than neuronal nuclei). The number of rat astrocytes was assessed by counting astrocyte cells containing fluorescent microspheres in the cytoplasm. Rat astrocytes represented approximately 18% of the total number of astrocytes in the coculture. Data were analyzed by ANOVA followed by Fisher's test. $*p<0.05$.

Acknowledgments

We thank Michael Hanna for his expert assistance with tissue culture procedures.

Author Contributions

Conceived and designed the experiments: OG JB. Performed the experiments: OG MT PH PC. Analyzed the data: OG MT PH PC JB. Wrote the paper: OG JB.

References

1. Benavides-Piccione R, Ballesteros-Yanez I, de Lagran MM, Elston G, Estivill X, et al. (2004) On dendrites in Down syndrome and DS murine models: a spiny way to learn. Prog Neurobiol 74: 111–126.
2. Marin-Padilla M (1972) Structural abnormalities of the cerebral cortex in human chromosomal aberrations: a Golgi study. Brain Res 44: 625–629.
3. Marin-Padilla M (1976) Pyramidal cell abnormalities in the motor cortex of a child with Down's syndrome. A Golgi study. J Comp Neurol 167: 63–81.
4. Ferrer I, Gullotta F (1990) Down's syndrome and Alzheimer's disease: dendritic spine counts in the hippocampus. Acta Neuropathol 79: 680–685.
5. Suetsugu M, Mehraein P (1980) Spine distribution along the apical dendrites of the pyramidal neurons in Down's syndrome. A quantitative Golgi study. Acta Neuropathol 50: 207–210.
6. Belichenko PV, Kleschevnikov AM, Salehi A, Epstein CJ, Mobley WC (2007) Synaptic and cognitive abnormalities in mouse models of Down syndrome: exploring genotype-phenotype relationships. J Comp Neurol 504: 329–345.
7. Belichenko PV, Masliah E, Kleschevnikov AM, Villar AJ, Epstein CJ, et al. (2004) Synaptic structural abnormalities in the Ts65Dn mouse model of Down Syndrome. J Comp Neurol 480: 281–298.
8. Kurt MA, Kafa MI, Dierssen M, Davies DC (2004) Deficits of neuronal density in CA1 and synaptic density in the dentate gyrus, CA3 and CA1, in a mouse model of Down syndrome. Brain Res 1022: 101–109.
9. Dierssen M, Ramakers GJ (2006) Dendritic pathology in mental retardation: from molecular genetics to neurobiology. Genes Brain Behav 5(Suppl 2): 48–60.
10. Haber M, Zhou L, Murai KK (2006) Cooperative astrocyte and dendritic spine dynamics at hippocampal excitatory synapses. Journal of Neuroscience 26: 8881–8891.
11. Murai KK, Nguyen LN, Irie F, Yamaguchi Y, Pasquale EB (2003) Control of hippocampal dendritic spine morphology through ephrin-A3/EphA4 signaling. Nature Neuroscience 6: 153–160.
12. Nishida H, Okabe S (2007) Direct astrocytic contacts regulate local maturation of dendritic spines. J Neurosci 27: 331–340.
13. Ventura R, Harris KM (1999) Three-dimensional relationships between hippocampal synapses and astrocytes. Journal of Neuroscience 19: 6897–6906.
14. Halassa MM, Fellin T, Takano H, Dong JH, Haydon PG (2007) Synaptic islands defined by the territory of a single astrocyte. J Neurosci 27: 6473–6477.
15. Haydon PG (2001) GLIA: listening and talking to the synapse. Nat Rev Neurosci 2: 185–193.
16. Pfrieger FW, Barres BA (1997) Synaptic efficacy enhanced by glial cells in vitro. Science 277: 1684–1687.
17. Ullian EM, Sapperstein SK, Christopherson KS, Barres BA (2001) Control of synapse number by glia. Science 291: 657–661.
18. Volterra A, Meldolesi J (2005) Astrocytes, from brain glue to communication elements: the revolution continues. Nat Rev Neurosci 6: 626–640.
19. Mauch DH, Nagler K, Schumacher S, Goritz C, Muller EC, et al. (2001) CNS synaptogenesis promoted by glia-derived cholesterol. Science 294: 1354–1357.
20. Christopherson KS, Ullian EM, Stokes CC, Mullowney CE, Hell JW, et al. (2005) Thrombospondins are astrocyte-secreted proteins that promote CNS synaptogenesis. Cell 120: 421–433.
21. Hama H, Hara C, Yamaguchi K, Miyawaki A (2004) PKC signaling mediates global enhancement of excitatory synaptogenesis in neurons triggered by local contact with astrocytes. Neuron 41: 405–415.
22. Busciglio J, Pelsman A, Wong C, Pigino G, Yuan M, et al. (2002) Altered metabolism of the amyloid beta precursor protein is associated with mitochondrial dysfunction in Down's syndrome. Neuron 33: 677–688.
23. Hering H, Sheng M (2001) Dendritic spines: structure, dynamics and regulation. Nat Rev Neurosci 2: 880–888.
24. Ziv NE, Smith SJ (1996) Evidence for a role of dendritic filopodia in synaptogenesis and spine formation. Neuron 17: 91–102.
25. Fiala JC, Spacek J, Harris KM (2002) Dendritic spine pathology: cause or consequence of neurological disorders? Brain Res Brain Res Rev 39: 29–54.
26. Asch AS, Leung LL, Shapiro J, Nachman RL (1986) Human brain glial cells synthesize thrombospondin. Proc Natl Acad Sci U S A 83: 2904–2908.
27. Adams JC, Tucker RP (2000) The thrombospondin type 1 repeat (TSR) superfamily: diverse proteins with related roles in neuronal development. Dev Dyn 218: 280–299.
28. DeFreitas MF, Yoshida CK, Frazier WA, Mendrick DL, Kypta RM, et al. (1995) Identification of integrin alpha 3 beta 1 as a neuronal thrombospondin receptor mediating neurite outgrowth. Neuron 15: 333–343.
29. O'Shea KS, Liu LH, Dixit VM (1991) Thrombospondin and a 140 kd fragment promote adhesion and neurite outgrowth from embryonic central and peripheral neurons and from PC12 cells. Neuron 7: 231–237.
30. Yu K, Ge J, Summers JB, Li F, Liu X, et al. (2008) TSP-1 secreted by bone marrow stromal cells contributes to retinal ganglion cell neurite outgrowth and survival. PLoS One 3: e2470.
31. Blake SM, Strasser V, Andrade N, Duit S, Hofbauer R, et al. (2008) Thrombospondin-1 binds to ApoER2 and VLDL receptor and functions in postnatal neuronal migration. EMBO J 27: 3069–3080.
32. O'Shea KS, Rheinheimer JS, Dixit VM (1990) Deposition and role of thrombospondin in the histogenesis of the cerebellar cortex. J Cell Biol 110: 1275–1283.
33. Liauw J, Hoang S, Choi M, Eroglu C, Sun GH, et al. (2008) Thrombospondins 1 and 2 are necessary for synaptic plasticity and functional recovery after stroke. J Cereb Blood Flow Metab 28: 1722–1732.
34. Chapleau CA, Carlo ME, Larimore JL, Pozzo-Miller L (2008) The actions of BDNF on dendritic spine density and morphology in organotypic slice cultures depend on the presence of serum in culture media. J Neurosci Methods 169: 182–190.
35. Gu J, Firestein BL, Zheng JQ (2008) Microtubules in dendritic spine development. J Neurosci 28: 12120–12124.
36. Lawler J, Sunday M, Thibert V, Duquette M, George EL, et al. (1998) Thrombospondin-1 is required for normal murine pulmonary homeostasis and its absence causes pneumonia. J Clin Invest 101: 982–992.
37. Deshpande A, Kawai H, Metherate R, Glabe CG, Busciglio J (2009) A role for synaptic zinc in activity-dependent Abeta oligomer formation and accumulation at excitatory synapses. J Neurosci 29: 4004–4015.
38. Deshpande A, Mina E, Glabe C, Busciglio J (2006) Different conformations of amyloid beta induce neurotoxicity by distinct mechanisms in human cortical neurons. J Neurosci 26: 6011–6018.
39. Deshpande A, Win KM, Busciglio J (2008) Tau isoform expression and regulation in human cortical neurons. FASEB J 22: 2357–2367.
40. Busciglio J, Yankner BA (1995) Apoptosis and increased generation of reactive oxygen species in Down's syndrome neurons in vitro. Nature 378: 776–779.
41. Kaufmann WE, Moser HW (2000) Dendritic anomalies in disorders associated with mental retardation. Cereb Cortex 10: 981–991.
42. Lovatt D, Sonnewald U, Waagepetersen HS, Schousboe A, He W, et al. (2007) The transcriptome and metabolic gene signature of protoplasmic astrocytes in the adult murine cortex. J Neurosci 27: 12255–12266.
43. Mori T, Buffo A, Gotz M (2005) The novel roles of glial cells revisited: the contribution of radial glia and astrocytes to neurogenesis. Curr Top Dev Biol 69: 67–99.
44. Oberheim NA, Tian GF, Han X, Peng W, Takano T, et al. (2008) Loss of astrocytic domain organization in the epileptic brain. J Neurosci 28: 3264–3276.
45. Tian GF, Azmi H, Takano T, Xu Q, Peng W, et al. (2005) An astrocytic basis of epilepsy. Nat Med 11: 973–981.
46. Wetherington J, Serrano G, Dingledine R (2008) Astrocytes in the epileptic brain. Neuron 58: 168–178.
47. Nagele RG, D'Andrea MR, Lee H, Venkataraman V, Wang HY (2003) Astrocytes accumulate A beta 42 and give rise to astrocytic amyloid plaques in Alzheimer disease brains. Brain Res 971: 197–209.
48. Nagele RG, Wegiel J, Venkataraman V, Imaki H, Wang KC (2004) Contribution of glial cells to the development of amyloid plaques in Alzheimer's disease. Neurobiol Aging 25: 663–674.
49. Takano T, Oberheim N, Cotrina ML, Nedergaard M (2009) Astrocytes and ischemic injury. Stroke 40: S8–12.
50. Nagai M, Re DB, Nagata T, Chalazonitis A, Jessell TM, et al. (2007) Astrocytes expressing ALS-linked mutated SOD1 release factors selectively toxic to motor neurons. Nat Neurosci 10: 615–622.
51. Yamanaka K, Chun SJ, Boillee S, Fujimori-Tonou N, Yamashita H, et al. (2008) Astrocytes as determinants of disease progression in inherited amyotrophic lateral sclerosis. Nature Neuroscience 11: 251–253.
52. Ballas N, Lioy DT, Grunseich C, Mandel G (2009) Non-cell autonomous influence of MeCP2-deficient glia on neuronal dendritic morphology. Nat Neurosci 12: 311–317.
53. Maezawa I, Swanberg S, Harvey D, LaSalle JM, Jin LW (2009) Rett syndrome astrocytes are abnormal and spread MeCP2 deficiency through gap junctions. J Neurosci 29: 5051–5061.

54. Jacobs S, Doering LC Astrocytes prevent abnormal neuronal development in the fragile x mouse. J Neurosci 30: 4508–4514.
55. Bambrick LL, Golovina VA, Blaustein MP, Yarowsky PJ, Krueger BK (1997) Abnormal calcium homeostasis in astrocytes from the trisomy 16 mouse. Glia 19: 352–358.
56. Bambrick LL, Yarowsky PJ, Krueger BK (2003) Altered astrocyte calcium homeostasis and proliferation in theTs65Dn mouse, a model of Down syndrome. J Neurosci Res 73: 89–94.
57. Sebastia J, Cristofol R, Pertusa M, Vilchez D, Toran N, et al. (2004) Down's syndrome astrocytes have greater antioxidant capacity than euploid astrocytes. European Journal of Neuroscience 20: 2355–2366.
58. Shukkur EA, Shimohata A, Akagi T, Yu W, Yamaguchi M, et al. (2006) Mitochondrial dysfunction and tau hyperphosphorylation in Ts1Cje, a mouse model for Down syndrome. Hum Mol Genet 15: 2752–2762.
59. Griffin WS, Stanley LC, Ling C, White L, MacLeod V, et al. (1989) Brain interleukin 1 and S-100 immunoreactivity are elevated in Down syndrome and Alzheimer disease. Proc Natl Acad Sci U S A 86: 7611–7615.
60. Jorgensen OS, Brooksbank BW, Balazs R (1990) Neuronal plasticity and astrocytic reaction in Down syndrome and Alzheimer disease. J Neurol Sci 98: 63–79.
61. Nelson PG, Fitzgerald S, Rapoport SI, Neale EA, Galdzicki Z, et al. (1997) Cerebral cortical astroglia from the trisomy 16 mouse, a model for down syndrome, produce neuronal cholinergic deficits in cell culture. Proc Natl Acad Sci U S A 94: 12644–12648.
62. Takashima S, Iida K, Mito T, Arima M (1994) Dendritic and histochemical development and ageing in patients with Down's syndrome. J Intellect Disabil Res 38(Pt 3): 265–273.
63. Dailey ME, Smith SJ (1996) The dynamics of dendritic structure in developing hippocampal slices. J Neurosci 16: 2983–2994.
64. Fiala JC, Feinberg M, Popov V, Harris KM (1998) Synaptogenesis via dendritic filopodia in developing hippocampal area CA1. J Neurosci 18: 8900–8911.
65. Papa M, Bundman MC, Greenberger V, Segal M (1995) Morphological analysis of dendritic spine development in primary cultures of hippocampal neurons. J Neurosci 15: 1–11.
66. Holtmaat AJ, Trachtenberg JT, Wilbrecht L, Shepherd GM, Zhang X, et al. (2005) Transient and persistent dendritic spines in the neocortex in vivo. Neuron 45: 279–291.
67. Zuo Y, Lin A, Chang P, Gan WB (2005) Development of long-term dendritic spine stability in diverse regions of cerebral cortex. Neuron 46: 181–189.
68. Marrs GS, Green SH, Dailey ME (2001) Rapid formation and remodeling of postsynaptic densities in developing dendrites. Nat Neurosci 4: 1006–1013.
69. Harris KM (1999) Structure, development, and plasticity of dendritic spines. Curr Opin Neurobiol 9: 343–348.
70. Wong WT, Wong RO (2000) Rapid dendritic movements during synapse formation and rearrangement. Curr Opin Neurobiol 10: 118–124.
71. Beattie EC, Stellwagen D, Morishita W, Bresnahan JC, Ha BK, et al. (2002) Control of synaptic strength by glial TNF alpha. Science 295: 2282–2285.
72. Dowell JA, Johnson JA, Li L (2009) Identification of astrocyte secreted proteins with a combination of shotgun proteomics and bioinformatics. J Proteome Res 8: 4135–4143.
73. Keene SD, Greco TM, Parastatidis I, Lee SH, Hughes EG, et al. (2009) Mass spectrometric and computational analysis of cytokine-induced alterations in the astrocyte secretome. Proteomics 9: 768–782.
74. Moore NH, Costa LG, Shaffer SA, Goodlett DR, Guizzetti M (2009) Shotgun proteomics implicates extracellular matrix proteins and protease systems in neuronal development induced by astrocyte cholinergic stimulation. J Neurochem 108: 891–908.
75. Booth GE, Kinrade EF, Hidalgo A (2000) Glia maintain follower neuron survival during Drosophila CNS development. Development 127: 237–244.
76. Guizzetti M, Moore NH, Giordano G, Costa LG (2008) Modulation of neuritogenesis by astrocyte muscarinic receptors. J Biol Chem 283: 31884–31897.
77. Hughes EG, Elmariah SB, Balice-Gordon RJ Astrocyte secreted proteins selectively increase hippocampal GABAergic axon length, branching, and synaptogenesis. Mol Cell Neurosci 43: 136–145.
78. Chen H, Herndon ME, Lawler J (2000) The cell biology of thrombospondin-1. Matrix Biol 19: 597–614.
79. Osterhout DJ, Frazier WA, Higgins D (1992) Thrombospondin promotes process outgrowth in neurons from the peripheral and central nervous systems. Dev Biol 150: 256–265.
80. Xu JY, Xiao N, Xia J (2010) Thrombospondin 1 accelerates synaptogenesis in hippocampal neurons through neuroligin 1. Nature Neuroscience 13: 22–24.
81. Lu ZJ, Kipnis J (2010) Thrombospondin 1-a key astrocyte-derived neurogenic factor. Faseb Journal 24: 1925–1934.
82. Caceres M, Suwyn C, Maddox M, Thomas JW, Preuss TM (2007) Increased cortical expression of two synaptogenic thrombospondins in human brain evolution. Cereb Cortex 17: 2312–2321.
83. Nishiwaki T, Yamaguchi T, Zhao C, Amano H, Hankenson KD, et al. (2006) Reduced expression of thrombospondins and craniofacial dysmorphism in mice overexpressing Fra1. Journal of Bone and Mineral Research 21: 596–604.
84. Olson LE, Richtsmeier JT, Leszl J, Reeves RH (2004) A chromosome 21 critical region does not cause specific Down syndrome phenotypes. Science 306: 687–690.
85. Richtsmeier JT, Baxter LL, Reeves RH (2000) Parallels of craniofacial maldevelopment in Down syndrome and Ts65Dn mice. Dev Dyn 217: 137–145.
86. Lawler J (2000) The functions of thrombospondin-1 and-2. Curr Opin Cell Biol 12: 634–640.
87. Greenwood JA, Pallero MA, Theibert AB, Murphy-Ullrich JE (1998) Thrombospondin signaling of focal adhesion disassembly requires activation of phosphoinositide 3-kinase. J Biol Chem 273: 1755–1763.
88. Giehl K, Graness A, Goppelt-Struebe M (2008) The small GTPase Rac-1 is a regulator of mesangial cell morphology and thrombospondin-1 expression. Am J Physiol Renal Physiol 294: F407–413.
89. Isenberg JS, Martin-Manso G, Maxhimer JB, Roberts DD (2009) Regulation of nitric oxide signalling by thrombospondin 1: implications for anti-angiogenic therapies. Nature Reviews Cancer 9: 182–194.
90. Jimenez B, Volpert OV, Crawford SE, Febbraio M, Silverstein RL, et al. (2000) Signals leading to apoptosis-dependent inhibition of neovascularization by thrombospondin-1. Nat Med 6: 41–48.
91. Lymn JS, Rao SJ, Clunn GF, Gallagher KL, O'Neil C, et al. (1999) Phosphatidylinositol 3-kinase and focal adhesion kinase are early signals in the growth factor-like responses to thrombospondin-1 seen in human vascular smooth muscle. Arterioscler Thromb Vasc Biol 19: 2133–2140.
92. Dawson DW, Pearce SF, Zhong R, Silverstein RL, Frazier WA, et al. (1997) CD36 mediates the In vitro inhibitory effects of thrombospondin-1 on endothelial cells. J Cell Biol 138: 707–717.
93. Eroglu C, Allen NJ, Susman MW, O'Rourke NA, Park CY, et al. (2009) Gabapentin receptor alpha2delta-1 is a neuronal thrombospondin receptor responsible for excitatory CNS synaptogenesis. Cell 139: 380–392.
94. Busciglio J, Andersen JK, Schipper HM, Gilad GM, McCarty R, et al. (1998) Stress, aging, and neurodegenerative disorders. Molecular mechanisms. Ann N Y Acad Sci 851: 429–443.
95. Helguera P, Pelsman A, Pigino G, Wolvetang E, Head E, et al. (2005) ets-2 promotes the activation of a mitochondrial death pathway in Down's syndrome neurons. J Neurosci 25: 2295–2303.
96. Pelsman A, Hoyo-Vadillo C, Gudasheva TA, Seredenin SB, Ostrovskaya RU, et al. (2003) GVS-111 prevents oxidative damage and apoptosis in normal and Down's syndrome human cortical neurons. Int J Dev Neurosci 21: 117–124.
97. Tran MD, Neary JT (2006) Purinergic signaling induces thrombospondin-1 expression in astrocytes. Proc Natl Acad Sci U S A 103: 9321–9326.
98. Roberts DD, Isenberg JS, Ridnour LA, Wink DA (2007) Nitric oxide and its gatekeeper thrombospondin-1 in tumor angiogenesis. Clin Cancer Res 13: 795–798.
99. Nickoloff BJ, Riser BL, Mitra RS, Dixit VM, Varani J (1988) Inhibitory effect of gamma interferon on cultured human keratinocyte thrombospondin production, distribution, and biologic activities. J Invest Dermatol 91: 213–218.
100. Franciotta D, Verri A, Zardini E, Andreoni L, De Amici M, et al. (2006) Interferon-gamma- and interleukin-4-producing T cells in Down's syndrome. Neurosci Lett 395: 67–70.
101. Guazzarotti L, Trabattoni D, Castelletti E, Boldrighini B, Piacentini L, et al. (2009) T lymphocyte maturation is impaired in healthy young individuals carrying trisomy 21 (Down syndrome). Am J Intellect Dev Disabil 114: 100–109.
102. Hallam DM, Capps NL, Travelstead AL, Brewer GJ, Maroun LE (2000) Evidence for an interferon-related inflammatory reaction in the trisomy 16 mouse brain leading to caspase-1-mediated neuronal apoptosis. J Neuroimmunol 110: 66–75.
103. Hallam DM, Maroun LE (1998) Anti-gamma interferon can prevent the premature death of trisomy 16 mouse cortical neurons in culture. Neurosci Lett 252: 17–20.
104. Iwamoto T, Yamada A, Yuasa K, Fukumoto E, Nakamura T, et al. (2009) Influences of interferon-gamma on cell proliferation and interleukin-6 production in Down syndrome derived fibroblasts. Arch Oral Biol 54: 963–969.
105. Tan YH (1976) Chromosome 21 and the cell growth inhibitory effect of human interferon preparations. Nature 260: 141–143.
106. Tan YH, Schneider EL, Tischfield J, Epstein CJ, Ruddle FH (1974) Human chromosome 21 dosage: effect on the expression of the interferon induced antiviral state. Science 186: 61–63.
107. Zihni L (1994) Down's syndrome, interferon sensitivity and the development of leukaemia. Leuk Res 18: 1–6.
108. Maroun LE (1996) Interferon action and chromosome 21 trisomy (Down syndrome): 15 years later. J Theor Biol 181: 41–46.
109. Murphy M, Friend DS, Pike-Nobile L, Epstein LB (1992) Tumor necrosis factor-alpha and IFN-gamma expression in human thymus. Localization and overexpression in Down syndrome (trisomy 21). J Immunol 149: 2506–2512.
110. Hattori M, Fujiyama A, Taylor TD, Watanabe H, Yada T, et al. (2000) The DNA sequence of human chromosome 21. Nature 405: 311–319.
111. Maheshwari RK, Banerjee DK, Waechter CJ, Olden K, Friedman RM (1980) Interferon treatment inhibits glycosylation of a viral protein. Nature 287: 454–456.
112. Kaech S, Banker G (2006) Culturing hippocampal neurons. Nat Protoc 1: 2406–2415.
113. Hayashi K, Ishikawa R, Ye LH, He XL, Takata K, et al. (1996) Modulatory role of drebrin on the cytoskeleton within dendritic spines in the rat cerebral cortex. J Neurosci 16: 7161–7170.
114. Kobayashi C, Aoki C, Kojima N, Yamazaki H, Shirao T (2007) Drebrin a content correlates with spine head size in the adult mouse cerebral cortex. J Comp Neurol 503: 618–626.

Triple Test Screening for Down Syndrome: An Egyptian-Tailored Study

Hazem S. Abou-Youssef*, Manal M. Kamal, Dina A. Mehaney

Clinical and Chemical Pathology Department, Faculty of Medicine, Cairo University, Cairo, Egypt

Abstract

Background: The incidence of Down syndrome (DS) in Egypt varies between 1:555 and 1:770 and its screening by triple test is becoming increasingly popular nowadays. Results, however, seem inaccurate due to the lack of Egyptian-specific information needed for risk calculation and a clear policy for programme implementation. Our study aimed at calculation and validation of the triple marker medians used in screening Egyptian females as well as to recommend programme conventions to unify screening in this country.

Methods: The study was conducted on 668 Egyptian women, in weeks 15–20 of pregnancy as proven by sonar. Chorionic gonadotropin (CG), α-fetoprotein (AFP) and unconjugated oestriol (uE3) were measured on Siemens Immulite analyzer. Medians of the three parameters were calculated, regressed against gestational age (GA) and weighted by the number of participants/week. Equations were derived to adjust each parameter to the maternal weight and were centered on the median Egyptian weight. Prisca software was fed with the above data, multiples-of-median (MoM) and DS risks were calculated and the screening performance was evaluated at a mid-trimester risk cutoff of 1:270.

Results: Log-linear [$AFP/uE3 = 10^{(A+B*GA)}$] and exponential equations [$CG = A*e^{(B*GA)}$] were derived and the regressed medians were found to follow similar patterns to other Asian and Western medians. Oestriol was always lowest (even halved) while CG and AFP were intermediate. A linear reciprocal model best fitted weight distribution among Egyptians and successfully adjusted each parameter to a weight of 78.2 kg. Epidemiological monitoring of these recommendations revealed satisfactory performance in terms of 6.7% initial positive rate and 1.00 grand MoM.

Conclusions: Adoption of the above recommendations is hoped to pave the way to a successful DS screening programme tailored to Egyptian peculiarities.

Editor: Tao Cai, NIDCR/NIH, United States of America

Funding: This work was supported by the Cairo University Research Fund. The funder had no role in study design, data collection and analysis, decision to publish, or preparation of the manuscript.

Competing Interests: The authors have declared that no competing interests exist.

* Email: hazem2000@kasralainy.edu.eg

Introduction

Down syndrome (DS) is the most common chromosomal aneuploidy in live born infants. The overall incidence of DS is approximately 1 in 800 births in the general population [1]. Figures in Egypt vary between 1 in 555 in one study [2] to 1 in 770 in another [3]. In 2007, the American College of Obstetricians and Gynecologists (ACOG) recommended that all pregnant women, regardless of their age, should be offered screening for DS. Those with high risk should be confirmed by an invasive diagnostic procedure like amniocentesis or chorionic villus sampling [4].

Second trimester screening is traditionally based on the "triple test". In this test, three maternal serum markers [α-fetoprotein (AFP), chorionic gonadotropin (CG) and unconjugated oestriol (uE3)] are measured and used to modify the women's prior risk (based on her age) to yield a patient specific DS risk [5]. In order to compensate for variation of these markers with gestational age, the measured concentrations are divided by the median marker levels in the relevant gestational week yielding "Multiples of the Median (MoM)". Furthermore, these MoMs are adjusted to compensate for factors, other than DS, that alter marker levels [6].

Most commercial software packages rely on the same algorithm (overlapping multivariate Gaussian distributions) for risk calculation. The quality of the results obtained depends therefore, among others, on the following variables: analytical performance of the immunoassays used [7]; accurate dating of pregnancy [8], proper choice of medians used to calculate the MoMs, and of valid factors for MoM adjustment and on the selection of suitable population parameters [9].

Despite the increasing number of triple test requests, risk calculations have not been tailored to the Egyptian peculiarities, leading to gross errors in risk prediction and a greater proportion of women unnecessarily exposed to invasive techniques. Aiming at

Table 1. Observed and regressed median values for the three measured triple marker parameters.

GA, wk	Mean GA	N	AFP, IU/ml		uE3, ng/ml		CG, mIU/ml	
			Obs	Reg	Obs	Reg	Obs	Reg
15	15.34	124	33.3	30.5	0.48	0.49	30 700	29 523
16	16.33	106	35.5	34.0	0.65	0.63	26 900	26 979
17	17.30	109	37.2	38.0	0.81	0.81	23 500	24 789
18	18.30	102	43.4	42.5	1.18	1.04	21 500	22 783
19	19.35	117	43.7	47.4	1.34	1.34	20 500	20 768
20	20.34	110	62.0	53.0	1.62	1.72	20 400	19 102

GA, gestational age in weeks; *N*, number; *AFP*, alpha fetoprotein; *uE3*, unconjugated oestriol; *CG*, chorionic gonadotropin; *Obs*, observed median, *Reg*, regressed weighted median.

bridging this serious gap in our practice, the current study was conducted.

Considering the economic situation of our region, adding a fourth test (quadruple testing) or combination with first trimester screening, though more efficient, was projected to decrease programme uptake. A wide-spread, less expensive but less efficient programme was thought to be more valuable to our community.

Materials and Methods

The study was conducted on 668 pregnant women spanning gestational weeks 15^{+0} to 20^{+6}. They were recruited from the Obstetric department of the Faculty of Medicine, Cairo University between December 2011 and November, 2012. Gestational dating for all women was based on biparietal diameter measurement, while dating based on last menstrual period (LMP) was only used to calculate the magnitude of error in dating and in subsequent risk calculation. Ultrasonography was also used to exclude multiple pregnancies and gross fetal anomalies. Blood samples were extracted from each participant and serum was separated and stored at $-20°C$ for a period that did not exceed 6 days to ensure analyte stability [10]. All participants signed informed consent accepting all the procedures to be done. The study was approved by the Research Ethics Committee of The Faculty of Medicine, Cairo University. All specimens were analysed for AFP, CG and uE3 using Immulite 2000 analyser (Siemens Medical Solutions Diagnostics) and their corresponding reagents and calibrators; catalogue numbers: L2KAP2, L2KCG2 and L2KUE32, respectively). The technique is a solid-phase, enzyme-amplified chemiluminescence immunoassay that was run fully-automated according to the manufacturer instructions. Strict adherence to quality assurance procedures were followed throughout the study including acceptable performance of a two-level quality control material introduced in each run. DS risk was calculated using Siemens PRISCA Prenatal Risk Calculation Software v. 4.0, catalogue Number: 402692. Calculations were based on the population parameter set of Cuckle [11]. The used version of Prisca does not allow selecting between different parameter sets.

Medians values of the three parameters were calculated for each completed gestational week. These medians were smoothened by regression against the gestational weeks (average decimal weeks). A log-linear model best fitted the relation between GA and both AFP and uE3 whereas CG was described by an exponential equation. These regression equations were weighted based on the square root of the number of samples in each week.

To derive adjustment factors for maternal weight, a linear reciprocal model [12] was found to best fit the weight distribution of Egyptian women. An equation was derived to adjust the MoMs of each of the three parameters to maternal weight. Prisca default adjustment factors for insulin-treated diabetes, smoking and in-vitro fertilization were accepted. Since the observed medians were calculated from a homogeneous subset of Egyptians belonging to the same ethnic origin (Arab panethnicity) [13], no correction was warranted for ethnicity. A priori DS risk was calculated according to the formula of Snijders et al [14]. Data were statistically analysed using IBM SPSS v. 20.

Results

The 668 studied females were fairly equally distributed among weeks 15 to 20, with no less than a hundred participants/week. Their ages at sampling time ranged between 15.3 and 47.7 years; median (interquartile range) were 27.8 (24.7–30.9) y with 93.3% younger than 35 y. Maternal weight ranged between 50 and

Table 2. Regression coefficients for the equations relating the three measured triple marker parameters to gestational age (in decimal weeks).

	AFP, IU/ml	uE3, ng/ml	CG, mIU/ml
A (SE)[1]	0.759 (0.167)	−1.938 (0.036)	111899.7 (1950)
B (SE)[2]	0.048 (0.009)	0.109 (0.002)	−0.087 (0.003)
r (R^2)[3]	0.928 (0.862)	0.990 (0.980)	0.984 (0.969)
P	0.007	<0.0005	<0.0005

[1] Intercept (standard error);
[2] Slope (standard error);
[3] Correlation coefficient (coefficient of determination).

103 kg; median: 78.2 (76.3–82.6) kg. None of them declared smoking and only 1.6% were on insulin treatment. Raw data are presented in table S1.

The observed medians of the three parameters are given in table 1. When regressed against the average GA for each week gestational age, the equations describing the relation of median AFP and uE3 to gestational age were log-linear having the general layout: AFP (IU/ml) or uE3 (ng/ml) = $10^{(A+B*GA)}$. For CG, the equation was exponential; CG (mIU/ml) = $A*e^{(B*GA)}$. These equations were weighted by the square root of the number of participants/week. Details of the equations are given in table 2. Using these median analyte values, the grand median MoM for each of the three parameters (without regard for the gestational week) was always 1.00. Figure 1 compares Egyptian medians with those in Korea [15] and a number of Western areas compiled by Vranken et al [16].

The linear reciprocal model for weight correction yielded the following general layout formula: *Weight-adjusted MoM* $= \frac{MoM}{F}$; where $F = a + \left(\frac{b}{Wt}\right)$, Wt is the maternal weight in kg, F for $AFP = 0.33 + \left(\frac{52.25}{Wt}\right)$, for $uE3 = 0.79 + \left(\frac{16.32}{Wt}\right)$ and for $CG = 0.49 + \left(\frac{39.42}{Wt}\right)$. Weight correction was centred on the median weight of the screened population (78.2 kg) and is

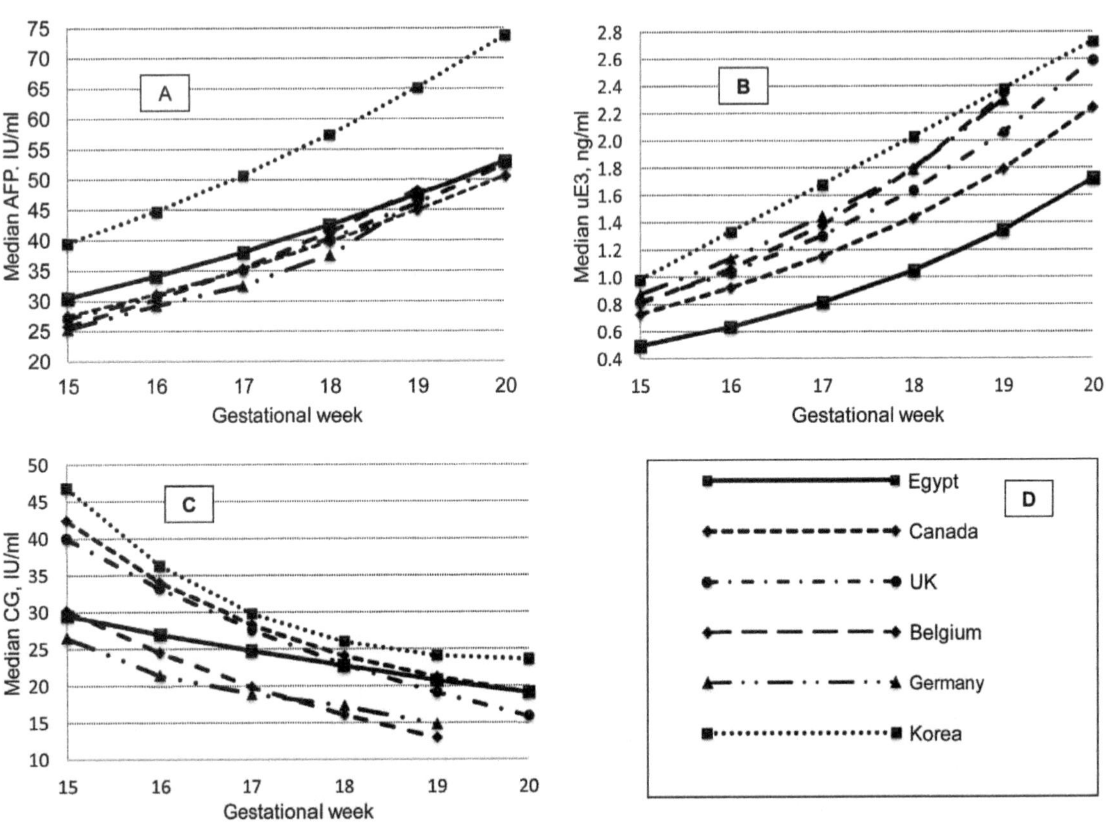

Figure 1. Comparison between median triple marker parameters in Egypt and different geographic regions. Panel A is AFP, B is uE3, C is CG and D is an explanatory legend.

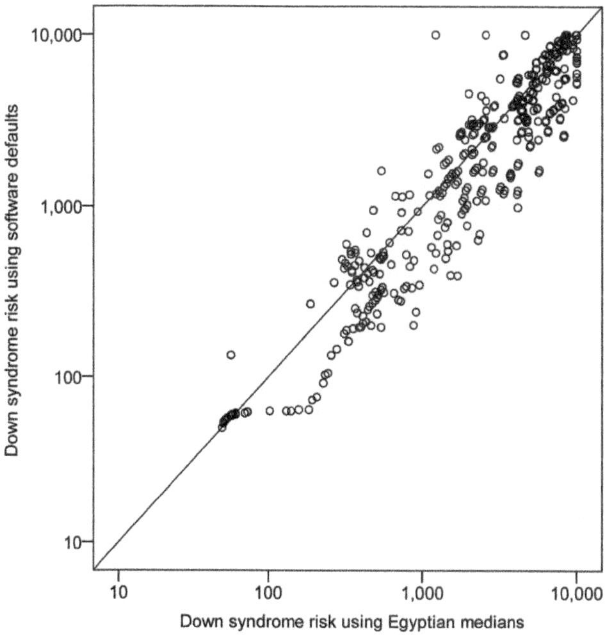

Figure 2. Comparison between risks (1:n) generated using Egypt-specific medians and software default medians.

applicable within the studied weight range (50 to 103 kg). Within this weight range, weight-correction factors ranged between 0.91–1.33 for AFP, 0.83–1.02 for uE3 and 0.93–1.25 for CG. Based on these correction factors, a woman's MoM value may increase up to 120.5% or decrease by 75.2%; particularly at the extremes of weights studied. Such factors were constantly 1.00 for the three analytes for women weighing 78.2 kg.

Using the Egyptian-specific medians and weight correction factors; the DS risk for 45 out of the 668 screened women exceeded the risk cutoff adopted (1:270 at sampling time). This figure equates to an initial positive rate (IPR) of 6.7%. When software default medians (European-based) were used, 76 cases were risky (IPR = 11.4%); including the 45 women identified risky when using Egyptian medians and extra 31 considered non-risky. In general, 67.7% of women were considered less risky when calculations were based on Egyptian medians, particularly in weeks 17 to 20. Figure 2 displays the general trend for overestimation of DS risk when default medians were blindly accepted.

Both prior (based on age) and posterior (based on Egyptian medians) risks were concordant (risk >1:270) in 596 (89.2%) of females and were <1:270 in 10 (1.5%) of them. The risks were discrepant in the remaining 62 (9.3%) participants; 27 (4.0%) were risky based on their ages only but turned-out to be non-risky after introducing biochemical markers into risk calculation, and 35 (5.3%) had an opposite scenario.

An error of at least 1 week was found in 8.5% of the studied females when last menstrual period was used for gestational dating. In half of them, the difference was 2 weeks or more. Such dating method caused doubling of initial positive rate from 6.7% to 13.9% compared to sonographic dating.

Discussion

Successful, wide-spread implementation of a national screening programme for DS in Egypt is hampered by a number of hurdles. Developing a set of median values for each biochemical marker in every week of gestation comes on top of the list. Reliance on medians originating from other communities or accepting software defaults undermine the philosophy of such a population-specific programme and is postulated to be the primary cause for poor performance in our country. Other obstacles exist and need to be rectified as well. The current study was planned to address these issues aiming at promulgating a screening policy worthwhile adoption in Egypt. The study was conducted on 668 Egyptian females making sure that at least a hundred participants were included in each week between 15 and 20 as has been recommended [17]. The American College of Medical Genetics and Genomics, *(ACMG)* technical standards and guideline for DS screening state that ideally 100 samples for each gestational week from 15 through 20 should be used to calculate medians [18]. Definition of gestational age was consistently based on measurement of fetal biparietal diameter to circumvent errors associated with last menstrual period calculations. A difference of at least one week was found in 57 (8.5%) females, 14 of them were 2–3 weeks and 15 were 3–5 weeks. This finding underscores the importance of objective gestational dating using sonar [19,20]; otherwise risk calculation would be erroneously based on analyte medians that belong to gestational ages 2–5 weeks away. Should this error be neglected in the current study, the initial positive rate was found to jump to 13.9%; more than double what sonographic age calculations furnished. It was calculated that an error of 3–4 days in gestational age can approximately double (or halve) the expected DS risk [17].

Median values for AFP, CG and uE3 were calculated for each week of the 2nd trimester. Appropriate weighted regression analysis was used to fit the observed data to the GA. These equations are used to predict "smoothened" medians for each week of gestation, minimizing the effect of outliers and giving less weight to weeks with smaller number of participants. When these medians were compared to other geographical regions (Canada, UK, Germany, Belgium and Korea), they showed similar pattern of variation with GA (Figure 1). AFP increased by a constant proportion of 11.7% per week (11.3%–23.5% in the other regions) and uE3 increased by 28.4% (compared to 14.7%–35.7% elsewhere). CG, on the other hand, showed least association with GA, decreasing by 8.0% to 8.8%/week (8.0% to 19.6% in other countries). Errors in GA dating will, then, have its greatest impact on uE3. On a week to week basis, Egyptian AFP medians were second highest among other geographical regions; following Korean medians. Oestriol was lowest all through, particularly when compared to Korean medians that were higher by a factor of 1.6 to 2.1. CG occupied an intermediate position between Korea, Canada and UK (below them) and Belgium and Germany (above both). Interestingly, CG curve showed the least steep decline with GA compared to the five regions. The observed difference in medians is not purely racial, because the quoted measurements were made on Beckman Coulter Access rather than Siemens Immulite used in the current study. Both techniques, however, are immuno-chemiluminescence-based. Asian women who were reported to have the highest AFP, CG and uE3 [21,22], are still leading even when compared to Egyptians.

Another potential source of error in DS risk calculation is the adjustment for maternal weight. Weight distribution in our community is different from that in Western, black or Asian communities, and needs to be considered when adjustments to MoMs are to be made. Three formulas were derived and served to adjust measured MoMs to a population median maternal weight of 78.2 kg (compared to 60 kg in a Caucasian-based study [23] and 57.2 kg in a Korean study) [15]. A difference in median weight as small as 2.5 kg was recommended to warrant formula modification to minimize errors in risk calculation [24]. This recommendation highlights the importance of using population-tailored equations. Neveux's linear reciprocal model better fitted weight distribution in our community than the log-linear model recommended by Reynolds et al [24].

Due to the small number of diabetics (only 11 women) and absence of smoking history in the 668 participants, default software correction factors for these potential confounders were accepted. Multiple pregnancies were excluded from the study to avoid "pseudo-risk" calculations. Other suggested covariates (as parity, in vitro fertilization, intra-uterine insemination, analyte concentrations in a previous pregnancy or sex of the fetus) were beyond the scope of the current study. The improvement in screening that can be achieved by incorporating additional clinical factors needs to be balanced against the practical realities involved with the data collection [17].

In addition to the above statistical findings, a number of conventions need to be agreed upon by policy makers in order to harmonize results and unify terms across the whole country. The first convention is the time at which risk is to be calculated and expressed; whether mid-trimester (i.e., at sampling-time) or term-risk. The former choice was adopted in the current study. Another decision is the choice of DS risk cut-off that warrants invasive diagnostic procedures. A risk cut-off was set at 1:270. It is equivalent to the risk of a 35-year old woman in the absence of serum screening. The risk cut-off of a screening test should be set specifically to each country in consideration of the cost and safety of invasive diagnostic procedures, the prevalence of DS, and the age distribution of pregnant women [15].

The appropriateness of findings and conventions recommended in the current study was assessed by epidemiological monitoring [25,26]. Our target was to keep the percentage of women considered screen positive to a figure less than 7%. This figure, often termed initial positive rate (IPR) reached 6.7% in our study; well below our target. In many US laboratories using the same risk cut-off, same test-combination (triple test) and same method of gestational age dating (sonar); IPR was reportedly 6.5% [27].

Another statistic calculated was the grand MoM for each of the three measured parameters. It is the median of all 668 MoMs of each parameter; without regard for the gestational week. The target was to keep the 3 grand MoMs as close to unity as possible. All three MoMs were exactly 1.00.

It's believed that a similar study has not been done in Egypt, nor in many countries in the Arab region and North Africa, and is hoped that implementation of the above medians, correction factors and conventions will pave the way to a successful national DS screening programme. Considering the ethnic similarities between most of the Arab women (Arab panethnicity), such recommendations can even extend to other countries in the region and would surely be a better option for some of them than accepting literature-based recommendations or software defaults.

Supporting Information

Data S1 Raw data.

Acknowledgments

We are grateful to Dr Moutaz El-Sherbini, lecturer of Obstetrics and Gynaecology, Faculty of Medicine, Cairo University; for his help in obstetric evaluation of many participants. The help of Asmaa Ismail, resident of Chemical Pathology in specimen and data collection is also acknowledged.

Author Contributions

Conceived and designed the experiments: HSA MMK DAM. Performed the experiments: HSA MMK DAM. Analyzed the data: HSA. Contributed reagents/materials/analysis tools: HSA MMK DAM. Contributed to the writing of the manuscript: HSA MMK DAM.

References

1. Cuckle HS, Wald NJ, Thompson SG (1987) Estimating a woman's risk of having a pregnancy associated with Down's syndrome using her age and serum alpha-fetoprotein level. BJOG 94: 387–402.
2. Hafez M, El-Tahan M, Zedan M, Eisa M (1984) Demographic trends of Down's Syndrome in Egypt. Human Biology 56: 703–712.
3. Temtamy SA, Abdel Meguid N, Mazen I, Ismael SR, Kassem NS, et al. (1998) A genetic epidemiological study of malformations at birth in Egypt. East Mediterr Health J 4: 252–259.
4. ACOG Practice Bulletin No 77 (2007) Screening for fetal chromosomal abnormalities. Obstet Gynecol 109: 217–227.
5. Palomaki GE, Haddow JE (1987) Maternal serum alpha-fetoprotein, age and Down syndrome risk. Am J Obstet Gynecol 156: 460–463.
6. Reynols TM, Penney MD (1990) The mathematical basis of multivariate risk screening: with special reference to screening for Down's syndrome associated pregnancy. Ann Clin Biochem 27: 425–428.
7. Wald NJ, Hackshaw AK, George LM (2000) Assay precision of serum alpha fetoprotein in antenatal screening for neural tube defects and Down's syndrome. J Med Screen 7: 74–77.
8. Bishop J, Dunstan FD, Nix BJ, Reynold TM (1995) The effects of gestation dating on the calculation of patient specific risks in Down's syndrome screening. Ann Clin Biochem 32: 464–477.
9. Reynolds T, Ellis A, Jones R (2004) Down's syndrome risk estimates demonstrate considerable heterogeneity despite homogeneity of input. Ann Clin Biochem 41: 464–468.
10. Messerlian GM, Eklund EE, Malone FD, Palomaki GE, Canick JA, et al. (2006) Stability of first- and second- trimester serum markers after storage and shipment. Prenat Diagn 26: 17–21.
11. Cuckle H (1995) Improved parameter for risk estimation in Down's syndrome screening. Prenat Diagn 15: 1057–1065.
12. Neveux LM, Palomaki GE, Larrivee DA, Knight GJ, Haddow LE (1996) Refinements in managing weight adjustment for interpreting prenatal screening results. Prenat Diagn 16: 1115–1119.
13. Nicholas SH, Saad Eddin I (1997) Arab society: class, gender, power, and development. Cairo: American University in Cairo Press. p6.
14. Snijders RJ, Sundberg K, Holzgreve W, Henry G, Nicolaides KH (1999) Maternal age- and gestation-specific risk for trisomy 21. Ultrasound Obestet Gynecol 13: 167–170.
15. Kwon LY, Park IY, Park YG, Lee Y, Lee G, et al. (2011) Korean-Specific Parameter Models for Calculating the Risk of Down Syndrome in the Second Trimester of Pregnancy. J Korean Med Sci 26: 1619–1624.
16. Vranken G, Reynold T, Van Nueten J (2006) Medians for second-trimester maternal serum markers: geographical differences and variation caused by median multiples-of-median equations. J Clin Pathol 59: 639–644.
17. Benn PA (2002) Advances in prenatal screening for Down syndrome: I. General principles and second trimester testing. Clinica Chemica Acta 323: 1–16.
18. Palomaki GE, Bradley LA, McDowell GA (2005) Down Syndrome Working Group; ACMG Laboratory Quality Assurance Committee. Technical standards and guidelines: prenatal screening for Down syndrome. Genet Med 7: 344–354.
19. Wald NJ, Cuckle HS, Densem JW, Kennard A, Smith D (1992) Maternal serum screening for Down's syndrome: the effect of routine ultrasound scan determination of gestational age and adjustment for maternal weight. Br J Obstet Gynaecol 99: 144–149.
20. Benn PA, Borgida A, Horne D, Briganti S, Collins R, et al. (1997) Down syndrome and neural tube defect screening: the value of using gestational age by ultrasonography. Am J Obstet Gynecol 176: 1056–1061.
21. O'Brien JE, Dvorin E, Drugan A, Johnson MP, Yaron Y, et al. (1997) Race-ethnicity-specific variation in multiple-marker biochemical screening: alpha-fetoprotein, hCG, and estriol. Obstet Gynecol 89: 355–358.
22. Wang YY, Luo J, Zhu MW, Liu LN, Ma X (2006) Second-trimester double or triple screening for Down syndrome: a comparison of Chinese and Caucasian populations. Int J Gynaecol Obstet 94: 67–72.
23. MacRae AR, Gardner HA, Allen LC, Tokmakelian S, Lepage N (2003) Outcome validation of the Beckman Coulter access analyzer in a second-trimester Down syndrome serum screening application. Clin Chem 49: 69–76.

24. Reynolds TM, Vranken G, Van Nueten J (2006) Weight correction of MoM values: which method? J Clin Pathol 59: 753–758.
25. Palomaki GE, Neveux LM, Haddow JE (1996) Can reliable Down's syndrome detection rates be determined from prenatal screening intervention trials? J Med Screen 3: 12–17.
26. Knight GJ, Palomaki GE (2003) Epidemiologic monitoring of prenatal screening for neural tube defects and Down syndrome. Clin Lab Med 23: 531–551.
27. Ashwood ER, Knight GJ (2012) Pregnancy and its disorders. In: Burtis CA, Ashwood ER, Bruns DE, editors. Tietz textbook of clinical chemistry and molecular diagnostics. 5th Ed. St. Louis: Elsevier Saunders. 1991–2044.

Incorporating DNA Sequencing into Current Prenatal Screening Practice for Down's Syndrome

Nicholas J. Wald*, Jonathan P. Bestwick

Wolfson Institute of Preventive Medicine, Barts and the London School of Medicine and Dentistry, London, United Kingdom

Abstract

Background: Prenatal screening for Down's syndrome is performed using biochemical and ultrasound markers measured in early pregnancy such as the Integrated test using first and second trimester markers. Recently, DNA sequencing methods have been introduced on free DNA in maternal plasma, yielding a high screening performance. These methods are expensive and there is a test failure rate. We determined the screening performance of merging the Integrated test with the newer DNA techniques in a protocol that substantially reduces the cost compared with universal DNA testing and still achieves high screening performance with no test failures.

Methods: Published data were used to model screening performance of a protocol in which all women receive the first stage of the Integrated test at about 11 weeks of pregnancy. On the basis of this higher risk women have reflex DNA testing and lower risk women as well as those with a failed DNA test complete the Integrated test at about 15 weeks.

Results: The overall detection rate was 95% with a 0.1% false-positive rate if 20% of women were selected to receive DNA testing. If all women had DNA testing the detection rate would be 3 to 4 percentage points higher with a false-positive rate 30 times greater if women with failed tests were treated as positive and offered a diagnostic amniocentesis, or 3 times greater if they had a second trimester screening test (Quadruple test) and treated as positive only if this were positive. The cost per women screened would be about one-fifth, compared with universal DNA testing, if the DNA test were 20 times the cost of the Integrated test.

Conclusion: The proposed screening protocol achieves a high screening performance without programme test failures and at a substantially lower cost than offering all women DNA testing.

Editor: Cees Oudejans, VU University Medical Center, The Netherlands

Funding: These authors have no support or funding to report.

Competing Interests: Nicholas Wald is a Director of Intema, which holds patents for the Integrated test as follows (Application No; Country; Filing Date; Patent No; Issue/Grant Date): 09/301,621; US; 29.04.99; 6,573,103; 03.06.03 36213/99; Australia; 29.04.99; 763171; 31.10.06 2330538; Canada; 29.04.99; 2330538; 11.09.07 99918188; Europe; 29.04.99;1076824; 14.06.06 139302; Israel; 29.04.99; 139302; 26.10.05. The subject matter in this paper has been submitted as an application for patents. With others he held a patent in connection with the use of uE3 as a second trimester screening marker in prenatal screening for Down syndrome, although this has now expired. He is Director of Logical Medical Systems Ltd, which produces software for the interpretation of Down's syndrome screening tests. There are no further patents, products in development or marketed products to declare.

* E-mail: n.j.wald@qmul.ac.uk

Introduction

The testing of cell-free DNA circulating in maternal plasma offers an effective means of screening for Down's syndrome with detection rates (proportion of affected pregnancies with positive results) of 98% or more and false-positive rates (proportion of unaffected pregnancies with positive results) of about 0.2% or less [1–7]. At present such DNA testing tends to be expensive (cited as being charged $795 to $2762 in the United States [6]) and requires specialist expertise available in only a few laboratories. In about 2–13% of pregnancies a result cannot be obtained for various reasons including insufficient fetal DNA in the maternal plasma. These can be referred to as test failures and tend to be ignored in describing the efficacy of the test. One study [1] reported 11.5% (compromised sample, haemolyzed sample, inadequate volume, failed quality control). Another reported a test failure rate of 3.4% (0.88% assay failure and 2.50% of samples inadequate [2]). A third study reported that 16 out of 532 pregnancies (3%) yielded insufficient fetal DNA and could not be tested and 4 out of 96 Down's syndrome pregnancies (4.2%; 3 mosaics) yielded an unidentifiable result as well as 24 out of 426 unaffected pregnancies (5.6%) suggesting a test failure rate of 7% [3]. A fourth study reported that in one group 5% did not meet "QC criteria", but none in a second group of the same size [4]. In a fifth study based on women undergoing routine screening, results were not obtained on 4.9% of samples [5]. In a sixth study, based on a mixture of women with positive conventional screening tests for Down's syndrome and women undergoing routine screening, 1.6% failed the quality control criteria [5]. In a seventh study 21 out of 166 samples did not pass the DNA quality test (13%) [7].

We here propose a screening protocol arising from, and improving on, an idea previously reported [8], that merges existing methods based on fetal ultrasound measurements and immunoassays with the newer DNA techniques in a way that would substantially reduce the cost compared with the cost of universal DNA testing and still achieve a high screening performance, that is, a high detection rate for a low false-positive rate.

The proposed protocol, which is outlined in Figure 1, uses the first trimester stage of an Integrated test (late first trimester measurement of the ultrasound marker nuchal translucency [NT] and the serum markers free β-human chorionic gonadotropin [hCG] and pregnancy associated plasma protein-A [PAPP-A] with maternal age; the Combined test) to determine which women would receive an automatic DNA sequencing test on the sample already collected. The automatic application of a second test in this way can be referred to as "reflex" DNA testing, ie. one triggered by the result of the first test. All women who do not receive a DNA test result proceed to have the second part of the Integrated test which includes the re-use of maternal age and the NT, free β-hCG and PAPP-A measurements together with early second trimester measurement of the serum markers alphafeto-protein [AFP], unconjugated estriol [uE_3] and inhibin-A. Typically the Integrated test uses an hCG (total or the free β) measurement in the second trimester, but in the proposed protocol it is measured in the first trimester instead.

The proposal provides a practical solution to the problem that while DNA testing is an effective screening method it is expensive and can be done only at a small number of laboratories. We offer a solution to this by using the existing screening tests based on serum markers and an ultrasound marker used at a very low false-positive rate to identify a higher risk group, such that only the higher risk women need to have the DNA testing. Importantly, this entails little loss in screening performance.

Methods

Screening performance of the protocol was estimated as follows. Multivariate Gaussian distribution parameters (means, standard deviations and correlation coefficients) of the screening markers from a large cohort study (the Serum Urine and Ultrasound Screening Study [SURUSS]) [9], revised to incorporate subsequent improvements [10], were used to simulate 500,000 Down's syndrome pregnancies and 500,000 unaffected pregnancies, each with a set of marker values (first trimester marker values measured at 11 completed weeks' gestation). Each simulated pregnancy was assigned a maternal age based on the distribution of maternities in England and Wales from 2006 to 2008 inclusive (the latest available at the time the study was performed) [11] and the maternal age-specific odds of an affected livebirth [12–14].

For each simulated pregnancy, a risk of being affected with Down's syndrome based on the first stage of the Integrated test (NT, free β-hCG and PAPP-A) was calculated by multiplying the maternal age-specific odds of having an affected live birth (adjusted to early second trimester by multiplying by 1/0.77 to allow for the general fetal loss in Down's syndrome pregnancies from this time in pregnancy until term [14]) by the likelihood ratio for being affected (for the simulated set of marker values) which was calculated from the multivariate Gaussian distributions of NT, free β-hCG and PAPP-A levels in affected and unaffected pregnancies. The risk cut-offs that yielded initial false-positive rates of 10%, 20%, 40%, 60%, 80% and 90% were determined. A DNA result for those with a risk greater than or equal to the calculated risk cut-off levels was generated. The test failure rate was taken as 3% (towards the lower range of estimates because in some instances a repeat sample may be obtained and provide a test result and these are not considered as test failures in our analyses). 97% were assigned a successfully completed DNA test and 3% were not. Of those in which DNA testing was assumed to have been successfully completed, screening performance was taken from Palomaki et al. [2] as being typically within the range of estimates, so 98.6% of the simulated Down's syndrome pregnancies and 0.2% of the simulated unaffected pregnancies were randomly classified as being screen positive based on DNA sequencing. For those initially classified low risk, and for those in whom DNA testing failed, an Integrated test risk of being affected with Down's syndrome was calculated re-using the first trimester markers together with the second trimester markers. Those with an Integrated test risk greater than 1 in 50 were classified as being screen positive. Overall detection and false-positive rates were estimated, and compared with estimates based on all women having a DNA test. The estimated screening performance was compared with universal DNA testing based on (i) offering women with failed tests a diagnostic test, treating them as screen positive, so yielding a 3.0% false-positive rate, which with the 0.2% test false-positive rate sums to 3.2% or (ii) offering women a second

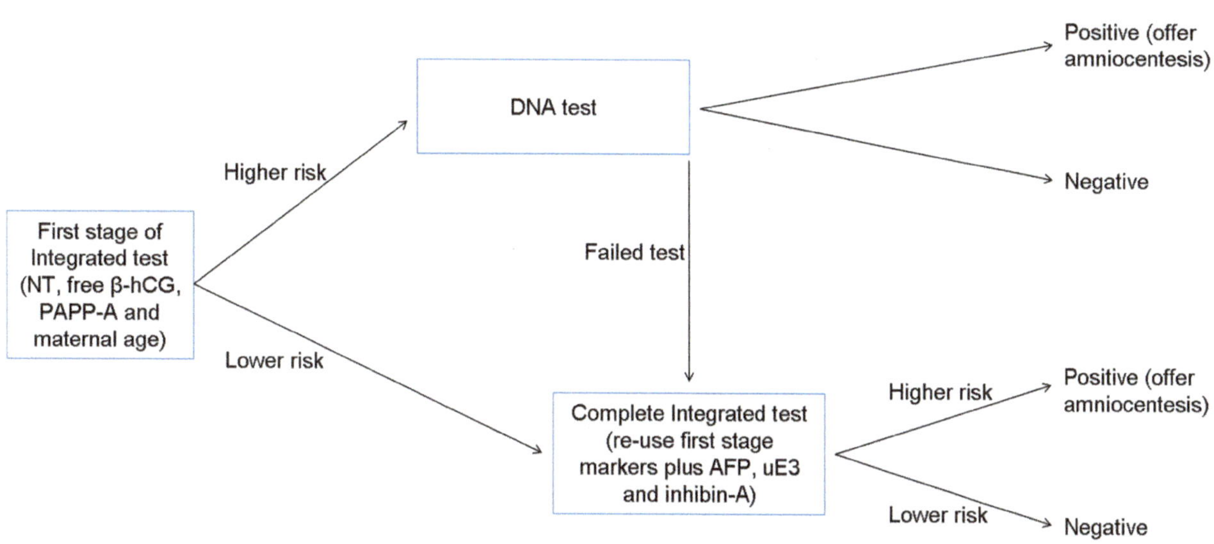

Figure 1. Protocol for reflex DNA testing in conjunction with Integrated test screening.

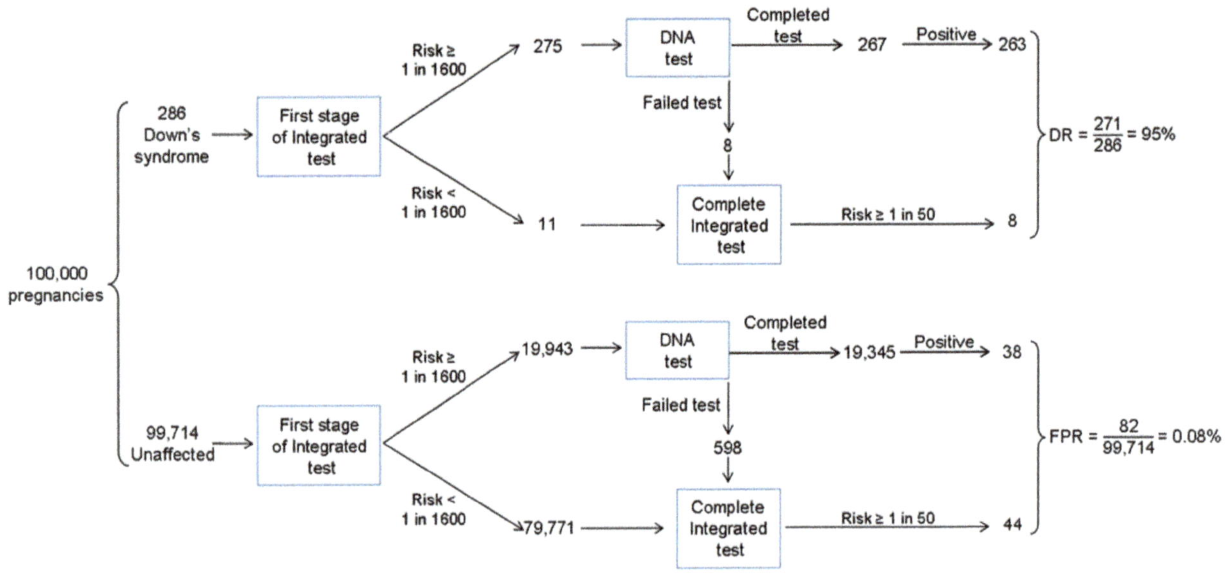

Figure 2. Protocol for reflex DNA testing in conjunction with Integrated test screening in which 20% of women at highest risk using NT, PAPP-A, and free β-hCG (first part of the Integrated test) receive a DNA sequencing test.

trimester Quadruple test (AFP, uE_3, hCG and inhibin-A; 85% detection rate for a 5% false-positive rate) [10]. A similar analysis was done based on using the Combined test (NT, free β-hCG and PAPP-A) only.

We estimated the cost of the screening protocol per woman as a multiple of the cost of an Integrated test. If C_{IT} is the cost of an Integrated test, C_{DNA} the cost of a DNA test, a the proportion of the Integrated test cost incurred in the first trimester, b the proportion of the Integrated test cost incurred in the second trimester and P the proportion of women who have DNA testing (i.e. the positive rate of the initial stage of the Integrated test), the cost per woman screened is:-

$$(a\times C_{IT})+(C_{DNA}\times P)+[b\times C_{IT}\times(1-P)]+(0.03\times b\times C_{IT}\times P),$$

i.e. the cost of the first stage of an Integrated test, plus the cost of a DNA test in women who have a DNA test plus the cost of the second stage of the Integrated test in women who do not have a DNA test plus the cost of the second stage of the Integrated test in women who have a DNA test, but the test failed.

Because $a+b=1$, $b=1-a$, and after dividing throughout by C_{IT} and rearranging, the cost per woman screened as a multiple of the cost of the Integrated test is given by the following equation

$$\frac{\textit{Cost per woman screened}}{C_{IT}}=1+[0.97\times P\times(a-1)]+P\times\frac{C_{DNA}}{C_{IT}}$$

So if a is 75%, P is 10% and the DNA test is 20 times more expensive than the Integrated test, the cost per woman screened as a multiple of the Integrated test cost is $1+[0.97\times0.1\times(0.75-1)]+20\times0.1=3.0$.

A similar analysis was performed using the protocol applied to the Combined test.

The cost per woman screened as a multiple of the Combined test is

$$\frac{\textit{Cost per woman screened}}{C_{CT}}=1+P\times\frac{C_{DNA}}{C_{CT}}$$

Results

Figure 2 is a flow diagram showing an example of the effect of DNA sequencing in conjunction with the Integrated test in 100,000 pregnancies (including 286 with Down's syndrome based on the early second trimester prevalence [11–15]). The first trimester risk cut-off to achieve an initial false-positive rate of 20% based on NT, free β-hCG, and PAPP-A was 1 in 1,600. Women with a risk estimate greater than or equal to this risk cut-off have a reflex DNA test. A test result is not reported at this stage. The remaining women continue to have the second part of the Integrated test. The figure shows 275 (96%) affected and 19,943 (20%) unaffected pregnancies have a reflex DNA test. For 3% of these women the DNA test fails (8 affected, 598 unaffected). These women have second trimester markers measured and an Integrated test risk is reported. Among women who have a completed DNA test, 263 affected and 38 unaffected pregnancies have a positive result. Among the women whose DNA test failed and the women who were not selected for DNA testing after the first trimester stage of the Integrated test, 8 affected and 44 unaffected pregnancies are positive based on the completed Integrated test (risk ≥1 in 50). The overall screening performance is an estimated detection rate of 95% (271/286) with a false-positive rate of 0.1% (82/99,714).

Table 1 shows the screening performance of this approach according to the percentage of women selected for a reflex DNA test based on the first stage of the Integrated test. As the percentage increases from 10% to 90% the detection rate increases from about 92% to 98% and the false-positive rate initially decreases from 0.11% (10% have a DNA test) to 0.08% (20% have a DNA test) then increases to 0.20% (90% have a DNA test). Table 1 also shows the screening performance of routine DNA testing without an Integrated test if (i) women with a DNA test failure have a diagnostic amniocentesis or (ii) women with a DNA test failure have a second trimester screening Quadruple test, the two practical options available. In the first case DNA test failures are regarded as screen-positive and the detection rate is 98.6% with a false-positive rate of 3.2%. In the second case, in which women with a failed test have a Quadruple test, the detection rate is 98.0% with a false-positive rate of 0.3%.

Table 2 shows, in a similar way to Table 1, the cost per woman screened expressed as a multiple of the cost of an Integrated test. As the percentage of women having reflex DNA testing increases from 10% to 90% the cost increases from double to ten-fold if the cost of the DNA test is ten times the cost of the Integrated test. Table 2 also shows how the cost per woman screened changes as the cost of the DNA test decreases. For example if the cost of the DNA test were 20 times the cost of the Integrated test, and 20% of women classified as higher risk at the first stage of the Integrated test, the cost per woman screened would be 5.0 times greater than the cost of the Integrated test. If the cost of the DNA test were 10 times the cost of the Integrated test, the cost per woman screened would be 3.0 times greater. The estimates in Table 2 are based on 75% of the cost of the Integrated test being incurred at the first trimester stage but are robust to different proportions. For example with the cost being split equally between the first and second trimesters the cost per woman screened would be 4.9 instead of 5.0 and 2.9 instead of 3.0 times greater in the examples above.

Figures S1 and S2 illustrate the effect of using the reflex DNA testing approach with the Combined test in the same way that figures 1 and 2 do with the Integrated test, and Tables S1 and S2 present the corresponding estimates in the same way as tables 1 and 2. The screening performance is similar to that with the Integrated test.

Discussion

The reflex DNA testing protocol proposed here, in which the first part of an Integrated test is used to determine who should receive a DNA test, has a number of advantages. First, it has a high screening performance; while the detection rate may be about five percentage points lower than routine DNA testing, the false-positive rate is about 30 times lower if DNA test failures are considered positive and these women have a diagnostic amniocentesis, or about 3 times lower if these women have a second trimester Quadruple test. Second, all women receive a screening result; there are no failed tests and there is no need to tell some women that they had a failed DNA test and needlessly cause them anxiety. Third, the cost of DNA sequencing for the programme is reduced by 80 or 90%, depending on which of the options is adopted. The cost of continuing the Integrated test would remain, which in a public service context is available at the Wolfson Institute of Preventive Medicine, London, for £35 (about $50), but at present this is substantially less than all women having a DNA test. Fourth, the very low false positive rate means that only about 3 per 1000 women screened would need a diagnostic amniocentesis and in about 2 in 3 a Down's syndrome pregnancy would be diagnosed. Fifth, such a protocol allows for the screening of other pregnancy complications such as pre-eclampsia, identified using immunoassays or heart defects using ultrasound markers.

In our analysis we used the results of Palomaki and colleagues (DNA test detection rate of 98.6% and false-positive rate of 0.2% [1]) and a DNA test failure rate of 3%. A sensitivity analysis showed that our estimated overall detection rate of 94.8% and overall false-positive rate of 0.08% is robust to reported variations in the DNA test detection rates, false-positive rates, and test failure rates. For DNA detection rates between 97.5% and 99.5%, and false-positive rates between 0.1% and 0.3%, and DNA test failure rates between 1% and 5%, the overall detection rates were between 93.6% and 95.8% and the overall false-positive rate between 0.05% and 0.12%.

In a typical Integrated test free β-hCG is not measured in the first trimester, but either total or free β-hCG is measured in the second trimester. In the proposed protocol, the overall screening performance is marginally better by measuring hCG earlier; if total hCG were measured in the second trimester and only an NT and PAPP-A measured in the first trimester, the overall detection rate would be 93.8% (instead of 94.8%) and the overall false-positive rate 0.12% (instead of 0.08%) if 20% of women were selected for a reflex DNA test. There is no advantage in measuring hCG in both the first and second trimesters. The measurement of additional markers such as serum placental growth factor, or ultrasound ductus venosus blood flow or nasal bone would improve the screening performance of the proposed protocol, but these are not routinely used, and therefore are not considered here.

Table 1. Screening performance of reflex DNA tests with the Integrated test according to percentage of women having reflex DNA test (Integrated test risk cut-off 1 in 50).

Women selected for reflex DNA test after first stage of Integrated test	Risk cut-off for first stage of Integrated test	Overall screening performance	
		Detection rate (%)	False-positive rate (%)
10%	1 in 630	92.4	0.11
20%	1 in 1600	94.8	0.08
40%	1 in 4900	96.9	0.10
60%	1 in 12000	97.7	0.14
80%	1 in 27000	98.1	0.18
90%	1 in 47000	98.2	0.20
All women have a DNA test (no Integrated test):-			
test failures classified as positive		98.6	3.19
test failures have a Quadruple test, risk cut-off 1 in 100		98.0	0.29

Table 2. Illustration of the cost per woman screened according to the cost of the DNA test, expressed as a multiple of the cost of an Integrated test, and the proportion of women who have a DNA test (i.e. positive based on a the first trimester stage of the Integrated test, 75% of the cost of the Integrated test incurred in the first trimester).

Women selected for reflex DNA test after first stage of Integrated test	DNA test cost as a multiple of Integrated test cost				
	2.5	5	10	20	40
10%	1.2	1.5	2.0	3.0	5.0
20%	1.5	2.0	3.0	5.0	9.0
40%	1.9	2.9	4.9	8.9	17
60%	2.4	3.9	6.9	13	25
80%	2.8	4.8	8.8	17	33
90%	3.0	5.3	9.8	19	37

Most of the published studies on DNA sequencing as a screening test for Down's syndrome were performed on women who were, for one reason or another, at higher than average risk, but this is not a source of bias as the detection rate and false-positive rate of screening tests using markers that are the consequence of the disorder are independent of the prevalence of the disorder.

As experience is gained with the screening protocol proposed in this paper, and if the cost of DNA testing falls, with a lower rate of failed tests, DNA testing could be offered to a larger proportion of pregnancies. At the same time the need for immunoassays and ultrasound measurements currently used to screen for Down's syndrome can be reviewed to assess their value in screening for other disorders such as pre-eclampsia.

Table 2 provides an indication of the costs of the proposed protocol with varying proportions having a DNA test. Expressing cost in multiples of the cost of the Integrated test makes the table generally applicable, so that, if a 4 to 5 fold greater cost per woman screened were acceptable, a 20% DNA testing percentage could be done if the DNA test were 20 times more costly than the Integrated test, or 40% if 10 times more costly. As can be seen from figure 2, the marginal cost of detecting the extra 4% (from 95% to 99%) of Down's syndrome pregnancies that would be detected if all women had DNA testing rather than adopting the proposed protocol would be extremely high, requiring about 80,000 extra DNA tests (100,000 – 20,000) for each extra Down's syndrome pregnancy detected (if 20% have reflex DNA testing). This would remain the case unless the cost of a DNA test were substantially reduced. Collecting plasma samples for DNA testing that may not be used is, of course, an expense, but a small one compared with routine DNA testing.

Reflex DNA testing with the Combined test rather than the Integrated test yields a similar screening performance (see Table S1) with a similar overall cost (see Table S2). The principal disadvantage in using reflex DNA testing with the first trimester Combined test instead of the first stage of the Integrated test is that it would generate a burden of anxiety in a significant number of women. This is because a negative Combined test result would be informed immediately if testing were done at the time of the ultrasound NT measurement or within a day or two if done in a central laboratory. However, because many would regard it to be wrong to artificially delay the reporting of a negative screening result, a "positive" would trigger a DNA test that would take 1–2 weeks, so if women did not receive a prompt result they would realize that they were in a higher risk category. If 20% were selected for a DNA test, as shown in Figure S2, this would apply to 20% of women in the population. If, however, as we suggest DNA testing were conducted together with the Integrated test the corresponding proportion would be substantially less than 1%.

A feature of the proposed screening protocol is that it applies equitably to all pregnant women with the cost averaged over all women screened, regardless of who has a DNA test. This is a practical approach in the context of a screening programme, which is the appropriate way of delivering the service to a population.

Our proposed protocol could usefully be linked to interpretive software that would automatically modify the proportion of women selected for reflex DNA testing and provide the appropriate risk cut-off to achieve this. Also, all women who have a DNA test could receive an estimate of the risk of having a Down's syndrome pregnancy, based on a combination of the DNA test result and the first stage of the Integrated test, so the results would be quantitative and not simply be based on a qualitative DNA result. In deriving this risk, the DNA result could be adjusted for relevant factors such as the fetal DNA fraction and maternal weight.

In summary, the proposed protocol combines current screening methods with the newer DNA sequencing methods to provide a cost effective strategy for all pregnant women with a very high level of efficacy and safety.

Supporting Information

Figure S1 Protocol for reflex DNA testing in conjunction with Combined test screening.

Figure S2 Protocol for reflex DNA testing in conjunction with Combined test screening in which 20% of women at highest risk using the Combined test receive a DNA sequencing test.

Table S1 Screening performance of reflex DNA tests with the Combined test according to percentage of women having reflex DNA test. (Combined test risk cut-off 1 in 50 for DNA test failures).

Table S2 Illustration of the cost per woman screened according to the cost of the DNA test, expressed as a multiple of the cost of a Combined test, and the

proportion of women who have a DNA test (i.e. positive based on the Combined test).

Author Contributions

Conceived and designed the experiments: NW. Performed the experiments: NW JB. Analyzed the data: NW JB. Wrote the paper: NW JB.

References

1. Chiu RWK, Akolekar R, Zheng YWL, Leung TY, Sun H, et al. (2011) Noninvasive prenatal assessment of trisomy 21 by multiplexed maternal plasma DNA sequencing: large scale validity study. *BMJ* 342:c7401.
2. Palomaki GE, Kloza EM, Lambert-Messerlian GM, Haddow JE, Neveux LM, et al. (2011) DNA sequencing of maternal plasma to detect Down syndrome: An international clinical validation study. *Genet Med* 13;913–920.
3. Bianchi DW, Platt LD, Goldberg JD, Abuhamad AZ, Sehnert AJ, et al. (2012) Maternal Blood IS Source to Accurately diagnose fetal aneuploidy (MELISSA) Study Group. Genome-wide fetal aneuploidy detection by maternal plasma DNA sequencing. *Obstet Gynecol* 119:890–901.
4. Sparks AB, Stuble CA, Wang ET, Song K, Oliphant A (2012) Noninvasive prenatal detection and selective analysis of cell-free DNA obtained from maternal blood: evaluation for trisomy 21 and trisomy 18. *Am J Obstet Gynecol* 206:319.e1–9.
5. Nicolaides KH, Syngelaki A, Ashoor G, Birdir C, Touzet G (2012) Noninvasive prenatal testing for fetal trisomies in a routinely screened first-trimester population. *Am J Obstet Gynecol* 207:374.e1–6.
6. Dan S, Wang W, Ren J, Li Y, Hu H, et al. (2012) Clinical application of massively parallel sequencing-based prenatal noninvasive fetal trisomy test for trisomies 21 and 18 in 11105 pregnancies with mixed risk factors. *Prenat Diag* 32:1225–1232.
7. Zimmerman B, Hill M, Gemelos G, Demko Z, Banjevic M, et al. (2012) Noninvasive prenatal aneuploidy testing of chromosomes 13, 18, 21, X and Y, using targeted sequencing of polymorphic loci. *Prenat Diagn* 32:1233–1241.
8. Wald NJ (2011) Community Corner: Opening the Pandora's box of prenatal genetic testing. Nature Medicine 17:250–251.
9. Wald NJ, Rodeck C, Hackshaw AK, Walters J, Chitty L, et al. (2003) First and Second trimester Antenatal screening for Down's syndrome: the results of the Serum, Urine and Ultrasound Screening Study (SURUSS). *J Med Screen* 10:56–104.
10. Wald NJ, Bestwick JP, Huttly WJ (2013) Improvements in antenatal screening for Down's syndrome. *J Med Screen* (in press).
11. Office for National Statistics (2008) Birth Statistics. England and Wales; 2006, 2007, 2008 (FM1, Nos 35–37). London: The Stationary Office.
12. Morris JK, Mutton DE, Alberman E (2002) Revised estimates of the maternal age specific live birth prevalence of Down's syndrome. *J Med Screen* 9:2–6.
13. Morris JK, Wald NJ, Mutton DE, Alberman E (2003) Comparisons of models of maternal age-specific risk for Down syndrome live births. *Prenat Diagn* 23:252–258.
14. Morris J, Mutton D, Alberman E (2005) Corrections to maternal age-specific live birth prevalence of Down's syndrome. *J Med Screen* 12:202.
15. Morris JK, Wald NJ, Watt HC (1999) Fetal loss in Down syndrome pregnancies. *Prenat Diagn* 19:142–145.

17

Mainstream and Special School Attendance among a Dutch Cohort of Children with Down Syndrome

Jacobus P. van Wouwe[1]*, Helma B. M. van Gameren-Oosterom[1], Paul H. Verkerk[1], Paula van Dommelen[2], Minne Fekkes[1]

1 Department of Child Health, Netherlands Organization for Applied Scientific Research TNO, Leiden, the Netherlands, **2** Department of Life Style, Netherlands Organization for Applied Scientific Research TNO, Leiden, the Netherlands

Abstract

Object: To determine the level of mainstream education in a nationwide cohort of adolescents with Down Syndrome (DS), and to find characteristics related to mainstream or special school attendance.

Method: Dutch children with DS born in 1992, 1993 or 1994, were assessed when 16–19 years old. Parents scored school enrolment between the age of 4–18 years, general characteristics and the levels of intellectual disability using the Dutch Social Competence Rating Scale. Associations between disability and years in mainstream school were assessed by ordinal logistic regression, adjusting for sex and parental education.

Results: We collected data from 170 boys and 152 girls (response 63%); mean age 18.3 years (ranges 16.8–19.9). Intellectual disability was mostly moderate (43%). Most children (74%) entered mainstream education between 4 and 6 years of age. At 13 years 17% was in mainstream school and 7% stayed in up to 16 years. From the age of 8 years onwards the majority was in special education, while 6% never attended school. Girls were more often in mainstream school and stayed in longer. Level of disability was significantly associated with number of years in mainstream education.

Conclusion: Three out of four Dutch children with DS entered mainstream primary education, however late entry and high dropout are common.

Editor: Karen Lidzba, University Children's Hospital Tuebingen, Germany

Funding: This study is financed by the Nederlandse Stichting voor het Gehandicapte Kind (NSGK, Dutch Foundation for Disabled Children). The funders had no role in study design, data collection and analysis, decision to publish, or preparation of the manuscript.

Competing Interests: The authors have declared that no competing interests exist.

* E-mail: ko.vanwouwe@tno.nl

Introduction

Down Syndrome (DS) is the most common genetic cause of intellectual disability. In the Netherlands, 245 infants with DS are live born annually [1] Their growth and development follow a specific pattern and an array of treatable concomitant medical conditions is recognized. Considerable efforts focus on early recognition and treatment of these conditions in order to guarantee their optimal health, growth and development, especially their motor and cognitive development [2]. In an era where survival has positively changed and these medical conditions are managed, social competence and functioning are factors to focus on now.

One of these issues is enrolment in mainstream education, as part of the increased focus on social participation. In the Netherlands, the Dutch Down Syndrome Foundation (SDS, parent organization) advocates a pro-active attitude and assists to communicate the special needs towards schools. Only a few studies focus on the advantages of mainstream vs. special education in children with DS. Achievements of teenagers with DS in mainstream education may improve some short term progress for communication, expressive language or literacy and reading skills [3]. Another study shows that mainstream education has a modest beneficial effect on academic scores, independently of the level of intellectual disability, although no comparison with special education was made [4]. A Dutch study showed that children with DS in mainstream education learn more academics, most pronounced for reading skills. However these advantages were also determined by other factors, such as parental educational level [5].

It is estimated that 56% of all Dutch children born since the 1990s start in mainstream school, and that 22% are still in at the age of 12 years [6]. In other countries the proportion of children entering mainstream education and staying in increased over the years [7]. In Norway nowadays it is common for children with DS to enter mainstream education [8]. The actual overall schooling (getting in and staying) of children with DS has not been studied in a nationwide cohort before. Therefore, in the present study we aim to investigate the actual school career in adolescents with DS nationwide and to find characteristics related to those in mainstream or special school. Hereby we focus on two issues: which type of schools have they visited and for how many years, and are cognitive disability and sex associated with type of education?

Methods

Data Collection

Data were collected from a nationwide cohort assessed at the age of 16–19 years [9]. This included children born in 1992, 1993, and 1994, living in the Netherlands. All known parents (n = 513) received a written request by the parent organization (SDS); no selection was made. Approximately 80% of all parents of a child with DS of this age in the Netherlands had joined this organization and was therefore invited to participate. Written informed consent was obtained from parents/next of kin of all participants. Permission of an ethical committee was not obtained because it is in the Netherlands not required for this type of study with anonymous data collection

School Enrolment

Parents were asked to score separately, the type of school their child had visited, from the age of 4 to 18 years for each year. The options were: no formal education, mainstream primary or secondary school, special primary or secondary school, other school type specified. Parents were invited to add comments. If only the name of a school was given the school type was classified by one of the authors (HvG-O). If more items were entered, the answer was counted in the category 'combinations and unknown'.

Cognitive Disability

Levels of cognitive disability were based on the Dutch Social Competence Rating Scale (SRZ). Its validity and reliability regarding practical daily skills in children and adults with DS has been reported to be good [10,11]. The SRZ contains 31 items that determine the level of intellectual disability. These represent the following skills: *profound intellectual disability* (hardly able to dress oneself, wash hands and face properly and use adequate toilet hygiene, just able to eat independently without the use of a knife, and nearly unable to speak), *severe intellectual disability* (can undress, able to wash hands and face, uses knife and fork, cleans up after dinner, speaks with incomplete sentences with unclear pronunciation, understood only by close caregivers or familiar people), *moderate intellectual disability* (dresses completely, washes hands and face properly, uses adequate toilet hygiene, uses knife and fork including cutting meat without bone, able to walk outside home without supervision, and speech is mostly understood by others), *mild intellectual disability* (dresses oneself completely also footwear, keeps complete personal hygiene, sets table properly, plates, cutlery, napkins, food, etc., permitted to walk several streets away from home without supervision, uses compound sentences, speech and language understood by unfamiliar people).

Statistical Analyses

General characteristics of the study population were determined. As our subjects varied in age between 16 and 19 year outcome measures were; the type of school at 16 years of age (special, mainstream or none), the overall presence in mainstream primary school (ever in mainstream) and the total years in mainstream and special school before the age of 17.

To evaluate differences between boys and girls, we applied *t*-tests for continuous and chi-square tests for categorical variables. Ordinal logistic regression analyses were performed to assess the association between intellectual disability and the years that children were in mainstream. Ordinal regression analysis with a complementary log-log link function was applied with the outcome measure of three categories years of enrolment in mainstream. The models were presented unadjusted and adjusted for parental education and sex. For all analyses, statistical tests were 2-tailed and significance was defined at $p<0.05$. The analyses were performed using Statistical Package for the Social Sciences, version 20.0 for Windows (SPSS Inc, Chicago, Illinois).

Results

Cross-sectional data were obtained from the nationwide cohort. Data from 322 subjects out of the 513 invited, were suitable for analysis (response 63%). Table 1 shows the general characteristics, stratified by sex; 53% of the subjects were boys, nearly all subjects were of Dutch descent. They were on average 18 years old (18.3 years, ranges 16.8 to 19.9). The vast majority lived at home and had practiced an early intervention program, such as the adapted version of the Macquarie/Portage Programs. The level of cognitive disability was mostly moderate, 43%, however the distribution was wide with 30% severe, 10% profound and 17% mild. No differences between boys and girls were noticed in age, residence or parental education. However, the level of cognitive disability varied. More girls scored a level of mild cognitive disabilities, while relatively more boys scored severe and profound cognitive disabilities.

The scores on actual school enrolment are summarized in Figure 1. Entry of school started between the ages of 4 and 6 years. The majority was enrolled in mainstream at the ages 4, 5, 6 and 7 years (48–63%). Dropout rate was high: from the age of 7 onwards, annually 3–6% of the children transferred out towards special education. At transition from primary to secondary school (at approximately 12–13 years), efflux was larger (6–10%). Only 17% of the children was in mainstream school at the age of 13 years. A group of 7% stayed in primary and secondary level mainstream up to the age of 17. An equal group of 6% had never attended any school, they were in residential care or daycare.

Data on overall presence in mainstream primary school, enrolment at the age of 16 years and average enrollment from 4

Table 1. General characteristics of the adolescents with Down syndrome (n = 322).

	Total		Boys		Girls		
General Characteristics	n	%	n	%	n	%	*p**
Number of Subjects	322	100	170	53	152	47	<0.001
Dutch Descent^	300	93	162	95	138	91	0.110
Age in Years (range)	16.8–19.9		16.9–19.9		16.8–19.8		
Age in Years (mean ± SD)	18.3±0.8		18.3±0.8		18.3±0.8		0.553
Living at Home	283	88	149	88	134	88	0.888
Early Stimulation Practiced	265	82	143	84	122	80	0.366
Parental Education							0.524
Low	39	12	23	14	16	11	
Medium	105	33	58	34	47	31	
High	177	55	89	52	88	58	
Level of Cognitive Disability							<0.001
Mild	54	17	16	9	38	25	
Moderate	139	43	73	43	66	44	
Severe	97	30	58	34	39	26	
Profound	31	10	23	14	8	5	

Abbreviation: SD – standard deviation.
* Boys with DS compared to girls with DS.
^Both parents born in the Netherlands.

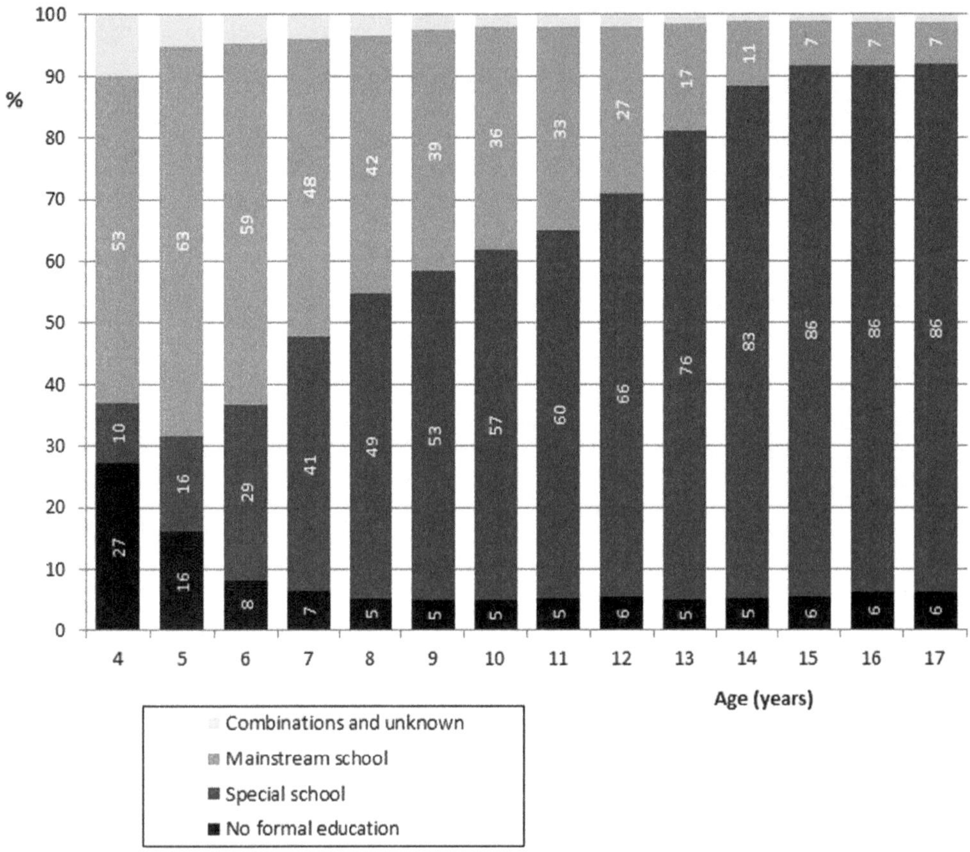

Figure 1. School enrolment of Dutch children with Down Syndrome by age, as retrospectively reported by their parents at the end of school career (n = 322).

to 16 years are presented in Table 2. A total of 74% of the children had entered mainstream. A majority (60%) was in mainstream for at least 3 years; girls more often and they stayed in longer. Boys were on average 5.5 years in mainstream, girls 7.0 years ($p = 0.001$). Boys were on average 8.9 years in special schools, girls 7.1 years ($p < 0.001$). It is more relevant to state that 60% stayed in three years or longer, since the distribution of total years of mainstream showed these four peaks; no mainstream school at all, three years (range 1–5 years), 9 years (range 6–11 years) and a small peak at 13 years (12–13 years, i.e. only mainstream). Therefore we made these four subgroups: only mainstream which equals 12–15 years mainstream, 6–11 years, 1–5 years and no mainstream. Figure 2 shows the proportion of boys and girls in these four categories by level of intellectual disability. Since the group with only mainstream school was small, the group was combined with those who were 6–11 years in mainstream school (Table 3). Therefore ordinal regression analysis was conducted with duration of mainstream schooling in three groups as outcome. As few children with profound disability entered mainstream education, their duration in mainstream school was shorter, however not significant. Children with severe intellectual disability stayed shorter in mainstream school than those with a moderate disability ($p = 0.021$). Those with a mild intellectual disability did not significantly stay in longer than those with a moderate disability. Parental education and sex was not associated with duration in mainstream school.

Discussion

Most Dutch children with DS, 74%, participated socially and entered mainstream primary school. They entered at a slower rate, at the appropriate age of 4 years 53% had started mainstream primary school, another 10% a year later. At special school 10% started at the age of 4, another 6% at 5 years of age, another 13% at 6 years. Moreover, dropout rate from mainstream to special school was high at the age of 6–7 years. In the end of primary school only 17% was still in mainstream at the age of 13 years. Just a small group of 7% stayed in throughout secondary mainstream education. Overall most children stayed in mainstream school for 3 years or longer (60%). Girls were more often in mainstream school and stayed in longer. As expected, there is a significant association between the level of intellectual disability and years in mainstream school: those with a moderate disability stay in longer than those with severe intellectual disability. Parental education and sex did not contribute to this association.

Our study has some limitations. Selection bias may be present. Parents with a more positive attitude towards their child may be more inclined to join the parent organization or participate in this study. Conversely it is possible that those with relatively more problems may seek support by joining a parent organization or are inclined to participate in order to be able to express their problems. Institutionalized children could be underrepresented as parents might be unable to answer our questions. Also our data were obtained from questionnaires reported by parents retrospectively. However, the specific questions dealing with the type of

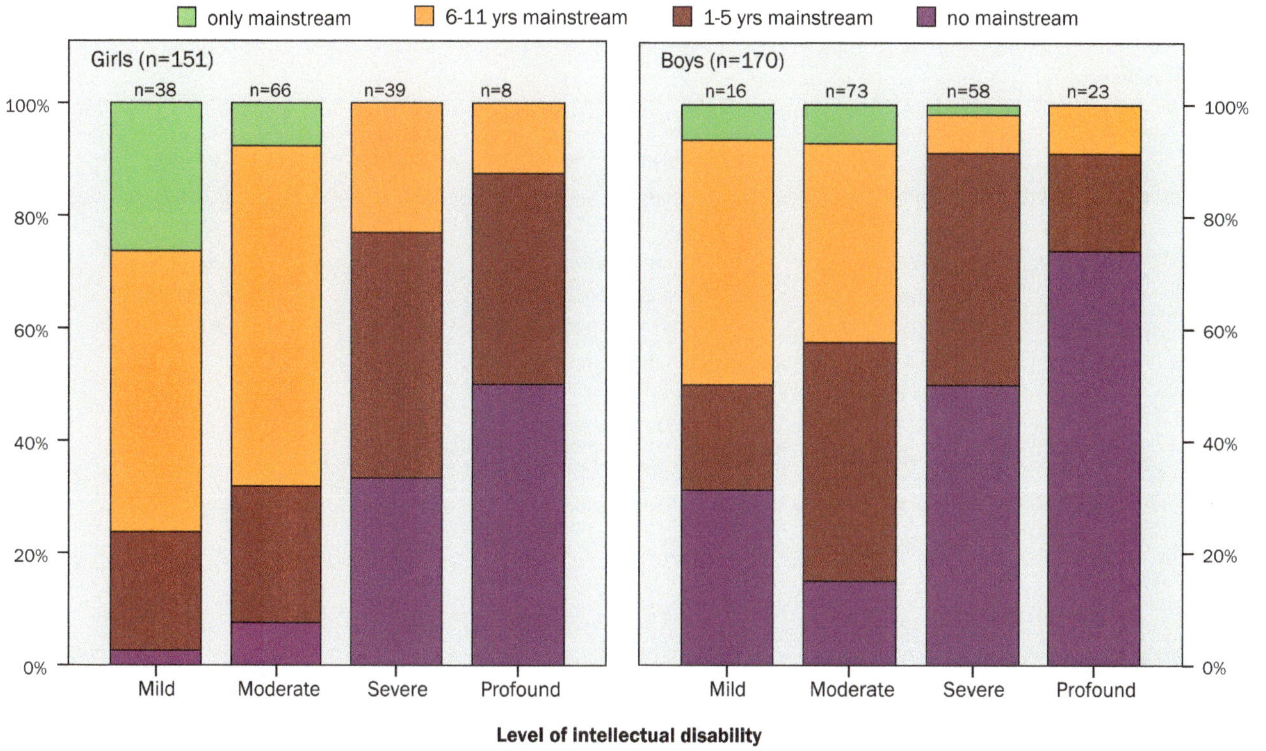

Figure 2. The proportion of resp. girls (n = 151) and boys (n = 170) in categories of years of mainstream school by level of intellectual disability.

school were directly answered or clarified in the comments (which made it easy to score missing data). We, therefore, think parents accurately answered such questions as Dolva also suggested [8]. We did not investigate the arguments of parents to choose for mainstream or special schooling, neither the actual possibility to be admitted to mainstream primary school, nor the reason to drop out. Some parents may not be able to find a mainstream school to admit their child with DS. Another limitation of our study is lack data on of academic performance. No information is available about repeating classes and degree of special support needed and whether this indeed had been offered. We studied the cohort up to 18 years, and report a 7% enrolment in mainstream secondary school, this is the likely lower estimate of children that has completed mainstream primary school with full academic levels. Up to the age of 13 years 17% attended mainstream primary school, the higher estimate of children with DS that completed mainstream primary. The results of our study gave a somewhat lower mainstream school participation compared to the estimates of De Graaf [6], who noticed a remarkable increase between 1984 and 2011. Because of differences in study design a close comparison cannot be made. Our cohort was born between 1992–1994, more recent year cohorts showed higher initial attendance rates of mainstream education.

Table 2. School enrolment* of Dutch children with Down syndrome (n = 319); arranged by sex.

	Total		Boys		Girls		
	n	%	n	%	n	%	*p*
Overall enrolment in mainstream primary school							
Ever in	237	73.6	108	63.5	129	84.9	<0.001
Enrolled at 16 years of age							0.002
Special School	276	86.5	142	84.5	134	88.7	
Mainstream Secondary School	23	7.2	8	4.8	15	10.0	
None	20	6.3	18	10.7	2	1.3	
Average school enrollment in years (mean ± SD)*							
Mainstream School (n = 237)	6.3±3.7		5.5±3.7		7.0±3.6		0.001
Special School (n = 285)	8.0±3.5		8.9±3.3		7.1±3.5		<0.001

*Data of school enrollment from 4 to 16 years were presented, since data on 17 and 18 years were not complete (some subjects are under 17 at the time of study).

The reason children with DS entered school after the age of 4 years may be due to their overall development. Dolva et al. [8] found that postponement of school entry was related to skills in self-care and social functioning. In Norway skills related to toileting, functional comprehension and expressive communication, problem solving and initiation of simple chores were lower at the age of 5 among children whose school entry was postponed compared to others. In the Netherlands mainstream schools refuse usually children not fully toilet trained. Other reasons for a late entry could be efforts to locate a school and willingness of the educational staff to accept a child with DS, time necessary to organize special facilities and parental hesitation to make the decision and formalize transition.

The majority of Dutch children started mainstream with a steady group opting out annually until the age of 13 years. At

Table 3. Univariate regression weights of the ordinal regression models in 16–19-year-olds with Down syndrome (n = 317]; positive weights indicate a higher probability of being longer in mainstream school (higher category of the outcome] compared to the reference.

		Unadjusted w° (95%CI]	Adjusted w† (95%CI]
Degree of Intellectual Disability^	Mild	0.447 (−0.127,1.022]	0.182 (−0.328,0.693]
	Moderate (reference]	0	0
	Severe	−0.514 (−0.897,−0.132]**	−0.441 (−0.815, −0.068]*
	Profound	−0.289 (−1.073,0.495]	−0.229 (−0.981,0.522]
Parental Education	Low	−0.374 (−0.896,0.147]	−0.129 (−0.609,0.350]
	Medium	−0.098 (−0.475,0.280]	−0.018 (−0.347,0.312]
	High (reference]	0	0
Sex	Girls	0.330 (−0.013,0.674]	0.146 (−0.164, 0.456]
	Boys (reference]		0

^Degree of intellectual disability is based on all items of the SRZ.
°Unstandardized regression weights.
†Unstandardized regression weights adjusted for parental education and sex.
* *p*-value<0.05.
** *p*-value<0.001.

transition to secondary education more children transfer out into special education. Transition could be difficult as parents may reconsider the optimal place for their child at puberty. Secondary schools are clustered and some became large institutions with various levels and large amount of pupils. This requires social skills in order to travel to and from school independently. It seems only a fraction of adolescents with DS master such practical skills. The vast majority (90%) of adolescents with DS experience significant problems in social functioning [9]. Children with DS are socially vulnerable and may require a special setting especially before entering puberty [12].

More girls entered mainstream primary school than boys and they stayed in longer (on average 7.0 years, compared to 5.5 years for boys). This sex difference is significant, and has not been reported in other cohorts of children with DS. Only one study speaks of "a female advantage for verbal abilities in the DS population", however this thesis has not been published [13]. It is not known what issues may attribute to the more favorable school career for girls with DS.

Also the high dropout rate needs to be confirmed. With all the efforts put into the enrolment of children with DS in mainstream school, some explanation of the high dropout needs to be studied. Is it merely an issue of cognitive and social development? The reported advantages of mainstream schooling for children with DS are more academic and language skills; especially some improvement in communication, expressive language or reading and literacy skills. To what extent are these effects of mainstream school enrolment on the overall development worthwhile? Adolescents with DS have limited abilities to perform relatively more complex tasks and experience serious difficulties in social functioning [14]. Serious problem behavior is also highly prevalent in them [9]. How could mainstream school improve effectively social functioning, behavior and the ability to perform more complex tasks? We hope future studies on mainstream school will also focus on overall social competence. We need to answer questions like; what determines a successful mainstream school career? what is the optimal education for individuals with DS? what is the most desirable curriculum? what long term goals do we need to set? Besides health, growth, development and cognition, pediatricians and other caretakers should discuss school choice in these perspectives. Their advice should aim to achieve optimal social competence and skills for independent living as well as the need for a focus on general behavior improvement and on the detection and treatment of specific psychopathology. Such an approach may improve the self-esteem of adolescents with DS. In this prospect school choice is relevant and should be discussed in wider perspective than just academic achievements.

Conclusions

It is common for Dutch children with DS to enter mainstream school, 74% does. Most children stayed in 3 or more years, however, dropout rate was considerably. There is a sex difference in mainstream schooling in favor of girls. A significant association was found between level of intellectual disability and years in mainstream: those with a moderate disability stay in longer than those with severe intellectual disability.

Author Contributions

Conceived and designed the experiments: JPVW HBMVG-O PV MF. Analyzed the data: JPVW HBMVG-O PVD MF. Wrote the paper: JPVW.

References

1. Van Gameren-Oosterom HBM, Buitendijk SE, Bilardo CM, Van der Pal-De Bruin KM, Van Wouwe JP, et al. (2012) Unchanged prevalence of Down syndrome in the Netherlands: results from an 11-year nationwide birth cohort. Prenat Diagn 32: 1035–1040.
2. Weijerman ME, De Winter JP (2010) Clinical practice. The care of children with Down syndrome. Eur J Pediatr 169 :1445–1452.
3. Buckley S, Bird G, Sacks B, Archer T (2006) A comparison of mainstream and special education for teenagers with Down syndrome: Implications for parents and teachers. Down Syndrome Research and Practice 89 :54–67.
4. Turner S, Alborz A, Gayle V (2008) Predictors of academic attainments of young people with Down's syndrome. J Intellect Disabil Res 52 :380–392.
5. De Graaf G, Van Hove G, Haveman M (2013) More academics in regular school? The effect of regular versus special school placement on academic skills

in Dutch primary school students with Down syndrome. J Intellect Disabil Res 57 :21–38.
6. De Graaf G, Van Hove G, Haveman M (2013) A quantitative assessment of educational integration of students with Down syndrome in the Netherlands. J Intellect Disabil Res [Epub ahead of print]. doi: 10.1111/jir.12060. Accessed 19 February 2014.
7. Cuckle P (1999) Getting in and staying there; children with Down syndrome in mainstream schools. Downs Syndr Res Pract6 :95–99.
8. Dolva A-S, Lilja M, Hemmingsson H (2007) Functional performance characteristics associated with postponing elementary school entry among children with Down syndrome. Am J Occup Ther 61 :414–420.
9. Van Gameren-Oosterom HBM, Fekkes M, Van Wouwe JP, Detmar SB, Oudesluys-Murphy AM, et al. (2013) Problem behavior of individuals with Down syndrome, assessed in a nationwide cohort at late-adolescence. J of Ped 163 :1396–1401.
10. Kraijer DW, Kema GN, De Bildt AA (2004) Social independence scale for mentally disabled children, manual [in Dutch]. 2nd ed. Amsterdam: Pearson Assessment and Information
11. Coppus AM, Evenhuis HM, Verberne GJ, Visser FE, Arias-Vasquez A, et al. (2008) The impact of apolipoprotein E on dementia in persons with Down's syndrome. Neurobiol Aging 29 :828–835.
12. Lightfoot L, Bond C (2013) An exploration of primary to secondary school transition planning for children with Down's syndrome. Educ Psychol Pract 29 :163–179.
13. Crombie MP (1994) Development of adolescents with Down syndrome: does early intervention have a long term effect? Unpublished doctoral dissertation. University of Queensland, Brisbane
14. Van Gameren-Oosterom HBM, Fekkes M, Reijneveld SA, Oudesluys-Murphy HM, Verkerk PH, et al. (2013) Practical and social skills of 16–19-year-olds with Down syndrome: independence still far away. Res Dev Disabil 34 :4599–4607.

18

Molecular Signatures of Cardiac Defects in Down Syndrome Lymphoblastoid Cell Lines Suggest Altered Ciliome and Hedgehog Pathways

Clémentine Ripoll[1], Isabelle Rivals[2], Emilie Ait Yahya-Graison[1], Luce Dauphinot[3], Evelyne Paly[1], Clothilde Mircher[4], Aimé Ravel[4], Yann Grattau[4], Henri Bléhaut[4], André Mégarbane[4,5], Guy Dembour[6], Bénédicte de Fréminville[7], Renaud Touraine[7], Nicole Créau[1], Marie Claude Potier[3], Jean Maurice Delabar[1]*

1 Univ Paris Diderot, Sorbonne Paris Cité, Unité de Biologie Fonctionnelle et Adaptative, EAC4413 CNRS, Paris, France, **2** Equipe de Statistique Appliquée, ESPCI ParisTech, Paris, France, **3** CRICM, CNRS UMR7225, INSERM UMR975, UPMC Hôpital de la Pitié-Salpêtrière, Paris, France, **4** Institut Médical Jérôme Lejeune et Fondation Jérome Lejeune, Paris, France, **5** Unité de Génétique Médicale, Faculté de Médecine, Université Saint-Joseph, Beirut, Lebanon, **6** Cardiologie pédiatrique, Cliniques Universitaires St Luc, Bruxelles, Belgique, **7** Service de Génétique, Centre Hospitalier Universitaire de Saint-Etienne, Saint-Etienne, France

Abstract

Forty percent of people with Down syndrome exhibit heart defects, most often an atrioventricular septal defect (AVSD) and less frequently a ventricular septal defect (VSD) or atrial septal defect (ASD). Lymphoblastoid cell lines (LCLs) were established from lymphocytes of individuals with trisomy 21, the chromosomal abnormality causing Down syndrome. Gene expression profiles generated from DNA microarrays of LCLs from individuals without heart defects (CHD^-; n = 22) were compared with those of LCLs from patients with cardiac malformations (CHD^+; n = 21). After quantile normalization, principal component analysis revealed that AVSD carriers could be distinguished from a combined group of ASD or VSD (ASD+VSD) carriers. From 9,758 expressed genes, we identified 889 and 1,016 genes differentially expressed between CHD^- and AVSD and CHD^- and ASD+VSD, respectively, with only 119 genes in common. A specific chromosomal enrichment was found in each group of affected genes. Among the differentially expressed genes, more than 65% are expressed in human or mouse fetal heart tissues (GEO dataset). Additional LCLs from new groups of AVSD and ASD+VSD patients were analyzed by quantitative PCR; observed expression ratios were similar to microarray results. Analysis of GO categories revealed enrichment of genes from pathways regulating clathrin-mediated endocytosis in patients with AVSD and of genes involved in semaphorin-plexin-driven cardiogenesis and the formation of cytoplasmic microtubules in patients with ASD-VSD. A pathway-oriented search revealed enrichment in the ciliome for both groups and a specific enrichment in Hedgehog and Jak-stat pathways among ASD+VSD patients. These genes or related pathways are therefore potentially involved in normal cardiogenesis as well as in cardiac malformations observed in individuals with trisomy 21.

Editor: Reiner Albert Veitia, Institut Jacques Monod, France

Funding: This work was supported by the European Union integrated AnEUploidy project (contract no. 037627). The funders had no role in study design, data collection and analysis, decision to publish, or preparation of the manuscript.

Competing Interests: The authors have declared that no competing interests exist.

* E-mail: delabar@univ-paris-diderot.fr

Introduction

Trisomy 21 (Ts21) or Down syndrome (DS) is the most common human chromosomal aneuploidy at birth, and the only one with long-term viability. Congenital heart defects (CHD) are present in about 40–60% of newborns with DS [1]. Neonatal detection of cardiac defects followed by cardiac surgery has contributed to increased life expectancy of individuals with DS.

Cardiac abnormalities in DS include atrioventricular septal defect (AVSD) (with or without other CHDs), ventricular septal defect (VSD) (with or without other CHDs), isolated secundum atrial septal defect (ASD), isolated persistent patent ductus arteriosus (PDA), and isolated tetralogy of Fallot (TOF). The reported frequency of each defect varies between studies of different populations, indicating that genetic background or consanguinity may affect the CHD phenotype [2–8]. Additionally, analysis of Ts21 fetal hearts [9], showing that CHD phenotypes may include the small anomaly called linear insertion of atrioventricular valves (LIAVV), suggest that the number of individuals with Ts21 and LIAVV may be underestimated. Most of the cardiovascular abnormalities associated with Down syndrome can be detected during fetal development; however, percentages of cardiac defects detected in fetuses, mostly AVSD and VSD, vary between studies [10,11]. Cardiac septal defects are typically observed during the first trimester and are frequently associated with an increase in nuchal translucency thickness.

The cellular and molecular events that control cardiac development are conserved among vertebrates. Heart development in humans occurs very early, from the third to eight weeks of gestation, beginning with a primitive tube that beats at 25 days gestation and ending in the four-chamber heart. Many steps occur after formation of the primitive heart tube, including looping, cell migration, cell transition, and septation events [12–14]. Many studies indicate that cardiac development is tightly regulated by a series of molecular signaling pathways and morphological events. However, many questions remain regarding the changes that occur to alter heart development in individuals with DS. For example, it is unclear to what extent secondary changes occur as a consequence of the aneuploid state, and which environmental factors combine with genetic causes to induce such changes.

Inter-individual differences in gene expression are likely to account for an important fraction of phenotypic differences, including susceptibility to common disorders. Recent studies have shown extensive variation in gene expression levels in humans and other organisms, and that a fraction of this variation is under genetic control [15].

Indeed, the genetic alterations in DS are not as simple as once believed: while genes on chromosome 21 (HSA21) are transmitted in 3 copies, all of those genes do not necessarily exhibit a straightforward 1.5-fold increase in expression. Gene expression may be regulated by dosage compensation such that only a subset of those genes exhibit the expected 50% increase in expression. A previous study using lymphoblastoid cell lines (LCLs) from diploid (2N) individuals and individuals with Ts21 showed that only 30% of HSA21 genes are significantly overexpressed [16]. For genes located on chromosomes other than 21, the effect of Ts21 could be relatively subtle or massively disruptive.

One hypothesis explaining the complicated genetics of DS proposes that gene expression changes on HSA21 are likely to affect the expression of genes on other chromosomes through the modulation of transcription factors, chromatin remodeling proteins, and related molecules or other targets. Thus, the dysregulation of pathways involved in heart development may cause the cardiac defects observed in DS. A second hypothesis implicating both environmental and genetic factors in DS phenotypes is supported by epidemiological studies of DS: specific cardiac defects were associated with smoking mothers (AVSD, TOF) [17,18], folate pathways and folate supplementation have been proposed to interfere with the incidence of AVSD [19,20], and an association between DS and CHD with global hypomethylation status has been found in a Dutch population-based case-control study [21].

We hypothesized that if the cardiac phenotypes observed in DS are caused, at least in part, by trisomy-induced gene dosage effects, it should be possible to genetically differentiate individuals with DS by their specific heart defects, as well as distinguishing those with heart defects from those without. Further, such genetic differences may be manifested in peripheral tissues: dermatoglyphic indicators used to characterize individuals with DS have been used to correctly classify them according to their heart status [22].

Several studies have suggested that LCLs can be used to detect biologically plausible correlations between candidate genes and various genetically-induced diseases. We collected blood samples from individuals with DS and controls (2N) and established an LCL biobank. From this cell bank, we selected LCLs from the following five types of donors: euploid individuals, individuals with DS and without CHD, individuals with DS and AVSD, individuals with DS and ASD, and individuals with DS and VSD. Microarrays and quantitative PCR were used to identify differentially expressed (DE) genes. Interestingly, principal component analysis was able to distinguish between cells from individuals with AVSD and those with ASD or VSD (combined group, hereafter ASD+VSD). Differential expression analyses allowed us to identify genes and pathways specifically dysregulated in AVSD and/or ASD+VSD.

Results

Cell lines and phenotypes of each group

Blood samples were collected at five different clinical centers to establish a Biobank from 190 controls and 550 individuals with DS. Recorded phenotypes included cardiac defects (AVSD, ASD, VSD, TOF, PDA, mitral valve prolapsus) and murmurs. To construct the CHD^- group individuals without murmurs were selected. For the CHD^+ group individuals with only one heart malformation were selected. For the expression study, samples were selected from caucasian individuals with DS with the same age distribution (23.05±2.4) for CHD^+ and (24.66±2.2) for CHD^-. These groups were also created with the same gender ratio (M/F = 1.1 for CHD^+; M/F = 1.2 for CHD^-). The same criteria (ethnicity, age, gender) were used to select a group of 2N controls.

Differential expression between AVSD and ASD +VSD

Using human pangenomic Illumina microarrays containing 48,701 probes, we obtained expression profiles from 43 samples: 21 from individuals with DS and with a heart defect (CHD^+: 7 AVSD, 8 ASD, 6 VSD) and 22 with DS and without heart defect (CHD^-). Among the 48,701 probes on the microarrays, 11,224 probes corresponding to 9,758 genes displayed significant expression in LCLs. Results from three independent experiments (43 total samples from people with DS) were analyzed to identify DE genes. Data were normalized using quantile normalization. A first comparison of gene expression profiles using principal component analysis (PCA) could not differentiate between the CHD^+ and the CHD^- groups. We thus performed a PCA on the CHD^+ group only. This analysis showed that individuals with DS and AVSD could be separated from a second group corresponding to individuals with DS and ASD or VSD (Figure 1). However, PCA failed to separate between the ASD and VSD groups, even in the subspace of the first three principal components. A second analysis of the CHD^+ group consisted of two-by-two t-tests with a global estimate of the common variance, leading to 249 transcripts with p-value below 0.01 for the AVSD/ASD comparison, 192 transcripts for the AVSD/VSD comparison, and 33 for the ASD/VSD comparison. We performed a classification of heart defects (CHD+) according to the distribution frequency of their p-values. We calculated the empirical cumulative distributions of p-values for the 2-by-2 Student tests A: AVSD/ASD; B: AVSD/VSD; C: ASD/VSD. Comparisons were obtained for 11 224 tests. The comparison to the uniform distribution shows that there is no overall differential expression between ASD and VSD (less small p-values than for an uniform distribution).This analysis indicated that there were no significantly DE genes between ASD and VSD, and validated our choice to group ASD with VSD for further analysis (ASD+VSD group) (Figure 2).

Analysis of the data was then performed using ANalysis Of Variance (ANOVA) on the three following groups: the CHD^- group, the AVSD group, and the ASD+VSD group. We considered genes with $p<0.05$ as DE, and, for the latter, we performed two-by-two comparisons with the CHD^- groups. This analysis revealed a group of DE genes in AVSD with respect to CHD^- (889) and a group of DE genes in ASD+VSD with respect to CHD^- (1016); the two groups exhibited a small overlap (119) (Table S1).

We also compared cells from 11 CHD^- individuals with DS to cells from 12 controls (2N individuals) and found 1,766 DE genes with $p<0.05$. DS phenotypic variability may be related to dysregulation of genes with a causative effect (inducing the defect) or with a protective effect (compensating other negative effects).

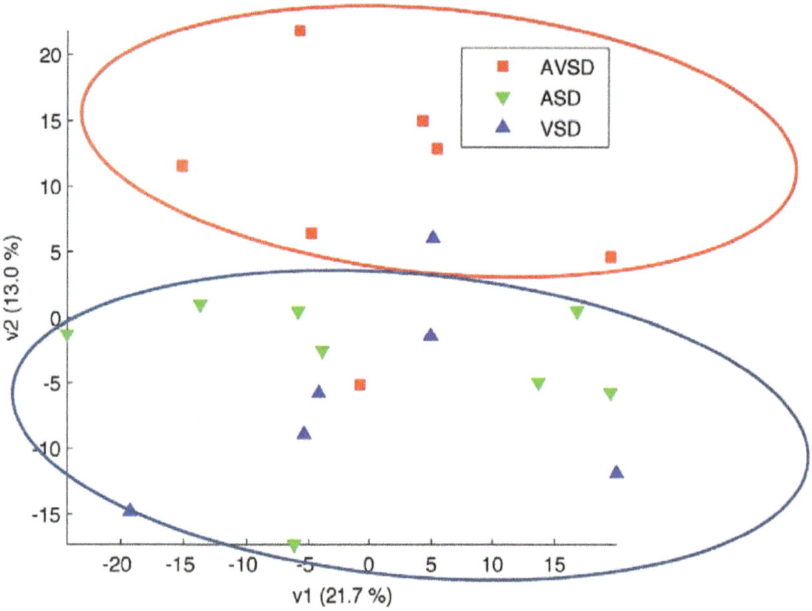

Figure 1. Principal component analysis of gene expression profiles of LCLs from individuals with DS and with CHD: red- AVSD (n = 7); green- ASD (n = 8); blue- VSD (n = 6). Red circle indicates AVSD, blue circle indicates ASD and VSD.

Detailed analysis of the two groups with heart defects (CHD^+ vs. CHD^-) allowed us to group the DE genes into two classes. The first class (I) contained genes DE in CHD^+ (AVSD or ASD+VSD) with a larger effect between CHD^+ and CHD^- than between CHD^- and 2N; we further divided this class into two sub-classes (IA, IB) to differentiate genes with similar expression (ratio interval between 0.95 and 1.05) between CHD^- and 2N individuals (i.e., genes that are not dysregulated in CHD^-). The second class (II) contained genes DE in CHD^+ with expression levels closer to the those observed in 2N individuals than to those found in the CHD^- group; we also divided this into two sub-classes (IIA, IIB) to differentiate genes that presented similar expression (ratio interval between 0.95 and 1.05) between CHD^+ and controls (Table 1 and Table S2).

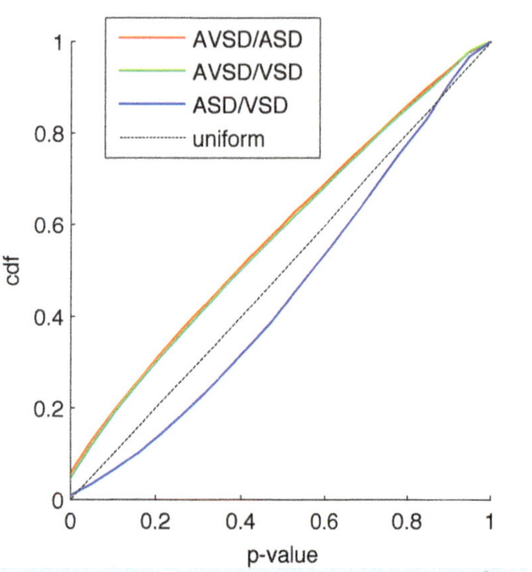

Figure 2. Classification of heart defects (CHD+) according to the distribution frequency of their p-values. Empirical cumulative distributions of p-values for the 2-by-2 Student tests A: AVSD/ASD; B: AVSD/VSD; C: ASD/VSD. Comparisons were obtained for 11 224 tests. The comparison to the uniform distribution shows that there is no overall differential expression between ASD and VSD (less small p-values than for an uniform distribution). Cdf: cumulative distribution function.

Validation by quantitative PCR

We then performed quantitative PCR on a set of LCLs including the ones analyzed in microarray experiments and LCLs from other individuals. Two reference genes were selected for these experiments: hypoxanthine phosphoribosyl transferase (HPRT) and polymerase (RNA) II (DNA directed) polypeptide A (POLR2A). Validation experiments were performed on genes showing high differential expression (ratio >1.3 or ratio <0.75), genes selected for their potential functional involvement in heart development, and genes from clusters on HSA21 (oligonucleotide sequences are listed in Table S3). We confirmed results obtained by microarray analysis both for genes with an increased expression in CHD^+ and for genes with a decreased expression in CHD^+ ($R^2 = 0.941$, $p<0.0001$) (Table 2).

Chromosomal localization

We then analyzed the chromosomal localization of DE genes. Interestingly, genes DE in AVSD as compared to CHD^- preferentially mapped to chromosomes 7, 11, 16, 19, and 20. In addition, we identified a cluster that contained three contiguous genes mapped to HSA21: *PIGP (DSCR5)*, *TTC3*, and *DSCR3*. A numerical simulation to compute the probability of finding a triplet on chromosome 21, assuming that gene expression and regulation are independent of localization, showed that the triplet found on HSA21 in the AVSD group was significant ($p = 0.039$) (Table S4). These three genes belonged to class IA (genes DE in AVSD as compared to CHD^- with a larger effect between AVSD and CHD^- than between CHD^- and 2N, see Table 1). When

Table 1. Classification of differentially expressed genes according to heart phenotype and relative expression in Ts21 compared to 2N.

CHD^+ categories	# DE genes:	group I genes:		group II genes:		Clusters on HSA21
		|CHD+−CHD−|>|CHD−−2N|		|CHD+−CHD−|<|CHD−−2N|		
		A	B	A	B	
	N probes/n genes	$CHD^- \neq 2N$	$CHD^- = 2N$	$CHD^+ \neq 2N$	$CHD^+ = 2N$	
	p<0.05	(p<0.05)	(p≥0.05)	(p<0.05)	(p≥0.05)	
AVSD	1006/889	295	336	64	0	PIGP-TTC3-DSCR3 (IA)
ASD+VSD	1136/1016	320	327	34	62	IFNAR1-GART-DONSON (IIA)

Group IA: $|CHD^+ - CHD^-| > |CHD^- - 2N|$ and $CHD^- \neq 2N$; Group IB : $|CHD^+ - CHD^-| > |CHD^- - 2N|$ and $CHD^- = 2N$; Group IIA: $|CHD^+ - CHD^-| < |CHD^- - 2N|$ and $CHD^+ \neq 2N$; Group IIB: $|CHD^+ - CHD^-| < |CHD^- - 2N|$ and $CHD^+ = 2N$.

Table 2. Transcriptome signature of heart defects.

genes	Transcriptome signature of heart malformations		
	array ratios	array ratios	qPCR ratios
	CHD−/2N	AVSD/CHD−	AVSD/CHD−
AUTS2	0.86 (NS)	1.83*	1.73*(11/10), 1.55*(10/10), 1.76* (16/16), 1.92*(18/18), 1.81*(18/18)
CNN2	0.9 (NS)	0.69*	0.82*(11/10)
DSCR3	1.21*	1.22*	1.27*(10/10), 1.19*(9/10)
DYNLT3	1.01(NS)	1.42*	1.68*(18/19), 1.71*(17/18)
NQO1	1.57*	0.62*	0.63*(20/19)
OFD1	0.99(NS)	1.39*	1.17 (NS)
PDIA4	1.14(NS)	0.74*	0.7*(11/10), 0.76*(17/17), 0.66*(20/20)
PIGP	1.31*	1.26*	1.35*(10/10), 2.2*(8/9), 1.22*(19/17), 1.31*(17/18)
TTC3	1.35*	1.24*	1.39(12/11), 1.35(10/19), 1.34*(11/12), 1.14*(18/20)
TUBB2B	1.01(NS)	1.79*	1.64*(18/18), 1.8*(18/18)
	CHD−/2N	ASD+VSD/CHD−	ASD+VSD/CHD−
ACTG1	0.96(NS)	0.63*	0.73*(11/11)
ALDOC	0.87(NS)	1.36*	1.56*(10/10), 1.56*(19/17), 1.54*(19/20)
CACYBP	1.07(NS)	0.73*	0.75*(11/10)
DTYMK	1.00(NS)	0.7*	0.76*(9/9), 0.74*(10/10), 0.8*(11/11)
ENO2	0.89(NS)	1.54*	1.34(NS)
GART	1.39*	0.83*	0.72*(11/11)
IFNAR1	1.21*	0.87*	0.78*(10/10), 0.58* (10/10)
PLTP	1.01(NS)	1.37*	1.32*(10/10)
RPL10A	0.84*	0.64*	0.71*(10/11)
TNFAIP2	1.02(NS)	1.49*	1.5*(9/9)

Comparison of ratios for DE genes up- or down-regulated in the AVSD or ASD+VSD group between (1) array ratio in the Ts21 CHD^- vs 2N, (2) array ratio in CHD^+ vs CHD^-, (3) q-PCR ratio from different experiments in CHD^+ vs CHD^- using additional samples (total number in parentheses). Gene nomenclature, *AUTS2*: autism susceptibility candidate 2; *CNN2*: calponin 2; *DSCR3*: Down syndrome critical region gene 3; *DYNLT3*: dynein, light chain, Tctex-type 3; *NQO1*: NAD(P)H dehydrogenase, quinone 1; *OFD1*: oral-facial-digital syndrome 1; *PDIA4*: protein disulfide isomerase family A, member 4; *PIGP*: phosphatidylinositol glycan anchor biosynthesis, class P; *TTC3*: tetratricopeptide repeat domain 3; *TUBB2B*: tubulin, beta 2B; *ACTG1*: actin, gamma 1; *ALDOC*: aldolase C, fructose-bisphosphate; *CACYBP*: calcyclin binding protein; *DTYMK*: deoxythymidylate kinase (thymidylate kinase); *ENO2*: enolase 2 (gamma, neuronal); *GART*: phosphoribosylglycinamide formyltransferase, phosphoribosylglycinamide synthetase, phosphoribosylaminoimidazole synthetase; *IFNAR1*: interferon (alpha, beta, and omega) receptor 1; *PLTP*: phospholipid transfer protein; *RPL10A*: ribosomal protein L10a; *TNFAIP2*: tumor necrosis factor, alpha-induced protein 2.

analyzing genes DE in ASD+VSD as compared to CHD^-, we found an enrichment of genes from chromosomes 11, 19, and 22. We also found a cluster of genes from HSA21, including *IFNAR1*, *CART*, and *DONSON*, mapping close to each other. These genes were from class IIA (genes with expression levels closer to the ones observed in 2N individuals than to the ones found in the CHD^- group, see Table 1). The triplet on chromosome 21 in the ASD+VSD group was not significant (Table S4).

Expression pattern, GO category and pathways enrichment analysis

A list of genes potentially expressed in fetal heart was built from the human and mouse microarray datasets from GEO. Although this list is not exhaustive, it allowed us to characterize expression in the heart as compared to other tissues. We compared this list to our list of DE genes, and found that 65% of DE genes in AVSD and 63% of DE genes in ASD+VSD were expressed in the heart with a significant enrichment ($p = 5 \times 10^{-3}$ for AVSD and $p = 0.01$ for ASD+VSD).

Gorilla software was used to calculate the enrichment of GO categories in DE genes. Comparison of genes expressed in LCLs (background set) with genes DE in AVSD as compared to CHD^- (target set) showed an enrichment of two GO categories corresponding to genes involved in the regulation of metabolic processes and zinc ion binding. Similar analysis performed on DE genes in ASD+VSD (as compared to CHD^-) indicated an enrichment of three GO categories: biosynthetic processes, demethylation, and regulation of transcription by glucose (Table 3).

Since pathway analysis is highly dependent on the gene annotations present in databases, we established lists of genes for pathways potentially related to heart development (Table S5), specifically the Wnt, Hedgehog, Notch, and Jak-stat pathways. In addition, we created lists of genes involved in angiogenesis/cardiogenesis and in the epithelial-to-mesenchymal transition, i.e., genes expressed in the progenitors of the mitral and tricuspid valves and the membranous interventricular septum since they are known to arise by an epithelial-mesenchymal cell transformation (EMT) from embryonic endothelial cells [23],[24]. Among genes DE in ASD+VSD as compared to CHD^-, we found a significant enrichment in genes belonging or connected to the Hedgehog pathway and to the Jak-Stat pathway (Table 4, in bold). Interestingly, we also found a highly significant enrichment in cilia genes known to be critical for organ laterality and heart development [25] (and listed from McClintock [26]) among DE genes in the ASD+VSD cases but also in the AVSD cases (Table 4).

Discussion

Identification of candidate genes or pathways involved in the occurrence of congenital heart defects in DS has been extensively pursued, but has failed to provide a clear picture of the genes responsible for the developmental anomalies observed in individuals with DS. In the mouse, the construction of models carrying partial trisomies for chromosomal regions orthologous to HSA21 have suggested that (1) trisomy of genes from HSA21—or their orthologs—may induce heart defects, as shown in Tc1 [27] and Ts65Dn [28],[29] mice, and (2) specific genes or regions may contribute heavily to heart defects [30],[31] in the murine models. In human, attempts to identify candidate genes have compared the transcriptomes of hearts from fetuses with or without DS [32–34]. However, these studies were performed either without screening

Table 3. GO categories in the CDH^+ DE genes.

Heart defects	GO Term	Description	P-value	Enrichment (N, B, n, b)
DE [AVSD/CHD^-]	GO:0008270	zinc ion binding (F)	7.22E-04	1.30 (8259,986,810,126)
	GO:0030665	clathrin coated vesicle membrane (C)	7.56E-04	3.71 (8259,22,810,8)
DE [ASD+VSD/CHD^-]	GO:0016043	cellular component organization (P)	3.14E-05	1.25 (8264,1736,888,234)
	GO:0071840	cellular component organization or biogenesis (P)	3.98E-05	1.25 (8264,1759,888,236)
	GO:0071822	protein complex subunit organization (P)	1.26E-04	1.56 (8264,393,888,66)
	GO:0006909	phagocytosis (P)	4.40E-04	3.92 (8264,19,888,8)
	GO:0043933	macromolecular complex subunit organization (P)	4.67E-04	1.42 (8264,551,888,84)
	GO:0071526	semaphorin-plexin signaling pathway (P)	6.06E-04	7.45 (8264,5,888,4)
	GO:0007411	axon guidance (P)	6.94E-04	1.90 (8264,132,888,27)
	GO:0051592	response to calcium ion (P)	9.90E-04	2.84 (8264,36,888,11)
	GO:0032774	RNA biosynthetic process (P)	9.97E-04	1.46 (8264,407,888,64)
	GO:0017154	semaphorin receptor activity (F)	1.33E-04	9.31 (8264,4,888,4)
	GO:0032991	macromolecular complex (-C)	2.97E-05	1.22 (8264,2220,888,290)
	GO:0043234	protein complex (-C)	3.26E-04	1.21 (8264,1789,888,233)
	GO:0005881	cytoplasmic microtubule (-C)	3.71E-04	3.64 (8264,23,888,9)
	GO:0005829	cytosol (-C)	8.17E-04	1.22 (8264,1521,888,199)
	GO:0005829	cytosol (-C)	4.43E-04	1.26 (8256,1388,804,170)

Analysis of the enrichment of GO categories for the genes DE in the comparison between AVSD or ASD+VSD set of genes and CHD^- set of genes compared to the genes expressed in LCLs. Analysis used GOrilla software with a p-value threshold at 10^{-3}. N - is the total number of genes, B - is the total number of genes associated with a specific null, n - is the number of genes in the group with heart defect, b - is the number of genes in the intersection.

Table 4. Pathways analysis of DE genes in the CHD$^+$.

	LCLs	AVSD/CHD$^-$		ASD+VSD/CHD$^-$	
pathways	N	n	enrichment p value	n	enrichment p value
notch	82	6	0.615	11	0.163
wnt	92	10	0.277	12	0.204
jak-stat	68	7	0.259	12	**0.008**
hedgehog	37	1	0.912	8	**0.012**
epithel-mesenchym	31	2	0.673	4	0.23
angiogenesis/cardiogenesis	17	2	0.703	2	0.428
ciliome	1134	134	**0.00017**	148	**0.00027**

N is the number of genes from the pathway in genes expressed in LCLs. n is the number of DE genes from the pathway in the AVSD or ASD+VSD set of genes. p is the p value for the enrichment calculated with 9,758 genes expressed in LCLs, 889 DE genes in AVSD group, and 1,017 DE genes in ASD/VSD group.

for heart defects or without differentiating between various heart defects for a small number of cases and did not lead to the identification of genes DE in individuals with DS with CHD as compared to individuals with DS without CHD.

Peripheral tissues carry signatures of heart defects

Using peripheral tissues for analysis of genetic changes allows a study to assess a larger number of individuals. Recent studies describe the use of LCLs to characterize expression changes in various genetic diseases including including Rett syndrome [35], nonspecific X-linked mental retardation [36], bipolar disorder [37], autism and fragile X syndrome [38]'[39], imprinting diseases [40], and cardiomyopathy [41]. A recent study of individuals with mosaicism for trisomy 21 showed that congenital heart defects were significantly correlated with the percentage of trisomy in lymphocytes [42]. Here, performing microarray experiments on RNAs extracted from LCLs of individuals with DS with and without CHD, we have shown that it was possible to classify DS carriers of heart defects.

Alteration of signaling pathways differs according to specific heart defects

Within the group with heart defects (CHD$^+$), it was possible to differentiate between the transcriptome of cells from individuals with DS carrying AVSD and those carrying ASD or VSD. With a p-value below 0.05, 889 genes were DE between AVSD and CHD$^-$ and 1,016 genes between ASD+VSD and CHD$^-$. The two groups had a modest overlap of 10–15%, indicating that, for the most part, different molecular causes contribute to these morphologically-different cardiac malformations.

Genes that exhibit stronger dysregulation in those with heart defects are good candidates to explain the defects, particularly considering alteration of the pathways including or associated with these genes. However, expression analysis also revealed, at least in LCLs, the presence of genes (group II) with an expression level closer to the expression observed in controls than in CHD$^-$: these results may suggest that over-dysregulation of these genes in CHD$^-$ exerts a protective effect against the dysregulation of other genes directly involved in heart defects.

Chromosomal localizations of dysregulated genes is not always random

Among DE genes located on HSA21, two clusters were identified: the AVSD cluster (*PIGP-TTC3-DSCR3*) and the ASD+VSD cluster (*IFNAR1-GART-DONSON*). These genes are included in the narrowed candidate region containing potentially relevant genes for heart defects in the trisomy 16 mouse models [31]. Moreover, SNP-to-expression associations have been found in *cis* for TTC3 and PIGP(DSCR5) [43]. Screening the chromosomal location of DE genes revealed an overrepresentation of genes located on specific chromosomes, specifically chromosomes 7, 11, 16, 19, and 20 for the AVSD group and 11, 19, and 22 for the ASD+VSD group. The presence of these contiguous clusters of genes points to possible common regulatory processes involved in CHD likely arising from local chromatin modifications.

Dysregulated genes or pathways are associated with cardiogenesis and/or cardiac defects

Among DE genes that can be considered as candidate genes there is a gene encoding an ubiquitin E3 ligase (*TTC3*). Interestingly, E3 ligases have been implicated in the etiology of human cardiovascular diseases: *FBXO25* targets cardiac transcription factors, indicating that cardiac protein homeostasis has a pivotal impact on cardiac development that is dependent on the ubiquitin-proteasome system [44]; increased levels of *TTC3* may interact with similar processes.

There also exist potential synergistic effects. For example, co-regulation of *TTC3* and *AUTS2* has been shown during the differentiation of human embryonic stem cells (hESC) into cardiomyocytes. *TTC3* and *AUTS2* are upregulated during the first step of differentiation of hESC-derived cardiomyocytes into beating embryoid bodies that highly express cardiac transcriptional regulator genes [45]. Interestingly, *TTC3* and *AUTS2*, which appear to be involved in common mechanisms, are both DE in cells from individuals with DS with AVSD.

GO analyses of differential expression in AVSD revealed an enrichment for genes linked to the formation of clathrin-coated vesicle membranes; clathrin-mediated membrane trafficking is essential for cell organisation and likely to be involved in various steps of heart formation. Additionally, we noted an enrichment in genes from the semaphorin-plexin signaling pathway for ASD+VSD: knockdown of semaphorin3D reduces the size of the primary heart field [46], and semaphorin3C appears to be regulated by *Tbx1*, *Pitx2*, and *Gata6*—critical regulators of secondary heart field development [47]; PlexinA1-SemaD6 interaction are involved in myocardial organization and growth [48].

Enrichment of DE genes in pathways that are known to be involved in the differentiation of the heart were analyzed more specifically than with the GO approaches. We developed lists of genes in involved pathways by compiling three different sources (AMIGO, KEGG, and SAB). We identified an enrichment in the Hedgehog pathway only in the ASD+VSD group. Hedgehog, and particularly the Sonic Hedgehog (Shh) pathway, is proposed to be involved in heart development. Many processes (proliferation/differentiation, migration, transition) and cell types participate in heart development, from the heart tube to the four-chamber heart. Of particular interest are the secondary heart field and neural crest [49],[50],[51], [52]. The secondary heart field, composed of different sub-domains, is the target of multiple signals that emerge from outside the cardiac progenitors. Among these signals, alteration in the level of Shh secreted by the pulmonary endoderm may affect the development of the atrial septum [53]'[54]. Interestingly, abnormal SHH expression has been observed in fetuses with DS presenting an increased nuchal translucency [55], a feature frequently associated with heart defects. Moreover, altered response to Shh is suggested to be associated to a deficit in neural crest development in Ts65Dn mice [56]. Thus, Shh signaling may contribute, via various cells, in the ASD or VSD anomalies observed in DS.

The Jak-stat pathway was also found to be dysregulated in the ASD+VSD group. A recent study using *Drosophila* as a model system found that Jak-stat controls the expression of *tin*, a member of the NK2 transcription factor family, and modulates heart precursor diversification [57]. Further, a study of proteins secreted by hESCs identified a potential role of the Jak-stat pathway in cardiogenesis [58]. Therefore, even subtle alterations in this pathway could modify very early heart development.

The primary cilium has recently been shown to play a crucial role in vertebrate development, including that of the heart [25],[59],[60]. Cilia also appear to be involved in Hedgehog signaling. Interestingly, although human mutations in cilia genes were first implicated in LR asymmetry inducing heterotaxy, they may also lead to heart defects including AVSD, ASD, or VSD, as in Ellis-van Creveld syndrome [61]. We therefore tested whether cilia genes were DE in cells from CHD^+ individuals as compared to CHD^-. Using the database constructed from mouse cilia genes [26], we found an enrichment in cilia genes for the two CHD^+ groups (AVSD and ASD+VSD), with an overlap of only 16 genes (12%) between the two sets. Interestingly, *TUBB2B* and *OFD1* (Table 2), as well as the HSA21 gene *TSGPA2/RSPH1* (or meichroacidin [62]) are upregulated in cells from AVSD cases.

Together, the results of this study highlight genes already known to participate in heart defects, suggest new involvement of specific pathways in heart morphogenesis, and open new perspectives to understanding cardiogenic alterations present in individuals with Down syndrome. Further studies on embryonic samples at different stages of development will be necessary to identify the mechanisms at the origin of these different cardiac defects.

Materials and Methods

Individuals and cell lines

LCLs were derived from peripheral blood lymphocytes collected from individuals with DS by Genethon platform. Parents of individuals with DS gave written informed consent, and the French biomedical ethics committees gave their approval for this study (Comité de Protection des Personnes dans la Recherche Biomédicale number 03025 and CPP SDE I agreement N° AC-2009-12). Heart phenotypes were established from the medical records either on surgery or echocardiography. Cell lines from control individuals were also obtained, with written informed consent, for comparison of chromosome 21 gene expression profiles. Immortalization was performed in Cell department of Genethon with the same EBV batch. All cell lines were karyotyped to confirm their trisomic or euploid status and to verify that immortalization by the Epstein-Barr virus (EBV) did not produce any additional chromosomal rearrangement beyond trisomy 21. Lymphoblastoid cells were grown in Opti-MEM supplemented with 5% fetal calf serum (Life Technologies) and antibiotics (Penicilline, Streptomycine).

RNA extraction

Frozen vials from previously immortalized cell lines were cultured in 5% fetal calf serum in a 5% CO_2 incubator. Cells were harvested at approximately 60% confluency by centrifugation to a cell pellet of on average 10^7 cells. The cell pellet was resuspended in lysis buffer and cell aggregates were dissociated by careful pipeting, and the Macherey-Nagel mini kit was used to extract total RNA. RNA was quantified using a NanoDrop and checked for quality using the Agilent Bioanalyser. Individual samples were randomised before RNA extraction, amplification, and hybridisation to Illumina Human WG-6 Sentrix BeadArray arrays. Arrays were hybridised with labelled cRNA material and scanned according to manufacturer's instructions.

Expression data

Expression data were obtained using Illumina Human-6 v2 expression beadchips with 47,701 probes (Illumina Inc., San Diego, CA) on cRNAs from 21 individuals with heart defects (CHD^+: 7 AVSD, 8 ASD, 6 VSD) and 22 without heart defects (CHD^-). In a second experiment, Illumina Human HT-12 v3 beadchips with 48,803 probes were used to compare 11 individuals with DS without heart defects (CHD^-) to 12 controls (2N individuals). For Illumina BeadArray assay, cRNA (500 ng) was synthesized with the Illumina RNA Amplification Kit (Ambion, Austin, TX, USA), purified, labeled, and hybridised according to the manufacturer's instructions. Then, arrays were scanned using the Illumina BeadArray reader (500GX, Illumina), and scanned images were imported in the BeadStudio software version 3.1.3.0 (Illumina). For the expression array, unprocessed data were collected from BeadStudio and processed using variance-stabilizing transformation (VST) method and quantile normalization with the R bead array package. Microarray data have been deposited in GEO database with the number GSE34459.

Pathways analysis

Gene content of pathways were defined according to three databases: AMIGO, KEGG, and SAB. Gene lists were constructed by including aliases (GeneCards V3 database, http://www.genecards.org/).

Real-time quantitative Reverse Transcription PCR

qRT-PCR was used to confirm the results obtained by expression arrays. The number of samples was increased in comparison with microarrays to increase the statistical power of the analysis. cDNAs were synthesized using 1 µg of total RNA with reverse transcriptase enzyme (Takara, Ozyme) in combination with oligo-dT and random hexamer priming, and qPCR was performed as described elsewhere (Roche 480). Primer details are in Table S3. Expression of the genes of interest was normalized by using the program. Two normalization genes were selected within this program: *HPRT* and *POLR2A*. Relative quantification was performed using standard curves, followed by adjustment with a normalization factor (REST 2009 v2.0.13). Average relative expression of genes of interest in studied groups was compared to controls (either 2N or CHD^-).

Statistical analysis

Because they were obtained on two different versions of the Illumina beadarrays, the expression data sets were analyzed separately. Both were normalized using quantile normalization, and expression levels were considered significant when their p-values were below 1%. Principal component analyses (PCA) were performed on the transcripts whose expression levels were significant.

In the data set of individuals with DS only, we first analyzed the subset of 21 individuals with heart defects (CHD^+: 7 AVSD, 8 ASD, 6 VSD) with ANOVA, followed by two-by-two t-tests with a global estimate of the common variance, on the 11,224 transcripts showing a significant expression level across at least 4 arrays in each of the three groups. For the ASD/VSD comparison, only 33 transcripts were found differentially expressed (DE), i.e., far less than expected under the global null hypothesis (112); therefore, the ASD and VSD group were merged into one, the ASD+VSD group. Then, a second ANOVA was conducted on the totality of the first data (22 CHD^-, 7 AVSD, and 14 ASD+VSD) again followed by two-by-two t-tests.

The data set with 11 CHD^- individuals with DS and 12 controls was analyzed with a t-test on the 14,649 transcripts showing significant expression across at least 9 arrays in each group.

Supporting Information

Table S1 Differentially expressed genes in LCLs from DS with and without heart defect.

Table S2 Classification of differentially expressed genes according to their relative level of expression in CHD+ as compared to CHD.

Table S3 Oligonucleotide sequences for qRTPCR. Gene nomenclature.

Table S4 Genomic localization of DE genes: Enrichment in DE genes from specific chromosomes and probability to find contiguous genes as doublets or triplets.

Table S5 List of genes involved in pathways associated with heart morphogenesis.

Acknowledgments

We thank all the personnel at each site, as well as the family recruiters and laboratory personnel from Institut médical Lejeune, département de Génétique du CHU de St Etienne, Unité de Génétique Médicale de l'Université Saint-Joseph, département de Cardiologie pédiatrique des Cliniques Universitaires St Luc. We thank the many families whose participation has made this study possible.

Author Contributions

Conceived and designed the experiments: JMD MCP. Performed the experiments: CR EAY-G LD EP. Analyzed the data: IR CR EAY-G NC MCP JMD. Contributed reagents/materials/analysis tools: CM AR YG HB BdF RT GD AM. Wrote the paper: NC MCP JMD.

References

1. Delabar JM, Aflalo-Rattenbac R, Creau N (2006) Developmental defects in trisomy 21 and mouse models. Scientific World Journal 6: 1945–1964.
2. Venugopalan P, Agarwal AK (2003) Spectrum of congenital heart defects associated with Down Syndrome in high consanguineous Omani population. Indian Pediatr 40: 398–403.
3. Kallen B, Mastroiacovo P, Robert E (1996) Major congenital malformations in Down syndrome. Am J Med Genet 65: 160–166.
4. Freeman SB, Taft LF, Dooley KJ, Allran K, Sherman SL, et al. (1998) Population-based study of congenital heart defects in Down syndrome. Am J Med Genet 80: 213–217.
5. Stoll C, Alembik Y, Dott B, Roth MP (1998) Study of Down syndrome in 238,942 consecutive births. Ann Genet 41: 44–51.
6. Torfs CP, Christianson RE (1998) Anomalies in Down syndrome individuals in a large population-based registry. Am J Med Genet 77: 431–438.
7. Freeman SB, Bean LH, Allen EG, Tinker SW, Locke AE, et al. (2008) Ethnicity, sex, and the incidence of congenital heart defects: a report from the National Down Syndrome Project. Genet Med 10: 173–180.
8. Vida VL, Barnoya J, Larrazabal LA, Gaitan G, de Maria Garcia F, et al. (2005) Congenital cardiac disease in children with Down's syndrome in Guatemala. Cardiol Young 15: 286–290.
9. Fredouille C, Baschet N, Morice JE, Soulier M, Liprandi A, et al. (2005) [Linear insertion of the atrioventricular valves without defect]. Arch Mal Coeur Vaiss 98: 549–555.
10. Hyett J, Moscoso G, Nicolaides K (1997) Abnormalities of the heart and great arteries in first trimester chromosomally abnormal fetuses. Am J Med Genet 69: 207–216.
11. Paladini D, Tartaglione A, Agangi A, Teodoro A, Forleo F, et al. (2000) The association between congenital heart disease and Down syndrome in prenatal life. Ultrasound Obstet Gynecol 15: 104–108.
12. Moorman A, Webb S, Brown NA, Lamers W, Anderson RH (2003) Development of the heart: (1) formation of the cardiac chambers and arterial trunks. Heart 89: 806–814.
13. Aanhaanen WT, Moorman AF, Christoffels VM (2011) Origin and development of the atrioventricular myocardial lineage: insight into the development of accessory pathways. Birth Defects Res A Clin Mol Teratol 91: 565–577.
14. Anderson RH, Webb S, Brown NA, Lamers W, Moorman A (2003) Development of the heart: (2) Septation of the atriums and ventricles. Heart 89: 949–958.
15. Deutsch S, Lyle R, Dermitzakis ET, Attar H, Subrahmanyan L, et al. (2005) Gene expression variation and expression quantitative trait mapping of human chromosome 21 genes. Hum Mol Genet 14: 3741–3749.
16. Ait Yahya-Graison E, Aubert J, Dauphinot L, Rivals I, Prieur M, et al. (2007) Classification of human chromosome 21 gene-expression variations in Down syndrome: impact on disease phenotypes. Am J Hum Genet 81: 475–491.
17. Torfs CP, Christianson RE (1999) Maternal risk factors and major associated defects in infants with Down syndrome. Epidemiology 10: 264–270.
18. Dolk H, Loane M, Garne E (2010) The prevalence of congenital anomalies in Europe. Adv Exp Med Biol 686: 349–364.
19. Locke AE, Dooley KJ, Tinker SW, Cheong SY, Feingold E, et al. (2010) Variation in folate pathway genes contributes to risk of congenital heart defects among individuals with Down syndrome. Genet Epidemiol 34: 613–623.
20. Bean LJ, Allen EG, Tinker SW, Hollis ND, Locke AE, et al. (2011) Lack of maternal folic acid supplementation is associated with heart defects in Down syndrome: a report from the National Down Syndrome Project. Birth Defects Res A Clin Mol Teratol 91: 885–893.
21. Obermann-Borst SA, van Driel LM, Helbing WA, de Jonge R, Wildhagen MF, et al. (2011) Congenital heart defects and biomarkers of methylation in children: a case-control study. Eur J Clin Invest 41: 143–150.
22. Durham NM, Koehler JL (1989) Dermatoglyphic indicators of congenital heart defects in Down's syndrome patients: a preliminary study. J Ment Defic Res 33 (Pt 4): 343–348.
23. Luna-Zurita L, Prados B, Grego-Bessa J, Luxan G, del Monte G, et al. (2010) Integration of a Notch-dependent mesenchymal gene program and Bmp2-driven cell invasiveness regulates murine cardiac valve formation. J Clin Invest 120: 3493–3507.
24. Fernandez B, Duran AC, Fernandez-Gallego T, Fernandez MC, Such M, et al. (2009) Bicuspid aortic valves with different spatial orientations of the leaflets are distinct etiological entities. J Am Coll Cardiol 54: 2312–2318.
25. Clement CA, Kristensen SG, Mollgard K, Pazour GJ, Yoder BK, et al. (2009) The primary cilium coordinates early cardiogenesis and hedgehog signaling in cardiomyocyte differentiation. J Cell Sci 122: 3070–3082.
26. McClintock TS, Glasser CE, Bose SC, Bergman DA (2008) Tissue expression patterns identify mouse cilia genes. Physiol Genomics 32: 198–206.
27. O'Doherty A, Ruf S, Mulligan C, Hildreth V, Errington ML, et al. (2005) An aneuploid mouse strain carrying human chromosome 21 with Down syndrome phenotypes. Science 309: 2033–2037.

28. Moore CS (2006) Postnatal lethality and cardiac anomalies in the Ts65Dn Down syndrome mouse model. Mamm Genome 17: 1005–1012.
29. Williams AD, Mjaatvedt CH, Moore CS (2008) Characterization of the cardiac phenotype in neonatal Ts65Dn mice. Dev Dyn 237: 426–435.
30. Dunlevy L, Bennett M, Slender A, Lana-Elola E, Tybulewicz VL, et al. (2010) Down's syndrome-like cardiac developmental defects in embryos of the transchromosomic Tc1 mouse. Cardiovasc Res 88: 287–295.
31. Liu C, Morishima M, Yu T, Matsui S, Zhang L, et al. (2011) Genetic analysis of Down syndrome-associated heart defects in mice. Hum Genet 130: 623–632.
32. Li CM, Guo M, Salas M, Schupf N, Silverman W, et al. (2006) Cell type-specific over-expression of chromosome 21 genes in fibroblasts and fetal hearts with trisomy 21. BMC Med Genet 7: 24.
33. Mao R, Wang X, Spitznagel EL Jr, Frelin LP, Ting JC, et al. (2005) Primary and secondary transcriptional effects in the developing human Down syndrome brain and heart. Genome Biol 6: R107.
34. Conti A, Fabbrini F, D'Agostino P, Negri R, Greco D, et al. (2007) Altered expression of mitochondrial and extracellular matrix genes in the heart of human fetuses with chromosome 21 trisomy. BMC Genomics 8: 268.
35. Schule B, Li HH, Fisch-Kohl C, Purmann C, Francke U (2007) DLX5 and DLX6 expression is biallelic and not modulated by MeCP2 deficiency. Am J Hum Genet 81: 492–506.
36. Laumonnier F, Shoubridge C, Antar C, Nguyen LS, Van Esch H, et al. (2010) Mutations of the UPF3B gene, which encodes a protein widely expressed in neurons, are associated with nonspecific mental retardation with or without autism. Mol Psychiatry 15: 767–776.
37. Iwamoto K, Kakiuchi C, Bundo M, Ikeda K, Kato T (2004) Molecular characterization of bipolar disorder by comparing gene expression profiles of postmortem brains of major mental disorders. Mol Psychiatry 9: 406–416.
38. Nishimura Y, Martin CL, Vazquez-Lopez A, Spence SJ, Alvarez-Retuerto AI, et al. (2007) Genome-wide expression profiling of lymphoblastoid cell lines distinguishes different forms of autism and reveals shared pathways. Hum Mol Genet 16: 1682–1698.
39. Torrioli M, Vernacotola S, Setini C, Bevilacqua F, Martinelli D, et al. (2010) Treatment with valproic acid ameliorates ADHD symptoms in fragile X syndrome boys. Am J Med Genet A 152A: 1420–1427.
40. Boyle J, Hawkins M, Barton DE, Meaney K, Guitart M, et al. (2011) Establishment of the first WHO international genetic reference panel for Prader Willi and Angelman syndromes. Eur J Hum Genet 19: 857–864.
41. Xu T, Yang Z, Vatta M, Rampazzo A, Beffagna G, et al. (2010) Compound and digenic heterozygosity contributes to arrhythmogenic right ventricular cardiomyopathy. J Am Coll Cardiol 55: 587–597.
42. Papavassiliou P, York TP, Gursoy N, Hill G, Nicely LV, et al. (2009) The phenotype of persons having mosaicism for trisomy 21/Down syndrome reflects the percentage of trisomic cells present in different tissues. Am J Med Genet A 149A: 573–583.
43. Stranger BE, Forrest MS, Clark AG, Minichiello MJ, Deutsch S, et al. (2005) Genome-wide associations of gene expression variation in humans. PLoS Genet 1: e78.
44. Jang JW, Lee WY, Lee JH, Moon SH, Kim CH, et al. (2011) A novel Fbxo25 acts as an E3 ligase for destructing cardiac specific transcription factors. Biochem Biophys Res Commun 410: 183–188.
45. Cao F, Wagner RA, Wilson KD, Xie X, Fu JD, et al. (2008) Transcriptional and functional profiling of human embryonic stem cell-derived cardiomyocytes. PLoS One 3: e3474.
46. Sato M, Tsai HJ, Yost HJ (2006) Semaphorin3D regulates invasion of cardiac neural crest cells into the primary heart field. Dev Biol 298: 12–21.
47. Parisot P, Mesbah K, Theveniau-Ruissy M, Kelly RG (2011) Tbx1, subpulmonary myocardium and conotruncal congenital heart defects. Birth Defects Res A Clin Mol Teratol 91: 477–484.
48. Toyofuku T, Zhang H, Kumanogoh A, Takegahara N, Yabuki M, et al. (2004) Guidance of myocardial patterning in cardiac development by Sema6D reverse signalling. Nat Cell Biol 6: 1204–1211.
49. de Lange FJ, Moorman AF, Anderson RH, Manner J, Soufan AT, et al. (2004) Lineage and morphogenetic analysis of the cardiac valves. Circ Res 95: 645–654.
50. Dyer LA, Kirby ML (2009) The role of secondary heart field in cardiac development. Dev Biol 336: 137–144.
51. Snider P, Olaopa M, Firulli AB, Conway SJ (2007) Cardiovascular development and the colonizing cardiac neural crest lineage. Scientific World Journal 7: 1090–1113.
52. Xu H, Baldini A (2007) Genetic pathways to mammalian heart development: Recent progress from manipulation of the mouse genome. Semin Cell Dev Biol 18: 77–83.
53. Goddeeris MM, Rho S, Petiet A, Davenport CL, Johnson GA, et al. (2008) Intracardiac septation requires hedgehog-dependent cellular contributions from outside the heart. Development 135: 1887–1895.
54. Hoffmann AD, Peterson MA, Friedland-Little JM, Anderson SA, Moskowitz IP (2009) sonic hedgehog is required in pulmonary endoderm for atrial septation. Development 136: 1761–1770.
55. de Mooij YM, van den Akker NM, Bekker MN, Bartelings MM, Wisse LJ, et al. (2009) Abnormal Shh and FOXC2 expression correlates with aberrant lymphatic development in human fetuses with increased nuchal translucency. Prenat Diagn 29: 840–846.
56. Roper RJ, VanHorn JF, Cain CC, Reeves RH (2009) A neural crest deficit in Down syndrome mice is associated with deficient mitotic response to Sonic hedgehog. Mech Dev 126: 212–219.
57. Johnson AN, Mokalled MH, Haden TN, Olson EN (2011) JAK/Stat signaling regulates heart precursor diversification in Drosophila. Development 138: 4627–4638.
58. LaFramboise WA, Petrosko P, Krill-Burger JM, Morris DR, McCoy AR, et al. (2010) Proteins secreted by embryonic stem cells activate cardiomyocytes through ligand binding pathways. J Proteomics 73: 992–1003.
59. Goetz SC, Anderson KV (2010) The primary cilium: a signalling centre during vertebrate development. Nat Rev Genet 11: 331–344.
60. Slough J, Cooney L, Brueckner M (2008) Monocilia in the embryonic mouse heart suggest a direct role for cilia in cardiac morphogenesis. Dev Dyn 237: 2304–2314.
61. Hills CB, Kochilas L, Schimmenti LA, Moller JH (2011) Ellis-van Creveld syndrome and congenital heart defects: presentation of an additional 32 cases. Pediatr Cardiol 32: 977–982.
62. Shetty J, Klotz KL, Wolkowicz MJ, Flickinger CJ, Herr JC (2007) Radial spoke protein 44 (human meichroacidin) is an axonemal alloantigen of sperm and cilia. Gene 396: 93–107.

Health Conditions and Their Impact among Adolescents and Young Adults with Down Syndrome

Terri J. Pikora[1], Jenny Bourke[1], Katherine Bathgate[1,2], Kitty-Rose Foley[1], Nicholas Lennox[3], Helen Leonard[1]*

1 Telethon Kids Institute, The University of Western Australia, Perth, Western Australia, Australia, 2 School of Public Health, Curtin University, Bentley, Western Australia, Australia, 3 Queeensland Centre for Intellectual and Developmental Disability, University of Queensland, South Brisbane, Queensland, Australia

Abstract

Objective: To examine the prevalence of medical conditions and use of health services among young adults with Down syndrome and describe the impact of these conditions upon their lives.

Methods: Using questionnaire data collected in 2011 from parents of young adults with Down syndrome we investigated the medical conditions experienced by their children in the previous 12 months. Univariate, linear and logistic regression analyses were performed.

Results: We found that in addition to the conditions commonly experienced by children with Down syndrome, including eye and vision problems (affecting 73%), ear and hearing problems (affecting 45%), cardiac (affecting 25%) and respiratory problems (affecting 36%), conditions also found to be prevalent within our young adult cohort included musculoskeletal conditions (affecting 61%), body weight (affecting 57%), skin (affecting 56%) and mental health (affecting 32%) conditions and among young women menstrual conditions (affecting 58%). Few parents reported that these conditions had no impact, with common impacts related to restrictions in opportunities to participate in employment and community leisure activities for the young people, as well as safety concerns.

Conclusion: There is the need to monitor, screen and provide appropriate strategies such as through the promotion of healthy lifestyles to prevent the development of comorbidities in young people with Down syndrome and, where present, to reduce their impact.

Editor: Takeo Yoshikawa, Rikagaku Kenkyūsho Brain Science Institute, Japan

Funding: The study was funded by an Australian Research Council Linkage Project LP0989847. The funders had no role in study design, data collection and analysis, decision to publish, or preparation of the manuscript.

Competing Interests: The authors have declared that no competing interests exist.

* E-mail: hleonard@ichr.uwa.edu.au

Introduction

With a relatively stable birth prevalence of almost one per 1000 live births in Western Australia over the past 20 years,[1] Down syndrome is the most common known cause of intellectual disability in developed countries.[2] Health-related problems occurring in children with Down syndrome include congenital heart[3,4,5] and gastrointestinal defects,[3,4,5] infections,[6,7] ear and hearing impairments,[6,8] thyroid disease,[7] childhood leukaemia,[9,10] and immune-related disorders.[11] Age-related disorders also begin earlier in Down syndrome than in the general population. Adults with Down syndrome are at increased risk for skin and hair changes, early-onset menopause, visual and hearing losses,[12] adult-onset seizure disorder,[13] thyroid dysfunction,[14] diabetes,[15] obesity,[16] and musculoskeletal problems.[17] As life expectancy for individuals with Down syndrome has increased in infancy, childhood[18] and adulthood[19,20] so has the incidence of dementia although development of Alzheimer's dementia is frequent but not inevitable.[21]. While research has investigated medical conditions among infants and children[4,6,22,23,24,25] and older adults,[7,26] medical issues among adolescents and young people with Down syndrome, who are at an important transition point in their lives, tend to have been neglected.

The aims of this paper were: to examine the prevalence of medical conditions and health service use among adolescents and young adults with Down syndrome; to describe the impact of these conditions upon the young person's daily life; and to explore the relationship between the presence of medical conditions and level of functioning in daily life.

Methods

As part of an Australian-wide study of young adults with intellectual disability transitioning from school, young adults with Down syndrome were identified through the Western Australian (WA) Down Syndrome population database which has been following children with Down syndrome in Western Australia since 1997.[22,23] In 2011 questionnaires were distributed to 223 families whose children were now young adults aged between 15 and 30 years. Approval for the study was granted by the Ethics Committee of Princess Margaret Hospital for Children.

The questionnaire included demographic information about the individual with Down syndrome and questions about the presence of current medical conditions and the extent that these conditions impacted on daily life. Information related to the use of health services in the previous 12 months, the number and reason for any hospitalisations in the previous year, and the type of illnesses experienced in the same time period was also collected. Body weight conditions were based on parental perceptions of the young person being either underweight or overweight/obese. The level of functioning in activities of daily living was measured using the Index of Social Competence (ISC).[27] With twelve subscales grouped into the domains of communication, self-care and community skills, this is an internally consistent measure of functioning which has been validated in a cohort of adults with intellectual disability.[28] Higher functioning scores indicate a higher level of functioning in daily life. The second section of the questionnaire asked mainly about family characteristics. Age was categorised into three groups: 16 to 20 years, 21 to 25 years, and 26 years and older.

Statistical analysis

Univariate analysis of current medical conditions by age group and gender were performed. The overall and within categories of age group and gender frequency distribution of individual medical condition, and the impact of specific health conditions on daily living were explored. Pearson chi-squared test was used to test for homogeneity of proportion. Linear regression analysis was used to investigate the effect of the presence of selected medical conditions, adjusted for age and gender, on the level of communication, community and self-care skills as measured by the ISC and logistic regression to investigate relationship between some selected co-morbidities. All data analyses were conducted using Stata version 12.[29]

Results

Of the 223 families who were invited to participate in the study, 197 (88.3%) responded. There were slightly more males (55.8%) than females in the Down syndrome sample and their median age was 23.6 years (range 16.3–31.9). Of those with living arrangements reported (n = 193), the majority (85.0%) of young adults were reported to be living with parents in the family home, 12 (6.2%) lived alone, six (3.1%) lived in a group home and six (3.1%) lived with other family or friends.

Medical conditions

A median of four (range 0–11) current medical conditions were reported for the young adults, with slightly fewer conditions being reported for those aged between 21 and 25 years than in the other age-groups (Table 1). Eye and vision conditions were most likely to be present (in 72.6%) followed by muscle or bone conditions (in 61.1%) and body weight conditions (in 57.4%) (see Table 2).

Females were reported to experience more medical conditions than their male counterparts even after excluding menstrual conditions which affected more than half (57.5%) of them (Table 1). As shown in Table 2, a higher proportion of females than males were reported to have a body weight condition (77.0% vs 41.8%) and a thyroid condition (41.4% vs 14.5%). However more males were reported to have a muscle or bone (74.5%) and skin (66.7%) conditions than females (66.7% and 49.4% respectively).

There were also differences in the prevalence of medical conditions according to age. A higher proportion of the younger age group were reported to have muscle or bone conditions (77.4%), while body weight (64.4%) and skin (58.9%) conditions were more common among the older age group. In addition, menstrual conditions were more commonly reported among females in the younger age group (65.4%) and a higher proportion (80.6%) of young people aged between 21 and 25 years were reported to have an eye or vision condition than the two other age groups.

Table 3 provides a breakdown of the specific medical conditions in each category and the impact reported on the young person's daily life. More than one specific type of medical condition could be reported per category. The most common eye and vision condition was short-sightedness reported for over a third (36.5%) and considered to have an impact upon the young person's daily life in over half (55.5%). Common impacts included issues to do with safety, such as "has difficulty with daily tasks, such as negotiating steps and crossing roads" (female aged 26 years) and "can't gauge distances like crossing roads etc." (male aged 19 years).

Foot problems were the commonest muscle and bone condition reported affecting nearly two thirds (63.4%) and these were frequently (in 65.6%) reported to be impacting upon the young person's daily life. Relevant comments referred to restrictions in employment opportunities, such as "requires work that need to be seated" (male aged 20 years), and with mobility, such as "slow walker with gait affecting body aches and pains" (male aged 22 years) and "flatfooted; poor posture – walks slightly stooped and a little stiff leggedly" (male aged 19 years).

All the young adults with a body weight condition were reported as being overweight or obese and two thirds (66.4%) of parents reported that this impacted upon the young person's daily life. Common issues raised were related to mobility, such as "harder for her to get around" (female aged 27 years), "gets puffed easily" (male aged 20 years), "trouble walking distances – tires quickly" (male aged 24 years) and reduced activities, such as "participation in activity" (female aged 21 years), "not flexible, slow walker, not interested in participating in active sports" (female aged 29 years) and "lack of motivation to exercise/participate in activities etc." (female aged 28 years). Other issues included concerns related to other medical conditions, such as "small skin lesions between thighs" (female aged 31 years) and "obesity caused his knee caps to dislocate, limping most of the time especially in winter" (male aged 28 years).

One half (55.8%) of parents reported that the young adult had a skin condition with 25.4% reporting fungal infections, 24.8% psoriasis and 22.8% acne (see Table 3). A slightly higher proportion (79.6%) of parents reported that psoriasis impacted on their young person's daily life compared with acne and fungal infections (65.9% and 64.0% respectively). Embarrassment issues were also raised for those with psoriasis, such as "wears long sleeves and pants due to embarrassment" (female aged 30 years).

While just over half (57.5%) of the young women were reported to have a menstrual condition, almost three quarters (72.0%) of parents reported that these conditions impacted on the young woman's life. Comments included issues related to attending employment, such as "has to have days off work" (female aged 25 years) and "sometimes not able to attend work" (female aged 19 years), to hygiene, such as "does not manage periods well – doesn't change pads often enough" (female aged 26 years), and to activities, such as "has low pain threshold sometimes misses activities" (female aged 19 years).

Although less than one third (31.0%) of the young people were reported as having a mental health condition, a large proportion (74.4% for anxiety and 73.9% for depression) of parents reported that this impacted upon the young person's daily life (Table 3). Comments from parents among young adults with anxiety include

Table 1. Number of current medical conditions by age group and gender.

	n	mean	sd	median	range
Overall	197	4.79	2.246	5	0–11
Age group:					
16–20 years	62	4.82	2.092	5	1–10
21–25 years	62	4.60	2.221	4	0–10
Older than 26 years	73	4.92	2.408	4	0–11
Gender:					
Male	110	4.33	2.037	4	0–10
Female	87	5.37	2.373	5	1–11

sd = standard deviation.

"extreme anxiety effects every aspect of life: work, leisure, friendships" (female aged 25 years), "anxious about future, often refusing to do things" (male aged 17 years), "worries a lot, gets headaches and does not sleep well" female aged 27 years), "dwells on things unnecessarily" (male aged 22 years), and "doesn't want to go out in public" (male aged 25 years). Among those reported to have depression comments included "unable to function without medication" (female aged 29 years) and "work hours reduced. Social activities reduced. General wellbeing flat" (male aged 24 years).

While one quarter (26.4%) of young people were reported to have hypothyroidism, young adults who were reported as being overweight or obese were 2.9 times more likely (OR 2.88; 95% CI 1.42–5.84) to have a thyroid condition than those who were not overweight or obese. Furthermore, females were four times more likely to have a reported thyroid condition (OR 4.15; 95% CI 2.10–8.19) than males. Over half (56.8%) of parents with young people with hypothyroidism reported that there was an impact upon the young person's daily life. Comments reported by parents included issues related to lethargy, such as "without taking the medication he would be too lazy to move around" (male aged 28 years). One parent reported a number of issues which highlights the complexity of providing care to this population "As he has a phobia of hospitals and needles, the only way we can get blood to test his levels is when he has an anaesthetic. He has not had blood levels done for 5 years as we are unable to restrain him despite large doses of lorazapam. His skin and hair are extremely dry. Constipation a problem. Falls asleep frequently during the day, but consultant reluctant to increase thyroxine further without blood levels." (male aged 25 years).

Level of functioning and health conditions

The young adult's level of functioning was measured using the ISC [28] and included three skills domains of communication (mean 5.66, sd 1.52, median 6, range 2–8), community (mean 11.05, sd 4.28, median 11, range 4–19) and self-care (mean 19.92, sd 4.18, median 20, range 7–26). After adjusting for gender and age, young adults with mental health conditions were more likely to score lower on communication skills (−0.57, 95% CI −1.02, −0.13), community skills (−1.36, 95% CI −2.63, −0.09) and self-care skills (−1.99, 95% CI −3.21, −0.78) than those without a mental health condition (Table 4). There were no other strong

Table 2. Medical conditions overall and by age and gender of young person.

Have condition	Overall	Male	Female	16 to 20 years	21 to 25 years	26 years & over
	% (n)	% (n)	% (n)	% (n)	% (n)	% (n)
Eye/vision	72.6 (143)	69.1 (76)	77.0 (67)	69.3 (43)	80.6 (50)	66.5 (50)
Muscle/bone	61.1 (140)	74.5 (82)	66.7 (58)	77.4 (48)	71.0 (44)	65.7 (48)
Menstrual[1]	57.5 (50)	-	-	65.4 (17)	53.6 (15)	54.5 (18)
Body weight[2]	57.4 (113)	41.8 (46)	77.0 (67)	48.4 (30)	58.1 (36)	64.4 (47)
Skin	55.8 (110)	60.9 (67)	49.4 (43)	54.4 (35)	51.6 (32)	58.9 (43)
Ear/hearing	44.7 (88)	47.3 (52)	41.4 (36)	45.2 (28)	41.9 (26)	46.6 (34)
Respiratory	36.0 (71)	36.4 (40)	35.6 (31)	41.9 (26)	29.0 (18)	37.0 (27)
Mental health	31.5 (62)	32.7 (36)	29.9 (26)	33.9 (21)	27.4 (17)	32.9 (24)
Bowel	28.4 (56)	28.2 (31)	28.7 (25)	35.5 (22)	22.6 (14)	27.4 (20)
Thyroid[1]	26.4 (52)	14.5 (16)	41.4 (36)	22.6 (14)	29.0 (18)	27.4 (20)
Heart	25.4 (50)	24.4 (28)	25.3 (22)	24.2 (15)	22.6 (14)	28.8 (21)
Diabetes	1.5 (3)	2.7 (3)	0	0	0	4.1 (3)

[1]only among females;
[2]difference between genders p≤0.000.

Table 3. Overall general condition and those with specific condition and the impact upon daily life.

Condition	Those with condition	Impact upon daily life[2]				
	Total	Major	Moderate	Minor	None	Missing
	% (n)[1]	% (n)	% (n)	% (n)	% (n)	% (n)
EYE & VISION	72.6 (143)					
Short-sightedness	36.5 (72)	8.3 (6)	22.2 (16)	25.0 (18)	16.7 (12)	27.8 (20)
Long-sightedness	23.3 (46)	6.5 (3)	21.7 (10)	34.8 (16)	19.6 (9)	17.4 (8)
Astigmatism	27.4 (54)	7.4 (4)	20.4 (11)	25.9 (14)	16.7 (9)	29.6 (16)
Strabismus	5.6 (11)	0	36.4 (4)	27.3 (3)	18.2 (2)	18.2 (2)
Other eye	17.3 (34)	8.8 (3)	11.8 (4)	26.5 (9)	11.8 (4)	41.2 (14)
MUSCLE & BONE	61.1 (140)					
Foot problems	63.4 (125)	5.6 (7)	24.8 (31)	35.2 (44)	12.8 (16)	21.6 (27)
Atlantoaxial instability	8.1 (16)	0	31.2 (5)	37.5 (6)	31.2 (5)	0
Scoliosis	7.1 (14)	0	7.1 (1)	64.3 (9)	21.4 (3)	7.1 (1)
Arthritis	4.6 (9)	33.3 (3)	22.2 (2)	22.2 (2)	0	22.2 (2)
Other muscle/bone	10.1 (20)	15.0 (3)	20.0 (4)	20.0 (4)	0	45.0 (9)
MENSTRUAL PROBLEMS[3]	57.5 (50)	10.0 (5)	32.0 (16)	30.0 (15)	0	28.0 (14)
BODY WEIGHT	57.4 (113)					
Obesity or overweight	57.4 (113)	9.7 (11)	29.2 (33)	27.4 (31)	8.0 (9)	25.7 (29)
Underweight	0					
SKIN	55.8 (110)					
Psoriasis	24.9 (49)	8.2 (4)	36.7 (18)	34.7 (17)	8.2 (4)	12.2 (6)
Acne	22.8 (45)	6.7 (3)	20.0 (9)	40.0 (18)	11.1 (5)	22.2 (10)
Fungal infections	25.4 (50)	4.0 (2)	26.0 (13)	34.0 (17)	12.0 (6)	24.0 (12)
EAR & HEARING	44.7 (88)					
Hearing loss	35.5 (70)	12.9 (9)	32.9 (23)	32.9 (23)	10.0 (7)	11.4 (8)
Glue ear, otitis media	15.7 (31)	6.4 (2)	29.0 (9)	35.5 (11)	12.9 (4)	16.1 (5)
Other ear	10.7 (21)	19.0 (4)	9.5 (2)	38.1 (8)	4.8 (1)	28.6 (6)
RESPIRATORY	36.0 (71)					
Sleep apnoea	23.9 (47)	14.9 (7)	19.1 (9)	36.2 (17)	6.4 (3)	23.4 (11)
Asthma	8.6 (17)	0	23.5 (4)	47.1 (8)	0	29.4 (5)
Other respiratory	9.6 (19)	5.3 (1)	21.0 (4)	26.3 (5)	10.5 (2)	36.8 (7)
MENTAL HEALTH	31.5 (62)					
Anxiety	22.3 (44)	18.2 (8)	27.3 (12)	29.5 (13)	0	25.0 (11)
Depression	11.7 (23)	21.7 (5)	21.7 (5)	30.4 (7)	0	26.1 (6)
Other mental health	10.7 (21)	38.1 (8)	9.5 (2)	9.5 (2)	0	42.9 (9)
BOWEL	28.4 (56)					
Constipation	23.3 (46)	8.7 (4)	37.0 (17)	43.5 (20)	0	10.9 (5)
Coeliac disease	3.0 (6)	33.3 (2)	16.7 (1)	33.3 (2)	16.7 (1)	0
Bowel other	6.1 (12)	25.0 (3)	25.0 (3)	8.3 (1)	0	41.7 (5)
THYROID	26.4 (52)					
Hypothyroidism	22.3 (44)	6.8 (3)	22.7 (10)	27.3 (12)	20.4 (9)	22.7 (10)
Hyperthyroidism	4.6 (9)	33.3 (3)	22.2 (2)	11.1 (1)	22.2 (2)	11.1 (1)
HEART	25.4 (50)					
Congenital heart disease	15.2 (30)	3.3 (1)	6.7 (2)	26.7 (8)	46.7 (14)	16.7 (5)
Cardiomyopathy	0.5 (1)	0	0	0	100 (1)	0
Other heart	10.1 (20)	0	5.0 (1)	35.0 (7)	40.0 (8)	20.0 (4)
DIABETES	1.5 (3)					
Type 1 diabetes	1.5 (3)	33.3 (1)	33.3 (1)	33.3 (1)	0	0
Type 2 diabetes	0					
OTHER MAJOR CONDITIONS	11.2 (22)					

Table 3. Cont.

Condition	Those with condition	Impact upon daily life[2]				
	Total	Major	Moderate	Minor	None	Missing
	% (n)[1]	% (n)	% (n)	% (n)	% (n)	% (n)
Leukaemia	1.0 (2)	0	0	0	100 (2)	0
Epilepsy	1.0 (2)	0	50.0 (1)	0	50.0 (1)	0

[1]add to more than 100% as more than one condition could be reported; [2]not all respondents chose to answer this question; [3]only among females.

relationships found between the remaining health conditions and level of functioning scores.

Recent illness, hospitalisations and health care provider visits

The most common acute illnesses reported in the previous 12 months were cold or influenza (experienced by 74.0%, median episodes 2, range 1–20) and ear infection (experienced by 22.7%, median 2, range 1–12). Thirty seven of the young adults (20.7%) had at least one hospital admission (median admission 2, range 1–3) and common reasons were for surgery (n = 8), dental treatment (n = 8) and eye treatment (n = 7).

A total of 174 (88.3%) young people had visited their general practitioner in the previous 12 months (median number of visits 3, range 1–15), 20 (10.1%) visited a psychologist (median 5, range 1–20) and 14 (7.1%) a mental health doctor (median 2, range 1–12). Information was also provided about other specialist services used by the young adults in the previous 12 months. A total of 92 (46.7%) had visited "other specialists" that included: 25 (12.7%) visiting an eye specialist, 24 (12.2%) an ear nose and throat specialist and 21 (10.7%) a dentist. A range of allied health professionals were also visited by 45 (22.8%) of whom 13 (6.6%) visited a podiatrist. Eighteen (9.1%) were reported having visited "alternative therapists" of which five visited a naturopath.

Discussion

This is the first paper to our knowledge to describe both the prevalence of medical conditions and their impact in a population of adolescents and young adults with Down syndrome. We previously examined the prevalence of medical conditions in school-aged children with Down syndrome in 1997[23] and 2004[22]. In 1997 we found that eye or visual problems were the commonest condition experienced by 75% with current problems in 43%, followed by ear or hearing problems experienced by 57% and with current problems in 23%. Cardiac problems had affected 40% but only 7% had current problems and bowel problems 21% with current problems also in 7%. Finally, thyroid disease was reported for 14% with current problems in only 6%. When we compared the 2004 with the 1997 data we found that in 2004, children with Down syndrome were less likely to have a current problem due to their cardiac condition but more likely to have a bowel condition reported but that there was an overall reduction in episodic illnesses and infections. If we compare the prevalence of health conditions in adolescents and young adults (from the current study) with that of school-aged children at the previous time point (2004)[22], as illustrated in Figure 1, the main differences we see are in the increased prevalence of musculoskeletal problems in young adults 61% compared with only 36% in the school-aged group and of thyroid problems 26% vs 13%. In contrast the main decreased prevalences we see are in respiratory conditions reported in 60% of the school-aged group but only in 36% of the young adults and in heart conditions from 46% in the school-aged to 25% in the young adults. In the school-aged surveys just over a third (39%) of families commented on difficulties in experiencing a healthy weight (unpublished data) compared with 57% of the young adults in the current study. We did not previously specifically ask questions about mental health but the figure of a prevalence of nearly a third in the current study is concerning. We also noted a decrease in episodes of acute illness. Only 74% were reported to have an episode of influenza compared with 85% in the 2004 school-aged cohort (unpublished data), 23% an ear infection compared with 30% and 21% a hospital admission compared with 31%.

Aside from the survey data obtained from our population cohort we have also previously studied the morbidity patterns in children

Table 4. Linear regression analysis of specific medical condition and level of functioning[1].

	Measures of functioning[2]					
	Communication skills		Community skills		Self-care skills	
Have condition	Coef.	95% CI	Coef.	95% CI	Coef.	95% CI
Mental health	−0.57	−1.02, −0.13	−1.36	−2.63, −0.09	−1.99	−3.21, −0.78
Respiratory	−0.49	−0.92, −0.05	−0.83	−2.06,0.40	−1.26	−2.45, −0.06
Ear/hearing	−0.49	−0.91, −0.08	−0.22	−1.41,0.98	−0.71	−1.87,0.45
Skin	−0.32	−0.74,0.10	−0.20	−1.39,0.99	−1.16	−2.31, −0.01
Bowel	−0.44	−0.90,0.03	−0.42	−1.74,0.90	−1.39	−2.66, −0.12

Coef. = Coefficient.
[1]Adjusted for gender and age; [2]Coefficients are not comparable between different domains of functioning due to the different scales of each domain.

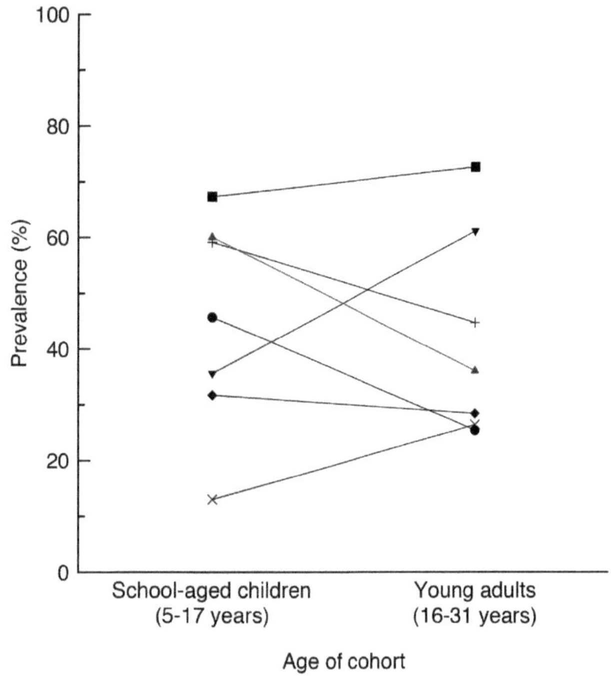

Figure 1. Prevalence of specific medical conditions in children with Down syndrome at school-age and young adults. Black dot: Cardiac. Black diamond: Bowel. Vertical line: Ear/hearing. Black square: Eye/vision. X: Thyroid. Upside-down black triangle: Musculoskeletal. Black triangle: Respiratory.

with Down syndrome through hospitalisation linked data.[30,31] Here we found that upper respiratory tract conditions affected the most children (58%) and accounted for 12% of all admissions. Other disorders, which affected a high percentage of children, were ear/hearing conditions (51%), lower respiratory tract conditions (37%) and disorders of the oral cavity (38%). Overall, we were able to demonstrate that children with Down syndrome were being hospitalised at a rate five times that of the general population. Therefore the health profile of the adolescents and young adults presented through this current study would appear to be somewhat different from that of their younger peers in that they probably have fewer acute episodes of illness, especially respiratory infections and less need for hospitalisations. However in contrast, they would appear to be developing more life style diseases such as obesity, mental health and musculoskeletal problems.

The high prevalence of overweight and obesity which we identified and has previously been reported[32] is of concern. In particular the impact of being overweight on motivation and ability to participate in physical activity, which would help prevent and manage weight gain, is worrisome. Overweight and obesity are linked with an increased risk of type 2 diabetes, commoner in Down syndrome[33] although not identified in our cohort, as well as cardiovascular disease and cancer. Obesity can also exacerbate some gastrointestinal and orthopaedic conditions, impacting further on quality of life among this group.[34] An association has been reported between a reduced body-mass index and lifestyle variables including satisfaction in friendships and access to social and recreational opportunities for adults with Down syndrome.[35] Recent research has emphasised that support workers can play a key role in encouraging participation in physical activity for this group.[36,37] It has also been suggested that, similar to many people without impairment, adults with Down syndrome often lack the motivation to exercise as well as being restricted due to medical and physiological factors. Research into factors impacting on the body composition of young people with Down syndrome is currently underway by our study team.

Consistent with previous research raising concerns about the mental health of people with intellectual disability,[38,39] we found mental health conditions to be almost four times higher than in the general WA population of similar age.[40] The prevalence of depression in our cohort was similar to that reported in previous studies of people with Down syndrome (16% for depression and/or anxiety;[41] 11% for one or more episodes of depressive illness;[42] and 22% for emotional problems[32]) but higher than reported among adults with Down syndrome based on clinical diagnostic criteria (3%).[43] In our study mental health conditions were reported to have an adverse impact on employment as well as leisure and social activities among the young adults. We also found that those with mental health problems scored lower on all three measures of functioning, although the directionality of this association is not able to be determined due to the cross-sectional study design. That is, we do not know whether mental health conditions impacted levels of functioning or whether level of functioning impacted on mental health conditions. Further research is needed to determine the prevalence, predictors and impact of mental health conditions in people with Down syndrome.

Muscle and bone conditions had double the prevalence in this young adult cohort compared with our findings in childhood and can be exacerbated further by obesity and inactivity.[22] Foot problems were the most common condition and their frequency appeared to be increasing. These conditions were reported to have an impact on both employment and mobility and yet only 7% of the total sample had been reported to visit a podiatrist in the previous year.

The prevalence of skin conditions in our cohort was much higher than reported previously among young people with Down syndrome aged between 0 and 29 years.[41] More than two thirds of our parents reported that these conditions impacted on the young person's daily life and those with skin conditions scored lower on self-care skills. There is a need for more research into both the treatment of skin conditions and the impact upon daily life.

There has been minimal research [44] into the prevalence and impact of menstrual conditions among young women with Down syndrome. Nevertheless, menstrual issues have important impacts upon daily activities including restrictions on employment and social participation, as well as issues related to hygiene needs among these young women. Furthermore, previous research among parents and carers of women with intellectual disability found that menstrual problems were no more common in this group than in the general population, but may be experienced more negatively and not always appropriately recognised.[45] Further research is needed to develop optimal strategies for menstrual management for young women with Down syndrome and other intellectual disability.

We have shown in our population-based Down syndrome cohort that the prevalence of thyroid disease increases with age at least into early adulthood. The prevalence of hypothyroidism among children with Down syndrome has been reported to range between 8% and 28%. [41,46,47] We also found gender differences with young women four times more likely to be reported to have a thyroid condition and those who were reported to be overweight and/or obese almost three times more likely. That there were impacts reported by parents for just over half of the young adults raises the question as to whether this condition is being adequately monitored and maintained for this group. These findings support the need for young people to have their thyroid levels regularly checked and treatment initiated and monitored if a thyroid condition is detected.

Overall there is limited research on the extent of health service use by other populations of young people with Down syndrome with which to compare our findings. However, In a US study using hospital records there was an average of two (range 1–3) health care sub-specialities being accessed by adults with Down syndrome transitioning from child to adult care.[48] When compared to the general Western Australian population aged between 15 and 24 years,[49] hospitalisations were higher in our Down syndrome cohort (21% versus 9%) while general practitioner visits were similar (72% versus 76%) and dentist visits were lower (11% versus 47%). In contrast, other sources report that between 50%[41] and 68%[50] of young adults with Down syndrome had visited a dentist in the previous year. However, dentists were not included as a separate medical specialist in the questionnaire and thus their visits may have been under-reported in our results.

While many of the conditions we identified among young adults with Down syndrome are also seen in the general population, these young people experience multiple conditions and, often, at a higher prevalence. Eye and vision, muscle and bone conditions, menstrual conditions among young women, body weight, skin, ear and hearing, respiratory and mental health conditions were each reported to affect one third or more of our cohort. Furthermore, some level of impact upon the young person's daily life was reported with few parents reporting no impact across these conditions. These parent-reported impacts included restrictions in opportunities to participate in employment and community leisure activities for the young people, as well as safety concerns although we did not demonstrate any impact of medical conditions on participation when we previously described friendships and leisure activities in children with Down syndrome.[51]

To our knowledge, this is the first study to report the comprehensive list of medical conditions experienced by young people with Down syndrome and the impact upon their daily lives. Furthermore, it is among the first to report on the use of medical and health services by this group. There has been no validation of the reported conditions with medical examinations or clinical measures and body weight conditions reported by parents were not validated with biometric measures. However from the health assessment literature it is clear that the identified health needs, be it morbidity or unmet health screening/promotion, exist and the level of comorbidity reported by the parents underestimate the real prevalence of disease experienced by this population.[52,53]

An additional strength of this study is the inclusion of a large representative cohort of community-living young Western Australians with Down syndrome with a good response fraction. However there are some limitations that require noting. While the questionnaire collected comprehensive information related to many aspects of the young person's life, it was long and could have resulted in respondent fatigue. There may also have been a level of recall error associated with retrospective parent-report although it was mostly related to fairly recent events. These two aspects may have contributed to missing data that limited the interpretation of some of the findings. Of note were the data missing in relation to the level of impact of medical conditions and, among those who did report, often there was no indication of how this was impacting. However, parents were encouraged to complete the questionnaire in their own time and at multiple sittings. They were also provided with options to complete a web-based or paper version of the questionnaire or by telephone or face-to-face with a research team member.

The cross-sectional nature of the study limits conclusions and directionality. As such, there is no indication of the influence of the functional scores upon the health conditions or whether the health conditions influenced the functional scores.

Conclusion

Monitoring and screening for health conditions among young adults with Down syndrome is important due to the number of conditions that occur among this group. This will assist with developing management plans and strategies to avoid long-term consequences of these conditions and to ensure that they do not act as barriers to participation in employment and social activities. There is also the need to develop and implement strategies and programs that promote healthy lifestyles among young people with Down syndrome.

Acknowledgments

We thank the families and carers for their participation and their ongoing support for research among young people with Down syndrome. We also thank the Disability Services Commission of WA for assisting with the distribution of questionnaires. We would like to acknowledge Down syndrome WA and the DSNOW consumer reference group for their continued support and advice with our research.

Author Contributions

Conceived and designed the experiments: HL TP JB. Performed the experiments: HL TP JB. Analyzed the data: TP. Wrote the paper: HL TP JB NL KB KF.

References

1. Bower C, Rudy E, Callaghan A, Quick J, Cosgrove P, et al. (2011) Western Australian Register of Developmental Anomalies 1980–2010. Perth, Western Australia: King Edward Memorial Hospital, Women's and Children's Health Service
2. Thomas K, Girdler S, Bourke J, Deshpande A, Bathgate K, et al. (2010) Overview of Health Issues in School-aged Children with Down Syndrome. In: Urbano R, C., editor. International Review of Research in Mental Retardation: Academic Press. pp. 67–106.
3. Cleves MA, Hobbs CA, Cleves PA, Tilford JM, Bird TM, et al. (2007) Congenital defects among liveborn infants with Down syndrome. Birth Defects Res A Clin Mol Teratol 79: 657–663.
4. Frid C, Anneren G, Rasmussen F, Sundelin C, Drott P (2002) Utilization of medical care among children with Down's syndrome. Journal of Intellectual Disability Research 46: 310–317.
5. Irving CA, Chaudhari MP (2012) Cardiovascular abnormalities in Down's syndrome: spectrum, management and survival over 22 years. Archives of Disease in Childhood 97: 326–330.
6. Fitzgerald P, Leonard H, Pikora T, Bourke J, Hammond G (2013) Hospital admissions in children with Down syndrome: experience of a population-based cohort followed from birth. Plos One 8: e70401.
7. Tenenbaum A, Chavkin M, Wexler ID, Korem M, Merrick J (2012) Morbidity and hospitalizations of adults with Down syndrome. Research in Developmental Disabilities 33: 435–441.
8. Määttä T, Kaski M, Taanila A, Iivanainen M (2006) Sensory impairments and health concerns related to the degree of intellectual disability in people with Down syndrome. Down Syndrome Research and Practice 11: 78–83.
9. Goldacre MJ, Wotton CJ, Seagroatt V, Yeates D (2004) Cancers and immune related diseases associated with Down's syndrome: a record linkage study. Archives of Disease in Childhood 89: 1014–1017.
10. Sullivan SG, Hussain R, Glasson EJ, Bittles AH (2007) The profile and incidence of cancer in Down syndrome. Journal of Intellectual Disability Research 51: 228–231.
11. Bergholdt R, Eising S, Nerup J, Pociot F (2006) Increased prevalence of Down's syndrome in individuals with type 1 diabetes in Denmark: A nationwide population-based study. Diabetologia 49: 1179–1182.

12. van Allen MI, Fung J, Jurenka SB (1999) Health care concerns and guidelines for adults with Down syndrome. Am J Med Genet 89: 100–110.
13. Puri BK, Ho KW, Singh I (2001) Age of seizure onset in adults with Down's syndrome. Int J Clin Pract 55: 442–444.
14. Prasher VP (1999) Down syndrome and thyroid disorders: a review. Downs Syndr Res Pract 6: 25–42.
15. Van Goor JC, Massa GG, Hirasing R (1997) Increased incidence and prevalence of diabetes mellitus in Down's syndrome. Archives of Disease in Childhood 77: 186.
16. van Schrojenstein Lantman-de Valk HMJ, Haveman MJ, Crebolder HFJM (1996) Comorbidity in people with Down's syndrome: a criteria-based analysis. Journal of Intellectual Disability Research 40: 385–399.
17. Hresko MT, McCarthy JC, Goldberg MJ (1993) Hip disease in adults with Down syndrome. J Bone Joint Surg Br 75: 604–607.
18. Leonard S, Bower C, Petterson B, Leonard H (2000) Survival of infants born with Down's syndrome: 1980–96. Paediatr Perinat Epidemiol 14: 163–171.
19. Coppus AM, Evenhuis HM, Verberne GJ, Visser FE, Oostra BA, et al. (2008) Survival in elderly persons with Down syndrome. J Am Geriatr Soc 56: 2311–2316.
20. Yang Q, Rasmussen SA, Friedman JM (2002) Mortality associated with Down's syndrome in the USA from 1983 to 1997: a population-based study. Lancet 359: 1019–1025.
21. Costa AC (2012) Alzheimer disease: Treatment of Alzheimer disease in Down syndrome. Nat Rev Neurol 8: 182–184.
22. Thomas K, Bourke J, Girdler S, Bebbington A, Jacoby P, et al. (2011) Variation over time in medical conditions and health service utilization of children with Down syndrome. Journal of Pediatrics 158: 194–200.
23. Leonard S, Bower C, Petterson B, Leonard H (1999) Medical aspects of school-aged children with Down syndrome. Dev Med Child Neurol 41: 683–688.
24. Schieve LA, Boulet SL, Boyle C, Rasmussen SA, Schendel D (2009) Health of children 3 to 17 years of age with Down syndrome in the 1997–2005 National Health Interview Survey. Pediatrics 123: e253–260.
25. Hodapp RM, Miodrag N, Goldman SE, Urbano RC (2010) Health outcomes of infants and toddlers with Down syndrome. International Review of Research in Mental Retardation 39: 37–66.
26. Bittles AH, Bower C, Hussain R, Glasson EJ (2007) The four ages of Down syndrome. Eur J Public Health 17: 221–225.
27. McConkey R, Walsh J (1982) An index of social competence for use in determining the service needs of mentally handicapped adults. Journal of Mental Deficiency Research 26: 47–61.
28. McConkey R, Mezza F (2001) Employment aspirations of people with learning disabilities attending day centres. Journal of Learning Disabilities 5: 309–318.
29. StataCorp (2011) Stata Statistical Software: Release 12. College Station, Texas: Stata Corporation LP.
30. Fitzgerald P, Leonard H, Pikora TJ, Bourke J, Hammond G (2013) Hospital admissions in children with down syndrome: experience of a population-based cohort followed from birth. PLoS One 8: e70401.
31. Leonard H, Glasson E, Bebbington A, Hammond G, Croft D, et al. (2013) Application of Population-Based Linked Data to the Study of Intellectual Disability and Autism. In: Urbano RC, editor. International Review of Research in Mental Retardation: Academic Press. pp. 281–327.
32. McGrath R, Stransky M, Cooley C, Moeschler J (2011) National profile of children with Down syndrome: Disease burden, access to care and family impact. Journal of Pediatrics 159: 535–540.
33. Cohen WI (1999) Health care guidelines for individuals with Down syndrome. Down Syndrome Quarterly 4: 1–15.
34. Grondhuis SN, Aman MG (2013) Overweight and obesity in youth with developmental disabilities: a call to action. J Intellect Disabil Res.
35. Fujiura GT, Fitzsimons N, Marks B, Chicoine B (1997) Predictors of BMI among adults with down syndrome: The social context of health promotion. Res Dev Disabil 18: 261–274.
36. Mahy J, Shields N, Taylor NF, Dodd KJ (2010) Identifying facilitators and barriers to physical activity for adults with Down syndrome. J Intellect Disabil Res 54: 795–805.
37. Curtin C, Bandini LG, Must A, Gleason J, Lividini K, et al. (2013) Parent support improves weight loss in adolescents and young adults with Down syndrome. J Pediatr 163: 1402–1408 e1401.
38. Honey A, Emerson E, Llewellyn G (2011) The mental health of young peope with disabilities: Impact of social conditions. Soc Psychiatr Epidemiol 46: 1–10.
39. Spendelow JS (2011) Assessment of mental health problems in people with Down syndrome: Key considerations. British Journal of Learning Disabilities 39: 306–313.
40. Australian Bureau of Statistics (2013) 4364.0.55.003 - Australian Health Survey: Updated Results, 2011–2012. Canberra Australian Bureau of Statistics
41. Maatta T, Maatta J, Tervo-Maatta T, Taanila A, Kaski M, et al. (2011) Healthcare and guidelines: A population-based survey of recorded medical problems and health surveillance for people with Down syndrome. Journal of Intellectual and Developmental Disability 36: 118–126.
42. Collacott R, Cooper S, McGrother C (1992) Differential rates of psychiatric disorders in adults with Down's syndrome compared with other mentally handicapped adults. British Journal of Psychiatry 161: 671–674.
43. Mantry D, Cooper S, Smiley E, Morrison J, Allan L, et al. (2008) The prevalence and incidence of mental ill-health in adults with Down syndrome. Journal Of Intellectual Disability Research 52: 141–155.
44. Kyrkou M (2005) Health issues and quality of life in women with intellectual disability. Journal of Intellectual Disability Research 49: 770–772.
45. Rodgers J, Lipscombe J, Santer M (2006) Menstrual problems experienced by women with learning disabilities. Journal of Applied Research in Intellectual Disabilities 19: 364–373.
46. Gibson PA, Newton RW, Selby K, Price DA, Leyland K, et al. (2005) Longitudinal study of thyroid function in Down's syndrome in the first two decades. Archives Of Disease In Childhood 90: 574–578.
47. Tüysüz B, Beker D (2001) Thyroid dysfunction in children with Down's syndrome. Acta Paediatr 90: 1389–1393.
48. Jensen K, Davis M (2013) Health care in adults with Down syndrome: a longitudinal cohort study. Journal of Intellectual Disability Research 57: 947–958.
49. Australian Bureau of Statistics (2013) 4364.0.55.002 - Australian Health Survey: Health Service Usage and Health Related Actions, 2011–12. Canberra: Australian Bureau of Statistics.
50. Faulks D, Collado V, de Freminville B, Newton JT, Hennequin M (2006) A controlled national survey in France of health-related challenges for persons with Down syndrome. Nursing Outlook 54: 345–352.
51. Oates A, Bebbington A, Bourke J, Girdler S, Leonard H (2011) Leisure participation for school-aged children with Down syndrome. Disabil Rehabil 33: 1880–1889.
52. Lennox N, Bain C, Rey-Conde T, Purdie D, Bush R, et al. (2007) Effects of a comprehensive health assessment programme for Australian adults with intellectual disability: A cluster randomized trial. Int J Epidemiol 36: 139–146.
53. Lennox N, Bain C, Rey-Conde T, Taylor M, Boyle F, et al. (2010) Cluster randomized-controlled trial of interventions to improve health for adults with Intellectual Disability who live in private dwellings. J Appl Res Intellect Disabil 23: 303–311.

20

Histone Deacetylase 3 Promotes RCAN1 Stability and Nuclear Translocation

Kyung Ah Han, Hye Seon Kang, Jee Won Lee, Lang Yoo, Eunju Im, Ahyoung Hong, Yun Ju Lee, Woo Hyun Shin, Kwang Chul Chung*

Department of Systems Biology, College of Life Science and Biotechnology, Yonsei University, Seoul, Korea

Abstract

Regulator of calcineurin 1 (*RCAN1*; also referred as *DSCR1* or *MCIP1*) is located in close proximity to a Down syndrome critical region of human chromosome 21. Although RCAN1 is an endogenous inhibitor of calcineurin signaling that controls lymphocyte activation, apoptosis, heart development, skeletal muscle differentiation, and cardiac function, it is not yet clear whether RCAN1 might be involved in other cellular activities. In this study, we explored the extra-functional roles of RCAN1 by searching for novel RCAN1-binding partners. Using a yeast two-hybrid assay, we found that RCAN1 (RCAN1-1S) interacts with histone deacetylase 3 (HDAC3) in mammalian cells. We also demonstrate that HDAC3 deacetylates RCAN1. In addition, HDAC3 increases RCAN1 protein stability by inhibiting its poly-ubiquitination. Furthermore, HDAC3 promotes RCAN1 nuclear translocation. These data suggest that HDAC3, a new binding regulator of RCAN1, affects the protein stability and intracellular localization of RCAN1.

Editor: Christopher Mark Norris, Univ. Kentucky, United States of America

Funding: This research was supported by grants from the Korea Healthcare Technology R&D Project (H09C1311 to KCC) through the Korea Health Industry Development Institute (KHIDI), funded by the Ministry of Health & Welfare, and from the National Research Foundation of Korea (NRF) (2007-0056092 to KCC) funded by the Ministry of Science, ICT & Future Planning (MSIP), Republic of Korea. This work was also partially supported by grants (NRF-2012R1A1A2021749, H11C1606, and H14C0093 to KCC). The funders had no role in study design, data collection and analysis, decision to publish, or preparation of the manuscript.

Competing Interests: The authors have declared that no competing interests exist.

* Email: kchung@yonsei.ac.kr

Introduction

Down syndrome (DS) is the most frequent genetic disorder and is caused by extra copies of all or part of chromosome 21, thus resulting in overexpression of a subset of resident genes [1]. Cytogenetic studies of patients with partial triplication have shown that the distal part of chromosome 21, called Down syndrome critical region (DSCR), is sufficient to cause many phenotypic abnormalities found in DS patients. *Regulator of calcineurin 1* (*RCAN1*; also called as *DSCR1, Adapt78, MCIP1 or calcipressin 1*) is located near DSCR and is thought to be responsible for diverse DS phenotypes [2]. DS patients display features, including mental retardation, various cardiac and gastrointestinal anomalies, immune system defects, and Alzheimer's disease [3].

RCAN1 is preferentially expressed in heart, skeletal muscle, and brain [4], and can bind to and inhibit calcineurin [5,6]. Ca^{2+}/calmodulin-dependent protein phosphatase calcineurin mediates many cellular responses including lymphocyte activation and neuronal and muscle development [7]. The RCAN1 gene consists of seven exons plus an alternative first one (exon 1 through 4) [4]. There are four possible transcripts but the major transcriptional products are isoforms that include exon 1 (RCAN1-1) or 4 (RCAN1-4). RCAN1-1 encodes a protein of 197 amino acids and is abundant primarily in fetal and adult brains [4]. A recent study revealed an additional start site upstream of exon 1, which produces RCAN1-1 with 252 amino acids [8]. In order to avoid confusion between these two products, the former is referred as RCAN1-1S (short form) and the latter as RCAN1-1L (long form).

Histone deacetylases (HDACs) catalyze the removal of acetyl groups from lysine residues in histones. They function in opposition to histone acetyltransferases (HATs) and induce transcriptional repression via chromatin condensation [9]. Studies have suggested that HDACs regulate cell cycle progression, cell proliferation, and differentiation, thereby modulating human cancer development [10,11]. There are 18 known human histone deacetylases that are grouped into four classes based on their accessory domain structures. Class I includes HDAC1, HDAC2, HDAC3, and HDAC8. Although HDACs 1, 2, and 3 are ubiquitously expressed, HDAC3 contains an intriguingly variable C terminus, with no apparent similarity to other HDACs. In addition, HDAC3, unlike the predominantly nuclear HDACs 1 and 2, can be found in the nucleus, cytoplasm, and at the plasma membrane [12,13]. These observations led to the hypothesis that HDAC3 may have unique properties and thus may not be completely redundant with other HDACs [9].

In addition to histones, many other nuclear proteins have been reported to be the substrates of HDACs. For example, HDAC3 can deacetylate non-histone proteins, such as MEF2 [14], NF-κB [15], and retinoblastoma protein (pRB) [16]. HDAC3 enzymatic activity can be regulated by phosphorylation/dephosphorylation [17,18] as well as indirectly regulated through phosphorylation of its associated proteins. For instance, IκB kinase α-mediated phosphorylation of RelA/p65 and SMRT on NF-κB-regulated promoters disrupts the complex and subsequently de-represses corresponding genes [19].

In the present study, we performed a yeast two-hybrid screen to determine RCAN1 (RCAN1-1S) binding regulators and/or its potential regulators. After screening a human fetal brain cDNA library, HDAC3 was identified as a RCAN1 binding target, suggesting that RCAN1 could be a potential substrate or functional modulator of HDAC3 or vice versa. Therefore, we examined how RCAN1 is functionally linked to HDAC3. We found that HDAC3 deacetylates RCAN1. Moreover, HDAC3 increases RCAN1 protein stability via inhibition of ubiquitin-proteasome system (UPS)-mediated RCAN1 degradation. In addition, HDAC3 induces RCAN1 nuclear translocation.

Materials and Methods

Materials

Dulbecco's modified Eagle's medium (DMEM), fetal bovine serum (FBS), LipofectAMINE PLUS reagent, and secondary goat anti-IgG horseradish peroxidase conjugated anti-rabbit and anti-mouse IgGs were purchased from Life Technologies (Grand Island, NY, USA). Protein A-Sepharose was obtained from GE Healthcare (Piscataway, NJ, USA). Enhanced chemiluminescence (ECL) reagent was purchased from Perkin-Elmer Life and Analytical Sciences (Waltham, MA, USA). Anti-rabbit and -mouse Flag antibodies, trichostatin A (TSA), and all other chemicals used were analytical grade commercial products purchased from Sigma-Aldrich (St. Louis, MO, USA). Anti-rabbit and -mouse HA and HDAC3 antibodies, anti-histone-H1, anti-tubulin, anti-ubiquitin, anti-Hsp90, and mouse immunoglobulins (IgGs) were purchased from Santa Cruz Biotechnology. Anti-histone and anti-acetylated lysine antibodies were purchased from Abcam and Cell Signaling, respectively. Clasto-lactacystin-lactone and MG132 were purchased from A.G. Scientific (San Diego, CA, USA). Mammalian expression vectors for HA-tagged human wild type RCAN1 (RCAN1-1S) and HA-tagged constitutively active calcineurin A (denoted as CnA or CaN) were kindly provided by S. de la Luna (Genomics Regulation Center, Barcelona, Spain) and B. A. Rothermel (University of Texas Southwestern Medical Center, Dallas, USA), respectively. The plasmid encoding Flag-tagged HDAC3 was provided by E. Seto (H. Lee Moffitt Cancer Center and Research Institute, Tampa, FL, USA). HA-tagged mammalian expression vectors encoding RCAN1 mutants with deletions spanning amino acids 1–95 ($RCAN1^{1\text{-}95}$), 1–125 ($RCAN1^{1\text{-}125}$), 30–197 ($RCAN1^{30\text{-}197}$), and 90–197 ($RCAN1^{90\text{-}197}$) were constructed as described previously [20].

Cell culture and cell lysate preparation

Human embryonic kidney 293 (HEK293) cells were maintained in DMEM containing FBS and 100 U/ml penicillin-streptomycin. DNA transfections were performed using the Lipofectamine Plus reagent according to the manufacturer's instructions. In order to prepare cell lysates, cells were rinsed twice with ice-cold phosphate-buffered saline, and solubilized in lysis buffer (50 mM Tris, pH 7.5, containing 1.0% Nonidet P-40, 150 mM NaCl, 10% glycerol, 1 mM Na_3VO_4, 1 μg/ml leupeptin, 1 μg/ml aprotinin, 1 mM EGTA, 1 mM EDTA,10 mM NaF, and 0.2 mM phenylmethylsulfonyl fluoride). Cells were scraped, and supernatants were collected after centrifugation for 20 min at 13,000× *g* at 4°C.

Immunoprecipitation and immunoblot assay

Appropriate antibodies (1 μg) were incubated overnight at 4°C with cell extracts (0.5 to 1 mg) prepared in cell lysis buffer. Protein A-sepharose beads (50 μl of 1:1 suspension) were added and incubated for 2 hr at 4°C with gentle rotation. Beads were pelleted and washed extensively in cell lysis buffer. Immunocomplexes were dissociated by boiling in SDS-PAGE sample buffer, separated by SDS-PAGE, and transferred to nitrocellulose membranes (Millipore, Japan). Membranes were blocked for 1 hr at room temperature in TBST buffer (20 mM Tris, pH 7.5, 137 mM NaCl, and 0.1% Tween 20) plus 5% nonfat dry milk, followed by overnight incubation at 4°C in TBST buffer with 3% nonfat dry milk and the appropriate primary antibody. Membranes were washed three times in TBST, and incubated for 1 hr at room temperature with appropriate secondary IgG-coupled horseradish peroxidase antibody. Membranes were washed three times with TBST and visualized using the ECL reagent.

Immunocytochemistry

HEK293 cells were seeded at 60% confluence onto cover glasses in P35 dishes and incubated overnight. Cells were transfected for 24 hr with HA-RCAN1 or/and Flag-HDAC3, washed with PBS, fixed for 20 min in 4% paraformaldehyde in PBS, and permeabilized for 30 min in 0.2% Triton X-100 in PBS. Cells were blocked for 30 min with 1% BSA in PBS and incubated overnight at 4°C with anti-mouse HA or anti-rabbit Flag antibodies. After washing three times with PBS, the cells were incubated for 2 h with Alexa Fluor 488-conjugated anti-mouse and Alexa Fluor 594-conjugated anti-rabbit antibodies (Molecular Probes). To stain the nuclei, cells were incubated for 5 min with 1 μg/mL DAPI in PBS. After washing with PBS three times, cells were analyzed using confocal microscopy (LSM700; Carl Zeiss).

Preparation of Triton X-100-soluble/insoluble fractions

Cells were solubilized in 1.0% Triton X-100, and the resulting cellular suspensions were fractionated by centrifugation at 15,000× *g* for 15 min. Supernatants (*i.e.*, the Triton X-100-soluble fractions) were mixed with 5× SDS sample buffer and boiled for 5 min. The resulting pellets (*i.e.*, the Triton X-100-insoluble fractions) were sonicated for 10 sec at 25% Amp, which generates the insoluble supernatants. The samples were ice-incubated for 20 min, mixed with 5× SDS sample buffer, and boiled.

Preparation of cytosolic and nuclear fractions

Cells were washed with ice-cold PBS and resuspended in hypotonic buffer (10 mM HEPES, pH 7.9, 1.5 mM $MgCl_2$, 10 mM KCl) supplemented with protease inhibitors (including dithiothreitol, aprotinin, and leupeptin) and incubated for 30 min on ice. Cells were lysed with a disposable syringe, followed by centrifugation at 1,000× *g* for 15 min at 4°C. Supernatants were used as the cytosolic fractions. Nuclear pellet fractions were washed with hypotonic buffer, and lysed in 1.0% NP-40 lysis buffer. Supernatants from each fraction were collected after centrifugation at 15,000× *g* for 15 min at 4°C.

Statistical analysis

Group means were compared using Student's *t*-tests. *P* values less than 0.05 were considered statistically significant.

Results

RCAN1 interacts with HDAC3

To investigate additional cellular roles for RCAN1, we performed a yeast two-hybrid screen of a human fetal brain cDNA library using full-length RCAN1 as bait [21]. In addition to RCAN1-binding partners including calcineurin, we identified several previously unreported binding proteins, including NF-κB-inducing kinase [21], Tollip [22], STAT2 [20], and HDAC3 (data not shown). To further evaluate the RCAN1 and HDAC3 interaction as well as to determine the functional role of this interaction, we investigated whether RCAN1 specifically associates with HDAC3 in mammalian cells. After HEK293 cells were transfected with HA-tagged RCAN1 and/or Flag-tagged HDAC3, cell extracts were immunoprecipitated with the anti-Flag or anti-HA antibody, followed by immunoblotting with the anti-HA or anti-Flag antibody. Co-immunoprecipitation assays revealed that ectopically expressed RCAN1 bound HDAC3 in HEK293 cells (Fig. 1A). Next, HEK293 cell lysates were immunoprecipitated with either preimmune IgG or anti-RCAN1 antibodies. Immunoblot analyses of the immunocomplexes using the anti-HDAC3 antibody revealed that endogenous RCAN1 associated with endogenous HDAC3 (Fig. 1B). When the co-immunoprecipitation assays were performed in a reverse order, we observed the same result (Fig. 1C). These results suggest that the RCAN1-HDAC3 interaction is not an artifact of DNA transfection but rather is a specific interaction in mammalian cells.

To determine which domain(s) within the RCAN1 protein is responsible for the interaction with HDAC3, co-immunoprecipitation/immunoblot assays were performed using several constructs encoding RCAN1 deletion fragments fused to HA (Fig. 2A). As shown in Figure 2B, immunoblot analyses of anti-HDAC3 immunocomplexes with anti-HA IgG revealed that HDAC3 bound to full length RCAN1 as well as several RCAN1 deletion peptides, including $RCAN1^{1\text{-}95}$, $RCAN1^{1\text{-}125}$, and $RCAN1^{30\text{-}197}$. However, it did not bind to $RCAN1^{96\text{-}197}$ (Fig. 2B). This result suggests that the N-terminal amino acid region of RCAN1 from amino acid 30–95 is critical for the HDAC3 interaction.

RCAN1 is a non-histone substrate of HDAC3

Next, we examined how the interaction between RCAN1 and HDAC3 affects the biochemical and functional activity of these two proteins, such as HDAC3 enzymatic activity and the inhibitory action of RCAN1 toward calcineurin A. We first checked whether RCAN1 could be a substrate of HDAC3. Co-immunoprecipitation assays of anti-acetyl-Lys immunocomplexes with the anti-HA antibody showed that exogenously expressed HA-tagged RCAN1 is considerably acetylated (Fig. 3). In addition, co-transfection of RCAN1 and HDAC3 caused a significant decrease of RCAN1 acetylation levels (Fig. 3). Moreover, compared with cells co-transfected with HDAC3 and RCAN1 alone, the presence of TSA, a HDAC class I and II inhibitor, significantly elevated RCAN1 acetylation levels (Fig. 3). Taken together, our data suggest that RCAN1 is a non-histone substrate of HDAC3.

HDAC3 increases RCAN1 protein stability

Based on the finding that acetylation of Lys-ε-NH_2 side chains and reversible deacetylation affect the biochemical and functional properties of target proteins such as their stabilities, intracellular localizations, and interactions with other proteins, we next examined whether HDAC3 affects RCAN1 protein stability or vice versa. As shown in Fig. 4A, HDAC3 co-transfection increased the steady state level of RCAN1, compared to cells transfected with RCAN1 alone. In addition, the stabilizing effect of RCAN1 was observed to be dose-dependent in HDAC3-transfected cells (Fig. 4A). Moreover, overexpressed HDAC3 caused the increase of endogenous RCAN1 levels (Fig. 4B).

Next we analyzed the effect of HDAC3 on the formation of insoluble RCAN1 aggregates. After DNA transfection, 1.0% Triton X-100-soluble and insoluble fractions were prepared from cell lysates and subjected to the immunoblotting with anti-HA antibody. As shown in the Fig. 4C, there was no insoluble RCAN1-1S aggregate after ectopic expression of RCAN1-1S alone, which is consistent with our previous finding [21]. Moreover, the presence of HDAC3 had no effect on the formation of insoluble RCAN1 aggregates, and there was no insoluble RCAN1 level (Fig. 4C). We additionally examined the effect of exogenous HDAC3 expression on the formation of endogenous RCAN1 aggregates or/and any change of its insoluble levels. These data also showed that there was no RCAN1 protein in the insoluble fraction and it remains unchanged under HDAC3 overexpression, whereas HDAC3 increases the levels of endogenous RCAN1 in soluble fraction (data not shown). These data demonstrate that the protein solubility of RCAN1 is unaffected by HDAC3.

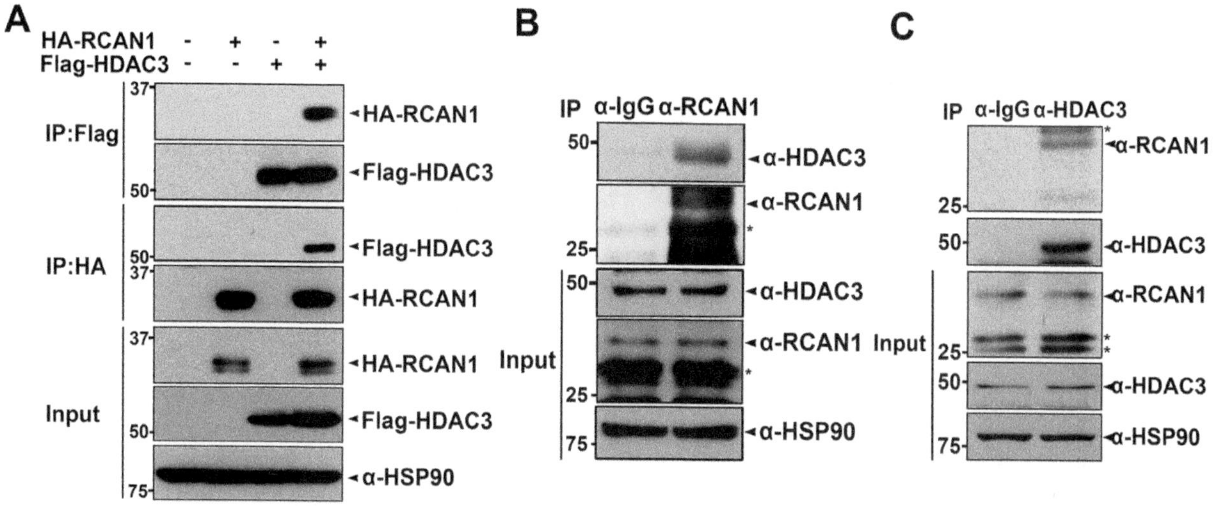

Figure 1. RCAN1 binds HDAC3 in HEK293 cells. (**A**) Where indicated, HEK293 cells were mock-transfected or transfected with plasmids encoding HA-tagged RCAN1 and/or Flag-tagged HDAC3 for 24 hr. Cell lysates were immunoprecipitated using anti-HA and anti-Flag antibodies, and immunocomplexes were analyzed by Western blotting using anti-HA or anti-Flag antibodies. Expression of transiently transfected proteins in cell lysates was identified using immunoblot analyses, as indicated. (**B, C**) HEK293 cell lysates were immunoprecipitated with anti-RCAN1 (**B**), anti-HDAC3 antibodies (**C**), or normal rabbit IgGs followed by immunoblotting using anti-HDAC3 and anti-RCAN1 antibodies, as indicated (*, nonspecific bands).

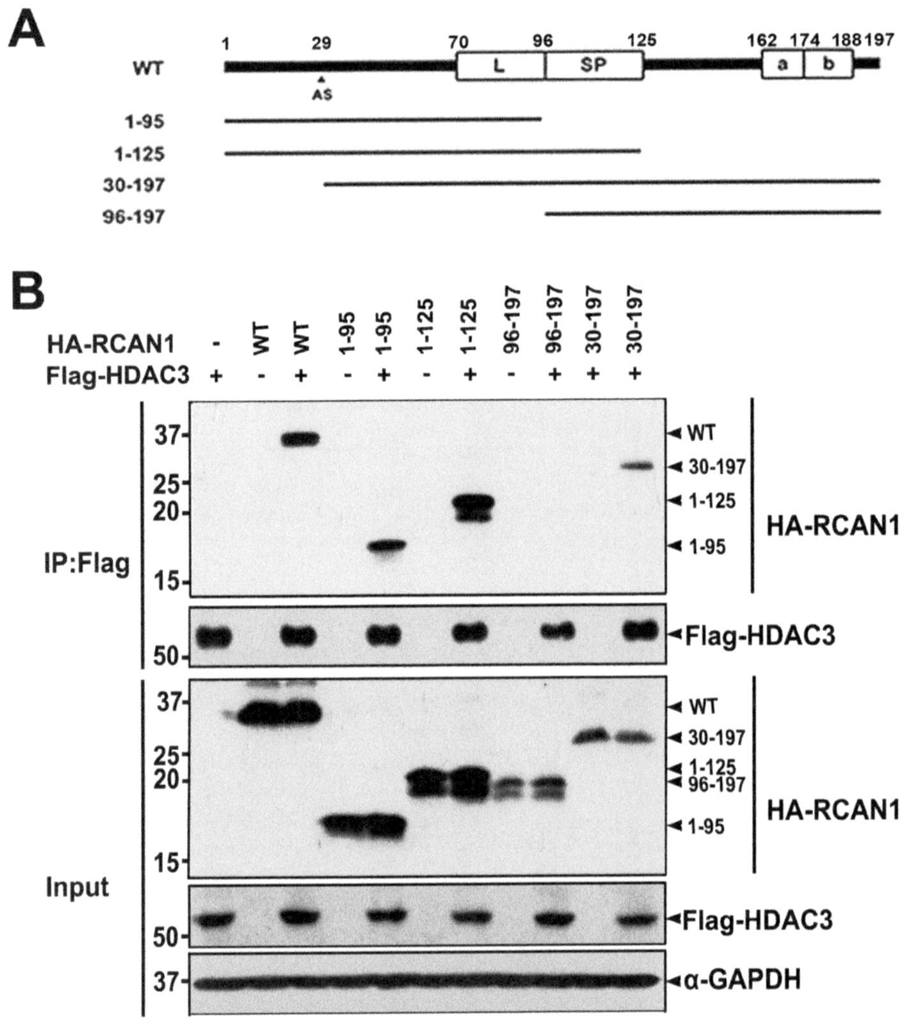

Figure 2. The N-terminal 30–95th amino acid region of RCAN1 is critical for HDAC3 binding. (**A**) Diagram of HA-tagged wild-type RCAN1 and its deletion mutants. RCAN1 consists of an N-terminal amphipathic leucine repeat (L) domain, a central span of 31 amino acids containing a serine-proline (SP) repeat, a C-terminal acidic region (a), and a cluster of basic amino acids (b). AS denotes the alternative splicing site of *RCAN1* between exon 1 or 4 and exon 5. (**B**) HEK293 cells were transfected for 24 hr with Flag-HDAC3 alone or in combination with various HA-tagged deletion RCAN1 mutants and treated for 6 hr with 10 μM MG132, as indicated. Total lysates and anti-Flag immunoprecipitates were analyzed by immunoblot using anti-HA or anti-Flag antibodies.

In contrast, the presence of RCAN1, as well as increasing doses of RCAN1, did not considerably affect HDAC3 levels (data not shown). Consistent with the binding pattern of RCAN1 to HDAC3, the stabilizing effect of HDAC3 toward RCAN1 was observed with wild type RCAN1, and the $RCAN1^{1\text{-}95}$, $RCAN1^{1\text{-}125}$, and $RCAN1^{30\text{-}197}$ fragments, but not in the $RCAN^{96\text{-}197}$ fragment (Fig. 5). Moreover, measurements of RCAN1 half-life using cycloheximide revealed that HDAC3 increases RCAN1 protein stability (Fig. 4D and E).

HDAC3 inhibits the poly-ubiquitination of RCAN1

To determine the underlying mechanism regarding how HDAC3 positively regulates RCAN1 levels, we examined the effect of HDAC3 on the extent of RCAN1-ubiquitination. HEK293 cells were co-transfected with plasmids encoding either HA-RCAN1 and/or Flag-HDAC3 in the presence of MG132. Cell extracts were subsequently immunoprecipitated using the anti-HA antibody, followed by immunoblotting using the anti-ubiquitin antibody. Although ectopically expressed RCAN1 was poly-ubiquitinated, upon HDAC3 co-expression RCAN1 ubiquitination was significantly decreased (Fig. 4F and G). These results indicate that the stabilizing effect of HDAC3 on RCAN1 results from inhibition of RCAN1 ubiquitination. Therefore, in the absence of ubiquitination, RCAN1 is not targeted for proteasomal degradation.

HDAC3 induces nuclear transport of RCAN1

We additionally evaluated whether the interaction between HDAC3 and RCAN1 affects their intracellular localization. After HEK293 cells were transfected with plasmids encoding HA-tagged RCAN1 or Flag-tagged HDAC3 alone or in combination for 24 hr, cells were fractionated into the cytoplasmic and nuclear fractions. As expected, HDAC3 was observed both in the nucleus and cytosol at a similar ratio (Fig. 6A). The presence of RCAN1 does not change the HDAC3 distribution pattern (Fig. 6A). In contrast, RCAN1 localized predominantly to the cytoplasmic

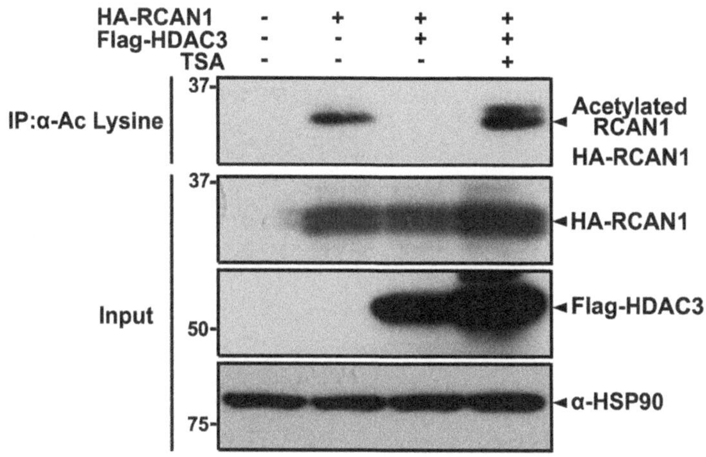

Figure 3. HDAC3 targets to and deacetylates RCAN1. Where indicated, HEK293 cells were transfected for 24 hr with HA-RCAN1 and/or Flag-HDAC3 (H3), and treated for 3 hr with 3 μM trichostatin A (TSA). Cell lysates were immunoprecipitated with anti-acetyl-Lys antibodies, followed by immunoblotting with anti-HA antiserum. Total lysates were analyzed by immunoblot using anti-HA or Flag antibodies. The HSP90 antibody was used as a loading control.

compartment (Fig. 6A). Furthermore, in the presence of HDAC3, RCAN1 was observed in the nucleus, accompanied by a decrease in cytosolic RCAN1 levels (Fig. 6A and B).

Immunocytochemical analysis of HEK293 cells transfected with HA-RCAN1 also showed that overexpressed RCAN1 was mainly localized within the cytosol in the absence of HDAC3, accompanying with its small amount inside nucleus. When cells were co-transfected with RCAN1 plus HDAC3, RCAN1 was mainly present within the nucleus (Fig. 6C). These results confirmed that HDAC3 overexpression causes the nuclear translocation of RCAN1.

Next we examined whether the nuclear transported RCAN1 is deacetylated or not. HEK293 cells were transfected HA-RCAN1 or/and Flag-HDAC3 for 24 h, and fractionated into the

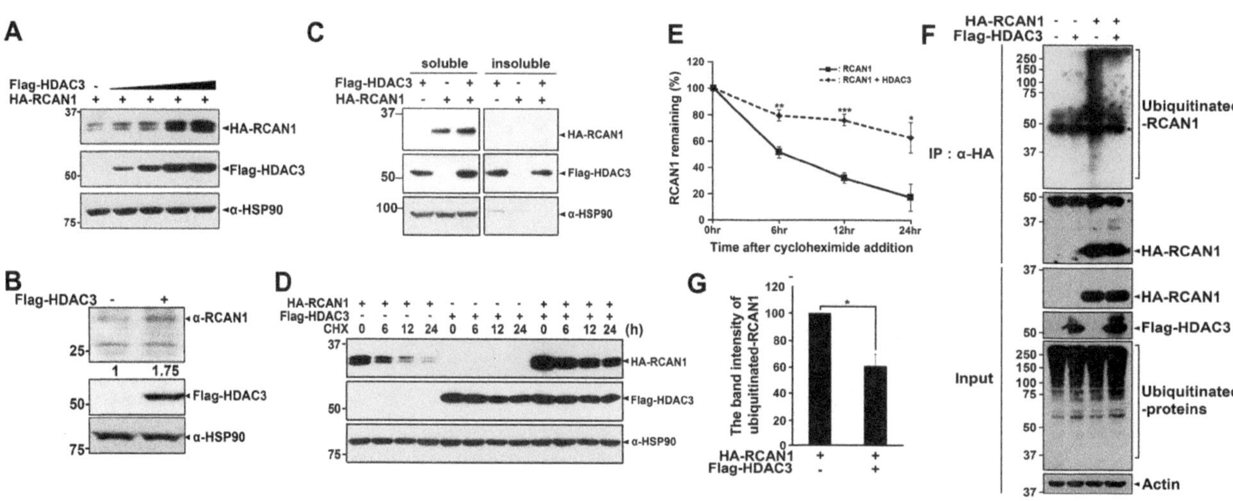

Figure 4. HDAC3 overexpression increases RCAN1 stability by inhibiting RCAN1 ubiquitination. (**A**) HEK293 cells were transfected for 24 hr with HA-tagged RCAN1 alone or in combination with increasing amounts of Flag-HDAC3. RCAN1 and HDAC3 levels were examined by immunoblotting with anti-HA and anti-Flag antibodies. The HSP90 antibody was used as a loading control. (**B**) HEK293 cells were mock-transfected or transfected with Flag-HDAC3 for 24 hr. Whole cell lysates were subjected to western blot analysis with anti-RCAN1, anti-Flag, and anti-HSP90 antibodies (*, nonspecific bands). (**C**) HEK293 cells were transfected for 24 hr with HA-RCAN1 and/or Flag-HDAC3 and cell extracts were lysed with Triton X-100 (soluble) and SDS (insoluble)-containing buffer. Each fraction was analyzed by immunoblotting with anti-HA or anti-Flag antibodies. To demonstrate equal loading, cell lysates were analyzed with anti-Hsp90 antibody, as indicated. (**D, E**) Where indicated, HEK293 cells were transfected for 24 hr with HA-RCAN1 or Flag-HDAC3 alone or in combination. Cells were treated with 100 μM cycloheximide (CHX) for the indicated times and harvested in PBS. RCAN1 levels in each sample were determined by western blot analyses using anti-HA antibodies (**D**). Data are representative of three independent experiments. Relative RCAN1 protein levels were quantified using the Multi Gauge V 3.1 program (*, $p<0.05$; **, $p<0.01$; ***, $p<0.001$; **E**). (**F, G**) HEK293 cells were transfected for 24 hr with HA-RCAN1 or Flag-HDAC3 alone or in combination and treated for 6 hr with 10 μM MG132, as indicated. Cell lysates were immunoprecipitated using anti-HA antibody and immunoblotted using anti-ubiquitin or anti-HA antibodies. Proper expression of ubiquitin, RCAN1, or HDAC3 in cell extracts was determined by immunoblotting with their antibodies (**F**). Data are representative of three independent experiments. Relative ubiquitinated RCAN1 protein levels were quantified using the Multi Gauge V 3.1 program (*, $p<0.05$; **G**).

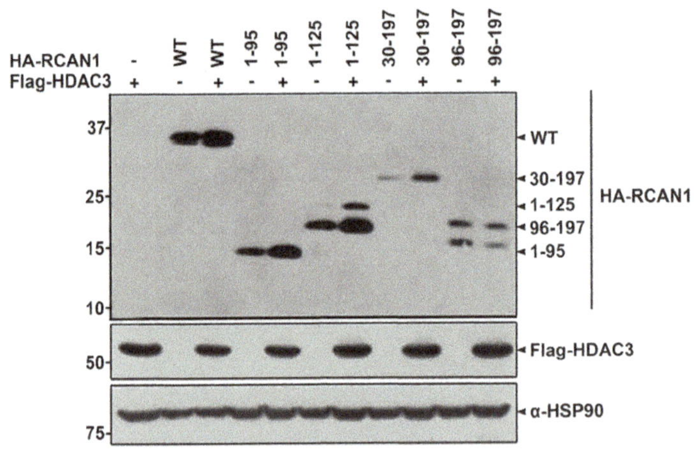

Figure 5. The stabilizing effect of HDAC3 is dependent on the RCAN1 N-terminal 30–95th amino acid. Where indicated, HEK293 cells were transfected for 24 hr with Flag-HDAC3 alone or together with HA-tagged wild-type RCAN1, RCAN11-95, RCAN11-125, RCAN130-197 or RCAN196-197 fragments. Cells were lysed in the lysis buffer containing 8 M urea, and immunoblot analyses were performed using HA and Flag antibodies. The HSP90 antibody was used as a loading control.

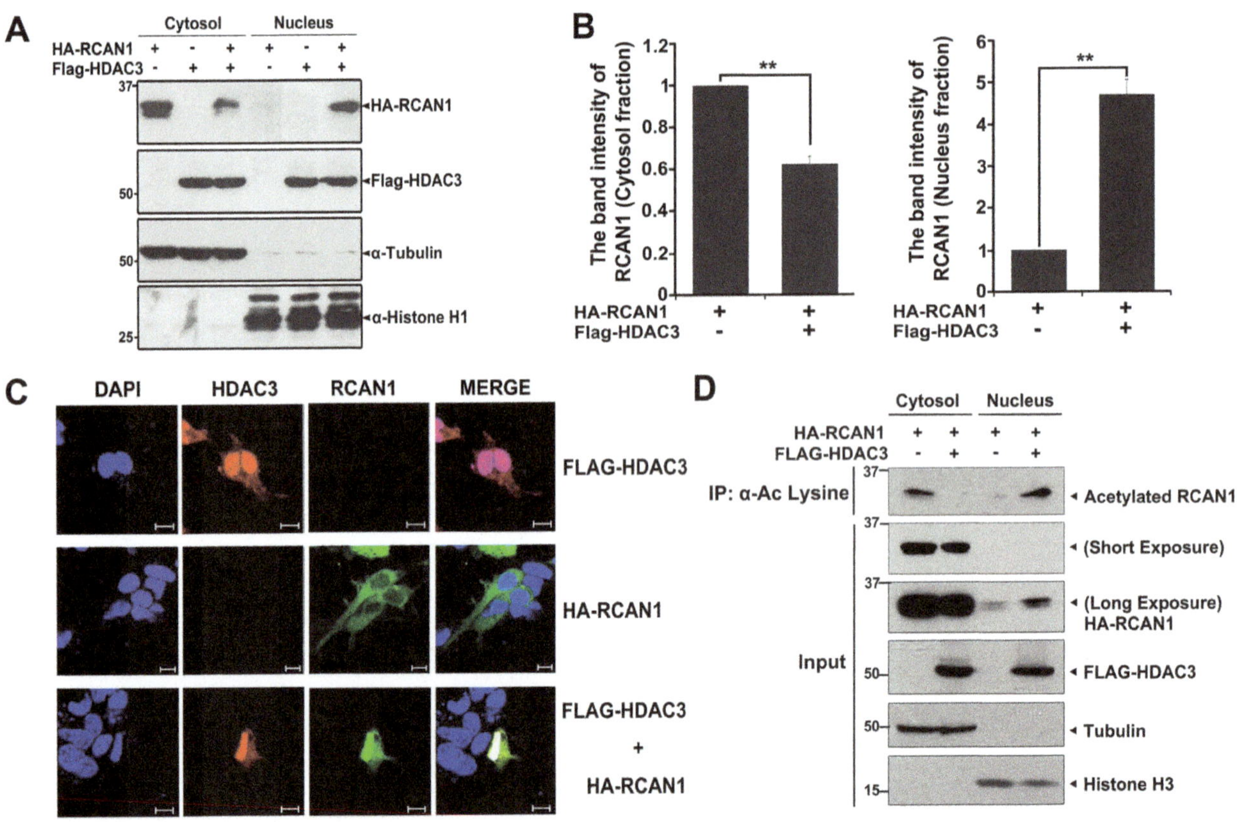

Figure 6. HDAC3 induces nuclear translocation of cytosolic RCAN1. (**A, B**) HEK293 cells were transfected for 24 hr with HA-RCAN1 and/or Flag-HDAC3 and fractionated into cytosolic and nuclear fractions. The fractions were analyzed by immunoblot using anti-HA or anti-Flag antibodies. The purity of each fraction was confirmed by immunoblotting with α-tubulin (cytosolic marker) or histone H1 (nuclear marker) (**A**). Data are representative of three independent experiments. Relative cytosolic RCAN1 and nuclear RCAN1 protein levels were quantified using the Multi Gauge V 3.1 program (**, $p<0.01$; **B**). (**C**) HEK293 cells were transfected for 24 hr with HA-RCAN1 or/and Flag-HDAC3, fixed and permeabilized, and labeled with anti-HA or Flag antibodies. The cells were then stained with Alexa Fluor 488-conjugated anti-mouse and Alexa Fluor 594-conjugated anti-rabbit secondary antibodies. Nuclei were counterstained with DAPI, and immunostained preparations were visualized by confocal microscopy. Scale bars: 10 μm (**D**) HEK293 cell were transfected for 24 hr with HA-RCAN1 and/or Flag-HDAC3, and fractionated into the cytosolic and nuclear fractions. These fractions were immunoprecipitated with anti-acetyl-Lys antibodies, followed by immunoblotting with anti-HA antiserum. The expression of exogenously added RCAN1 or HDAC3 protein in each fraction was analyzed by immunoblotting anti-HA or Flag antibodies. The purity of each fraction was confirmed by immunoblotting with α-tubulin (cytosolic marker) or histone H3 (nuclear marker).

cytoplasmic and nuclear fractions. These fractions were then immunoprecipitated with anti-acetyl-Lys antibodies, followed by the immunoblotting with anti-HA antibody. As shown in Fig. 6D, cells expressing RCAN1 alone exhibited that the acetylated RCAN1 was mainly localized in the cytosolic fraction. In addition, co-transfection of RCAN1 plus HDAC3 promoted the deacetylation of RCAN1 in the cytosolic fraction (Fig. 6D). However, co-transfection of RCAN1 and HDAC3 caused a significant increase of RCAN1 acetylation levels within the nucleus (Fig. 6D). As the increased levels of acetylated RCAN1 within the nucleus appear to be similar to the levels of nuclear-localized RCAN1, these results indicated that HDAC3-mediated nuclear translocation of RCAN1 and RCAN1 deacetylation are not linked together, but occur independently.

Discussion

There have been reports that, in addition to histones, HDAC3 can deacetylate non-histone proteins, such as MEF2 [14], NF-κB [15], and pRB [16]. HDAC3 also interacts with many nuclear and cytosolic proteins, including nuclear receptor co-repressors 1 and 2, the zinc finger transcription factor YY1, GATA1 and 2, RELA, peroxisome proliferator-activated receptor-γ and -δ, MAPK11, cyclin D1, RUNX2, and ubiquitin [24]. Here we report that HDAC3 physically and functionally interacts with RCAN1. Interestingly, exogenously expressed RCAN1 proteins were highly acetylated in resting condition, and it becomes a non-histone substrate of HDAC3. Since lysine side chains are cationic at physiological pH, N-acetylation of Lys-ε-NH_2 side chains would quench the positive charges, whereas deacetylation produces the positive charge again. Alternatively, the acetyl groups would provide additional link and acetylated lysine side chains can be specifically recognized, for example by bromodomains in partner proteins. Like other HAT/HDAC substrates, deacetylation also changes RCAN1 protein stability and intracellular address.

RCAN1 biochemical and functional activity is regulated by many types of post-translational modification modes. The most prominent regulatory mechanism is phosphorylation, and a number of protein kinases negatively or positively regulate RCAN1. For example, phosphorylation of the FLISPP motif within RCAN1 increases the calcineurin-inhibition effect of RCAN1 [8]. In addition, PKA and Dyrk1A increase the calcineurin inhibitory effect of RCAN1 [25,26]. In contrast, the MEK5-MEKK3-BMK signaling cascade, GSK-3β, and TAK1 phosphorylate RCAN1 and suppress its inhibition effect on calcineurin activity [23,27–29]. In addition to phosphorylation, RCAN1 was shown to be a target of ubiquitin and ubiquitin-like modifiers. Recently, we have shown that covalent conjugation of NEDD8 to RCAN1 increases the inhibitory effect of RCAN1 to the calcineurin-NF-AT pathway [30]. Furthermore, several reports have attempted to decrease RCAN1 expression levels via activation of its degradation signaling. Stimulation of H_2O_2-induced SCFβ-TrCP-mediated ubiquitination of RCAN1 resulted in RCAN1 degradation [31]. In addition, CREB, depending on its transcriptional activation, was also reported to activate RCAN1 degradation [32]. Our results show that RCAN1 is a target of HDAC3-mediated deacetylation, which consequently increases RCAN1 protein stability. In a similar way, class I HDACs regulate substrate protein stabilities. For example, HDAC3-mediated deacetylation increases cyclin A stability [33]. HDAC1 also deacetylates HIF-1 at Lys-709 residue, which results in the decrease of HIF-1 stability [34].

RCAN1 protein levels are also regulated by several degradation pathways, including the UPS and lysosomal pathway [32,35,36]. Specifically, FBW7 [37], SCFβ-TrCP [31], and Nedd4-2 [38] have been reported to covalently modify RCAN1 through poly-ubiquitination to trigger RCAN1 degradation. We have previously shown that STAT2 facilitates ubiquitin-dependent RCAN1 degradation and its action is mediated through FBW7 E3 ligase [22]. Furthermore, we demonstrated that FBW7-mediated RCAN1 degradation is enhanced by IFN-α treatment [22]. Based on these reports, it would be interesting to examine whether HDAC3 affects these enzymes. We also recently demonstrated that similar to STAT2, CREB can activate RCAN1 degradation, depending on its transcriptional activation [32]. Like the UPS, the chaperone-mediated autophagy pathway can also degrade RCAN1 [36].

The present study also revealed that HDAC3 promotes RCAN1 nuclear translocation. According to a previous report, the C-terminal 33 amino acid region of RCAN1 is important for nuclear localization [39]. It has been also reported that phosphorylation of the Thr-192 residue changes RCAN1 localization [26]. Regarding HDAC3, its deacetylase activity is critical for its modulatory action of intracellular substrate localization. For example, HDAC3-mediated deacetylation of RelA, a subunit of NF-κB promotes its nuclear export, which is depends on IκB during ES cell-derived endothelial cell differentiation [40]. In addition, acetylation of eIF5A [41], POP-1 [42], pRB [43], and PKM2 [44] changes the intracellular localization of protein. These examples suggest that HDAC3-mediated deacetylation may also trigger RCAN1 nuclear transport. However our results showed that the nuclear-localized HDAC3 is not deacetylated, suggesting that HDAC3-mediated nuclear transport of RCAN1 occurs irrelevant of its deacetylase activity. The biological and physiological roles of RCAN1 within the nucleus have not been clarified yet. Moreover, the detailed mechanism regarding when and how cytosolic RCAN1 is translocated into nucleus and vice versa is largely unknown, and more experiments are required to answer these questions.

In summary, the present work shows that HDAC3 and RCAN1 interact. RCAN1 is a deacetylation substrate of HDAC3. In addition, HDAC3 inhibits RCAN1 degradation via UPS as well as stimulates its nuclear translocation.

Acknowledgments

The authors thank S. de la Luna, B.A. Rothermel, and E. Seto for providing plasmids.

Author Contributions

Conceived and designed the experiments: KAH HSK JWL KCC. Performed the experiments: KAH HSK JWL LY EI AH YJL WHS. Analyzed the data: KAH HSK JWL LY EI KCC. Wrote the paper: KAH HSK KCC.

References

1. Roizen NJ, Patterson D (2003) Down's syndrome. Lancet 361: 1281–1288.
2. Fuentes JJ, Pritchard MA, Planas AM, Bosch A, Ferrer I, et al. (1995) A new human gene from the Down syndrome critical region encodes a proline-rich protein highly expressed in fetal brain and heart. Hum Mol Genet 4: 1935–1944.
3. Epstein CJ (1995) Epilogue: toward the twenty-first century with Down syndrome—a personal view of how far we have come and of how far we can reasonably expect to go. Prog Clin Biol Res 393: 241–246.
4. Fuentes JJ, Pritchard MA, Estivill X (1997) Genomic organization, alternative splicing, and expression patterns of the DSCR1 (Down syndrome candidate region 1) gene. Genomics 44: 358–361.

5. Fuentes JJ, Genesca L, Kingsbury TJ, Cunningham KW, Perez-Riba M, et al. (2000) DSCR1, over-expressed in Down syndrome, is an inhibitor of calcineurin-mediated signaling pathways. Hum Mol Genet 9: 1681–1690.
6. Rothermel B, Vega RB, Yang J, Wu H, Bassel-Duby R, et al. (2000) A protein encoded within the Down syndrome critical region is enriched in striated muscles and inhibits calcineurin signaling. J Biol Chem 275: 8719–8725.
7. Rusnak F, Mertz P (2000) Calcineurin: form and function. Physiol Rev 80: 1483–1521.
8. Genescà L, Aubareda A, Fuentes JJ, Estivill X, De La Luna S, et al. (2003) Phosphorylation of calcipressin 1 increases its ability to inhibit calcineurin and decreases calcipressin half-life. Biochem J 374: 567–575.
9. Yang WM, Yao YL, Sun JM, Davie JR, Seto E (1997) Isolation and characterization of cDNAs corresponding to an additional member of the human histone deacetylase gene family. J Biol Chem 272: 28001–28007.
10. Marks PA, Miller T, Richon VM (2003) Histone deacetylases. Curr Opin Pharmacol 3: 344–351.
11. Marks PA, Richon VM, Kelly WK, Chiao JH, Miller T (2004) Histone deacetylase inhibitors: Development as cancer therapy. Novartis Found Symp 259: 269–281.
12. Takami Y, Nakayama T (2000) N-terminal region, C-terminal region, nuclear export signal, and deacetylation activity of histone deacetylase-3 are essential for the viability of the DT40 chicken B cell line. J Biol Chem 275: 16191–16201.
13. Longworth MS, Laimins LA (2006) Histone deacetylase 3 localizes to the plasma membrane and is a substrate of Src. Oncogene 25: 4495–4500.
14. Grégoire S, Xiao L, Nie J, Zhang X, Xu M, et al. (2007) Histone deacetylase 3 interacts with and deacetylates myocyte enhancer factor 2. Mol Cell Biol 27: 1280–1295.
15. Chen LF, Fischle W, Verdin E, Greene WC (2001) Duration of nuclear NF-kappa B action regulated by reversible acetylation. Science 293: 1653–1657.
16. Nicolas E, AitSiAli S, Trouche D (2001) The histone deacetylase HDAC3 targets RbAp48 to the retinoblastoma protein. Nucleic Acids Res 29: 3131–3136.
17. Zhang X, Ozawa Y, Lee H, Wen YD, Tan TH, et al. (2005) Histone deacetylase 3 (HDAC3) activity is regulated by interaction with protein serine/threonine phosphatase 4. Genes Dev 19: 827–839.
18. Jeyakumar M, Liu XF, ErdjumentBromage H, Tempst P, Bagchi MK (2007) Phosphorylation of thyroid hormone receptor-associated nuclear receptor corepressor holocomplex by the DNA-dependent protein kinase enhances its histone deacetylase activity. J Biol Chem 282: 9312–9322.
19. Hoberg JE, Popko AE, Ramsey CS, Mayo MW (2006) IκB kinase α-mediated derepression of SMRT potentiates acetylation of RelA/p65 by p300. Mol Cell Biol 26: 457–471.
20. Lee JW, Kang HS, Lee JY, Lee EJ, Rhim H, et al. (2012) The transcription factor STAT2 enhances proteasomal degradation of RCAN1 through the ubiquitin E3 ligase FBW7. Biochem Biophy Res Commun 420: 404–410.
21. Lee EJ, Seo SR, Um JW, Park J, Oh Y, et al. (2008) NF-κB-inducing kinase phosphorylates and blocks the degradation of Down syndrome candidate region 1. J Biol Chem 283: 3392–3400.
22. Lee JY, Lee HJ, Lee EJ, Jang SH, Kim H, et al. (2009) Down syndrome candidate region-1 protein interacts with Tollip and positively modulates interleukin-1 receptor-mediated signaling. Biochim Biophys Acta 1790: 1673–1680.
23. Hilioti Z, Gallagher DA, LowNam ST, Ramaswamy P, Gajer P, et al. (2004) GSK-3 kinases enhance calcineurin signaling by phosphorylation of RCNs. Genes Dev 18: 35–47.
24. Moser MA, Hagelkruys A, Seiser C (2014) Transcription and beyond: the role of mammalian class I lysine deacetylases. Chromosoma 123: 67–78.
25. Kim SS, Oh Y, Chung KC, Seo SR (2012) Protein kinase A phosphorylates Down syndrome critical region 1 (RCAN1). Biochem Biophys Res Commun 418: 657–661.
26. Jung MS, Park JH, Ryu YS, Choi SH, Yoon SH, et al. (2011) Regulation of RCAN1 protein activity by Dyrk1A protein-mediated phosphorylation. J Biol Chem 286: 40401–40412.
27. Abbasi S, Su B, Kellems RE, Yang J, Xia Y (2005) The essential role of MEKK3 signaling in angiotensin II-induced calcineurin/nuclear factor of activated T-cells activation. J Biol Chem 280: 36737–36746.
28. Abbasi S, Lee JD, Su B, Chen X, Alcon JL, et al. (2006) Protein kinase-mediated regulation of calcineurin through the phosphorylation of modulatory calcineurin-interacting protein 1. J Biol Chem 281: 7717–7726.
29. Liu Q, Busby JC, Molkentin JD (2009) Interaction between TAK1-TAB1-TAB2 and RCAN1-calcineurin defines a signaling nodal control point. Nat Cell Biol 11: 154–161.
30. Noh EH, Hwang HS, Hwang HS, Min B, Im E, et al. (2012) Covalent NEDD8 conjugation increases RCAN1 protein stability and potentiates its inhibitory action on calcineurin. PLoS One 7: e48315.
31. Asada S, Ikeda A, Nagao R, Hama H, Sudo T, et al. (2008) Oxidative stress-induced ubiquitination of RCAN1 mediated by SCFβ-TrCP ubiquitin ligase. Int J Mol Med 22: 95–104.
32. Seo SR, Chung KC (2008) CREB activates proteasomal degradation of DSCR1/RCAN1. FEBS Lett 582: 1889–1893.
33. Vidal-Laliena M, Gallastegui E, Mateo F, Martínez-Balbás M, Pujol MJ, et al. (2013) Histone deacetylase 3 regulates cyclin A stability. J Biol Chem 288: 21096–21104.
34. Geng H, Liu Q, Xue C, David LL, Beer TM, et al. (2012) HIF1α protein stability is increased by acetylation at lysine 709. J Biol Chem 287: 35496–35505.
35. Park J, Oh Y, Chung KC (2009) Two key genes closely implicated with the neuropathological characteristics in Down syndrome: DYRK1A and RCAN1. BMB Rep 42: 6–15.
36. Liu H, Wang P, Song W, Sun X (2009) Degradation of regulator of calcineurin 1 (RCAN1) is mediated by both chaperone-mediated autophagy and ubiquitin proteasome pathways. FASEB J 23: 3383–3392
37. Kishi T, Ikeda A, Nagao R, Koyama N (2007) The SCF^{Cdc4} ubiquitin ligase regulates calcineurin signaling through degradation of phosphorylated Rcn1, an inhibitor of calcineurin. Proc Natl Acad Sci U S A 104: 17418–17423.
38. Kim SS, Seo SR (2010) Nedd4-2 ubiquitin ligase interacts with RCAN1 (DSCR1) for the proteasomal degradation. Genes & Genomics 32: 578–582.
39. Pfister SC, MachadoSantelli GM, Han SW, Henrique-Silva F (2002) Mutational analyses of the signals involved in the subcellular location of DSCR1. BMC Cell Biol 3: 24.
40. Greene WC, Chen LF (2004) Regulation of NF-κB action by reversible acetylation. Novartis Found Symp 259: 208–217.
41. Ishfaq M, Maeta K, Maeda S, Natsume T, Ito A, et al. (2012) Acetylation regulates subcellular localization of eukaryotic translation initiation factor 5A (eIF5A). FEBS Lett 586: 3236–3241.
42. Gay F, Calvo D, Lo MC, Ceron J, Maduro M, et al. (2003) Acetylation regulates subcellular localization of the Wnt signaling nuclear effector POP-1. Genes Dev 17: 717–722.
43. Pickard A, Wong PP, McCance DJ (2010) Acetylation of Rb by PCAF is required for nuclear localization and keratinocyte differentiation. J Cell Sci 123: 3718–3726.
44. Lv L, Xu YP, Zhao D, Li FL, Wang W, et al. (2013) Mitogenic and oncogenic stimulation of K433 acetylation promotes PKM2 protein kinase activity and nuclear localization. Mol Cell 52: 340–352.

FAST-SeqS: A Simple and Efficient Method for the Detection of Aneuploidy by Massively Parallel Sequencing

Isaac Kinde*, Nickolas Papadopoulos, Kenneth W. Kinzler*, Bert Vogelstein

The Ludwig Center for Cancer Genetics and Therapeutics and The Howard Hughes Medical Institute, Johns Hopkins Kimmel Cancer Center, Baltimore, Maryland, United States of America

Abstract

Massively parallel sequencing of cell-free, maternal plasma DNA was recently demonstrated to be a safe and effective screening method for fetal chromosomal aneuploidies. Here, we report an improved sequencing method achieving significantly increased throughput and decreased cost by replacing laborious sequencing library preparation steps with PCR employing a single primer pair designed to amplify a discrete subset of repeated regions. Using this approach, samples containing as little as 4% trisomy 21 DNA could be readily distinguished from euploid samples.

Editor: Reiner Albert Veitia, Institut Jacques Monod, France

Funding: This work was supported by The Virginia and D.K. Ludwig Fund for Cancer Research, the National Institutes of Health (CA62924, CA43460, and CA57345), and by a UNCF-Merck Graduate Fellowship to I.K. The funders had no role in study design, data collection and analysis, decision to publish, or preparation of the manuscript.

Competing Interests: The authors declare the following competing interests. This study was partially funded by a UNCF-Merck Graduate Fellowship (to I.K.). N.P., K.W.K, and B.V. are co-founders of Inostics and Personal Genome Diagnostics and are members of their Scientific Advisory Boards. N.P., K.W.K, and B.V. own Inostics and Personal Genome Diagnostics stock, which is subject to certain restrictions under The Johns Hopkins University policy. I.K., N.P., K.W.K, and B.V. have submitted a patent application entitled "Prenatal Aneuploidy Testing through Compressed Genome Sequencing of Maternal Plasma" covering the work presented in this manuscript. The terms of these arrangements are managed in accordance with University conflict-of-interest policies.

* E-mail: ik@jhmi.edu (IK); kinzlke@jhmi.edu (KWK)

Introduction

A major chromosomal abnormality is detected in approximately 1 of 140 live births [1] and in a much higher fraction of fetuses that do not reach term or are still-born [2]. The most common aneuploidy is trisomy 21 (Down syndrome), which currently occurs in 1 of 730 births [1]. Though less common than trisomy 21, trisomy 18 (Edwards Syndrome) and trisomy 13 (Patau syndrome) occur in 1 in 5,500 and 1 in 17,200 live births, respectively [1]. A large variety of congenital defects, growth deficiencies, and intellectual disabilities are found in children with chromosomal aneuploidies, and these present life-long challenges to families and societies [3]. For these reasons, much effort has been devoted to detecting chromosome abnormalities during early fetal life, at a time when therapeutic abortions can be offered as an option to prospective parents.

There are a variety of prenatal tests that can indicate increased risk for fetal aneuploidy, although invasive diagnostic tests such as amniocentesis or chorionic villus sampling are the current gold standard [4] and are associated with a non-negligible risk of fetal loss. More reliable, non-invasive tests for fetal aneuploidy have therefore long been sought. The most promising of these are based on the detection of fetal DNA in maternal plasma, as pioneered by Lo's group [5]. It has recently been demonstrated that massively parallel sequencing of libraries generated from maternal plasma can reliably detect chromosome 21 abnormalities [6,7]. In the most comprehensive study to date [8], 98.6% of fetuses with trisomy 21 were detected in maternal plasma, with a false positive rate of 0.2 percent. In an additional 0.8 percent of samples, the test failed to give a result. These exciting studies promise a new era of non-invasive prenatal testing.

Currently, almost half of trisomy 21 babies are born to mothers less than 35 years of age, as more than 80% of pregnant women are under 35 [9,10]. Though the risk of invasive procedures is thought to outweigh the benefit of invasive testing for eligible young mothers, it is clear that the vast majority of births associated with chromosomal aneuploidies could be safely identified with reliable non-invasive tests that could be administered to all pregnant women. Prenatal testing is an extraordinarily stressful exercise for pregnant mothers and their families, and the more rapid the process, the better.

To achieve this goal with circulating fetal DNA testing, decreases in cost and increases in throughput will be necessary. There are three major components of plasma DNA testing: preparation of DNA libraries for loading on the sequencing instrument, the sequencing of these libraries, and their analysis. The second component is being addressed by instrument manufacturers, who have made remarkable progress over the last few years. Potential improvements in the first and third components are the subject of the current study.

The only commercially available tests for circulating fetal DNA aneuploidy [8,11] involve the preparation of whole genome libraries and the analysis of a sufficient number of sequences on the relevant chromosomes to reliably detect small differences in copy number. The preparation of whole genome libraries involves several sequential steps - including end-repair, 5′-phosphorlyation, addition of a terminal dA nucleotide to the 3′ ends of the fragments, ligation of the fragments to adapters, and PCR amplification of the ligated products - many of which require intervening purifications. The PCR products are then quantified and loaded on the sequencing instrument. Following the sequencing run, the tags are aligned to the human genome and assessed with Digital Karyotyping [12], i.e., the number of tags per genomic locus is used to construct a virtual karyotype. Another recently described test involves fewer, but still a large number of, steps to prepare libraries for sequencing [13,14].

We reasoned that this process could be simplified if a defined number of fragments from throughout the genome could be amplified using a single primer pair, obviating the need for end-repair, terminal 3′-dA addition, or ligation to adapters. Furthermore, the smaller number of fragments to be assessed (compared to the whole genome) would streamline the genome matching and analysis processes. Here we detail our approach, which we have named "Fast Aneuploidy Screening Test-Sequencing System (henceforth FAST-SeqS).

Materials and Methods

Templates

Control DNA was obtained from normal spleen, peripheral blood white blood cells (WBCs), or plasma from patients (Table S1) giving written informed consent after approval by the institutional review board of The Johns Hopkins University. Fibroblast DNA from five individuals with trisomy 21 (NA02767, NA04616, NG05120, NG05397, and NG07438), two with trisomy 18 (NA03623 and NG12614), and one with trisomy 13 (NA03330), all with karyotype-confirmed aneuploidies, were purchased from the Coriell Institute for Medical Research (Camden, New Jersey). A total of 33 ng of DNA was used for each experiment. All templates were quantified by OD, except for the mixing experiments in which the templates were quantified by Digital PCR [15] to achieve a more accurate estimate of concentration.

Sequencing Library Preparation

The most significant time savings in FAST-SeqS is afforded by the replacement of currently used, laborious library preparation steps with an amplification using a single primer pair designed to amplify a discrete subset of repeated regions (see 'Results and Discussion' section). Templates were amplified as described by Kinde *et al.* [16] in which individual template molecules are tagged with a unique identifier DNA sequence. Though the unique identifier sequences turned out to be not necessary for FAST-SeqS (see 'Results and Discussion' section), we included them in the initial experimental design and continued to use them once they were observed to provide robust PCR products in our initial experiments. Briefly, FAST-1 amplification primers each contained a different 5′ universal primer sequence (UPS) followed by sequences allowing amplification of well-dispersed, repeated elements (see 'Results and Discussion' section and Table S2). Additionally, the forward primer contained either a stretch of 16 or 20 degenerate bases immediately 3′ to its UPS (Table S2). PCR was performed using Phusion Hot Start II Polymerase (Thermo Scientific, cat. no. F-549 L) in a total of 50 μL of 1× Phusion HF buffer containing 0.5 μM each primer and two units of polymerase under the following cycling conditions: 98°C for 120 s, followed by two cycles of 98°C for 10 s, 57°C for 120 s, and 72°C for 120 s. The initial amplification primers were removed with AMPure XP beads (Beckman Coulter Genomics, cat. no. A63880) according to the manufacturer with the exception that the beads were added at only 1.4× the PCR volume and the elution volume was reduced to 10 μL of TE. The elution was used directly for a second round of amplification using primers that annealed to the UPS site introduced by the first round primers and that additionally contained the 5′ grafting sequences necessary for hybridization to the Illumina flow cell (Table S2). Further, we introduced one of five indexes ("barcodes") (Table S2) to each sample in the reverse primer to later allow multiplexed sequencing. The second round of PCR was performed using Phusion Hot Start II Polymerase in a total of 50 μL of 1× Phusion HF buffer containing 0.5 μM each primer and two units of polymerase under the following cycling conditions: 98°C for 120 s, followed by 13 cycles of 98°C for 10 s, 65°C for 15 s, and 72°C for 15 s. Amplification products were again purified with AMPure XP beads and were quantified by spectrophotometry, real time PCR or on an Agilent 2100 Bioanalyzer; all methods of quantification yielded similar results. All oligonucleotides were purchased from IDT (Coralville, Iowa).

Sequence Tag Filtering and Alignment

Thirty-seven base sequence tags passing the Illumina chastity filter and containing at least three correct terminal bases of the amplification primer were filtered for quality by masking any base with a quality score <20 with an N using a custom script. Thus, tags with low quality bases were given the opportunity to align by considering only their most reliable bases. After quality masking, only the distinct sequences were aligned to the human genome (hg19 [17]) using Bowtie 0.12.7 [18]. When building the reference index for Bowtie, we included unresolved or unplaced contigs [19] to ensure the most accurate alignments. Sequences that aligned uniquely with up to one mismatch (using the flags –m 1 and –v 1, respectively) were retained and their alignments were matched back to the original data. Because tag alignment to a discrete set of chromosomal positions is simpler than alignment to the entire genome, the post-sequencing analysis process was very rapid. In fact, this mapping plus subsequent statistical analysis could be completed in less than 30 min per sample with a single computer housing two six-core CPUs (Intel Xeon X5680).

Normalization

Massively parallel sequencing will generate a different number of sequence tags from each sample, as well as from different sequencing runs of the same sample, due to stochastic and experimental variations. Thus, it is essential to normalize the data to make meaningful comparisons of the type used here. Although it would be most straightforward to simply express tag counts as a fraction of the total number of tags sequenced in an experiment, this normalization is too simplistic and is highly susceptible to systemic biases that frequently plague next generation sequencing of both DNA and RNA templates. For example, normalization for local GC content is routinely used in Digital Karyotyping [12] analyses such as that used for the diagnosis of trisomy 21 [8,20].

Because of the bimodal size distribution of the amplicons obtained with the FAST-1 primer pair (see 'Results and Discussion' section), we predicted that the majority of bias in FAST-1 amplifications would be due to the potential over-representation of the smaller-sized fragments. This bias could either be introduced during library preparation or during solid-phase bridge PCR on the Illumina flow cell. We found that an appropriate normalization for this distribution could be obtained using the quantile method [21], used extensively within the microarray community. By organizing our data into a list of

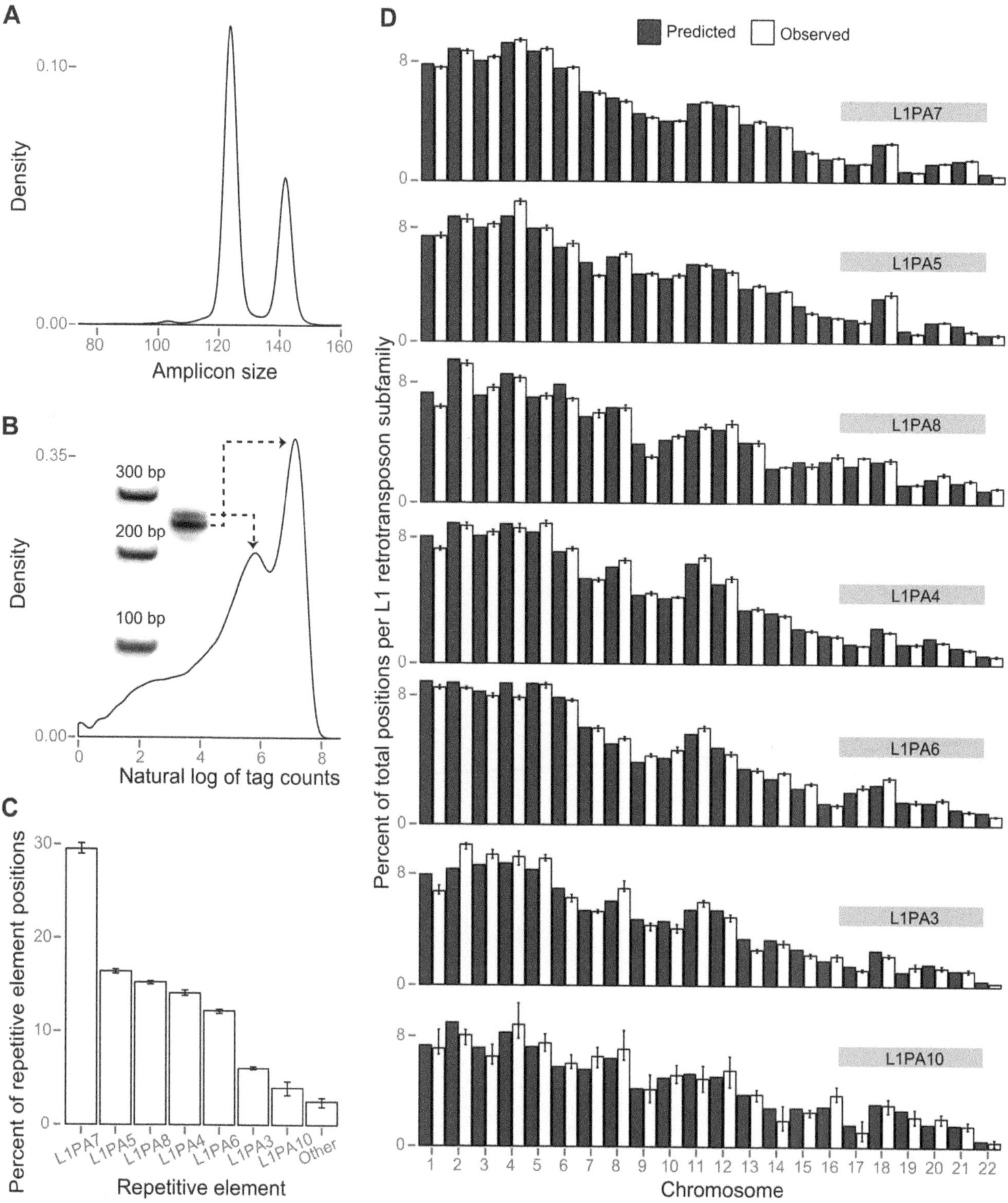

Figure 1. Comparison of observed and predicted distributions of FAST-SeqS amplification products. (A) A density plot of the expected distribution of fragment lengths, with peaks at 124 and 142 bp. (B) A density plot of the actual tag counts obtained in eight normal plasma DNAs. The 124 bp fragments are preferentially amplified compared to the 142 bp fragments, likely due to an amplification bias towards smaller fragments. Inset: polyacrylamide gel of a representative FAST-SeqS sequencing library. Note: the amplification products contain an additional ~120 bp of flanking sequence to facilitate sequencing (Table S2). (C) The average representation of the most frequently observed L1 retrotransposon subfamilies in eight normal plasma samples. Roughly 97% of uniquely aligning tags arise from positions representing only seven L1 retrotransposon subfamilies. (D) A detailed examination of the average number of observed positions per chromosome from eight normal plasma DNAs compared with the number predicted by RepeatMasker for each of the seven L1 retrotransposon subfamilies noted in (C). Error bars in each panel depict the range.

positions (equivalent to probes in microarray data), each associated with a tag count (equivalent to intensities in microarray data), we were able to apply standard quantile normalization to FAST-SeqS data. To best approximate the microarray data format, we chose to only analyze positions that were shared within each experimental group (e.g., the data from eight normal plasma samples). As the FAST-1 primers amplified a highly reproducible set of positions, this generally only eliminated <1% of the data. To maximize reproducibility, we excluded positions aligning to unresolved or unplaced contigs and those aligning to sex chromosomes, although inclusion of these chromosomes only marginally increased variability between experiments (e.g., in eight normal plasma samples, the maximum z-score from any chromosome rose from 1.9 to 2.3). The inclusion of sex chromosomes could be useful for other applications, such as detecting aneuploidies involving chromosome X or determining the gender of a sample (i.e., by the presence or absence of sequences aligning to chromosome Y).

We implemented the quantile normalization [21] for each experimental group (each of which contained multiple samples; Table S3) by performing the following steps:

1) generating a table of tag counts for each sample where each row represents a unique position (note that all tables will be of equal length as only the shared positions in each experiment were analyzed);
2) sorting the rows in each table based on tag counts, resulting in each table having a different order of positions;
3) determining the mean tag count for each row across all samples;
4) replacing an individual sample's tag count with the mean tag count for all samples at each row; and
5) sorting the tag counts for each sample's table back to their original order based on position.

The raw distribution of our data was always negatively skewed (see 'Results and Discussion' section). We excluded the positions falling within the left tail of each experiment's distribution (the positions containing the smallest number of tags) from our analysis by:

1) estimating the distribution of normalized values (see 'Results and Discussion' section);
2) determining the inflection point between the two peaks of the bimodal distribution; and
3) considering the positions that had a relative density below the inflection point as the left tail.

Once the left tail was determined and positions within it discarded, the quantile normalization was repeated. Through this process, each sample within an experimental group had the same sum total of tags and an identical distribution of counts, so direct comparisons could be made. We automated the quantile normalization in R [22]. The entire normalization procedure routinely took less than a few minutes to complete.

Quantitative Determination of Aneuploidy Status

A common method of determining the aneuploidy status of a particular sample in Digital Karyotyping-based [12] assays is by comparison of z-scores [6,11,23,24]. Through this method, one determines the mean and standard deviation of tag counts lying within a chromosome of interest in a group of reference samples (e.g., samples with known euploid content), and then creates a standardized score (i.e., z-score) for a chromosome of interest for

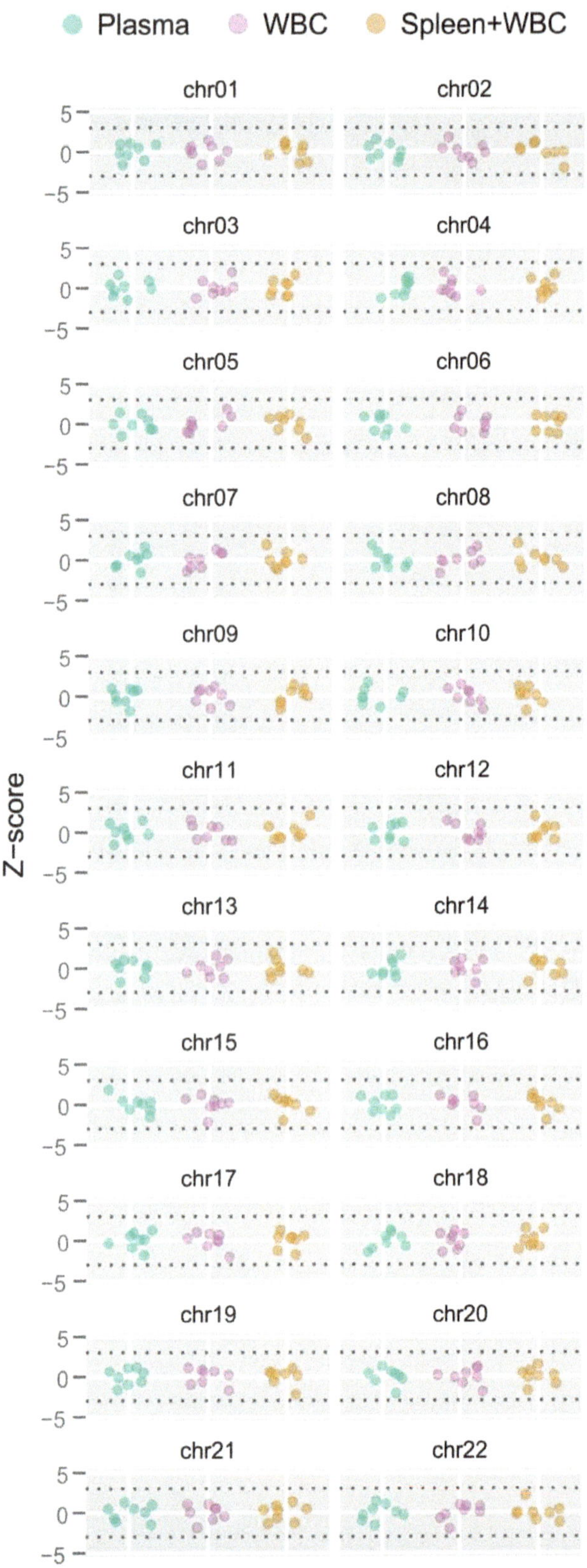

Figure 2. Demonstration of FAST-SeqS reproducibility among different samples, sequencing instruments, and sequencing depth. FAST-SeqS was performed on eight normal plasma DNA samples, their corresponding matched peripheral blood white blood cell (WBC) DNA, and on the splenic or WBC DNA of an additional eight unrelated individuals. The eight samples within each experiment

constituted the reference group (see 'Materials and Methods' section) from which the plotted z-scores were calculated. No autosome in any sample had a z-score outside the range of −3.0 and 3.0 (dotted lines). Despite 3-fold less sequencing of the splenic or WBC samples, the z-scores (range: −2.2 to 2.1) were similar to those obtained from the plasma (range: −2.1 to 1.9) and matched WBC DNA samples (range: −2.2 to 1.9).

each sample as follows:

$$\text{z-score}_{i,\,chrN} = (chrN_i - \mu_{chrN})/sd_{chrN},$$

where i represents the sample to be standardized, chrN represents the normalized tag count of the sample's chromosome, and μ_{chrN} and sd_{chrN} represent the mean and standard deviation of the normalized tag counts, respectively, of chrN in the reference group. When all samples are standardized in this way, outliers are easily detected because they have a z-score >3.0. This indicates that the normalized tag count of the outlier exceeds the mean of the reference group by at least three standard deviations.

Results and Discussion

Primer Selection and *in silico* Analysis

The key innovation behind FAST-SeqS, which increases throughput and lowers cost compared to traditional whole-genome sequencing fetal aneuploidy screening tests, is the use of specific primers that anneal to a subset of repeated regions dispersed throughout the genome. For maximum utility, we sought to target regions with enough similarity so that they could be amplified with a single pair of primers, but sufficiently unique to allow most of the amplified loci to be distinguished.

We began by searching a ~6.8 Mb region of chromosome 21 (hg19 [17] coordinates 35,888,786 to 42,648,523), containing the Down syndrome critical region [25], for sequence blocks of ~150 bp that were similar but not identical to those present on all chromosomes. To identify such blocks, we queried sequences obtained from 150 bp sliding windows incremented by 50 bp (135,186 sequences of 150 bp in length) with the BLAST-Like Alignment Tool (BLAT) algorithm [26]. We also required that the queried sequence be similar to at least three other blocks on chromosome 21, in addition to the one within the ~6.8 Mb region described above.

Out of the 135,186 queried blocks, we found only 56 that met the following criteria:

1) contained at least 11 variant bases from the query sequence, to aid in distinguishing amplified loci;
2) contained no more than 30 variant bases from the query sequence, to increase the chance of uniform amplification; and
3) spanned no more than a total of 180 bases, to be compatible with the analysis of degraded DNA [8].

We then manually scanned the BLAT alignments of these 56 blocks to search for those that had highly similar 5′ and 3′ ends. At least three of the 56 sequences met our criteria and we designed primers for them. *In Silico* PCR [27] predicted that each primer pair would amplify many distinct sequences from every nuclear chromosome.

Sequences that were too similar could pose a problem during alignment because of the inevitable errors introduced during library preparation or sequencing. We therefore wrote a custom script to assess how many distinct sequences would remain after

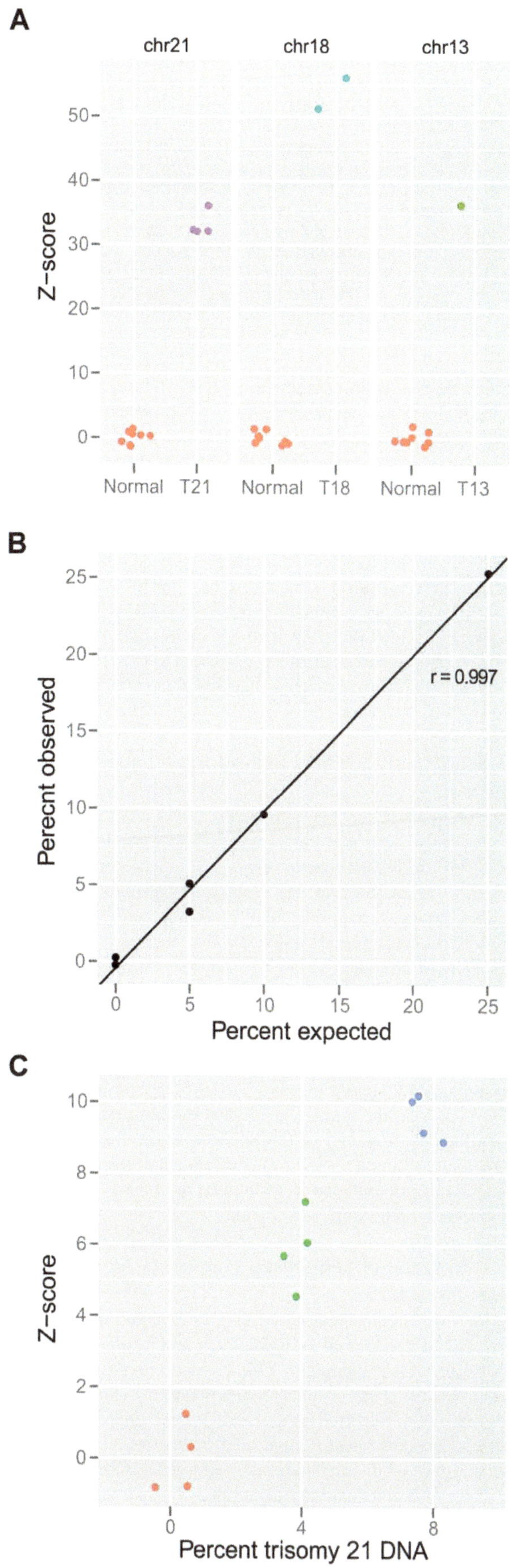

Figure 3. Accurate discrimination of euploid DNA samples from those containing trisomic DNA. (A) Comparison of z-scores from patients with trisomy 21 (n = 4), trisomy 18 (n = 2), and trisomy 13 (n = 1) with eight normal spleen or peripheral blood white blood cell (WBC) DNAs. The z-scores displayed represent the relevant chromosome for the comparison. The maximum z-score observed for any of the compared normal chromosomes was 1.9 (chr13). (B) Control WBC DNA was analyzed alone (n = 2) or when mixed with DNA from a patient with trisomy 21 at 5% (n = 2), 10% (n = 1), or 25% (n = 1) levels. A tight correlation existed between the expected and observed fractions of extra chromosome 21 (r = 0.997 by Pearson correlation test, n = 6). (C) Control WBC DNA was analyzed alone (z-score range: −0.8 to 1.3) or when mixed with DNA from a patient with trisomy 21 at 4% (z-score range: 4.5 to 7.2) or 8% (z-score range: 8.9 to 10.) levels. Each experiment in (C) was performed in quadruplicate.

allowing one, two, or three errors in each ~150 bp sequence. The theoretical amplification products of one primer pair (FAST-1) greatly outperformed the other two, and the superiority of FAST-1 was confirmed in pilot sequencing experiments.

The FAST-1 primer pair was predicted to amplify subfamilies of long interspersed nucleotide element-1 (L1 retrotransposons) in a primarily bimodal distribution of amplicon sizes, with the majority of amplicons having an average size of 124 or 142 bp (Fig. 1A). L1 retrotransposons, like other human repeats, have spread throughout the genome via retrotransposition, particularly in AT-rich regions [28]. As it is generally more difficult to uniformly amplify and sequence regions that vary widely in their GC content [8,20], we expected that this differential localization would work in our favor.

FAST-SeqS Yields a Highly Reproducible Subset of Sequences

An average of 38% of tags across all samples could be uniquely assigned to a genomic position (range: 31% to 45%; Table S3). As opposed to traditional whole genome amplification libraries, where the vast majority of tags align to the genome in unique positions and thus requiring that each tag be independently aligned, FAST-SeqS yielded sequences that aligned to an average of only 21,676 positions (Table S3). The number of positions to which the sequences aligned varied little compared to the range of sequence data obtained across all experiments. Though the number of uniquely aligned tags per experiment spanned a 12-fold range (1,343,382 to 16,015,347) the number of positions varied only by 0.25-fold (range: 18,484 to 24,562 positions; Table S3). Not only was the number of aligned positions similar among samples, but the identities of the positions were also remarkably similar: among samples within an experimental group, <1% of aligned tags were eliminated when limiting the analysis to positions shared among each sample.

The Distribution of Sequenced Fragments Agrees with *in silico* Predictions

Though we only sequenced 37 bases, we could estimate the relative size of the original PCR fragment and its unique position in the genome after alignment. This exercise provided additional evidence that the actual amplification products matched those that were predicted and alerted us to a preferential amplification bias towards sequences arising from smaller fragments.

We transformed the tag counts per uniquely aligned position to a log scale – a transformation frequently performed to this class of data to induce symmetry [29] – for each group of experiments (Table S3). Next, we used a nonparametric method to estimate a smoothened distribution (a kernel density estimator, implemented in R [22] using the density function), which made it straightforward to visualize the modality of our data. After plotting the distribution using ggplot2 [30] (an R [22] package), we observed that each group of experiments showed a similar clustering of tag counts per position, consistent with a primarily bimodal distribution with a negative skew. Tags originating from smaller PCR fragments were observed to have higher average tag counts, likely due to amplification biases. A representative plot is displayed in Figure 1B.

Autosomal Representation after Performing FAST-SeqS is Highly Reproducible

As an initial test of the performance of FAST-SeqS, we examined the representation of each autosome from different biologic sources (Table S1) using different sequencing instruments and depth (Table S3).

We first examined the representation of each autosome in the plasma DNA of seven normal females, including one biologic replicate (a total of eight samples), using only 37 cycles of sequencing in one-quarter of a lane on an Illumina HiSeq 2000 instrument. We recovered an average of 31,547,988 high quality tags per individual (range: 27,179,424 to 36,048,017 tags; Table S3). An average of 35% of these tags (range: 31 to 37%) could be uniquely mapped to one of an average of 23,681 unique chromosomal positions (range: 22,589 to 24,562 positions) when allowing up to one mismatch during alignment to hg19 [17] using Bowtie [18]. Of the uniquely aligned tags, 99.1% aligned to positions predicted to be repetitive DNA by RepeatMasker (http://www.repeatmasker.org), 97.5% of which fell into just seven L1 retrotransposon subfamilies (Fig. 1C). Additionally, as depicted in Fig. 1D, the distribution of each subfamily was not statistically distinguishable from that predicted by RepeatMasker (p = 1 for each of the seven L1 retrotransposon subfamilies when comparing the observed mean percentage of positions per chromosome with the predicted number; correlated two-tailed *t*-test).

Most importantly, the relative fraction of tags mapping to each chromosome was remarkably similar among the individual samples after normalizing [21] to compare chromosome tag counts among different samples (see 'Materials and Methods' section). In particular, the fraction of tags that matched to any of the autosomes in any of the eight samples studied never deviated from the average by a z-score >3.0 (Fig. 2). Of particular note, the maximum z-scores observed among the eight samples for chromosomes 21, 18, and 13 were 1.3, 1.4, and 1.0, respectively.

In the next experiment, we analyzed DNA from peripheral blood white blood cells (WBCs) from the same seven individuals who contributed plasma, including the biologic replicate (eight total samples). Four samples were sequenced on a single lane of an Illumina HiSeq 2000, yielding a mean of 10,835,559 uniquely aligned tags per sample (range: 4,905,067 to 16,015,347 tags). The maximum z-scores for any of the samples were 1.0, 1.2, and 1.6 for chromosomes 21, 18, and 13, respectively (Fig. 2).

Finally, we analyzed splenic or WBC DNA from an additional eight individuals using one-half of a lane of an Illumina GA IIx instrument, designed to yield fewer tags per sample than achieved above. Despite almost 3-fold less sequencing (average of 4,013,951 uniquely aligned tags per sample), the maximum z-scores among the samples were still only 1.3, 1.5, and 1.9 for chromosomes 21, 18, and 13, respectively, well below the widely used cutoff of 3.0 (Fig. 2).

FAST-SeqS Readily Identifies Samples Containing Trisomic DNA, Even when Present in Low Proportions

Given the tight distributions of tags evident in Figure 2, we expected it would be straightforward to distinguish the DNA of patients with trisomies from those of normal individuals with euploid chromosome constitutions. The data depicted in Figure 3A demonstrate that this expectation was realized in each of four patients with trisomy 21. The z-scores among these trisomy 21 patients ranged from 32 to 36, while the maximum z-score among eight normal individuals was 1.3. Similarly, the z-scores of DNA from two patients with trisomy 18 and one from trisomy 13 were 51, 56, and 36, respectively, far exceeding the maximum z-scores for these chromosomes in normal individuals (Fig. 3A).

Fetal DNA accounts for a geometric mean of 13.4% of maternal DNA, depending largely on maternal weight rather than gestational age [8]. To investigate whether FAST-SeqS could distinguish samples that contained mixtures of disomic and trisomic DNA, we performed mixing experiments using DNA from patients with trisomy 21 and normal individuals. In a first experiment of this type, we mixed 5% ($n = 2$), 10% ($n = 1$), and 25% ($n = 1$) trisomy 21 DNA into normal WBC DNA alongside two controls (Fig. 3B), and found a tight correlation between the expected and observed fractions of extra chromosome 21 ($r = 0.997$ by Pearson correlation test, $n = 6$). In a second experiment, we evaluated mixtures that contained 4% or 8% trisomy 21 DNA. As shown in Figure 3C, there was a clear distinction between the samples containing 4% trisomy 21 DNA vs. those from normal individuals ($p = 2\times10^{-4}$ as determined by uncorrelated two-tailed *t*-test, $n = 4$ in each group). The samples containing 8% trisomy 21 DNA were of course even more easily distinguishable ($p = 4\times10^{-6}$ when compared to the euploid group and $p = 1\times10^{-3}$ when compared to the 4% trisomy 21 samples, both by uncorrelated two-tailed *t*-test with $n = 4$ for each group).

Precise Template Counting

Finally, we evaluated whether precisely counting template molecules could further increase reproducibility. By incorporating degenerate bases at the 5′ end of one of the two FAST-1 primers (Table S2), it is possible to uniquely identify each template molecule giving rise to a PCR product [16]. This could potentially increase accuracy by minimizing the chance that the same template molecule was counted more than once in the final tally for each chromosome. In contrast, we found that the maximum z-score for any chromosome was subtly increased from 1.9 to 2.0 when using precise counting. By performing an uncorrelated two-tailed *t*-test on the absolute values of the z-scores for all autosomes, we found that the difference between the two methods was not statistically significant ($p = 0.759$, $n = 22\times8$ for each group).

Conclusions

FAST-SeqS was capable of detecting aneuploidies in a reproducible fashion in our pilot experiments. It has advantages over unbiased whole genome sequencing in ease of implementation, cost, analysis time, and throughput. Whether it will perform as well as whole genome sequencing for fetal aneuploidy testing in the clinic can only be determined by future large-scale studies in which a large number of pregnant women are analyzed by both testing procedures.

Supporting Information

Table S1 Samples analyzed in this FAST-SeqS study.

Table S2 Oligonucleotides used to prepare and sequence FAST-SeqS samples.

Table S3 Sequencing characteristics of FAST-SeqS experiments.

Author Contributions

Conceived and designed the experiments: IK NP KWK BV. Performed the experiments: IK NP BV. Analyzed the data: IK NP KWK BV. Contributed reagents/materials/analysis tools: IK NP KWK BV. Wrote the paper: IK NP KWK BV.

References

1. Hsu L (1998) Prenatal diagnosis of chromosomal abnormalities through amniocentesis. In: Milunsky A, editor. Genetic Disorders and the Fetus. 4 ed. Baltimore: The Johns Hopkins University Press. 179–180.
2. Staebler M, Donner C, Van Regemorter N, Duprez L, De Maertelaer V, et al. (2005) Should determination of the karyotype be systematic for all malformations detected by obstetrical ultrasound? Prenat Diagn 25: 567–573.
3. Jones KL (2006) Smith's recognizable patterns of human malformation. Philadelphia: Elsevier Saunders.
4. American College of Obstetricians and Gynecologists (2007) ACOG Practice Bulletin No. 88, December 2007. Invasive prenatal testing for aneuploidy. Obstet Gynecol 110: 1459–1467.
5. Lo YM, Tein MS, Lau TK, Haines CJ, Leung TN, et al. (1998) Quantitative analysis of fetal DNA in maternal plasma and serum: implications for noninvasive prenatal diagnosis. Am J Hum Genet 62: 768–775.
6. Chiu RW, Chan KC, Gao Y, Lau VY, Zheng W, et al. (2008) Noninvasive prenatal diagnosis of fetal chromosomal aneuploidy by massively parallel genomic sequencing of DNA in maternal plasma. Proc Natl Acad Sci U S A 105: 20458–20463.
7. Fan HC, Blumenfeld YJ, Chitkara U, Hudgins L, Quake SR (2008) Noninvasive diagnosis of fetal aneuploidy by shotgun sequencing DNA from maternal blood. Proc Natl Acad Sci U S A 105: 16266–16271.
8. Palomaki GE, Kloza EM, Lambert-Messerlian GM, Haddow JE, Neveux LM, et al. (2011) DNA sequencing of maternal plasma to detect Down syndrome: an international clinical validation study. Genet Med 13: 913–920.
9. Cleary-Goldman J, Malone FD, Vidaver J, Ball RH, Nyberg DA, et al. (2005) Impact of maternal age on obstetric outcome. Obstet Gynecol 105: 983–990.
10. Resta RG (2005) Changing demographics of advanced maternal age (AMA) and the impact on the predicted incidence of Down syndrome in the United States: Implications for prenatal screening and genetic counseling. Am J Med Genet A 133A: 31–36.
11. Bianchi DW, Platt LD, Goldberg JD, Abuhamad AZ, Sehnert AJ, et al. (2012) Genome-Wide Fetal Aneuploidy Detection by Maternal Plasma DNA Sequencing. Obstet Gynecol.
12. Wang TL, Maierhofer C, Speicher MR, Lengauer C, Vogelstein B, et al. (2002) Digital karyotyping. Proc Natl Acad Sci U S A 99: 16156–16161.
13. Ashoor G, Syngelaki A, Wagner M, Birdir C, Nicolaides KH (2012) Chromosome-selective sequencing of maternal plasma cell-free DNA for first-trimester detection of trisomy 21 and trisomy 18. Am J Obstet Gynecol 206: 322 e321–325.
14. Sparks AB, Wang ET, Struble CA, Barrett W, Stokowski R, et al. (2012) Selective analysis of cell-free DNA in maternal blood for evaluation of fetal trisomy. Prenat Diagn.
15. Vogelstein B, Kinzler KW (1999) Digital PCR. Proc Natl Acad Sci U S A 96: 9236–9241.
16. Kinde I, Wu J, Papadopoulos N, Kinzler KW, Vogelstein B (2011) Detection and quantification of rare mutations with massively parallel sequencing. Proc Natl Acad Sci U S A 108: 9530–9535.
17. Fujita PA, Rhead B, Zweig AS, Hinrichs AS, Karolchik D, et al. (2011) The UCSC Genome Browser database: update 2011. Nucleic Acids Res 39: D876–882.
18. Langmead B, Trapnell C, Pop M, Salzberg SL (2009) Ultrafast and memory-efficient alignment of short DNA sequences to the human genome. Genome Biol 10: R25.
19. International Human Genome Sequencing Consortium (IHGSC), Lander ES, Linton LM, Birren B, Nusbaum C, et al. (2001) Initial sequencing and analysis of the human genome. Nature 409: 860–921.
20. Fan HC, Quake SR (2010) Sensitivity of noninvasive prenatal detection of fetal aneuploidy from maternal plasma using shotgun sequencing is limited only by counting statistics. PLoS One 5: e10439.

21. Bolstad BM, Irizarry RA, Astrand M, Speed TP (2003) A comparison of normalization methods for high density oligonucleotide array data based on variance and bias. Bioinformatics 19: 185–193.
22. R Development Core Team (2011) R: A language and environment for statistical computing. R Foundation for Statistical Computing.
23. Ehrich M, Deciu C, Zwiefelhofer T, Tynan JA, Cagasan L, et al. (2011) Noninvasive detection of fetal trisomy 21 by sequencing of DNA in maternal blood: a study in a clinical setting. Am J Obstet Gynecol 204: 205 e201–211.
24. Sehnert AJ, Rhees B, Comstock D, de Feo E, Heilek G, et al. (2011) Optimal detection of fetal chromosomal abnormalities by massively parallel DNA sequencing of cell-free fetal DNA from maternal blood. Clin Chem 57: 1042–1049.
25. Rahmani Z, Blouin JL, Creau-Goldberg N, Watkins PC, Mattei JF, et al. (1989) Critical role of the D21S55 region on chromosome 21 in the pathogenesis of Down syndrome. Proc Natl Acad Sci U S A 86: 5958–5962.
26. Kent WJ (2002) BLAT–the BLAST-like alignment tool. Genome Res 12: 656–664.
27. Kuhn RM, Karolchik D, Zweig AS, Trumbower H, Thomas DJ, et al. (2007) The UCSC genome browser database: update 2007. Nucleic Acids Res 35: D668–673.
28. Smit AF (1999) Interspersed repeats and other mementos of transposable elements in mammalian genomes. Curr Opin Genet Dev 9: 657–663.
29. Tukey J (1977) Exploratory Data Analysis. Reading: Addison-Wesley.
30. Wickham H (2009) ggplot2: elegant graphics for data analysis. New York: Springer.

Adaptive and Maladaptive Correlates of Repetitive Behavior and Restricted Interests in Persons with Down Syndrome and Developmentally-Matched Typical Children: A Two-Year Longitudinal Sequential Design

David W. Evans[1,2]*, F. Lee Kleinpeter[3], Mylissa M. Slane[1], K. B. Boomer[4]

1 Developmental Neuropsychology Laboratory, Geisinger-Bucknell Autism and Developmental Medicine Institute, Lewisburg, Pennsylvania, United States of America, 2 Department of Neuroscience, Bucknell University, Lewisburg, Pennsylvania, United States of America, 3 Department of Psychology, River Parishes Community College, Sorrento, Louisiana, United States of America, 4 Department of Mathematics, Bucknell University, Lewisburg, Pennsylvania, United States of America

Abstract

We examined the course of repetitive behavior and restricted interests (RBRI) in children with and without Down syndrome (DS) over a two-year time period. Forty-two typically-developing children and 43 persons with DS represented two mental age (MA) levels: "younger" 2–4 years; "older" 5–11 years. For typically developing younger children some aspects of RBRI increased from Time 1 to Time 2. In older children, these aspects remained stable or decreased over the two-year period. For participants with DS, RBRI remained stable or increased over time. Time 1 RBRI predicted Time 2 adaptive behavior (measured by the Vineland Scales) in typically developing children, whereas for participants with DS, Time 1 RBRI predicted poor adaptive outcome (Child Behavior Checklist) at Time 2. The results add to the body of literature examining the adaptive and maladaptive nature of repetitive behavior.

Editor: Karen Lidzba, University Children's Hospital Tuebingen, Germany

Funding: The authors have no support or funding to report.

Competing Interests: The authors have declared that no competing interests exist.

* E-mail: dwevans@bucknell.edu

Introduction

Seemingly diverse neurodevelopmental and neuropsychiatric disorders share many features in their respective behavioral phenotypes, and even their possible underlying genotypes [1]. Further, many clinical syndromes are characterized by behaviors that are common in the typical population. Sharp boundaries have historically divided the study of normative and pathological behavior, but developmental psychologists have long noted the benefit of a continuous approach to development and psychopathology [2–4]. Such approaches rely on quantitative measures that capture the clinical severity of a given class of behaviors while maintaining sufficient sensitivity so as to examine their distribution in the general population. In this study we examine the similarities and differences in repetitive behaviors and restricted interests (RBRI) in typically developing children and children with Down syndrome (DS). In doing so, we highlight both the normative nature of RBRI, and important differences in the functions and developmental trajectory of RBRI in typically-developing (TD) children and children with a genetically-distinct subtype of intellectual disability – Down syndrome.

The theoretical and empirical attention paid to the study of RBRI pales in comparison to work examining the cognitive, social, and communication deficits associated with neurodevelopmental and neuropsychiatric disorders. RBRI comprise a broad range of behaviors such as compulsions, tics, and stereotypic, self-directed and self-injurious behaviors [5–9]. Such behaviors are prominent in a variety of disorders, including autism spectrum disorder (ASD), obsessive-compulsive disorder (OCD), tic disorders, attention deficit/hyperactivity, and a host of other developmental brain dysfunctions [5,10–16].

In a large scale collaborative study on a sample with autism spectrum disorders (ASD) [13] some restricted and repetitive behaviors abated with age, whereas others persisted, indicating that various kinds of repetitive behaviors may have different developmental trajectories. Other work reports that self-injury, insistence on sameness, restricted interests, and compulsions are more frequent among older than younger children with ASD [17,18]. Such findings illustrate the importance of placing the study of repetitive behaviors in a developmental context – one that transcends chronological age.

RBRI have been examined in several specific genetic copy number variation syndromes. Persons with Prader-Willi syndrome (PWS) for example, engage in compulsive behavior to such a degree that obsessive-compulsive (OC) behaviors may be considered a core aspect of the syndrome [19]. Children with PWS exhibit similar degrees of repetitive and ritualistic behaviors as do children with autism [20,21] although other work suggests that children with autism exhibit significantly more repetitive behavior, stereotypies, and compulsions relative to children with other developmental disabilities[5].

Children with DS also engage in restricted behaviors and rituals [15]. A preliminary cross-sectional study revealed that children with DS with mental ages (MA) between 2–5 years engaged in similar levels of RBRI relative to MA-matched typically developing children, differing only in the number of sensory-perceptual symptoms that they exhibited [15,22]. Older children with DS (MAs >6) engaged in fewer RBRI overall suggesting that children with DS may still "grow out" of their repetitive behaviors, albeit more slowly than typically developing children do [15]. Similar results have been reported on stereotypic motor movements in a heterogeneous sample of children with disabilities, where the development of repetitive motor movements has a delayed trajectory relative to typically-developing children [10]. Unlike the RBRI of typically developing children, however, the RBRI of children with DS was related to other maladaptive behaviors such as internalizing symptoms [15].

A study compared the repetitive behavior questionnaire (RBQ) across several genetic syndromes including Angelman, Cornelia de Lange, Cri-du-Chat, Fragile X, Prader-Willi, Lowe, and Smith-Magenis [23]. Angelman syndrome was associated with relatively few RBRI, whereas Prader-Willi, Cri-du-Chat, and Smith-Magenis syndromes exhibited unique profiles of RBRI [23]. So while RBRI are common across various syndromes, specific genotypes may exhibit differing kinds or degrees of RBRI. The profiles of RBRI are likely to change over development, and different RBRI may be differentially related to adaptive/maladaptive outcomes.

Normative Repetitive Behavior

RBRI are not limited to neurodevelopmental disorders. Indeed repetitive behavior and restricted interests are part of the behavioral repertoire of many, if not all, typically developing children [7,9,16,24–29]. Little is known about the normal development of repetitive behavior; its longitudinal course is not well understood, and we know little about the adaptive and maladaptive correlates of repetitive behavior [14,30].

In childhood, normal and pathological variants of RBRI may not be easy to distinguish. Typically-developing children exhibit a broad range of rituals, routines, and circumscribed interests that bear an uncanny resemblance to the OC behaviors of OCD and the rigid routines of ASD [16,24,25,28,30]. Bedtime rituals may include saying goodnight in a certain order to specific people or objects around the house, reading a special book in a certain manner over and over, arranging stuffed animals or other objects in a certain order, and leaving the light on and the door placed ajar with exactness. At mealtimes, the same bowl and cup may have to be used; foods may have to be presented in a certain way, with different foods not touching each other, or sandwiches cut in a certain shape [16,31,32].

Cross-sectional research indicates that RBRI are highly prevalent, with as many as 85% of children engaging in RBRI [16]. Preschool-aged children engage in significantly more RBRI than children less than 2 and older than 5 years, although such behaviors remain relatively prevalent throughout the 6th year, and persist to some degree throughout childhood [33,35]. Children's normative RBRI may be relatively frequent and intense, and may even be associated with some subjective distress [36], making them difficult to distinguish from pathological states.

Although these normative manifestations of RBRI may resemble clinical phenomena, many prominent developmentalists have noted the possible adaptive significance of repetitive, compulsive-like behaviors, such as mastery motivation [31], sensory-motor adaptation in early development [37], and self-regulation [38]. Normative rituals may be linked to magical thinking and may also serve to quell the fears and anxieties that accompany normative development [3]. Empirical efforts support some of these developmental predictions: children's rituals are related to magical beliefs [39,40] and to normally developing fears and phobias [36]. The development of RBRI is also associated with executive function ability [33,34,41,42] and cortical brain activity [43], suggesting a possible role of neurobiological maturation in the development of RBRI [26,41,43,44].

Normally-developing RBRI have been examined across a variety of cultures using the Childhood Routines Inventory [7,16,22,35], noting high prevalence rates of RBRI in young children in the UK [7], Israel [35], Sweden [21], and Turkey [45]. Animal models provide evidence that repetitive behaviors are common across a variety of species and have both normative and pathological variants that are related to behavioral inhibition and cognitive perseveration [41,42,44,46–50].

Common across these research efforts is evidence that RBRI a) are part of normal development; b) are particularly salient early in development (peaking in the preschool years); c) may differentially serve as adaptive or maladaptive functions at different points in development and in different populations. The first goal of this study is to examine the two year course of compulsive-like behavior in typically developing children, and its links to adaptive and maladaptive behaviors. Second, as questions remain as to whether compulsive-like behaviors are part of the behavioral phenotype associated with DS, or whether they reflect a delayed developmental process, we examine changes in RBRI over a two year period in children with and without DS, across two mental age groups. We do so using a quantitative measure of RBRI (the Childhood Routines Inventory [16]) that is sensitive to both the clinical presentation of RBRI, and to the normal distribution of RBRI in typical children. Third, we also examine the adaptive and maladaptive correlates of compulsive-like behaviors in typically-developing children and children with DS; specifically, our goal is to examine whether compulsive-like behaviors early in development predict later adaptive behavior – as would be suggested by a developmental perspective – or whether they reflect prodromal phases of later maladaptive compulsive or autistic-like behavior, and whether such patterns differ for persons with and without DS.

Methods

Ethics Statement

This research was approved by the institutional review board of the University of New Orleans. Written consent from all parents and verbal assent from all minors was obtained prior to testing.

Participants

Participants were two groups of children – with and without DS —tested at two time points separated by 24 months. Each diagnostic group was separated into 2 mental age (MA) groups. Forty-two typically developing children (24 males, 18 females) comprised two MA groups. The majority of the participants were involved in a previous study[15] on repetitive behavior, which served as Time 1. Seven of the original 50 participants tested at Time 1 relocated, but 2 participants at Time 1 (who were excluded from the original study because they did not meet the age criterion for that study) were included in the present study. At Time 1 the chronological ages ranged from 20 to 86 months (M = 53.76, SD = 20.45), and at Time 2, from 43 to 112 months (M = 77.02, SD = 19.31). The mean difference between age at Time 1 and Time 2 was 23.26 months (SD = 2.55 months). Children's cognitive abilities were assessed with the Stanford-Binet 4th edition. For children less than 30 months of age (at Time 1), the

Bayley Scales of Infant Development-II was administered. The mean IQs at Time 1 and Time 2 were nearly identical (Mean at Time 1 = 111.24 (SD = 9.28); Time 2 Mean was 110.76 (SD = 10.39); T1 and T2 IQ $r(42) = .69$, $p<.001$).

The participants were recruited from several sites in an urban region in the Southeastern United States – both public and private schools, and daycare centers. Parents of the participants completed a demographic form including information on parental education, marital status, ethnicity, religion, child's health status, gender, and sibling(s) [if any] as well as sibling's age and gender. The two groups were comparable in terms of the distribution of the demographic variables (all $p>.40$) with the following exceptions: Maternal education of the typical parents was higher than for the parents of DS participants ($p = .04$) and maternal ($p<.001$) and paternal ($p<.001$) ages were higher for the parents of the participants with DS.

For analyses, children were placed into one of two age levels based on Time 1 mental age (CA*IQ/100): We designate as "younger children" those children with MAs 22 to 59 (M = 43.01, SD = 12.76; n = 23) months and "older children" with MAs 60–109 months (M = 79.83, SD = 13.83; n = 19). These age cutoffs were derived from empirical work noting the peak prevalence of RBRI between two and five years of age [16]. The theoretical work of Werner and Gesell highlight the importance of this developmental period as being particularly marked by RBRI.

The group with DS was comprised of 43 persons (18 males, 25 females). These participants were matched on mental age (MA) to the typically developing group at Time 1. The younger group included children with DS whose mental ages ranged between 25 and 59 months (M = 44.71, SD = 10.17; n = 24). Older children ranged in MA from 60.68 to 134 months (M = 74.97, SD = 17.36; n = 19). Chronological ages ranged from 48–253 months at Time 1 (M = 143 months) and from 70–274 (M = 167) months at Time 2. The Time 1 mental ages of the typical children and the children with DS did not differ ($t(83) = 0.34$, $p = .74$). The Typical and DS groups did not differ on the distribution of male and female participants ($\chi^2(1) = 1.99$, $p = .159$). Participants with DS were also tested with either the Stanford-Binet 4th Ed or the Bayley Scales II: Time 1 IQ, M = 42.02 (*SD* = 7.44) (range = 36–72) and Time 2 IQ, M = 41.70 (SD = 6.49) (range = 36–57); intraclass $r(43) = .75$, $p<.001$(See Table 1).

Procedures

Parents received a written description of the proposed study, along with informed consent and several inventories. Willing participants were asked to return the signed consent forms and completed inventories to their child's school, or to the researcher. Children were tested individually at the site of their school, daycare, or home. Parents were then administered a phone interview concerning their child's adaptive behavior level.

Measures

The Childhood Routines Inventory. (CRI) [16] is a 19-item parental report questionnaire that asks parents to indicate the degree to which their child engages in repetitive, ritualistic, behaviors and circumscribed interests along a 5-point scale (frequency/intensity). Unlike other measures of RBRI, the CRI is a quantitative measure that is sensitive to the normal distribution of repetitive behavior in the general population. The CRI has good internal consistency (Cronbach's Alpha = .89), and comprises two factors: "Just Right" phenomena and "Repetitive Behaviors" [16]. The "Just Right" factor includes the items: "prefers to have things done in a particular order or certain way;" "arranges objects or performs certain behaviors until they are just right;" "lines up objects in straight lines or symmetrical patterns;" "insists on having certain belongings around the house in their place;" and "seems very aware of how certain clothes feel." The repetitive behaviors include: "prefers the same household activities every day;" "acts out the same thing in pretend play;" "engages in elaborate bedtime rituals;" "repeats certain actions over and over;" and "has strong preferences for certain foods" [16]. The CRI yields three indices that reflect mean frequency/intensity scores of the 1–5 Likert scale: the mean Just Right factor (Mean Just Right), the mean Repetitive Behavior factor (Mean Repeat), and the mean frequency/intensity of the overall CRI (Mean CRI). Scale reliability was conducted for the TS and DS samples in the present study. For TD participants Cronbach $\alpha = .90$; for DS, $\alpha = .89$.

The Child Behavior Checklist. (CBCL) [51] is a 112-item parent-report checklist that assesses child problem behaviors on a 3-point scale. The CBCL has extensive normative data and excellent reliability [51]. The items on the CBCL are factor analyzed into 2 broad-band categories: internalizing (withdrawal/depression) and externalizing (aggressive/delinquent). Two comparable versions of the CBCL were used: one for children less than 4 years old (CBCL/2–3), and the checklist for children 4 years and older (CBCL/4–18). For each scale, raw and standard scores (T scores) are derived.

The Vineland Adaptive Behavior Scales. (VABS) Screener [52] is an extension of a widely used measure of adaptive functioning [53]. The VABS Screener, like the VABS survey edition, is a semi-structured interview that assesses the child's current adaptive functioning in four domains: Communication, Daily Living Skills, Socialization, and Motor Skills. The VABS has extensive normative data and excellent psychometric properties. The VABS yields standard scores (M = 100; SD = 15) for each domain, as well as an overall adaptive behavior composite. The screener version of the VABS is correlated highly ($r = .95$) with the full Vineland Survey form [53] and has excellent inter-rater reliability ($\alpha = .98$).

Results

The first set of analyses examines the stability of the CRI variables as well as the Vineland and CBCL scales across the two time periods. For each diagnostic group and each MA Level Time 1 and Time 2 correlations are presented. For typically developing younger children, the T1–T2 Mean CRI ($r(23) = .53$, $p = .009$) and Repetitive Behaviors ($r(23) = .57$, $p = .005$) were correlated, but "Just Right" Behaviors were not (although they approached significance at $p = .051$). None of the Vineland scales were correlated across T1 and T2 but both the Internalizing and Externalizing CBCL scales were positively correlated from T1 to T2. (For this MA Level, not all CBCL narrow band scales are directly comparable from T1 to T2 since the CBCL has two slightly different versions for preschool and school age children).

For the older typically developing children, all CRI scores were highly correlated from T1 to T2 (Mean CRI $r = .79$; Just Right $r = .74$; Repetitive $r = .76$, all $ps<.001$). The VABS were correlated across time (Daily Living: $r(19) = .71$, $p = .001$; Socialization: $r(18) = .46$, $p = .053$; Communication: $r(19) = .77$, $p<.001$; Composite: $r(19) = .80$, $p<.0001$. The T1–T2 Internalizing ($r(19) = .58$, $p = .010$) and Externalizing ($r(19) = .68$, $p = .001$) CBCL scales were positively correlated.

For younger children with DS considerable stability was demonstrated for the CRI scales (Mean CRI $r(24) = .63$, $p = .001$; Just Right and Repetitive, $r(24) = .59$, $p = .002$ for both scales). VABS were correlated from T1 to T2 (Composite:

Table 1. Mental Age (MA), IQ, Vineland (VABS) and Child Behavior Checklist (CBCL-Total) Scores at Time 1 and Time 2 for Typically Developing (TD) and DS groups by MA Group.

		MA	IQ	VABS[1]	CBCL[2]	N
TD, Younger						
	(T1)	43(13)	111(9)	102(15)*	52(7)	23
	(T2)	70(14)	111(11)	103(17)	50(9)	23
TD, Older						
	(T1)	80(14)	111(9)	96(13)	50(7)	19
	(T2)	103(14)	110(10)	98(20)	52(9)	19
DS, Younger						
	(T1)	45(10)	44(8)	44(15)	55(7)	24
	(T2)	54(12)	43(7)	37(10)	57(8)	24
DS, Older						
	(T1)	75(17)	39(5)	35(11)	55(7)	19
	(T2)	86(20)	40(6)	33(9)	55(7)	19

Note: Mean values are presented with standard deviations in parentheses.
*N = 20 for T1 VABS Score.
[1]Vineland Adaptive Behavior Composite Score; [2]Child Behavior Checklist Total Problems Score.

$r(24) = .88$, $p < .0001$; Communication ($r(24) = .87$, $p < .0001$; Daily Living ($r(24) = .71$, $p < .0001$; Socialization ($r(24) = .82$, $p < .0001$). The Internalizing CBCL scale was not correlated from T1 to T2, but the Externalizing band was correlated ($r(24) = .72$, $p < .0001$).

Finally, for the older group with DS, all T1–T2 CRI scores were correlated (Mean CRI $r(19) = .72$, $p = .001$; Just Right $r(19) = .76$, $p < .001$; Repetitive $r(19) = .52$, $p = .022$). The VABS Communication ($r(19) = .52$, $p = .022$) and Socialization ($r(19) = .56$, $p = .012$) scores were positively correlated, but the overall Composite and the Daily Living scales were not. The Internalizing ($r(19) = .65$, $p = .002$) and Externalizing ($r(19) = .72$, $p < .001$) CBCL scales were positively correlated over the two time periods.

There is a risk of bias when comparing scores at two separate time points if the variances at these time points are not equal. However, the sample standard deviations for the dependent variables did not differ by more than a factor of 2 (a standard benchmark threshold) across the two time points. Thus we can assume equal variances.

Linear Mixed Modeling of RBRI

The main goal of this study was to examine differences in RBRI over time in two age cohorts in participants with and without DS. ID Group by MA level linear mixed multivariate models were performed for each of the three constructs measured by the CRI using a compound, symmetric covariance structure. Levene's tests indicated no significant differences in error variances (all $p > .05$). The first analysis examined the overall mean score of the CRI. Neither the main effects, nor the 2-way or 3-way interactions were significant indicating relative stability in mean CRI scores across the two year span for both children with DS and typically developing children. Thus, mean CRI score trajectories are similar across both ID groups when accounting for MA level. See Figure 1.

In the mixed model, the "Just Right" factor of the CRI revealed a three-way interaction (Wilks' Lambda $F(1,81) = 4.26$, $p < .05$). Conducted for the separate diagnostic groups, for the typical children, the interaction effect (Age Level X Time) was significant ($F(1,40) = 5.91$, $p < .05$). For the group with DS, this interaction was not significant ($p > .05$), indicating that the overall variance was contributed by changes over time (decreases in Just Right behavior) in the typical children, and relative stability for the children with DS. See Figure 2.

Regarding the Repetitive Behavior factor, the 3-way and 2-way interactions were not significant. The main effects for both MA Level ($F(1,81) = 4.60$, $p < .05$) and for ID group ($F(1,81) = 9.55$, $p < .01$) were significant, indicating that Repetitive Behaviors are more frequent/intense in the younger cohort of children than for the older cohort and, overall, differ between typically-developing children and children with DS, such that persons with DS are reported to engage in repetitive behaviors with greater frequency and intensity. When analyzing the diagnostic groups separately, there was a significant main effect of MA group for typically developing children ($F(1,40) = 5.30$, $p < .05$) indicating decreases in RB with increasing age group. No other results were significant. See Figure 3.

Predicting Adaptive and Maladaptive Behaviors with the CRI

Next, multiple regression analyses tested whether the three CRI indices predict later adaptive and/or maladaptive behaviors. Analyses were conducted within age level and diagnostic groups. For the first series of analyses, each Time 2 standard score from the Vineland Adaptive Behavior Scales was a criterion variable, and each of the three CRI variables from Time 1 served as predictor variables. In this way we examined whether RBRI at Time 1 predict later adaptive behaviors.

None of the CRI variables at Time 1 predicted the overall Vineland Adaptive Behavior Composite score, for either age level or for either diagnostic group. However several significant predictors emerged for the Vineland Domain scores. For older typical children the mean "Just Right" CRI score at Time 1 predicted significant variance in the Vineland Communication Domain at Time 2 ($R^2 = .27$, $F(1,17) = 6.15$, $p < .05$). Similarly, Time 1 Repetitive Behaviors was a significant predictor of Time 2 Vineland Daily Living Skills ($R^2 = .27$, $F(1,17) = 6.16$, $p < .05$). For older children with DS, Time 1 Mean Repetitive Behaviors predicted Time 2 Vineland Daily Living Skills ($R^2 = .28$, $F(1,17) = 6.50$, $p < .05$). The Beta (−.53) reveals that Time 1 repetitive behaviors are inversely related to Time 2 Daily Living

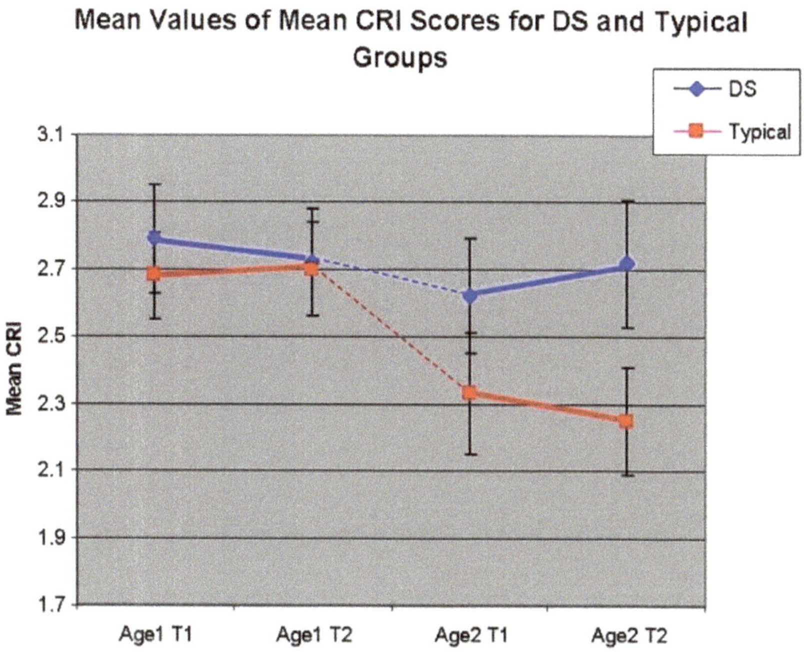

Figure 1. Trajectory of Mean CRI Scores by MA Group and Dx Group.

Skills, whereas the predictor variables for the typical children were positively related to the Time 2 adaptive criterion variables.

Next, regressions explored whether Time 1 CRI variables predicted later maladaptive behavior as assessed by the CBCL (Internalizing and Externalizing broad band scales). For typically developing younger children, Mean CRI scores at Time 1 predicted significant variance in Time 2 Internalizing scores ($R^2 = .24$, $F(1,21) = 6.68$, $p < .05$). For older children with DS, Mean "Just Right" behaviors at Time 1 predicted Internalizing symptoms at Time 2 ($R^2 = .40$, $F(1,17,) = 11.43$, $p < .01$.).

To gain a better sense of how early rituals may predict maladaptive behaviors for children with and without DS, we explored the predictive validity of early rituals on T2 narrow band scales of the CBCL (Anxiety, Social Problems, Thought Problems, Attention Problems and Aggression). For younger typically developing children, the Time 1 Mean CRI score predicted significant variance in Time 2 Attention problems ($R^2 = .34$,

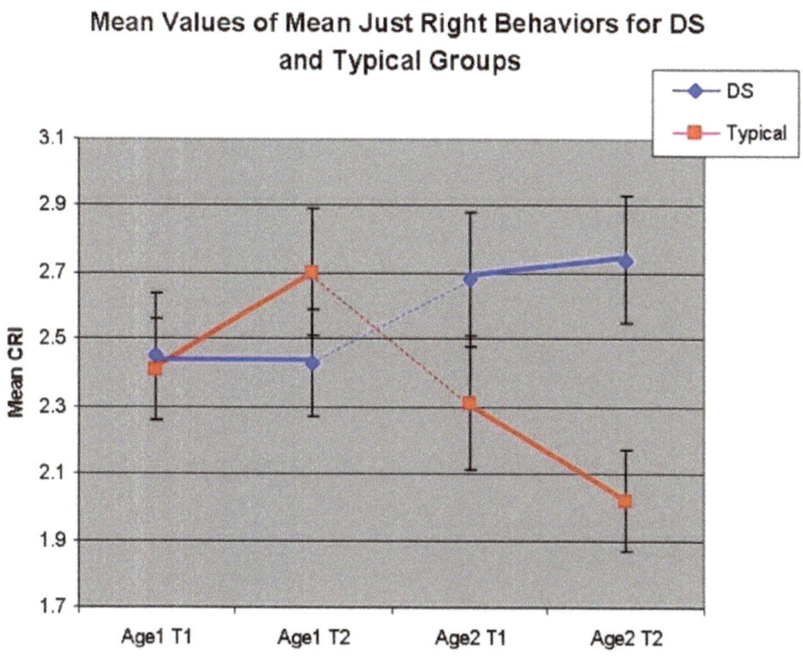

Figure 2. Trajectory of Mean "Just Right" Behaviors by MA Group and Dx Group.

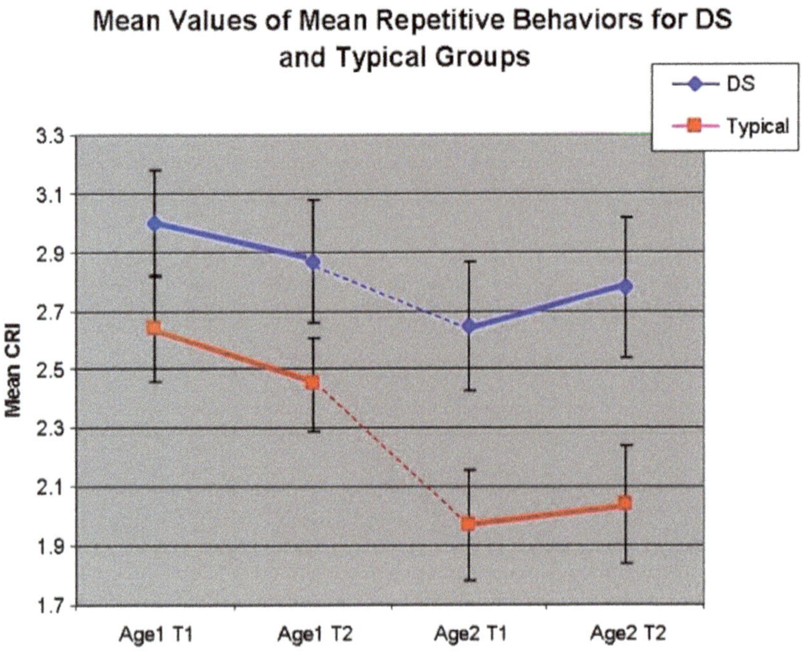

Figure 3. Trajectory of Mean Repetitive Behaviors by MA Group and Dx Group.

$F(1,17) = 8.72$, $p<.01$). No other CRI variables at Time 1 predicted Time 2 maladaptive behaviors for the typical children. For younger children with DS, the Time 1 Mean CRI score predicted Time 2 anxiety ($R^2 = .25$, $F(1,22) = 7.18$, $p<.05$). For older children with DS, the Time 1 mean "Just Right" score predicted significant variance in Time 2 Thought Problems ($R^2 = .26$, $F(1,17) = 6.06$, $p<.05$). No other Time 1 CRI scores predicted Time 2 CBCL narrow band scales.

Discussion

This two-year sequential design examined the development of RBRI and its relation to adaptive and maladaptive behavior in typically developing children and children with Down syndrome. This study extended previous cross-sectional research noting decreases in RBRI in typically developing children [16], and a relative "leveling off" of RBRI in persons with DS [15]. Thus the data elucidate a) our understanding of typical development and possible functions of RBRI; b) the role of cognitive development in the trajectory of RBRI; and c) the ways that RBRI develop as part of the behavioral phenotype of Down syndrome.

As predicted, typically developing children evidence a relatively sharp increase in "Just Right" behaviors throughout the preschool years, followed by significant decreases – both cross-sectionally at the older age levels, and longitudinally (note the significant decrease in "Just Right" behaviors between Time 1 and Time 2 for the older children). For children with Down syndrome, however, "Just Right" behaviors are relatively consistent across the age levels and over time. Children with DS do not experience the normative decreases in frequency/intensity of "Just Right" behaviors that is seen in typically developing children. Indeed, for children with DS, these behaviors persist well throughout childhood and well into adolescence – reaching a delayed asymptote. These findings are consistent with reports of delayed development of other repetitive movements, such as stereotypies and self-injurious behaviors in children with a variety of developmental disabilities [10,13,17,23].

Some repetitive behavior reflects cognitive and behavioral rigidity that precludes more flexible (i.e., adaptive) means of self-regulating and responding to a changing environment [34]. Typical children undergo important developments throughout the preschool and school age years that allow for more flexible and adaptive responses to their environments [54]. As development occurs, new tasks and expectations emerge requiring increasingly flexible and adaptive cognitive and behavioral responses, while maintaining structure and organization. In persons with developmental delays, rituals and routines may persist as the primary means for self-regulation [15,21]. In typical development, on the other hand, rituals and other compulsive-like behaviors presumably wane with the development of more conceptual and abstract means of self-regulation. Rituals do not disappear with development. Rather, under normal circumstances they become incorporated into relatively more complex and adaptive ways of organizing and regulating the self and the environment [14].

How, then, do early RBRI relate to later development? Some speculate that early developmental rituals may be associated with later behavior problems [28]. An alternative hypothesis suggests that since compulsive-like behaviors are common during early development they likely serve an adaptive function — at least in typically developing children. To date, however, no longitudinal studies have explored these hypotheses.

In the present study, we examined the longitudinal development of RBRI and adaptive/maladaptive behaviors in children with and without Down syndrome. For typically developing children, Time 1"Just Right" behavior predicted later Vineland Adaptive Communication Domain for the older MA level (MA = 5–11 years). The directionality of the findings suggests that early "Just Right" behaviors augur well for later adaptive behavior in the domain of communication. Similarly, for this same age cohort, early repetitive behaviors significantly predicted Vineland Daily Living Skills two years later. In typically developing children early RBRI are not only statistically normative but also appear to serve some adaptive function later in development. This is rather in contrast to the belief that early RBRI are a risk factor for later symptoms of OCD or ASD, although more research is needed.

For the same MA-matched cohort of children with DS, the Time 1 Repetitive Behavior factor on the CRI also predicted Daily Living Skills two years later. Unlike the finding with typically developing children, the more repetitive behavior a child with DS engaged in at Time 1, the lower his or her Daily Living score two years later. Overall, children with DS in this age cohort engaged in more repetitive behaviors relative to their typical MA-matched cohort. Children with DS may exhibit similar repetitive behaviors in a manner that is perhaps more circumscribed and thus more likely to interfere with, rather than enhance, later adaptive behaviors. This suggests a threshold effect such that, beyond a certain degree, repetitive behaviors are a risk factor for later poor Daily Living Skills. These findings support the ideas put forth by developmentalists such as Gesell [31,32], Piaget [37], and Werner [3,57] that for typically developing children repetitive behavior serves as an adaptive mechanism for mastering the environment. Yet early RBRI also predicted maladaptive (i.e., internalizing and externalizing) behaviors in children with and without DS. For the youngest typically developing children, Time 1 CRI scores predicted internalizing behaviors and attention problems two years later. Therefore early rituals and habits seem to predict a combination of adaptive and maladaptive behaviors. Adaptive and maladaptive behaviors are not mutually exclusive. It is quite reasonable to assume that certain kinds of repetitive behaviors may serve some adaptive function while also being linked to anxiety and/or inattention. Such findings may even suggest involvement of neurobiological structures and their development, linking striatal, limbic, and cortico-frontal brain regions that serve as the predominant model of pathogenesis in disorders like OCD [14].

While none of the CRI scores predicted variance in the CBCL broad-band scales for the younger children with DS, the Mean CRI score predicted Time 2 anxiety problems (narrow band). For the older cohort of children with DS, Time 1 Mean "Just Right" Score predicted Time 2 Internalizing symptoms. Regarding the CBCL narrow band factors, the Time 1 Mean CRI "Just Right" score predicted significant variance in Time 2 Thought Problems in the older cohort of children with DS.

In contrast to the findings in typically developing children, where early RBRI appeared to predict a combination of adaptive and maladaptive behaviors later in development, the RBRI of children with DS seem to predict only problem behavior. Children with DS engage in more RBRI than their MA-matched typically developing cohort – particularly at the older MA Level at Time 2 – but these behaviors appear to be more symptomatic. It is possible that repetitive behaviors in persons with DS arise from striatal activation and development, but they are perhaps less organized, integrated and coordinated by frontal-cortical regions, but such interpretation is speculative and merits further investigation.

The results from this study hold some theoretical and practical promise. From a theoretical standpoint, the results speak to continuities and discontinuities in the varieties of repetitive behavior in typically and atypically developing populations. The results may serve as practical information for parents and pediatricians alike who work to distinguish those behaviors that represent the behavioral phenotype of the disability from behaviors that reflect normal developmental processes in persons who are not otherwise experiencing developmental disability [5]. The results of this study suggest that earlier in development, the RBRI of children with DS may be difficult to distinguish from typically developing RBRI and, in this sense, may not be noteworthy. Later in development, RBRI may be considered part of the DS behavioral phenotype rather than a reflection of the typical developmental processes since RBRI predict later problems and disruptions in the acquisition of certain adaptive skills in communication and daily living skills.

The study is not without limitations. Comparing TD children with participants with intellectual disabilities presents special challenges in terms of matching. While matching on developmental constructs such as mental age as we did here is consistent with a developmental approach to disabilities [3], such approaches do not control for experiential or biological factors that may impact behavior in important ways. This approach is unavoidable when comparing individuals with neurodevelopmental disorders to neurotypical groups. Still, future work is needed to evaluate the differential roles of cognitive and biological factors in the development of RBRI. Indeed there is a significant body of work that points to the role of neural structures, such as the basal ganglia, in RBRI [8,14,26,33,44]. However, there is also evidence linking RBRI with deficits in cognitive control and executive function [14,26,34]. So while the repetitive behaviors themselves are strongly influenced by neural structure and function, it is the job of the cognitive systems governing executive functions and self-regulation, more generally, to regulate these behaviors. It is for this reason that we examined groups matched on cognitive level, rather than chronological age.

It is the case that different genetic subtypes of neurodevelopmental disabilities present with varied profiles of RBRI [20,23] and will likely respond differently to interventions aimed at RBRI to foster better overall adaptive behavior. For this reason, we suggest that future work examines RBRI in specific rare copy number variations associated with NDDs. Other limitations include the use of the Vineland Screener, which though highly correlated with the Survey edition, may yield different results; the necessity of using different measures to assess cognitive ability across age groups may also present bias, although the measures of cognitive development are regarded as comparable.

Conclusions

For typically developing children, relatively frequent and intense RBRI may be viewed as predictors of later adaptation, albeit with some link to later internalizing symptoms, especially anxiety and inattention. The association between early repetitive behavior and later anxiety/inattention suggests at least some continuity between the normative manifestations of RBRI and those associated with many clinical conditions which may in turn suggest some common underlying neurobiological mechanisms [14,26].

It is intriguing that some amount of RBRI persists well into childhood when the rigid and circumscribed behaviors are thought to give way to more flexible, adaptive behavior [56,57]. While RBRI do appear to be more common in children with disabilities and may be considered symptomatic (DS, ASD, PWS [19–21]), it is also the case that some repetitive behavior remains part of the repertoire of typical children and adults across cultures [58,59], possibly representing vestiges of an earlier and once effective means of understanding, organizing, and adapting to a changing environment [14,55]. This perspective is supported by work examining repetitive behavior in non-human animals as well [41,49,60]. Understanding the contextual and organismic factors that determine adaptive and maladaptive manifestations of various kinds of repetitive behavior will serve both theoretical and clinical endeavors.

Understanding the nature and development of RBRI is necessary in order to distinguish those behaviors that may be symptomatic and warranting clinical attention from those that are conspicuous by virtue of their relative asynchrony with other markers of developmental level. Long-term longitudinal studies of both typically developing and non-typically developing children will be necessary to fully understand the developmental nature of repetitive behavior.

Author Contributions

Conceived and designed the experiments: DWE FLK. Performed the experiments: DWE FLK. Analyzed the data: DWE MMS KBB. Contributed reagents/materials/analysis tools: DWE FLK. Wrote the paper: DWE FLK MMS KBB. Statistical consultation: MMS KBB.

References

1. Moreno De Luca A, Myers SM, Challman TD, Evans DW, Ledbetter DH (2013) Developmental brain dysfunction: revival and expansion of old concepts based on new genetic evidence. The Lancet Neurology 12: 406–414.
2. Cicchetti D (1984) The emergence of developmental psychopathology. Child Development 55: 1–7.
3. Werner H (1948) Comparative psychology of mental development. (Revised. Ed.). New York: Follett.
4. Zigler E (1967) Familial mental retardation: A continuing dilemma. Science 20: 292–298.
5. Bodfish J, Symons F, Parker D, Lewis M (2000) Varieties of repetitive behavior in autism: Comparisons to mental retardation. Journal of Autism and Developmental Disorders 30: 237–243.
6. Leekam S, Prior M, Uljarevic M (2011) Restricted and repetitive behaviors in autism spectrum disorders: A review of research in the last decade. Psychological Bulletin 137: 562–593.
7. Leekam S, Tandos J, McConachie H, Meins E, Parkinson K, et al. (2007) Repetitive behaviors in typically developing 2-year-olds. Journal of Child Psychology and Psychiatry 48: 1131–1138.
8. Schultz R, Evans DW, Wolff M (1999) Neuropsychological models of childhood obsessive-compulsive disorder. Child and Adolescent Psychiatric Clinics of North America, 8: 513–531.
9. Turner M (1999) Annotation: Repetitive behavior in autism: A review of psychological research. Child Psychology and Psychiatry and Allied Disciplines 40: 839–849.
10. Berkson G (2002) Early development of stereotyped and self-injurious behaviors: II. Age trends. American Journal on Mental Retardation 106: 468–477.
11. Boyd BA, Baranek GT, Sideris J, Poe MD, Watson LR, et al. (2010) Sensory features and repetitive behaviors in children with autism and developmental delay. Autism Research 3: 78–87.
12. Boyd BA, McBee M, Holtzclaw T, Baranek GT, Bodfish J (2009) Relationships among repetitive behaviors, sensory features, and executive functions in high functioning autism. Research in Autism Spectrum Disorders 3: 959–966.
13. Esbensen A, Seltzer M, Lam K, Bodfish J (2009) Age-related differences in restricted repetitive behaviors in autism spectrum disorders. Journal of Autism and Developmental Disorders 39: 57–66.
14. Evans DW, Leckman JF (2006) Origins of obsessive-compulsive disorder: Developmental and evolutionary perspectives. In D. . Cicchetti, Dante & D.J. . Cohen (Eds); Developmental psychopathology, Vol 3: Risk, disorder, and adaptation (2nd ed.). John Wiley & Sons, Hoboken, N., Pp. 404–435.
15. Evans DW, Gray FL (2000) Compulsive-like behaviors in typically developing children and individuals with and without Down syndrome: Its relation to MA, adaptive and maladaptive behavior. Child Development 71: 288–300.
16. Evans DW, Leckman JF, Carter A, Reznick JS, Henshaw D, et al. (1997) Ritual, habit and perfectionism: the prevalence and development of compulsive -like behavior in young children. Child Development 68: 58–68.
17. Bishop SL, Richler J, Lord C (2006) Association between restricted and repetitive behaviors and nonverbal IQ in children with autism spectrum disorders. Child Neuropsychology 12: 247–267.
18. Militerni R, Bravaccio C, Falco C, Fico C, Palermo MT (2002) Repetitive behaviors in autistic disorder. European Child & Adolescent Psychiatry 11: 210–218.
19. Dykens E, Shah B (2003) Psychiatric Disorders in Prader-Willi Syndrome: Epidemiology and Management. CNS-Drugs 17: 167–178.
20. Greaves N, Prince E, Evans DW, Charman T (2005) Repetitive and ritualistic behavior in children with Prader-Willi syndrome and children with autism. Journal of Intellectual Disability Research 50: 92–100.
21. Wigren M, Hansen S (2003) Rituals and compulsivity in Prader-Willi syndrome: Profile and stability. Journal of Intellectual Disability Research 47: 428–438.
22. Glenn S, Cunningham C (2006) Typical or pathological? Routinized and compulsive-like behaviors in children and young people with Down syndrome. Intellectual and Developmental Disabilities 45: 246–256.
23. Moss J, Oliver C, Arron K, Burbridge C, Berg K. (2009) The prevalence and phenomenology of repetitive behavior in genetic syndromes. Journal of Autism and Developmental Disorders 39: 572–588.
24. Bolton D (1996) Annotation: Developmental issues in obsessive compulsive disorder. Journal of Child Psychology and Psychiatry and Allied Disciplines 37: 131–137.
25. King R, Noshpitz JD (1991) Pathways of growth: Essentials of child psychiatry. NY: Wiley.
26. Evans DW, Lewis MD, Iobst E (2004) The role of the orbitofrontal cortex in normally-developing compulsive-like behaviors and obsessive-compulsive disorder. Brain and Cognition 55: 220–234.
27. Niler ER, Beck SJ (1989) The relationships among guilt, dysphoria, anxiety and obsessions in a normal population. Behavior Research and Therapy 27: 213–220.
28. Leonard H, Goldberger EL, Rapoport JL, Cheslow BS, Swedo S (1990) Childhood rituals: Normal development or obsessive-compulsive symptoms? Journal of the American Academy of Child and Adolescent Psychology and Psychiatry 29: 17–23.
29. Thelen E (1979) Rhythmical stereotypies in normal human infants. Animal Behavior 27: 699–715.
30. Marks I (1987) Fears, phobias and rituals. Oxford: Oxford University Press.
31. Gesell A (1928) Infancy and human growth. Oxford University Press.
32. Gesell A, Ames LB, Ilg FL (1974) Infant and the child in the culture today. NY: Harper and Row.
33. Pietrefesa A, Evans DW (2007) Affective and neuropsychological correlates of children's rituals and compulsive-like behaviors: Continuities and discontinuities with obsessive-compulsive disorder. Brain and Cognition 65: 36–46.
34. South M, Ozonoff S, Mcmahon W (2007) The relationship between executive functioning, central coherence, and repetitive behaviors in the high-functioning autism spectrum. Autism 11: 437–451.
35. Zohar AH, Bruno R (1997) Normative and pathological obsessive-compulsive behavior and ideation in childhood: a question of timing. Journal of Psychology and Psychiatry 38: 993–999.
36. Evans DW, Gray FL, Leckman JF (1999) The rituals, fears and phobias of young children: insights from developmental, psychopathology and neurobiology. Child Psychiatry and Human Development 29: 261–276.
37. Piaget J (1952) The origins of intelligence in the child. NY: Basic.
38. Kagan J (1981) The second year. Cambridge, MA: Harvard University Press.
39. Bolton D, Dearsley P, Madropnal-Luque R, Baron-Cohen S (2002) Magical thinking in childhood and adolescence: Development and relation to obsessive compulsion. British Journal of Developmental Psychology 20: 479–494.
40. Evans DW, Milanak M, Medeiros B, Ross J (2002) Magical beliefs and rituals in young children. Child Psychiatry and Human Development 33: 43–58.
41. Judge P, Evans DW, Schroepfer KK, Gross A (2011) Reversal learning perseveration correlates to repetitive behavior in non-human primates. Behavioural Brain Research 222: 54–61.
42. Tregay J, Gilmour J, Charman T (2009) Childhood rituals and executive functions. British Journal of Developmental Psychology 27: 283–296.
43. Evans DW, Maliken A (2011) Cortical activity and children's rituals habits and other repetitive behavior: A visual P300 study. Behavioural Brain Research 224: 174–179.
44. Lewis M, Kim SJ (2009) The pathophysiology of restricted repetitive behavior. Journal of Neurodevelopmental Disorders 1: 114–132.
45. Çevikaslan A, Evans DW, Dedeoğlu C, Kalaça S, Yazgan Y (2013) A cross-sectional survey of repetitive behaviors and restricted interests in a typically-developing Turkish population. Child Psychiatry and Human Development [ePub ahead of print].
46. Garner JP (2005) Stereotypies and other abnormal repetitive behaviors: potential impact of validity, reliability and replicability of scientific outcomes. ILAR J 45: 106–117.
47. Garner JP, Mason GJ (2002) Evidence for a relationship between cage stereotypy and behavioral disinhibition in laboratory rodents. Behavioural Brain Research 136: 83–92.
48. Garner JP, Mason GP, Smith R (2003) Stereotypic route-tracing in experimentally-caged songbirds correlates with general behavioral disinhibition. Animal Behavior 66: 711–727.
49. Lewis MH, Tanimura Y, Lee LW, Bodfish JW (2007). Animal models of restricted repetitive behavior in autism. Behavioural Brain Research 176: 66–74.
50. Lutz C, Well A (2003) Stereotypic and self-injurious behavior in rhesus macaques: A survey and retrospective analysis of environment and early experience. American Journal of Primatology 60: 1–15.
51. Achenbach T, Edelbrock C (1991) The Manual of the Youth Self Report Symptom Behavior Checklist. Burlington, VT: University of Vermont.
52. Sparrow S, Carter A, Cicchetti D (1993) The Vineland Screener: Overview, Validity, Reliability, Administration and Scoring New Haven, CT: Yale University Child Study Center.
53. Sparrow S, Balla D, Cicchetti D (1984) The Vineland Adaptive Behaviors Scales—Survey Edition. Circle Pines, MN: The Psychological Corporation.
54. Zelazo P, Jacques S (1996) Children's rule use: Representation, reflection and cognitive control. In R. . Vasta (Ed). Annals of child development: A research annual 12: 119–176. London, England: Jessica Kingsley Publishers.
55. Evans DW (2000). Rituals and other syncretic tools: Insights from Werner's comparative psychology. In D.W. . Evans (Guest Editor.), Heinz Werner and his

relevance for research and theory in the 21st century, Special issue, Journal of Adult Development 7: 49–61.
56. Janowsky J, Carper R (1996) Is there a neural basis for cognitive transitions in school-age children? In A. . Sameroff & M.M. . Haith (Eds). The five to seven year shift: The age of reason and responsibility. University of Chicago Press.
57. White S (1996) The child's entry into the "age of reason". In A. . Sameroff & M.M. . Haith (Eds) The five to seven year shift: The age of reason and responsibility. University of Chicago Press.
58. Dulaney S, Fiske A (1994) Cultural rituals and obsessive-compulsive disorder: Is there a common psychological mechanism? Ethos 22: 243–283.
59. Fiske A, Halsam N (1997) Is obsessive-compulsive disorder a pathology of the human disposition to perform socially meaningful rituals? Evidence of similar content. Journal of Nervous and Mental Disease 185: 211–222.
60. Eilam D, Zor R, Szechtman H, Hermesh H (2006) Rituals, stereotypy and compulsive behavior in animal and humans. Neuroscience and Biobehavioral Reviews 40: 456–471.

Antenatal Screening for Down Syndrome Using Serum Placental Growth Factor with the Combined, Quadruple, Serum Integrated and Integrated Tests

Nicholas J. Wald*, Jonathan P. Bestwick, Lynne M. George, Wayne J. Huttly

Wolfson Institute of Preventive Medicine, Barts and the London School of Medicine and Dentistry, Queen Mary University of London, London, United Kingdom

Abstract

Objective: To estimate the value of first or second trimester placental growth factor (PlGF) as an additional antenatal screening marker for Down syndrome.

Design: Nested case-control study.

Setting: Antenatal screening service.

Population or Sample: 532 Down syndrome pregnancies and 1,155 matched unaffected pregnancies.

Methods: Stored maternal serum samples (−40°C) were assayed for PlGF. Monte Carlo simulation was used to estimate the screening performance of PlGF with the Combined, Quadruple, serum Integrated and Integrated tests.

Main Outcome Measures: Median PlGF levels in affected and unaffected pregnancies and screening performance (detection rates [DR] for specified false-positive rates [FPR] and *vice versa*).

Results: First trimester median PlGF was 15%, 28% and 39% lower in Down syndrome than unaffected pregnancies at 11, 12 and 13 completed weeks' gestation respectively (all $p<0.001$). Second trimester median PlGF was 31% lower at 14 weeks ($p<0.001$), and the difference decreased (6% lower at 17 weeks). At a 90% DR with first trimester markers measured at 13 weeks, adding PlGF decreased the FPR from 11.1 to 5.1% using the Combined test, 9.3% to 4.5% using the serum Integrated test, and 3.4% to 1.5% using the Integrated test (or 1.5 to 1.4% with first trimester markers measured at 11 weeks). Adding PlGF to the Quadruple test (measured at 15 weeks) decreased the FPR from 10.0% to 9.6% at a 90% DR.

Conclusions: First trimester PlGF measurements improve the performance of antenatal screening for Down syndrome using the Combined, serum Integrated and Integrated tests. Second trimester PlGF measurements are of limited value.

Editor: Olga Y. Gorlova, The University of Texas M. D. Anderson Cancer Center, United States of America

Funding: PerkinElmer provided the PlGF assay kits free of charge. No additional external funding was received for this study. The funders had no role in study design, data collection and analysis, decision to publish, or preparation of the manuscript.

Competing Interests: The authors have the following interests: PerkinElmer provided the PlGF assay kits free of charge. N. Wald has a patent for the Integrated test as follows: Application No.; Country; Filing Date; Patent No.; Issue/Grant Date 09/301,621; US; 29.04.99; 6,573,103; 03.06.03 36213/99; Australia; 29.04.99; 763171; 31.10.06 2330538; Canada; 29.04.99; 2330538; 11.09.07 99918188; Europe; 29.04.99; 1076824; 14.06.06 139302; Israel; 29.04.99; 139302; 26.10.05 With others, he held a patent in connection with the use of uE3 as a second trimester screening marker in prenatal screening for Down syndrome, although this has now expired. He is Director of Logical Medical Systems Ltd, which produces software for the interpretation of Down syndrome screening tests. There are no further patents, products in development or marketed products to declare.

* E-mail: n.j.wald@qmul.ac.uk

Introduction

Placental growth factor (PlGF) is an angiogenic hormone which has been shown to be useful in late first trimester and early second trimester antenatal screening for pre-eclampsia. First trimester levels were found to be 36% lower in women who developed early pre-eclampsia compared to unaffected controls [1] and early second trimester levels were 30% lower. [2] The value of PlGF in screening for Down syndrome is less clear. Five studies have reported results on PlGF measured in the late first trimester (11 to 13 weeks' gestation). Four of these showed, on average, reduced PlGF levels in Down syndrome compared with unaffected pregnancies (22% [3], 24% [4], 29% [5] and 38% [6] lower based on 91, 70, 90 and 42 affected pregnancies respectively) and one study found a higher level in affected pregnancies (26% higher based on 45 affected pregnancies [7]). In the *second trimester* three studies reported PlGF results; one showed reduced levels (33% lower based on 24 affected prengnancies [8]), one increased levels (42% higher based on 36 affected pregnancies [9]) and one no material difference in Down syndrome compared with unaffected pregnancies (1% higher based on 39 affected pregnancies [10]).

Table 1. Number of pregnancies classified according to screening test, gestational age when screened, and selected characteristics of the Down syndrome and unaffected pregnancies.

	Down syndrome (N = 532)	Unaffected (N = 1,152)
Screening test received		
Combined test	289	576
Quadruple test	217	433
Integrated test	26	143
Median gestational age (days)		
First trimester	88	88
Second trimester	114	114
Median maternal age at EDD	37	37
Median maternal weight (kg)	66	66
Smoking (%)	5.8	7.7
Ethnicity (%)		
Afro-Caribbean	9.2	10
White	72	73
South Asian	6.5	5.7
Oriental	2.6	3.3
Other	10.2	8.3

EDD: expected date of delivery.

The uncertain value of PlGF in antenatal screening for Down syndrome prompted us to investigate the matter further by comparing the screening performance with and without (i) first trimester PlGF measurements added to the Combined test (nuchal translucency [NT], free β-human chorionic gonadotrophin [hCG] and pregnancy associated plasma protein A [PAPP-A] measured between 11 and 13 weeks' gestation), (ii) second trimester PlGF measurements added to the early second trimester Quadruple test (alphafetoprotein [AFP], unconjugated oestriol [uE_3], free β-hCG and inhibin-A measured between 14 and 22 weeks' gestation), (iii) first trimester PlGF measurements added to the Integrated test (first trimester NT and PAPP-A and second trimester AFP, uE3 free β-hCG and Inhibin-A) and serum Integrated test (Integrated test without NT) and (iv) early second trimester PlGF measurements added to the Integrated and serum Integrated tests.

Methods

According to guidelines from the National Research Ethics Committee, our research does not require research ethics committee approval as serum samples were collected as part of a routine antenatal screening programme. Women are informed of the possible subsequent use of samples in research or screening programme audits, so they could indicate to the programme staff that they did not want their samples used. The research analysis was conducted on anonymised samples and data.

We identified 532 Down syndrome singleton pregnancies screened at the Wolfson Insititute of Preventive Medicine between February 2000 and May 2010 from the screening service records and by linkage to data from the National Cytogenetic Register held at the Wolfson Institute. Among the 532 affected pregnancies, 289 were screened using the Combined test (from February 2005), 217 using the Quadruple test and 26 using the Integrated test (from March 2003). Each affected pregnancy was matched with 2 (Combined and Quadruple test) or 5 (Integrated test) unaffected control pregnancies for gestational age (same day), maternal age (in 5 year categories) and length of storage (in six-month categories).

Frozen (−40°C) stored samples were thawed and assayed for placental growth factor using the AutoDELPHIA® PlGF kit (Perkin Elmer). The samples were assayed "blind" i.e. without knowledge of whether the samples were from a Down syndrome or unaffected pregnancy. The inter-assay coefficient of variation was 7.5% and intra-assay coefficient of variation 3.9%. Serum from women screened using the Combined and Integrated tests was used to assess first trimester PlGF, and serum from women screened using the Quadruple and Integrated tests was used to assess second trimester PlGF.

PlGF concentrations were expressed as multiples of the median (MoM) for unaffected pregnancies of the same gestational age by performing a regression of the log median PlGF against the median gestational age in 2-day categories for first trimester measurements and weekly categories for second trimester measurements (weighted by the number of women in each category) and dividing PlGF concentrations by the regressed (i.e. expected) concentration for the same gestational age. MoM values were adjusted for maternal weight by performing a regression of the log median MoM values against weight in unaffected pregnancies and dividing MoM values by the regressed value for the same weight. Associations between weight adjusted PlGF MoM values and maternal smoking and ethnicity were also determined and MoM values further adjusted as required. The change in median MoM in Down syndrome pregnancies was investigated by performing a regression of the median PlGF MoM against the median gestational age in 2-day categories for first trimester measurements and weekly categories for second trimester measurements (weighted by the number of women in each category; 19 to 22 weeks were combined into one category due to the small numbers of Down syndrome pregnancies with PlGF measurements beyond 18 weeks' gestation). Probability plots and, if appropriate, the approximate point of risk reversal (to ensure risk estimation is a monotonic function of the marker value [11]) were used to specify truncation limits within which the range of values for PlGF approximately followed log-Gaussian distributions in affected and unaffected pregnancies.

Median PlGF MoM values were used as the measure of central tendency to avoid the influence of outliers and their log values as estimates of the means. Standard deviations (log) were calculated by regression of the points on the probability plot between the 10th and 90th centiles and correlation coefficients with the standard Down syndrome screening markers (first trimester NT, free β-hCG and PAPP-A and second trimester AFP, uE3 free β-hCG and Inhibin-A) were calculated after excluding points more than 3.5 standard deviations from the mean (correlations between first trimester PlGF and second trimester markers, and second trimester PlGF and first trimester markers were estimated using data from women screened using the Integrated test). Log means and standard deviations of the standard Down syndrome screening markers and correlation coefficients were taken from the SURUSS report.[12–15].

Monte Carlo simulation was used to estimate screening performance instead of numerical integration as used previously[12–15] (because Monte Carlo simulation is computationally faster). Hypothetical random samples of 250,000 Down syndrome and 250,000 unaffected pregnancies were generated based on the specified Gaussian distributions. Each simulated pregnancy was assigned a maternal age based on the maternal age distribution of

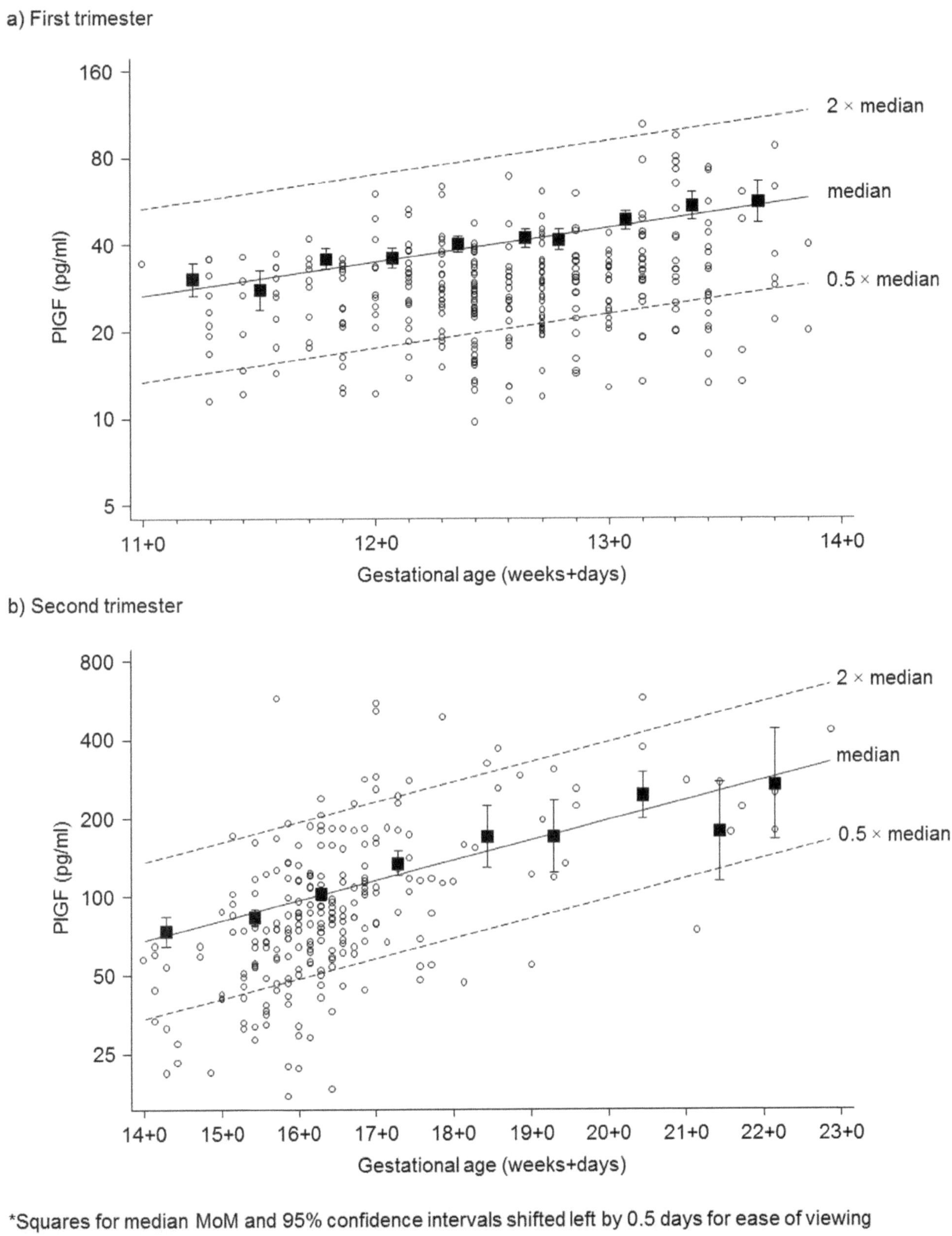

Figure 1. First trimester (a) and second trimester (b) placental growth factor (PlGF) according to gestational age in Down syndrome pregnancies (circles) and medians in 2-day intervals* (a) and weekly intervals (b) in unaffected pregnancies (squares, with 95% confidence intervals) together with expected (regressed) median in unaffected pregnancies.

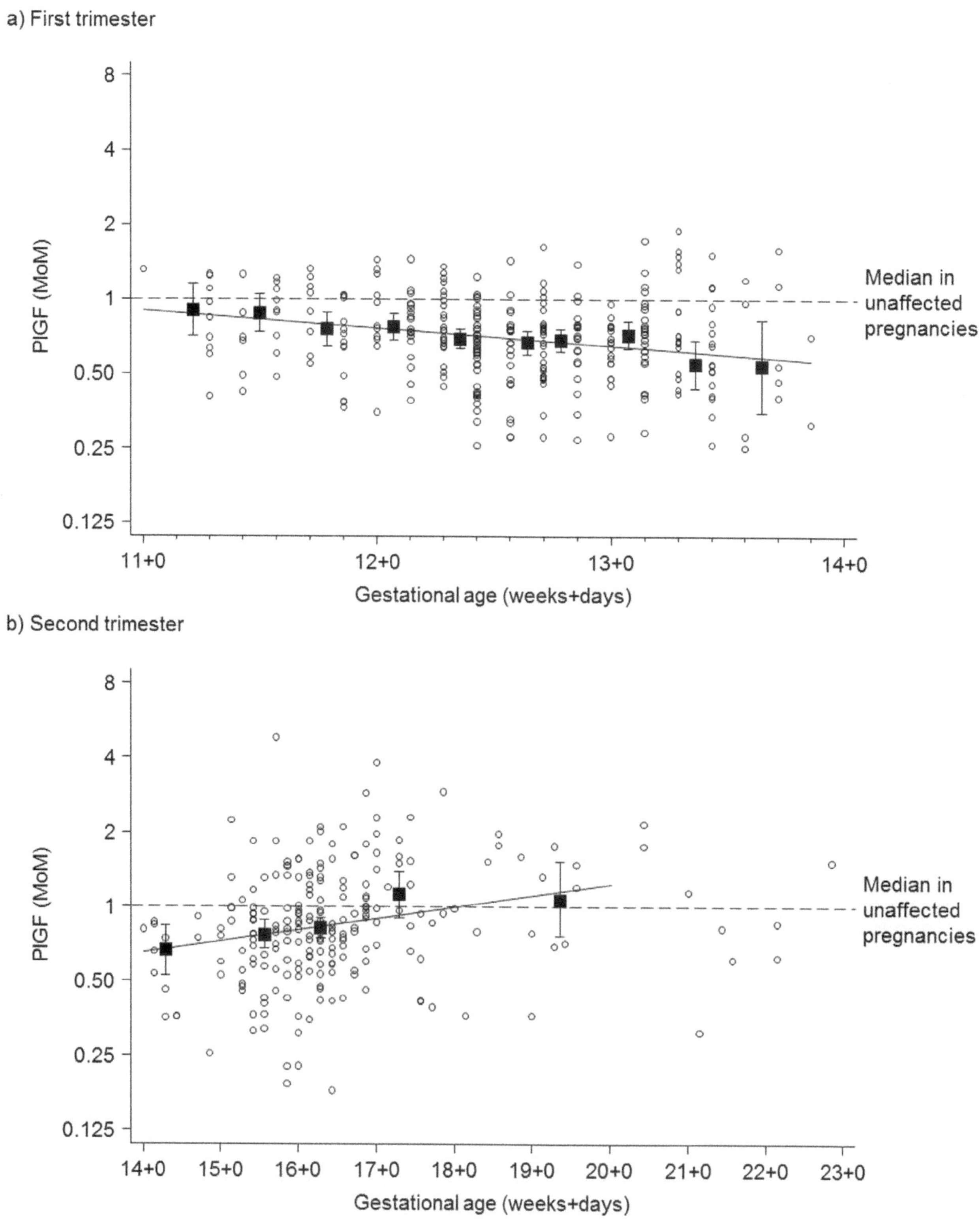

*Squares for median MoM and 95% confidence intervals shifted left by 0.5 days for ease of viewing

Figure 2. First trimester (a) and second trimester (b) placental growth factor (PlGF) maternal weight, smoking and ethnicity adjusted MoM values according to gestational age and medians (squares, with 95% confidence intervals) in 2-day intervals* (a) and weekly intervals (b) in Down syndrome pregnancies together with expected (regressed) median.

Table 2. Observed and regressed median PlGF MoM in Down syndrome pregnancies according to gestational age.

Completed week of gestation	Number of affected pregnancies	Observed	Regressed	
		Median MoM	Median MoM (95% CI)*	p-value
First trimester				
11	48	0.82	0.85 (0.76 to 0.95)	0.011
12	164	0.71	0.72 (0.68 to 0.76)	<0.001
13	89	0.68	0.61 (0.55 to 0.67)	<0.001
Second trimester				
14	13	0.66	0.69 (0.54 to 0.89)	0.019
15	63	0.77	0.77 (0.65 to 0.91)	0.016
16	97	0.82	0.85 (0.75 to 0.97)	0.031
17	27	1.12	0.94 (0.80 to 1.12)	0.368
18–22	24	1.06	1.15 (0.82 to 1.62)**	0.279

*Median MoM at completed week (week+3 days).
**Regressed median MoM at 135.5 days gestation (median gestational at 18–22 completed weeks).

maternities in England and Wales 2006–2008 [16] (instead of 1996–1998 as used previously, so screening performance figures of tests without PlGF will be expected to be a little different from those previously reported.[12–15]) and the maternal age-specific odds of an affected livebirth. [17,18] For each simulated pregnancy, the predicted risk of having a pregnancy with Down syndrome in the early second trimester was calculated by multiplying the maternal age specific odds of having an affected live birth adjusted to early mid-trimester by multiplying by 1/0.77 to allow for the general fetal loss in Down syndrome pregnancies from this time in pregnancy until term [19] by the likelihood ratio (for a given set of marker values) obtained from the overlapping multivariate Gaussian distributions of marker levels in affected and unaffected pregnancies. A woman was classified as screen positive if her risk of having a pregnancy affected with Down syndrome was greater than or equal to a specified risk cut-off level. Screening performance estimates were calculated as the detection rate (DR) for false-positive rates (FPR) of 1, 3 and 5%, the FPR for DR's of 85, 90 and 95% and the DR and FPR for early second trimester risk cut-offs of 1 in 100, 1 in 150 and 1 in 200.

Results

Table 1 shows the number of pregnancies screened classified according to test, gestational age when screened, and selected characteristics of the Down syndrome and unaffected pregnancies. The distributions of the variables in the two groups were similar.

Figure 1a shows the concentration of late first trimester (11–13 completed weeks) PlGF in affected pregnancies according to gestational age together with the expected (regressed) median concentration in unaffected pregnancies. The median PlGF in unaffected pregnancies increased by 31% per week of gestation ($p<0.001$). Figure 1b shows the corresponding data for early second trimester PlGF (14–22 completed weeks). The median PlGF in unaffected pregnancies increased by 19% per week of gestation ($p<0.001$). In unaffected pregnancies, first trimester PlGF MoM values decreased by 1.3% per 5 kg increase in maternal weight ($p=0.031$) and second trimester PlGF MoM values decreased by 3.1% per 5 kg increase ($p=0.002$);

Smokers had higher weight adjusted PlGF MoM values than non-smokers; 32% higher in the first trimester (95% confidence interval 25% to 61%) and 36% higher in the second trimester (95% confidence interval 11% to 59%). First trimester PlGF MoM values were 18% higher in Afro-Caribbean women compared with white women (95% confidence interval 7% to 35%) and second trimester MoM values 30% higher (95% confidence interval 9% to 54%). First trimester weight adjusted PlGF MoM values were therefore divided by 1.32 in smokers and by 1.18 in Afro-Caribbean women; second trimester MoM values by 1.36 in smokers and 1.30 in Afro-Caribbean women. There were no significant increases or decreases in either first or second trimester weight adjusted PlGF MoM values in other ethnic groups.

Figure 2a shows the first trimester PlGF MoM values (after adjustment for maternal weight, smoking and Afro-Caribbean ethnicity) in Down syndrome pregnancies according to gestational age together with the expected (regressed) median MoM and the corresponding results for second trimester PlGF. The median MoM values decreased by 15% per week ($p=0.003$), with the median MoM at 11, 12 and 13 completed weeks' gestation being 0.85 (95% confidence interval, CI 0.76 to 0.95), 0.72 (95% CI 0.68 to 0.76) and 0.61 (95% CI 0.55 to 0.67) respectively. Table 2 shows the observed and regressed median MoM values at each completed week of gestation.

Figure 2b and table 2 show that the median second trimester MoM increased by 11% per week ($p<0.001$), with the median MoM at 14, 15, 16 completed weeks' gestation being 0.69 (95% CI 0.54 to 0.89), 0.77 (95% CI 0.65 to 0.91) and 0.85 (95% CI 0.75 to 0.97) respectively. The median MoM at 17, completed weeks' gestation was 0.94 (95% CI 0.80 to 1.12) and at 18–22 weeks was 1.15 (95% CI 0.82 to 1.62); neither statistically significantly different from the median in unaffected pregnancies (1.0 MoM). Therefore, screening performance estimates for PlGF were not considered for measurements of PlGF beyond 16 weeks' gestation.

Inspection of probability plots of PlGF MoM values in Down syndrome and unaffected pregnancies showed that the distributions were reasonably Gaussian between 0.4 to 2.5 MoM (see figure in Appendix S1). The standard deviations of the first and second trimester log PlGF MoM values were, respectively, 0.1705 and 0.2243 in affected pregnancies and 0.1556 and 0.1786 in unaffected pregnancies. As a single marker the PlGF detection rates for a 5% false-positive rate were 14%, 26% and 41% at 11, 12 and 13 completed weeks respectively and 27%, 21% and 16% at 14, 15 and 16 weeks.

Table 3. Screening performance according to detection and false-positive rates of the Combined, Quadruple and Integrated tests with and without the addition of first or second trimester placental growth factor (PlGF) according to gestational age markers are measured.

	Gestational age first trimester markers measured (completed weeks)	DR (%) for FPR of:-			FPR (%) for DR of:-		
Test		**1%**	**3%**	**5%**	**85%**	**90%**	**95%**
Comined							
Without PlGF	11	76	84	88	3.2	6.7	16.6
	12	74	83	86	4.2	8.6	19.8
	13	70	79	84	5.9	11.1	23.0
With PlGF	11	77	85	89	2.9	6.1	15.3
	12	77	85	89	2.8	6.1	14.9
	13	78	86	90	2.4	5.1	12.4
Quadruple							
Without PlGF	–	64	77	83	5.9	10.0	19.6
With PlGF at 15 completed weeks	–	66	78	84	5.7	9.6	18.9
Serum Integrated							
Without PlGF	11	72	83	87	3.8	7.2	15.4
	12	69	81	86	4.7	8.4	17.3
	13	67	79	84	5.3	9.3	18.6
With first trimester PlGF	11	73	84	88	3.4	6.5	13.9
	12	73	84	88	3.4	6.1	12.9
	13	76	87	91	2.5	4.5	9.7
With second trimester PlGF at 15 completed weeks	11	74	84	88	3.3	6.4	14.1
	12	71	82	87	4.1	7.6	16.0
	13	69	81	86	4.7	8.5	17.2
Integrated							
Without PlGF	11	88	93	95	0.6	1.5	5.0
	12	86	92	94	0.8	2.2	6.6
	13	82	89	92	1.5	3.4	9.1
With first trimester PlGF	11	88	93	95	0.5	1.4	4.5
	12	88	93	95	0.6	1.5	4.6
	13	88	94	96	0.6	1.5	4.2
With second trimester PlGF at 15 completed weeks	11	89	94	95	0.5	1.3	4.4
	12	87	92	94	0.7	1.8	5.8
	13	84	90	93	1.3	2.9	8.1

Table 3 shows the screening performance of the Combined, Quadruple, serum Integrated and Integrated tests with and without the addition of PlGF at specified detection rates and at specified false-positive rates. The addition of a *first trimester* measurement of PlGF improves the screening performance of the Combined test; at a 90% detection rate the false-positive rate decreased from 6.7% to 6.1% with markers measured at 11 completed weeks of gestation and from 11.1% to 5.1% at 13 completed weeks' gestation. The addition of a *second trimester* PlGF measurement to the Quadruple test had little influence on screening performance; for example, at a 90% detection rate the false-positive rate decreased from 10.0% to 9.6% if PlGF is measured at 15 completed weeks' gestation. Results with PlGF measured at 14 and 16 completed weeks' gestation are similar [9.4% and 9.7% respectively] and so second trimester screening performance estimates are not shown in the Table.

Table 3 shows that at a 90% detection rate the addition of *first trimester* PlGF measurement to the Integrated test reduces the false-positive rate from 1.5% to 1.4% at 11 completed weeks' gestation and from 3.4% to 1.5% at 13 completed weeks. The addition of a *second trimester* PlGF measurement at 15 completed weeks' gestation to the Integrated test reduces the false positive rate from 1.5% to 1.3% when first trimester markers are measured at 11 completed weeks' gestation and from 3.4% to 2.9% when first trimester markers are measured at 13 completed weeks. The results are similar if PlGF is measured at 14 or 16 completed weeks' gestation.

Table 4. Screening performance according to risk cut-off of the Combined, Quadruple and Integrated tests with and without the addition of first or second trimester placental growth factor (PlGF) according to gestational age markers are measured.

Test	Gestational age first trimester markers measured (completed weeks)	Risk cut-off (early second trimester)								
		1 in 100			1 in 150			1 in 200		
		DR (%)	FPR (%)	OAPR	DR (%)	FPR (%)	OAPR	DR (%)	FPR (%)	OAPR
Comined										
Without PlGF	11	82	2.0	1:9	84	3.0	1:12	86	3.9	1:16
	12	80	2.1	1:9	83	3.0	1:13	85	3.9	1:16
	13	77	2.3	1:11	81	3.5	1:15	83	4.6	1:19
With PlGF	11	82	1.9	1:8	85	2.8	1:12	87	3.7	1:15
	12	82	1.9	1:8	85	2.7	1:11	87	3.6	1:15
	13	83	1.9	1:8	86	2.8	1:11	88	3.5	1:14
Quadruple										
Without PlGF	–	78	3.2	1:14	82	4.6	1:19	85	5.8	1:24
With PlGF at 15 completed weeks	–	78	3.0	1:13	82	4.2	1:18	85	5.5	1:23
Serum Integrated										
Without PlGF	11	81	2.5	1:11	85	3.6	1:15	87	4.6	1:19
	12	80	2.7	1:12	83	3.9	1:16	86	5.0	1:20
	13	79	2.9	1:13	83	4.2	1:18	85	5.4	1:22
With first	11	82	2.5	1:11	85	3.6	1:15	87	4.6	1:18
trimester PlGF	12	83	2.6	1:11	86	3.7	1:15	88	4.7	1:19
	13	85	2.4	1:10	88	3.4	1:14	90	4.3	1:17
With second	11	82	2.3	1:10	85	3.3	1:14	87	4.3	1:17
trimester PlGF at 15	12	81	2.5	1:11	84	3.6	1:15	86	4.7	1:19
completed weeks	13	80	2.6	1:12	83	3.9	1:16	85	4.9	1:20
Integrated										
Without PlGF	11	89	1.3	1:5	91	1.9	1:7	92	2.4	1:9
	12	88	1.4	1:6	90	2.0	1:8	91	2.6	1:10
	13	86	1.6	1:7	88	2.4	1:10	89	3.0	1:12
With first	11	90	1.3	1:5	91	1.8	1:7	92	2.3	1:9
trimester PlGF	12	89	1.3	1:5	91	1.9	1:7	92	2.4	1:9
	13	90	1.4	1:5	91	1.9	1:7	93	2.4	1:9
With second	11	89	1.2	1:5	91	1.7	1:7	92	2.2	1:8
trimester PlGF at 15	12	88	1.3	1:5	90	1.9	1:7	91	2.4	1:9
completed weeks	13	86	1.5	1:6	88	2.2	1:9	90	2.8	1:11

As with the Integrated test, the addition of a first trimester PlGF measurement to the serum Integrated test improves screening performance but a second trimester PlGF has little effect (Table 3). Table 4 shows, in a similar way to Table 3, results according to risk cut-off. Table 5 shows the overall screening performance (first trimester markers measured at 11–13 weeks' gestation) with and without the addition of first and second trimester PlGF to the Combined, Serum Integrated and Integrated tests assuming equal numbers of women screened at each week of gestation in the first trimester. The addition of a first trimester PlGF measurement decreases the overall false-positive rate by about one third. For example, at a 90% detection rate, the overall Combined test false-positive rate decreases from 8.8% to 5.8% and the overall Integrated test false-positive rate from 8.3% to 5.7%.

Probability plots of PlGF MoM values and the statistical parameters (means standard deviations, correlation coefficients and truncation limits) used in this study for the estimation of screening performance are shown in the Appendix S1.

Discussion

In the late first trimester our results show that PlGF levels are reduced in Down syndrome pregnancies at 11, 12 and 13 completed weeks of gestation. The levels are lower at 12 than 11 weeks and lower at 13 than at 12 weeks. Correspondingly, the improvement in screening performance due to the addition of

Table 5. Screening performance according to detection and false-positive rates of the Combined, Quadruple and Integrated tests with and without the addition of first trimester (11–13 weeks[1]) or second trimester placental growth factor (PlGF).

	DR (%) for FPR of:-			FPR (%) for DR of:-		
Test	**1%**	**3%**	**5%**	**85%**	**90%**	**95%**
Combined						
Without PlGF	73	82	86	4.4	8.8	19.8
With PlGF	77	85	89	2.7	5.8	14.2
Serum Integrated						
Without PlGF	69	81	86	4.6	8.3	17.1
With first trimester PlGF	74	85	89	3.1	5.7	12.2
With second trimester PlGF	71	82	87	4.0	7.5	15.8
Integrated						
Without PlGF	85	91	94	1.0	2.4	6.9
With first trimester PlGF	88	93	95	0.6	1.5	4.4
With second trimester PlGF	87	92	94	0.8	2.0	6.1

[1]Average of the individual estimates with first trimester markers measured at 11, 12 and 13 completed weeks of gestation (see Table 3), assuming equal numbers of women screened at each week.

PlGF to the Combined, serum Integrated and Integrated tests increases over these weeks. For example, with the Combined test, the addition of PlGF at 11 completed weeks' of pregnancy decreases the false-positive rate at a 90% detection rate by 0.6 percentage points (6.1% v 6.7%) but by 6 percentage points at 13 weeks (5.1% v 11.1%). Other first trimester studies on PlGF do not report results by individual weeks. Their overall results are consistent with ours in four studies[3–6], but not in one. [7].

The screening performance of the Combined (and also the serum Integrated test) is best if the first trimester markers, including PlGF, are measured at 13 completed weeks. However, the performance of the Integrated test is similar when the first trimester markers, including PlGF, are measured at 11, 12 or 13 completed weeks; the addition of PlGF thus removes the advantage of performing the first stage of an Integrated test at 11 weeks compared with 12 or 13 weeks.

In the early second trimester of pregnancy PlGF values in Down syndrome pregnancies tend to be reduced, but increase towards the normal median with increasing gestation, possibly increasing above the median and the standard deviation of second trimester values is greater than that of first trimester values. Both of these effects mean that the measurement of PlGF in the second trimester does not offer a clinically significant improvement in screening performance.

We used a linear regression model in the first trimester and a separate linear regression in the second trimester to quantify the PlGF levels in affected pregnancies according to gestational age; both regression models fitted the data reasonably well (see Figure 2), and fitted better than a single quadratic regression using all the data together. Separate linear regressions also have the advantage of being more stable.

PlGF has been shown to be a useful marker in prenatal screening for pre-eclampsia in both the first and second trimesters of pregnancy. [1,2] A first trimester PlGF measurement could be used as part of the Combined, serum Integrated or Integrated tests for Down syndrome as well as in screening for pre-eclampsia. There is some benefit for a second trimester measurement of PlGF if women book too late for a Combined, serum Integrated or Integrated test even though the improvement in the performance of antenatal screening for Down syndrome is small.

In estimating screening performance using first trimester markers alone compared with that using the Integrated test markers, there can be bias if the first trimester markers are associated with miscarriage at about 10–14 weeks. This, for example, affects PAPP-A, in which low values are associated with miscarriage as well as with Down syndrome. [12] Any effect of PlGF being associated with miscarriage in this period is likely to be small, if present at all, because in our data there wase no significant difference in the median PlGF MoM in affected pregnancies tested using the Combined test and those tested using the Integrated test (0.70 and 0.66 respectively, $p = 0.35$).

The financial cost of including first trimester PlGF measurement in the Combined, Serum Integrated and Integrated tests depends on when the first trimester markers are measured. If measured at 11 weeks, the cost per Down syndrome pregnancy diagnosed is about £300 more expensive with the Combined test and £600 more expensive with the Integrated test. Measured at 12 weeks, costs are £2,500 less for the Combined test and £100 less for the Integrated test; if measured at 13 weeks, the amounts are £7,100 and £1,700 less respectively. These estimates are based on using the unit costs given in SURUSS[12] increased by 25% to allow for inflation. Overall, therefore, the addition of PlGF at 11–13 weeks is probably worthwhile, given the improvement in screening performance with little or no increased cost per Down syndrome pregnancy diagnosed.

Conclusion

This study, based on 532 Down syndrome pregnancies, is the largest to have investigated the value of PlGF in antenatal screening for Down syndrome. It shows that PlGF is a useful Down syndrome screening marker in the late first trimester of pregnancy but of little value when measured in the early second trimester. Women having a Combined, serum Integrated or Integrated test should have PlGF measured in the first trimester and women having the Quadruple test need only have PlGF measured in the second trimester if the intention is to screen for pre-eclampsia as well as for Down syndrome.

Supporting Information

Appendix S1 PlGF probability plots and statistical parameters.

Acknowledgments

We thank PerkinElmer for providing the PlGF assay kits free of charge.

Author Contributions

Conceived and designed the experiments: NW. Performed the experiments: NW JB LG WH. Analyzed the data: NW JB. Wrote the paper: NW JB LG WH.

References

1. Akolekar R, Syngelaki A, Sarquis R, Zvanca M, Nicolaieds KH (2011) Prediction of early, intermediate and late pre-eclampsia from maternal factors, biophysical and biochemical markers at 11–13 weeks. Prenat Diagn 31: 66–74.
2. Wald NJ, Bestwick JP, George LM, Wu T, Morris JK (2012) Screening for pre-eclampsia using serum placental growth factor and endoglin measurement with Down's syndrome Quadruple test markers. J Med Screen 19: 60–67.
3. Koster MPH, Wortelboer EJ, Stoutenbeek P, Visser GHA, Schielen PCJI (2011) Modeling Down syndrome screening performance using first-trimester serum markers. Ultrasound Obstet Gynecol 38: 134–139.
4. Cowans NJ, Stamatopoulou A, Spencer K (2010) First trimester maternal serum placental growth factor in trisomy 21 pregnancies. Prenat Diagn 30: 449–453.
5. Zaragoza E, Akolekar R, Poon LCY, Pepes S, Nicolaides KH (2009) Maternal serum placental growth factor at 11–13 weeks in chromosomally abnormal pregnancies. Ultrasound Obstet Gynecol 33: 382–386.
6. Pandya P, Wright D, Syngelaki A, Akolekar R, Nicolaides KH (2012) Maternal serum placental growth factor in prospective screening for aneuploidies at 8–13 weeks' gestation. Fetal Diagn Ther 31: 87–93.
7. Spencer K, Liao AW, Ong CYT, Geerts L, Nicolaides KH (2001) First trimester maternal serum placenta growth factor (PlGF) concentrations in pregnancies with fetal trisomy 21 or trisomy 18. Prenat Diagn 21: 718–722.
8. Debieve F, Moiset A, Thomas K, Pampfer S, Hubinont C (2001) Vascular endothelial growth factor and placental growth factor concentrations in Down's syndrome and control pregnancies. Molecular Human Reproduction 7: 765–770.
9. Su YN, Hsu JJ, Lee CN, Cheng WF, Kung CCS, et al. (2002) Raised maternal serum placenta growth factor concentration during the second trimester is associated with Down syndrome. Prenat Diagn 22: 8–12.
10. Lambert-Messerlian GM, Canick JA (2004) Placenta growth factor levels in second-trimester maternal serum in Down syndrome pregnancy and in the prediction of preeclampsia. Prenat Diagn 24: 876–880.
11. Morris JK, Wald NJ (2005) Graphical presentation of distributions of risk in screening. J Med Screen 12: 155–160.
12. Wald NJ, Rodeck C, Hackshaw AK, Walters J, Chitty L, et al. (2003) First and Second trimester Antenatal screening for Down's syndrome: the results of the Serum, Urine and Ultrasound Screening Study (SURUSS). J Med Screen 10: 56–104.
13. Wald N, Rodeck C, Rudnicka A, Hackshaw A (2004) Nuchal translucency and gestational age. Prenat Diagn 24: 150–1.
14. Wald NJ, Rodeck C, Hackshaw AK, Walters J, Chitty L, et al. (2006B) Correction to the SURUSS report. J Med Screen 13: 51–52.
15. Bestwick JP, Huttly WJ, Wald NJ (2010) Distribution of nuchal translucency in antenatal screening for Down's syndrome. J Med Screen 17: 8–12.
16. Office for National Statistics 2008. Birth Statistics Series FM1 Numbers 35–37. HMSO: London, 2006, 2007, 2008.
17. Morris JK, Mutton DE, Alberman E (2002) Revised estimates of the maternal age specific live birth prevalence of Down's syndrome. J Med Screen 9: 2–6.
18. Morris JK, Wald NJ, Mutton DE, Alberman E (2003) Comparison of models of maternal age-specific risk for Down syndrome live births. Prenat Diagn 23: 252–8.
19. Morris JK, Wald NJ, Watt HC (1999) Fetal loss in Down syndrome pregnancies. Prenat Diagn 19: 142–145.

Healthy Growth in Children with Down Syndrome

Helma B. M. Van Gameren-Oosterom[1,2]*, Paula Van Dommelen[2], Anne Marie Oudesluys-Murphy[3], Simone E. Buitendijk[4], Stef Van Buuren[2,5], Jacobus P. Van Wouwe[1]

1 Department of Child Health, Netherlands Organization for Applied Scientific Research (TNO), Leiden, The Netherlands, **2** Department of Life Style, Netherlands Organization for Applied Scientific Research (TNO), Leiden, The Netherlands, **3** Department of Pediatrics, Leiden University Medical Centre, Leiden, The Netherlands, **4** Leiden University Medical Centre, Leiden, The Netherlands, **5** Department of Methodology and Statistics, FSS, University of Utrecht, Utrecht, The Netherlands

Abstract

Objective: To provide cross-sectional height and head circumference (HC) references for healthy Dutch children with Down syndrome (DS), while considering the influence of concomitant disorders on their growth, and to compare growth between children with DS and children from the general population.

Study design: Longitudinal growth and medical data were retrospectively collected from medical records in 25 of the 30 regional hospital-based outpatient clinics for children with DS in the Netherlands. Children with Trisomy 21 karyotype of Dutch descent born after 1982 were included. The LMS method was applied to fit growth references.

Results: We enrolled 1,596 children, and collected 10,558 measurements for height and 1,778 for HC. Children with DS without concomitant disorders (otherwise healthy children) and those suffering only from mild congenital heart defects showed similar growth patterns. The established growth charts, based on all measurements of these two groups, demonstrate the three age periods when height differences between children with and without DS increase: during pregnancy, during the first three years of life, and during puberty. This growth pattern results in a mean final height of 163.4 cm in boys and 151.8 cm in girls (−2.9 standard deviation (SD) and −3.0 SD on general Dutch charts, respectively). Mean HC (0 to 15 months) was 2 SD less than in the general Dutch population. The charts are available at www.tno.nl/growth.

Conclusions: Height and HC references showed that growth retardation in otherwise healthy children with DS meanly occurs in three critical periods of growth, resulting in shorter final stature and smaller HC than the general Dutch population shows. With these references, health care professionals can optimize their preventive care: monitoring growth of individual children with DS optimal, so that growth retarding comorbidities can be identified early, and focusing on the critical age periods to establish ways to optimize growth.

Editor: Stephen D. Ginsberg, Nathan Kline Institute and New York University School of Medicine, United States of America

Funding: The study is financially supported by grant 150020031 from the Netherlands Organization for Health Research and Development (ZonMw) and by the Tamarinde foundation (Stichting Tamarinde). An additional funding is received for open access publication from the Netherlands Organisation for Scientific Research (NWO). The funders had no role in study design, data collection and analysis, decision to publish, or preparation of the maunscript.

Competing Interests: The authors have declared that no competing interests exist.

* E-mail: helma.vangameren@tno.nl

Introduction

Appropriate, up-to-date growth charts are necessary for evaluation of physical growth and provision of optimal health care. The World Health Organization has produced a global standard chart describing how children, under optimal conditions, grow worldwide. [1] This is based on the idea that all humans are more or less equal. Health care workers, on the other hand, often wish to use growth charts of a well defined reference group closely related to the subpopulation they serve, since these charts provide a more accurate evaluation for an individual child. [2] Growth charts are available for various ethnic groups at specific moments in time. [3,4] Specific growth references have also been developed for children with various disorders known to interfere with growth, such as Turner and Down syndrome (DS). [5–9] Since growth assessment depends on the growth pattern characteristic for these conditions, disorder specific charts are desirable. Growth references for American children with DS have been constructed making it possible to accurately identify concomitant disorders known to influence growth. [6] Growth charts for Dutch children with DS were first published in 1996: they are shorter than children in the general Dutch population, but taller than their US peers with DS. [8]

In order to take the secular trend into account, growth references for height and head circumference (HC) need to be updated regularly. [3] Children with DS are at high risk of many disorders known to influence growth. Such disorders are generally regarded as exclusion criteria in growth studies: all children diagnosed with growth disorders or on medication known to interfere with growth are usually excluded. [3] However, in studies on growth in children with DS such exclusion criteria are usually not applied. [5–8,10] Only two recent growth studies in children with DS (in Japan and in the UK and Ireland) excluded children with various diagnoses known to affect growth. [11,12] In addition, no previous studies have investigated in which particular age periods height growth in otherwise healthy children with DS is relatively most delayed, by comparing their growth with that of healthy controls from the general population.

Therefore, the aim of the present study is to provide updated height and new HC growth references by a large nationwide sample, reflecting healthy growth in Dutch children with DS, and to compare their growth pattern with data from a recent nationwide study among children from the general Dutch population with focus on periods during which relative height differences increases. We think it is essential to establish new growth references for children with DS in the Netherlands, whereby a strict selection on their health status will be applied. Only with such references health care professionals can monitor growth of individual children with DS optimally, and can identify growth retarding comorbidities at an early stage.

Methods

Data source

To collect representative nationwide data, all specialized regional pediatric outpatient clinics for children with DS in the Netherlands were approached (n = 30). These hospital-based clinics provide standard medical care for children with DS, according to the guideline of the Pediatric Association of the Netherlands. [13] All children with DS, who live in the service area of these clinics, are eligible to participate in this standard care by specialized pediatricians that includes screening for congenital cardiac defects, thyroid dysfunction, celiac disease, hearing and visual disorders as well as motor development and growth monitoring. Youth health care physicians working in special education and looking after older children with DS were also approached. Names of all participating clinics, pediatricians and youth health care physicians are mentioned in the acknowledgement.

At the clinics all data were retrospectively collected from medical records, between July 2009 and February 2010, by the first author, who is a trained physician. The de-identification was also completed by the first author, using study numbers. Additional data from the youth health care physicians caring for older children with DS in special education were collected by completing standard forms. All measurements were carried out according to protocol. [14] Height was measured using a recumbent length device or a stadiometer and HC by using a measuring tape (fiberglass or other non-expanding material). Data concerning medical conditions and treatment of each subject, and specifically those conditions known to interfere with growth, were gathered from medical records, as well as specific background information. Children were considered to be of Dutch descent if both parents were born in the Netherlands, as reported in the medical records. If medical or background information was not available, subjects were excluded.

Inclusion/exclusion

Children with Trisomy 21 karyotype were selected, and those with DS caused by mozaïcisme or translocation were excluded (verified by karyotype). All children born after 1982 were included (aged up to 26 years). We collected semi-longitudinal data on growth over the previous 10 years, recording data from 2000 onwards. We selected only the first recorded observation per interval: from an infant (age of 0 to 1 year old) one observation in each month, from a toddler (age 1 to 3 years old) one observation in each three months period, and one observation in each six months in childhood and adolescence (age up to 26 years old). Measurements of HC were selected only from full-term children (born ≥37 weeks gestation) up to the age of 5 year. If gestational age was not specifically mentioned, children were considered to be born at term.

Health status

The children were categorized according to their health status in 4 groups: healthy, with only mild CHD, with only severe CHD or with other (multiple) concomitant disorders. Table 1 describes the characteristics of the various health categories and details of the criteria used for these categories.

Permission of an Ethical Committee or informed consent is not obtained, as not required in the Netherlands for this type of study or data collection, since the data were analyzed anonymously.

Statistical Analysis

Data cleansing was performed by excluding duplicate cases and outliers. Duplicate cases have arisen when children were seen at

Table 1. Characteristics of the various health categories in the study population of children with Down syndrome.

Healthy
Children without concomitant disorders that could possibly interfere with growth
Children were negatively screened for CHD, celiac disease and hypothyroidism
For example: children with cataract were included and children with musculoskeletal disorders were excluded
Mild CHD
Children with CHD not needing surgical intervention or medication and without pulmonary vascular disease
For example: children with an atrial septal defect or patent foramen ovale without complaints
Severe CHD
Children with CHD needing surgical intervention, medication, or with pulmonary vascular disease
For example: children with an atrioventricular septal defect or Tetralogy of Fallot
Other disorders
Children with other disorders and treatments known to interfere with growth, and children with multiple concomitant disorders
For example: children positively screened for hypothyroidism or celiac disease, children with congenital gastrointestinal disorders, children on anti-epileptic medication or corticosteroids (including inhalation medication)

Abbreviation: CHD – congenital heart defect.

multiple centers and were identified by comparing sex, date of birth and background information such as nationality, and medical condition. Outliers were defined using height and HC standardized by age and sex according to the reference charts of the general Dutch population, calculated in standard deviation scores (SDS). [3] Cutoff values >2 or <−6 for height SDS and HC SDS were used. If a child had one measurement outside the cutoff values, all measurements of this child were excluded. Moreover, the longitudinal growth pattern of each subject was checked by plotting them and excluding values outlying the plot. Data were analyzed separately for boys and girls.

The difference in mean height SDS and HC SDS between healthy children with DS and children with DS and a mild or severe CHD were tested by linear mixed-effects models. To correct for possible differences in the prevalence rates of sex and mean age, we adjusted these analyses by age and sex. Furthermore, growth references for boys and girls with DS were fitted for body height by age (range 0 to 21 years) and HC by age (range 0 to 15 months) using the LMS method. Growth references were fitted in R Version 2.9.0 using Generalized Additive Models for Location Scale and Shape (GAMLSS). [15] The LMS method summarizes the distribution by three age-dependent smooth curves representing skewness (L curve), median (M curve) and coefficient of variation (S curve). [16] The LMS method is based on the principle that after a transformation the data have to follow a standard normal distribution. The following transformations of age were tested to expand the ages where growth velocity is high and compress age where growth velocity is low: the age transformation proposed by Cole, a square root transformation, a log transformation and a cube root transformation. [17] Worm plots were used as a diagnostic tool to visualize the fit to the data. [18] These plots check the residuals for different age levels and indentify locations at which the fit can be improved. We fitted charts with lines of the −2.5, −2.0,−1.0, 0, 1.0, 2.0 and 2.5 SD (corresponding with 0.6, 2.3, 15.9, 50, 84.1, 97.7 and 99.4 percentile). The choice of these SD-lines is in agreement with the latest reference charts for the general Dutch population. We did not fit growth charts for the health category 'other disorders', because of the wide variety of data and medical conditions of the children in this category. Also, growth charts for subgroups in this category – like children with hypothyroidism or celiac disease – were not fitted, because of the small number of children included in our study.

In addition to the reference charts for height, formulas for Target Height (TH) for children with DS were calculated. [19] The TH was calculated by the method of Hermanussen and Cole, which takes into account two correlations (assortative mating r(P,P) and the parent-offspring correlation r(P,O)). [20] For this calculation, the data from three nationwide sources have been applied. The correlations were obtained from the latest growth study in the general Dutch population (2009) and were r(P,P) = 0.19 and r(P,O) = 0.58. [21] The calculation for the paternal and maternal height SD was based on the results from the previous national growth study (1997); final height of children measured in this study corresponds with final height of this generation of parents. [3] For the calculation of the TH SDS the mean and SD of final height of the children with DS observed in this study were used.

The established growth references for height and HC were compared with the most recent reference charts for the general Dutch population, by calculating SDS. [21]

Results

Pediatricians working in 25 hospital-based clinics (83% of all Dutch DS clinics) and 14 youth health care physicians caring for older children with DS in special education agreed to participate in this study. After exclusion of 7 children with a growth pattern outside the cut-off values, a total of 1,843 children with Trisomy 21 were indentified. Of these, 1,596 are of Dutch origin: 891 boys (55.8%) and 705 girls (44.2%). The sample provided 10,558 measurements for height and 1,778 for HC in the age range 0 to 5 years and born at term (418 HC measurements from children born pre-term in this age range were excluded). Of all height measurements, 98% were derived from the DS clinics and 2% from the youth health care physicians in special education. The HC measurements were only derived from the DS clinics. Table 2 provides total number of subjects and measurements of height and HC, split according to sex and to various health categories. In our sample, 26.6% was categorized as healthy, 15.0% had only a mild CHD and 16.9% only a severe CHD. The remaining group, 41.5%, was categorized as having various other disorders; most of them (over 60%) had multiple concomitant disorders.

Growth of children with DS within various health categories

Growth of healthy children with DS and those who suffer from mild CHD showed no difference in mean height SDS (p = 0.832) and HC SDS (p = 0.790). Both girls and boys with DS and severe CHD had significant lower mean height SDS and HC SDS compared to healthy children with DS or children with DS with mild CHD (both p-values<0.001). Mean height is observed to be 0.4 SD lower. This growth retardation arises in the first year of life; during childhood no further deflection neither catch-up growth was observed.

Growth references

Data for growth references of height and HC were derived by combining the groups of healthy children with DS and children with DS and mild CHD (664 children for height, and 223 for HC (see Table 2). The number of measurements of these selected groups, arranged by age en sex, are shown in Table 3. By fitting the growth references for height, the cube root transformation of age showed the best fit and was selected. Table 4 summarizes mean height and SD, arranged by age and sex. Mean birth length was 48.9 cm in boys and 48.4 cm in girls with DS. Mean final height was 163.4 cm in boys and 151.8 cm in girls. These new reference charts are available at www.tno.nl/growthhttp://www.tno.nl/growth.

Table 2. Number of subjects and measurements for height and head circumference of 1,596 Dutch subjects with Trisomy 21, specified by the health categories.

	Subjects				Measurements			
	Height		HC[1]		Height		HC	
Health category	Boys	Girls	Boys	Girls	Boys	Girls	Boys	Girls
Healthy	257	167	71	57	1,378	938	202	139
Mild CHD	130	110	49	46	751	661	169	147
Severe CHD	114	155	38	50	738	997	134	187
Other disorders	390	273	140	88	2,970	2,125	443	357
Total	891	705	298	241	5,837	4,721	948	830

Abbreviations: HC – head circumference, CHD – congenital heart defect.
[1]Only children born full-term up to the age of 5 years were included.

Table 3. Frequencies of measurements for height used for plotting the reference curves for Dutch children with Down syndrome, arranged by age and sex.

	Height[1]		
Age (years)	Male	Female	Total
0	474	392	866
1	241	201	442
2	201	147	348
3	178	129	307
4	151	101	252
5	132	96	228
6	117	86	203
7	83	89	172
8	105	66	171
9	86	49	135
10	72	52	124
11	62	46	108
12	68	37	105
13	52	29	81
14	36	28	64
15	31	12	43
16	20	14	34
17	8	6	14
≥18	12	19	31
Total	2129	1599	3728
	Head circumference[2]		
Age (years)	**Male**	**Female**	**Total**
0	244	199	443
1	69	50	119
2	22	18	40
3	19	10	29
4	17	9	26
Total	371	286	657

[1]Height measurements of the children categorized as healthy or with only mild CHD (n = 664).
[2]Head circumference of the children categorized as healthy or with only mild CHD, born at term (n = 223).

Table 4. Mean height (cm) and standard deviation (SD) of the new references for length/height of Dutch children with Down syndrome, arranged by age and sex.

	Boys		Girls	
Age (weeks)	Mean	SD*	Mean	SD*
0	48.9	2.5	48.4	2.1
2	50.4	2.6	49.8	2.2
4	51.9	2.6	51.3	2.2
6	53.4	2.6	52.6	2.2
8	54.8	2.6	54.0	2.2
10	56.2	2.6	55.3	2.2
12	57.5	2.6	56.5	2.3
16	60.0	2.6	58.7	2.3
20	62.2	2.6	60.7	2.3
24	64.1	2.7	62.6	2.4
28	65.8	2.7	64.2	2.4
32	67.3	2.7	65.7	2.4
36	68.6	2.7	67.0	2.5
40	69.8	2.7	68.2	2.5
44	70.9	2.8	69.3	2.5
48	71.9	2.8	70.3	2.6
52	73.0	2.8	71.3	2.6
Age (years)				
1.5	78.3	3.0	76.4	2.8
2.0	82.6	3.1	80.8	3.0
2.5	86.4	3.3	84.6	3.2
3.0	89.8	3.5	88.1	3.5
3.5	93.1	3.7	91.6	3.7
4.0	96.4	3.9	95.2	3.9
4.5	99.7	4.0	98.6	4.1
5.0	102.9	4.2	101.7	4.3
6.0	109.0	4.5	107.2	4.6
7.0	114.7	4.8	113.0	4.9
8.0	119.9	5.0	118.7	5.2
9.0	125.2	5.3	124.0	5.5
10.0	130.8	5.5	129.3	5.8
11.0	136.8	5.7	134.4	6.1
12.0	142.9	5.8	139.1	6.3
13.0	148.7	5.9	142.9	6.5
14.0	153.5	6.0	145.9	6.6
15.0	157.2	6.1	147.9	6.8
16.0	159.8	6.2	149.4	6.9
17.0	161.8	6.2	150.5	7.0
18.0	163.0	6.2	151.2	7.1
19.0	163.4	6.2	151.6	7.2
20.0	163.4	6.2	151.8	7.3
21.0	163.4	6.2	151.8	7.3

*Individual height SDS can be calculated by: SDS = (height (cm) − mean height (cm))/SD (cm).
Abbreviations: SD – standard deviation, SDS – standard deviation score.

Growth references for HC were established for up to the age of 15 months. We did not have enough measurements to construct growth references after the age of 15 months. By fitting HC references for boys no transformation of age and for girls the age transformation proposed by Cole was applied. [17] Table 5 summarizes the LMS-values, arranged by age and sex. At birth mean HC was 33.8 cm in boys and 32.9 cm in girls with DS; at the age of 15 months this was 45.0 cm and 43.7 cm respectively.

Target Height

The calculated formulas for TH of children with DS are:

$$\text{TH boys DS(cm)} = 41.8 + 0.328 \times (\text{paternal height}) + 0.359 \times (\text{maternal height})$$

Table 5. New head circumference (cm) references for 0–15 months in Dutch children with Down syndrome: values of L (skewness), M (median), and S (coefficient of variation)*, categorized by age and sex.

	Boys			Girls		
Age (weeks)	L	M	S*	L	M	S*
0	2.96	33.8	.0349	1	32.9	.0267
2	2.65	34.6	.0343	1	33.8	.0272
4	2.34	35.3	.0336	1	34.7	.0277
6	2.03	36.1	.0330	1	35.5	.0280
8	1.72	36.8	.0324	1	36.4	.0281
10	1.42	37.5	.0319	1	37.1	.0279
12	1.12	38.2	.0313	1	37.8	.0276
16	0.54	39.4	.0302	1	38.8	.0270
20	−0.01	40.4	.0292	1	39.7	.0265
24	−0.52	41.2	.0283	1	40.4	.0261
28	−0.99	42.0	.0274	1	41.0	.0259
32	−1.41	42.6	.0266	1	41.5	.0257
36	−1.80	43.1	.0258	1	42.0	.0255
40	−2.14	43.5	.0250	1	42.3	.0254
44	−2.45	43.9	.0243	1	42.7	.0252
48	−2.72	44.2	.0237	1	42.9	.0251
52	−2.97	44.4	.0231	1	43.2	.0249
56	−3.19	44.6	.0225	1	43.3	.0248
60	−3.40	44.8	.0221	1	43.5	.0247
65[a]	−3.64	45.0	.0216	1	43.7	.0245

[a]Corresponding with 15 months.
*Individual head circumference SDS can be calculated by: $SDS = \{(\text{height (cm)}/M)^L - 1\}/L*S$, $L \neq 0$ (if $L = 0$: $SDS = \ln(\text{height (cm)}/M)/S$).

$$\text{TH SDS boys DS(SD)} = (\text{TH boys DS} - 163.4)/6.2$$

$$\text{TH girls DS(cm)} = 8.64 + 0.387 \times (\text{paternal height}) + 0.422 \times (\text{maternal height})$$

$$\text{TH SDS girls DS(SD)} = (\text{TH girl DS} - 151.8)/7.3.$$

Comparison to the general Dutch population

In comparison with the currently used reference charts for the general Dutch population, a markedly shorter stature was found in children with DS. [21] Mean height revealed a deflection in the first 3 years of life from −1.1 SD at birth to −2.2 SD at 3 years, for boys as well as girls. During the age interval of 3 to 12 years average growth remained stable at −2.2 SD, and deflected again during puberty to a final height at −2.9 SD (20.4 cm shorter) for boys and −3.0 SD (18.9 cm shorter) for girls (Figure 1). [21] For HC, between birth and 15 months, mean values for boys and girls with DS are on average 1.8 SD lower (range −1.3 to −2.0) compared to the general Dutch population. [3]

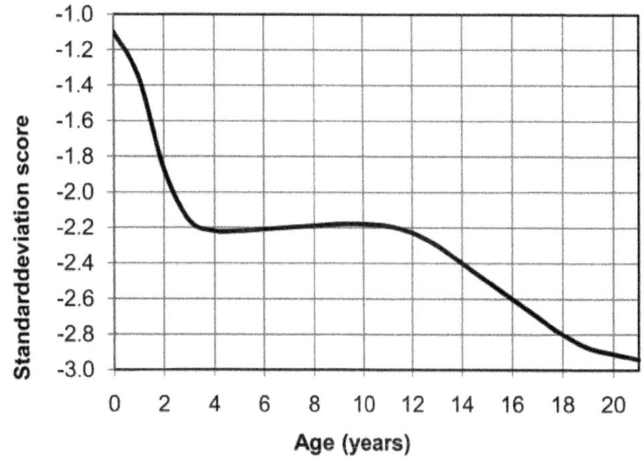

Figure 1. Mean height (SDS) of the Dutch children with Down syndrome compared to the general population. Comparison is made to the mean height of the national Dutch growth study (2009), calculated in standard deviation score (SDS).

Discussion

This study yields new charts of healthy growth of children with DS. Growth patterns were analyzed in 1,596 Dutch children with DS, with 10,558 height measurements and 1,778 HC measurements. All children were selected nationwide from pediatric hospital-based outpatient clinics specialized in the standard care of children with DS. Selection based on health complaints or influenced by financial restrictions was avoided, since all children with DS in the Netherlands were invited to avail of this care without financial barriers, as encouraged by the Dutch Down Syndrome Foundation (largest Dutch parent supporting organization). The result is a nationwide representative sample.

Our new reference charts for Dutch children with DS are unique. No previous studies on growth in DS made such a stringent selection of subjects with respect to their health. All children have received high quality medical care according to the guideline of the Pediatric Association of the Netherlands and underwent standard screening at regular intervals, provided by the regional hospital-based outpatient clinics for children with DS. [13] This screening programme provided confidence that children categorized as healthy in fact have no undiagnosed concomitant disorders, such as hypothyroidism, mild CHD and celiac disease. To illustrate the stringent selection: children with positive screening results for hypothyroidism and celiac disease were excluded (even though appropriate treatment was started early), because there is no evidence that growth could not be affected already.

The children with severe CHD showed growth retardation during the first year of life. After this period they had growth velocities similar to the healthy children with DS. In the Netherlands the surgical correction of significant CHD takes place preferably at the age of 2–4 months. [22] This early treatment may result in normal growth after the age of 1 year without further deflection. Cronk et al.also described growth retardation caused by CHD in children with DS. [6] However, they were unable to evaluate the effects of different types of cardiac lesions (those which healed spontaneously or those treated by corrective surgery) on growth. The present study provided appropriate data to make this distinction.

When comparing mean final heights of children with DS with other countries, we should take into account the different inclusion and exclusion criteria (Table 6). However, it is probably reasonable to conclude that Dutch children with DS are relatively tall among children with DS. Growth charts are available for West-European children with DS in Sweden, the UK and Ireland, and Northeastern France. [5,12,23]

Our study is the first to propose formulas to estimate the expected final height in children with DS. The TH formulas were derived under the assumption that the correlation between mid parental height SD and child height SD in Dutch children with DS is identical to the general Dutch population. Further research is needed to investigate whether this assumption is justified.

We compare HC in our population with values published by others. Reference charts for HC are also available for children with DS from Sweden, Northeastern France, Sicily, UK and Ireland, the USA, Egypt and Saudi Arabia, suitable for use in these countries. [5,10,12,23–26] Benefits of our study are the LMS-values presented, whereby for each individual the deviation exactly can be calculated. Comparing HC showed the Swedish children with DS have an average HC of 33 cm at birth, similar to our children with DS. [5] This mean values at birth corresponds with −0.5 SD on the reference charts for the general Swedish population, however with −1.5 SD for the general Dutch population. At 15 months mean HC is also identical in Swedish and Dutch children with DS. Since the other studies do not present enough details of their observations, we were unable to make further comparisons.

What are the main differences in growth pattern between DS and the general population? Mean birth length in DS is 1 SD lower than in the general population, indicating that children with DS already show retarded growth during pregnancy. Also, during the first three years of life they grow slower compared to the general population; the gap stays relatively constant during the age interval 3–12 years. After the age of 12 year a further deflection in growth is observed. This pattern is observed to be the same in boys and girls with DS. The mentioned three periods are already described by Karlberg et al. in the infant-childhood-puberty (ICP) model, which described during infancy (from birth up to about 3 years of age) and during puberty higher growth velocity than during childhood. [27] So, the children with DS show growth retardation just during the critical periods of growth when the highest growth velocity occurs. This finding indicate the age periods in which further health benefit may be obtained. Health care professionals should focus on these critical periods when providing preventive care to children with DS with the aim to establish ways to optimize growth during these specific periods. Either the observed growth retardation may be due to their genetic makeup or it may be caused by physical problems they encounter, such as feeding problems. In puberty an early or short growth spurt also limits final growth. Further research is needed to explain our observations and to provide physiological clarification on the nature of this growth retardation. All in all, these effects result in a substantial difference in final height (boys: 20.4 cm; girls: 18.9 cm).

Body weight will be reported separately. Because of the current increase in the proportion of children with obesity, it is not desirable to reflect the present distribution of weight in this population. Therefore, the increase in the proportion of children with obesity and the need for normative charts for weight deserve special attention. [21,28]

A limitation of our study is that the measurements of height and HC were retrospectively collected. This methodology may lead to more variation in the measurements compared to studies that used prospectively collected data, as all general Dutch growth studies did. We were however unable to detect such increased measurement variability in the data. The S-curves (which model the coefficient of variation) were quite similar in our growth charts and the charts of the general Dutch population (established in 2009). So, we do not expect that the used methodology had an impact on the variability in the growth charts. A benefit of the applied methodology is the larger and timelier data set. Similar methods were used in other growth studies in children with DS. [5,12,23]

The longitudinal data resulted in a varied number of measurements per child. To determine the possible influence of this variation, the statistical analyses were repeated where data points were weighted – whereby a weighting factor was calculated as the inverse of the number of measurements per child – in order to prevent over-representing children with a large number of measurements. This solution was almost the same as the unweighted analysis; differences in mean height were smaller than 0.1 SD.

For the interpretation of individual growth curves plotted on a reference chart, criteria are needed to define abnormal growth. No specific criteria for the charts for children with DS have been proposed. The utility of the referral criteria for the general Dutch population as presented in the guideline 'Detection and referral criteria in short stature' has not been tested for growth in children with DS. Further research is necessary to see whether such referral criteria are equally suitable for children with DS. [29,30] For the moment, we tentatively suggest to use the criteria for the general population (which are all framed in SDS) for children with DS.

Implications

The availability of appropriate up-to-date growth charts, that reflect healthy growth of height and HC in Dutch children with DS, will potentially improve the medical care they receive. Using

Table 6. Growth studies presenting mean final height (cm) of children with Down syndrome, with the applied inclusion and exclusion criteria, by country of origin.

		Inclusion	Exclusion criteria	Boys	Girls
The Netherlands	This study	T21	All concomitant disorders known to interfere with growth; separate analyses of mild and severe CHD	163.4	151.8
Sweden [5]	2002	DS	Treatment with growth hormone	161.5	147.5
UK, Ireland [12]	2002	DS	Coexistent major pathology such as severe CHD or preterm birth	157	146
Japan [11]	2003	T21	Complications that might affect natural growth	153.2	141.9
France [23]	1999	T21	Severe CHD	154	140
USA [6]	1988	T21	Separate analyses of moderate and severe CHD (if information is available)	153	146

Abbreviations: T21 – Trisomy 21, DS – Down syndrome (including DS caused by Trisomy 21, mozaïcisme or translocation), CHD – congenital heart defect.

these charts secondary growth abnormalities may be detected more accurately. For example, limited growth of height may be a symptom of hypothyroidism and a relative large HC may be caused by hydrocephalus. The charts were based on a large sample that is stringently selected on the basis of their health status, and therefore we will encourage research to investigate the suitability of these charts for international application.

In children with DS with severe CHD growth is decelerated during the first year of life, in comparison to reference growth in the healthy infants with DS. During childhood no catch-up growth is noticed in these children with DS and severe CHD, neither does their growth decline further. Future research should focus on the exact qualities of the observed deflections in growth of otherwise healthy children with DS: is their growth spurt restricted with a lower velocity or do other phenomena play a role. Lack of significant catch up growth in children with DS and severe CHD could be the result of similar failure to spurt. We can only hypothesis on the full nature of growth retardation in otherwise healthy children with DS: as their growth is primarily restricted by Trisomy 21 the mechanism is unknown. Is it primarily metabolic, hormonal or chondrocyte dysfunction? Or could it be explained by further advanced genome-wide analysis?

Conclusions

Growth patterns in otherwise healthy Dutch children with DS were established based on data from a large nationwide population. Growth in healthy children with DS differ from children with DS and severe CHD (0.4 SD). The established growth charts demonstrate the three age periods when height differences between children with and without DS increase: during pregnancy, during the first three years of life, and during puberty. This growth pattern results in a mean final height of 163.4 cm in healthy boys with DS and 151.8 in girls (a difference of 3 SD in comparison to the general population), and mean HC at birth of 33 cm and 44 cm at the age of 15 months (almost 2 SD less than in the general Dutch population). All in all, with these new growth charts, that reflect healthy growth in children with DS, health care professionals can monitor growth of individual children with DS optimal. In this way, early identification of growth retarding comorbidities will be enabled and ultimately the health of children with DS will be improved.

Acknowledgments

The following pediatricians (most on behalf of the Down Syndrome Medical Interest Group of the Pediatric Association of the Netherlands) are thanked for their co-operation in providing their data: C.D. Aarts-Tesselaar, MD (Amphia Ziekenhuis, Breda); A.J.I.W. Bergman-van Emous, MD (Ziekenhuis Rivierenland, Tiel); L.A. Bok, MD (Maxima Medisch Centrum, Veldhoven); W.E.A. Bolz, MD, PhD (Elkerliek Ziekenhuis, Helmond); M.E. Doornbos, MD (Albert Schweitzer Ziekenhuis, Sliedrecht); S.E. Elkerbout, MD (Rijnland Ziekenhuis, Leiderdorp); W. Goudsmit-Meijer, MD (BovenIJ Ziekenhuis, Amsterdam); A.A.M. Haagen, MD (VieCuri Medisch Centrum, Venlo); J.N. Jansen, MD (Lievensberg Ziekenhuis, Bergen op Zoom); G.J.M. Janssen, MD (Maasziekenhuis Pantein, Boxmeer); A.C.M. van Kessel, MD (Diaconessenhuis, Meppel); E.S.T. Knots, MD (Catharina Ziekenhuis, Eindhoven); E.H.G. van Leer, MD, PhD (Groene Hart Ziekenhuis, Gouda); S.A. de Man, MD, PhD (Amphia Ziekenhuis, Breda); K.M.E.J. Oberndorff, MD (Orbis Medisch Centrum, Sittard-Geleen); J. Potjewijd, MD (Diaconessenhuis, Meppel); W.P.M. Rijnvos, MD (TweeSteden Ziekenhuis, Tilburg); H.G.H. Thijs, MD (Gelre Ziekenhuizen, Zutphen); A.J.C.M. van der Velden, MD (Franciscus Ziekenhuis, Roosendaal); E. de Vries, MD, PhD (Jeroen Bosch Ziekenhuis, 's Hertogenbosch); M.E. Weijerman, MD (VU Medisch Centrum, Amsterdam); A.M. van Wermeskerken, MD (Flevoziekenhuis, Almere); H. Van Wieringen, MD (St. Antonius Ziekenhuis, Utrecht); J.P. de Winter, MD, PhD (Spaarne Ziekenhuis, Hoofddorp); I.I.C. Wymenga, MD (Martini Ziekenhuis, Groningen); P.H.T. van Zwieten, MD (HagaZiekenhuis, Juliana Kinderziekenhuis, Den Haag). Also the physicians for Intellectually Disability Medicine were thanked for providing data: A.M.W. Coppus, MD (Elkerliek Ziekenhuis, Deurne) and P.T.H. Vos, MD (Jeroen Bosch Ziekenhuis, Boxtel).

The following youth health care physicians, caring for children in special education are also thanked for their co-operation in providing data: H.A.G. van Domselaar-Renting, MD (GGD Gelre-IJssel); P.J.G.A.M. van Eeden, MD (GGD Zuid-Holland Zuid); V.J.J.M. Gijsen-Mol, MD (GGD Zuid Limburg); A. Goessen-Ickenroth, MD (GGD Zuid Limburg); M.W.G. Govaerts, MD (GGD Zuid Limburg); E. van Hoorn, MD (GGD Zaanstreek-Waterland); M.A.J. van Keulen, MD (GGD IJsselland); J. Lemij-Van Egmond, MD (GGD Hollands Midden); N.P. Meester, MD (GGD Zuid-Holland West); W.M. Nagelsmit, MD (GGD Kennemerland); I.T. Schramel, MD (GGD Midden Nederland); A.A.M. Sluiter-Van Nies, MD (GGD Gelre-IJssel); M.E.T. van Strien-Leloux, MD (GGD Kennemerland); M.G.A. van der Voort-Van Soest, MD (GGD Zuid Limburg).

Author Contributions

Conceived and designed the experiments: HVGO PVD JVW. Performed the experiments: HVGO. Analyzed the data: HVGO PVD. Contributed reagents/materials/analysis tools: PVD SVB. Wrote the paper: HVGO PVD AMOM SEB SVB JVW.

References

1. World Health Organization (WHO) Multicentre Growth Reference Study Group (2006) WHO Child Growth Standards based on lenght/height, weight and age. Acta Paediatr 450: 76–85.
2. van Buuren S, Van Wouwe JP (2008) WHO Child Growth Standards in action. Arch Dis Child 93: 549–551.
3. Fredriks AM, van Buuren S, Burgmeijer RJ, Meulmeester JF, Beuker RJ, et al. (2000) Continuing positive secular growth change in The Netherlands 1955–1997. Pediatr Res 47: 316–323.
4. Fredriks AM, van Buuren S, Jeurissen SE, Dekker FW, Verloove-Vanhorick SP, et al. (2004) Height, weight, body mass index and pubertal development references for children of Moroccan origin in The Netherlands. Acta Paediatr 93: 817–824.
5. Myrelid A, Gustafsson J, Ollars B, Anneren G (2002) Growth charts for Down's syndrome from birth to 18 years of age. Arch Dis Child 87: 97–103.
6. Cronk C, Crocker AC, Pueschel SM, Shea AM, Zackai E, et al. (1988) Growth charts for children with Down syndrome: 1 month to 18 years of age. Pediatrics 81: 102–110.
7. Cronk CE (1978) Growth of children with Down's syndrome: birth to age 3 years. Pediatrics 61: 564–568.
8. Cremers MJ, van de Tweel I, Boersma B, Wit JM, Zonderland M (1996) Growth curves of Dutch children with Down's syndrome. J Intellect Disabil Res 40(Pt 5): 412–420.
9. Lyon AJ, Preece MA, Grant DB (1985) Growth curve for girls with Turner syndrome. Arch Dis Child 60: 932–935.
10. Meguid NA, El-Kotoury AI, bdel-Salam GM, El-Ruby MO, Afifi HH (2004) Growth charts of Egyptian children with Down syndrome (0–36 months). East Mediterr Health J 10: 106–115.
11. Kimura J, Tachibana K, Imaizumi K, Kurosawa K, Kuroki Y (2003) Longitudinal growth and height velocity of Japanese children with Down's syndrome. Acta Paediatr 92: 1039–1042.
12. Styles ME, Cole TJ, Dennis J, Preece MA (2002) New cross sectional stature, weight, and head circumference references for Down's syndrome in the UK and Republic of Ireland. Arch Dis Child 87: 104–108.
13. Van Wouwe JP, Siderius EJ, Borstlap R, Nijenhuis TA, Hirasing RA (2001) [Optimal medical care for children with Down syndrome and their parents]. Ned Tijdschr Geneeskd 145: 1617–1621.
14. Fredriks AM, Buuren van S, Burgmeijer RJF, Verloove-Vanhorick SP, Wit JM (2002) [Growth charts. Manual to measure and weigh children and recording of growth charts]. Leiden: TNO/LUMC.
15. Rigby RA, Stasinopoulos DM (2005) Generalized additive models for location, scale and shape. Appl Statist 54: 507–554.
16. Cole TJ, Green PJ (1992) Smoothing reference centile curves: the LMS method and penalized likelihood. Stat Med 11: 1305–1319.
17. Cole TJ, Freeman JV, Preece MA (1998) British 1990 growth reference centiles for weight, height, body mass index and head circumference fitted by maximum penalized likelihood. Stat Med 17: 407–429.
18. Buuren van S, Fredriks M (2001) Worm plot: a simple diagnostic device for modelling growth reference curves. Stat Med 20: 1259–1277.

19. Dommelen van P, Schonbeck Y, Buuren van S (2011) A simple calculation of the target height. Arch Dis Child doi:10.1136/archdischild-2011-301095.
20. Hermanussen M, Cole J (2003) The calculation of target height reconsidered. Horm Res 59: 180–183.
21. Talma H, Schönbeck Y, Bakker B, Hirasing RA, Buuren van S (2010) [Growth charts 2010: manual to measure and weigh children and recording of growth charts]. Leiden: TNO, Quality of Life.
22. Weijerman ME, de Winter JP (2010) Clinical practice. The care of children with Down syndrome. Eur J Pediatr 169: 1445–1452.
23. Toledo C, Alembik Y, Aguirre JA, Stoll C (1999) Growth curves of children with Down syndrome. Ann Genet 42: 81–90.
24. Piro E, Pennino C, Cammarata M, Corsello G, Grenci A, et al. (1990) Growth charts of Down syndrome in Sicily: evaluation of 382 children 0–14 years of age. Am J Med Genet Suppl 7: 66–70.
25. Palmer CG, Cronk C, Pueschel SM, Wisniewski KE, Laxova R, et al. (1992) Head circumference of children with Down syndrome (0–36 months). Am J Med Genet 42: 61–67. 10.1002/ajmg.1320420114 [doi].
26. Al Husain M (2003) Growth charts for children with Down's syndrome in Saudi Arabia: birth to 5 years. Int J Clin Pract 57: 170–174.
27. Karlberg J (1987) On the modelling of human growth. Stat Med 6: 185–192.
28. Cole TJ, Roede MJ (1999) Centiles of body mass index for Dutch children aged 0–20 years in 1980- a baseline to assess recent trends in obesity. Ann Hum Biol 26: 303–308.
29. Grote FK, van Dommelen P, Oostdijk W, de Muinck Keizer-Schrama SM, Verkerk PH, et al. (2008) Developing evidence-based guidelines for referral for short stature. Arch Dis Child 93: 212–217.
30. Kamphuis M, Heerdink-Obenhuijsen N, Dommelen van P, Buuren van S, Verkerk PH (2010) [Guideline: Detection and referral criteria in short stature]. Ned Tijdschr Geneeskd 154: A2366.

Altered Expression of Immune-Related Genes in Children with Down Syndrome

Bruna Lancia Zampieri[1], Joice Matos Biselli-Périco[1], Jorge Estefano Santana de Souza[2,3,4], Matheus Carvalho Bürger[2,3,4], Wilson Araújo Silva Júnior[2,4], Eny Maria Goloni-Bertollo[1], Érika Cristina Pavarino[1]*

1 Unidade de Pesquisa em Genética e Biologia Molecular, Departamento de Biologia Molecular, Faculdade de Medicina de São José do Rio Preto (FAMERP), São José do Rio Preto, São Paulo, Brazil, **2** Department of Genetics and, Ribeirão Preto Medical School University of São Paulo, São Paulo, Brazil, **3** Institute of Bioinformatics and Biotechnology (2bio), São Paulo, Brazil, **4** National Institute of Science and Technology in Stem Cell and Cell Therapy and Center For Cell Based Therapy, Ribeirao Preto, São Paulo, Brazil

Abstract

Individuals with Down syndrome (DS) have a high incidence of immunological alterations with increased susceptibility to bacterial and viral infections and high frequency of different types of hematologic malignancies and autoimmune disorders. In the current study, we profiled the expression pattern of 92 immune-related genes in peripheral blood mononuclear cells (PBMCs) of two different groups, children with DS and control children, to identify differentially expressed genes that might be of pathogenetic importance for the development and phenotype of the immunological alterations observed in individuals with DS. PBMCs samples were obtained from six DS individuals with karyotypically confirmed full trisomy 21 and six healthy control individuals (ages 2–6 years). Gene expression was profiled in duplicate according to the manufacturer's instructions provided by commercially available TaqMan Human Immune Array representing 92 immune function genes and four reference genes on a 96-plex gene card. A set of 17 differentially expressed genes, not located on chromosome 21 (HSA21), involved in immune and inflammatory pathways was identified including 13 genes (*BCL2, CCL3, CCR7, CD19, CD28, CD40, CD40LG, CD80, EDN1, IKBKB, IL6, NOS2* and *SKI*) significantly down-regulated and four genes (*BCL2L1, CCR2, CCR5* and *IL10*) significantly up-regulated in children with DS. These findings highlight a list of candidate genes for further investigation into the molecular mechanism underlying DS pathology and reinforce the secondary effects of the presence of a third copy of HSA21.

Editor: Tim Thomas, The Walter and Eliza Hall of Medical Research, Australia

Funding: This work was supported by funding from FAPESP (2010/00153-3). BLZ and JMBP were the recipients of fellowships from CAPES. The funders had no role in study design, data collection and analysis, decision to publish, or preparation of the manuscript.

Competing Interests: The authors have declared that no competing interests exist.

* Email: erika@famerp.br

Introduction

Down syndrome (DS) is the most common chromosomal disorder and is associated with many medical conditions. Individuals with DS have a high incidence of immunological alterations with increased susceptibility to bacterial and viral infections and high frequency of different types of hematologic malignancies and autoimmune disorders. Leukemia, respiratory tract infections and autoimmune phenomena such as acquired hypothyroidism, celiac disease and diabetes mellitus, occur at higher frequency compared with non-DS individuals [1–4]. Even though improved medical care and progress in treatment, including the development of vaccines and antibiotics, have led to increased life expectancies of individuals with DS, they continue to have major health concerns associated with immunological impairment [5,6].

Although differences between the immune system of children with DS and that of the general population have been described and investigated over the years, the etiologic basis of the immunological alterations observed in these individuals remains unclear. A number of gene expression studies using a variety of methods, including microarrays, quantitative real-time PCR (qPCR) and serial analysis of gene expression (SAGE) and a variety of human DS tissues have been conducted [7–11] but very few attempted to investigate a selected network associated to a specific DS feature such as immune impairment. Considering that the activation of immune system is reflected in changes in gene expression profiles of immune competent blood cells, and these changes are detectable in peripheral blood [12,13], in the present study, we performed gene expression profiling of 92 immune-related genes in peripheral blood of children with DS and in control children, aiming to highlight a list of candidate genes and pathways associated with the immune abnormalities characteristically seen in DS individuals. As result, the comparison of gene expression in children with DS and controls showed 17 differentially expressed genes.

Materials and Methods

Ethics Statement

The study was approved by the Research Ethics Committee of São José do Rio Preto Medical School (CEP-FAMERP), State of

São Paulo. Written informed consent was obtained from the parents or legal guardians of all study participants.

Samples and groups

Blood samples drawn into EDTA collection tubes were obtained from six DS children with karyotypically confirmed full trisomy 21 (three male and three females) with a mean age of 4.00±1.41 years and 6 healthy control children (two male and four females) with a mean age of 3.82±1.09 years. Subjects that had personal history of chronic infection such as bronchitis, asthma and recurrent pneumonia, or clinical manifestations suggestive of acute infection including the flu, cough, fever and/or were under antibiotic treatment within 10 days preceding blood drawing did not meet the inclusion criteria for the study. Children with DS enrolled were attending routine follow-up at Genetics and Down syndrome Outpatient Pediatric Clinic at Hospital de Base de São José do Rio Preto (HB). Blood samples of control children were obtained from children attending routine follow-up at Outpatient Pediatric Clinic at HB and children from the day care center at Instituto de Biociências, Letras e Ciências Exatas - Universidade Estadual Paulista "Júlio de Mesquita Filho" (IBILCE-UNESP). During blood drawn an extra small amount of blood was collected for blood hemogram profiling.

Total RNA isolation

Peripheral blood mononuclear cells (PBMCs) were freshly isolated by Ficoll Paque Plus (Sigma-Aldrich, St Louis, Missouri, USA) density gradient centrifugation of venous blood. Total RNA was extracted using TRIzol reagent (Invitrogen, Carlsbad, California, USA) following the manufacturer's protocol and RNA purity (A260/280 nm) was assessed using NanoDrop ND-1000 (NanoDrop Technologies, Wilmington, Delaware, USA). RNA integrity was evaluated by an Agilent 2100 Bioanalyzer (Agilent Technologies, Foster City, California, USA) and only samples with preserved 18S and 28S peaks and RNA integrity number (RIN) values equal or greater than 5 were selected for gene expression analysis.

Quantitative real-time PCR

First, cDNA samples were prepared from total RNA samples using the High Capacity cDNA Reverse Transcription kit (Applied Biosystems, Carlsbad, California, USA). For each sample qPCR reactions were carried out in duplicate using 6.25 ng of cDNA and a 96-plex gene card, TaqMan Array Human Immune, Fast 96-Well Plate (Applied Biosystems, Carlsbad, California, USA), representing 92 immune-related genes and four reference genes (Table S1) according to the manufacturer's instructions. These reactions were performed using a StepOnePlus Real-Time PCR System (Applied Biosystems, Carlsbad, California, USA).

Statistical analysis

A chi-square analysis was performed between the groups for gender comparison. For age and hemogram analysis, data characterized by a normal distribution were expressed as mean ± standard deviation and parameters without such distribution were expressed as median with range. Student's *t* test (normally distributed data) or the Mann-Whitney test (non-normally distributed data) was used for comparing the two groups. These statistical analyses were performed using the Minitab for Windows (Release 14) program and p-values less than 0.05 were considered statistically significant. Regarding the gene expression, normalization and fold change were calculated with the ΔΔCq method standardized by the geometric averaging of the expression level of the four reference genes [14,15]. Genes with Cq value (quantification cycle, representing the cycle number in which the PCR products reach the threshold) equal 36 or lower were considered as detected. The relative gene expression levels were calculated based on the $2^{-\Delta\Delta Cq}$ method [14]. All expression analyses were performed in R statistical environment [16] using packages freely available under Bioconductor project [17]. The package HTqPCR [18] was used to preprocess the data and as an interface to other packages using as input the PCR data. The identification of differentially expressed genes was addressed using linear models for microarray data (LIMMA) [19]. In order to reduce the risk of false-positive, p-values were adjusted for multiple testing issues using Benjamini and Hochberg's method to control the false discovery rate (FDR) [20] and a gene was considered differentially expressed when the corresponding adjusted p-value was less than 0.05. Data from genes expressed in 50% or less of the samples in each group did not fit our criteria (i.e. be detected in at least four samples of each group) to be considered for statistical analyses.

To explore the degree of overlap between the dysregulated genes in our study with other gene expression studies, we downloaded available GEO datasets (http://www.ncbi.nlm.nih.gov/geo) and supplementary data of the 17 differentially expressed genes observed in our study from three of the latest gene expression profiling studies in DS: Lockstone et al. [8] (human adult DS brain), Li et al. [9] (PBMC) and Letourneau et al. [11] (fetal fibroblasts). For each gene, $\log_2$ expression fold change ($\log_2$[FC]) was determined by calculating the ratio of normalized expression values between the trisomic and the euploid samples (that is, a positive $\log_2$[FC] reflects the up-regualtion of the gene in the trisomic sample and a negative $\log_2$[FC] the down-regulation, with a 1.5 fold-change cut-off).

Results

Age and sex distribution were similar among the groups indicating the homogeneity of these data in the total sample ($P \geq 0.05$). Hemogram analysis demonstrated that individuals with DS have significantly lower absolute count of total typical lymphocyte ($P < 0.0001$) and leukocytes ($P = 0.002$) cells compared with control (Table 1).

Comparison of gene expression in children with DS and controls resulted in 17 differentially expressed genes that met threshold for significance after correction for multiple testing. Four of them, BCL2-like 1 (*BCL2L1*), chemokine (C-C motif) receptor 2 (*CCR2*), chemokine (C-C motif) receptor 5 (gene/pseudogene) (*CCR5*) and interleukin 10 (*IL10*), were up-regulated, while 13 genes, B-cell CLL/lymphoma 2 (*BCL2*), chemokine (C-C motif) ligand 3 (*CCL3*), chemokine (C-C motif) receptor 7 (*CCR7*), CD19 molecule (*CD19*), CD28 molecule (*CD28*), CD40 molecule, TNF receptor superfamily member 5 (*CD40*), CD40 ligand (*CD40LG*), CD80 molecule (*CD80*), endothelin 1 (*EDN1*), inhibitor of kappa light polypeptide gene enhancer in B-cells, kinase beta (*IKBKB*), interleukin 6 (interferon, beta 2) (*IL6*), nitric oxide synthase 2, inducible (*NOS2*) and v-ski sarcoma viral oncogene homolog (avian) (*SKI*), were down-regulated (Table 2). Regarding the comparison between our data and that from Lockstone et al. [8], Li et al. [9] and Letourneau et al. [11] little overlap was observed (Table 3).

Discussion

Individuals with DS have increased susceptibility to infections, hematological malignancies and are more likely to develop certain autoimmune disorders compared with non-DS individuals [3]. In

Table 1. Absolute count of immune cells in children with Down syndrome (DS) compared with controls.

	DS individuals	Control individuals	P value
Leukocytes	5,483±1,535	9,172±1,317	0.002[a]
Neutrophils	2,734±792	3,240±796	0.298[a]
Basophils	32.73±9.30	31.60±22.4	0.909[a]
Typical lymphocytes	2,128±931	4,912±796	<0.0001[a]
Monocytes	468±121	590±297	0.388[a]
Eosinophils	109 (62.2–187.0)	221 (90.0–926.0)	0.1282[b]

[a] Data are expressed as mean ± standard deviation, and two-tailed t test was used for comparisons.
[b] Data is expressed as median (interquartile range), and Mann-Whitney test was used.

Table 2. Immune-related genes differentially expressed in peripheral blood mononuclear cells of individuals with Down syndrome compared with controls.

Gene	Description	Location	FC	P-value*	Important biological processes	Reference
BCL2	B-cell CLL/lymphoma 2	18	0.53062	0.00051	Survival of mature lymphocytes and memory B cells	[28]
BCL2L1	BCL2-like 1	20	1.44879	0.00588	Survival of immature lymphocytes	[35]
CCL3	Chemokine (C-C motif) ligand 3	17	0.30759	0.00084	Chemotaxis induction of immune cells; T-helper cells differentiation; eosinophil degranulation induction; histamine release from mast cells	[36]
CCR2	Chemokine (C-C motif) receptor 2	3	2.49185	0.00034	Monocyte chemotaxis mediation	[37]
CCR5	Chemokine (C-C motif) receptor 5 (gene/pseudogene)	3	1.35093	0.04714	Regulation of trafficking and effector functions of memory/effector T cells, macrophages and immature dendritic cells	[38]
CCR7	Chemokine (C-C motif) receptor 7	17	0.43481	0.01015	Thymocytes generation; central and peripheral tolerance; regulatory T cell function; T cell homeostasis	[39]
CD19	CD19 molecule	16	0.50585	0.04625	Modulation of signal transduction through B cell antigen–receptor complex; peripheral B cells activation and proliferation	[40]
CD28	CD28 molecule	2	0.58229	0.02596	Homeostasis of regulatory T cells (CD28/CD80); activation and optimal function of T cells; peripheral tolerance	[41,42]
CD40	CD40 molecule, TNF receptor superfamily member 5	20	0.73739	0.04977	T cell-dependent immunoglobulin class switching; memory B cell development; germinal center formation	[43]
CD40LG	CD40 ligand	X	0.52433	0.00650	Regulation of B cell function	[43]
CD80	CD80 molecule	3	0.52103	0.00767	T cell proliferation; cytokine production	[44]
EDN1	Endothelin 1	6	0.29025	0.00319	Macrophages activation	[45–47]
IKBKB	Inhibitor of kappa light polypeptide gene enhancer in B-cells, kinase beta	8	0.61495	0.01943	Activation of the NFKB pathway	[48]
IL6	Interleukin 6	7	0.30417	0.00128	Antibody and autoantibody production; T cells activation; B cell differentiation; hematopoiesis	[49]
IL10	Interleukin 10	1	2.00380	0.00767	Secretion of cytokines like IL6, IL2 and interferon, gamma (IFNG); macrophages and B and T cells activation, differentiation and proliferation	[50]
NOS2	Nitric oxide synthase 2, inducible	17	0.45730	0.04625	Nitric oxide synthesis (microbicidal, antiviral, antiparasital and antitumoral effects)	[51]
SKI	V-ski sarcoma viral oncogene homolog (avian)	1	0.72524	0.04977	Regulation of transforming growth factor-beta (TGFB1) signaling	[52]

FC, fold change.
*Adjusted P-value (Benjamini-Hochberg multiple testing correction).

Table 3. Overlap between the 17 differentially expressed genes observed in our study with other gene expression studies.

	Mean log_2(fold-change)					
Gene symbol	**Lockstone et al.[8]**	**Li et al. [9][a]**	**Li et al. [9][b]**	**Li et al. [9][c]**	**Letourneau et al.[11]**	**Current study**
BCL2	0.01	0.64	0.76	0.35	0.04	−0.91
BCL2L1	0.15	−1.91	0.25	1.27	−0.80	0.53
CCL3	NA	NA	NA	NA	2.29	−1.70
CCL3/CCL3L1/CCL3L3	−0.38	NA	NA	NA	NA	NA
CCR2	−0.01	0.26	0.10	0.48	−0.99	1.32
CCR5	−0.06	NA	NA	NA	−1.84	0.43
CCR7	−0.17	0.18	0	−0.33	0.44	−1.20
CD19	−0.14	0.03	0.12	−0.71	−0.08	−0.98
CD28	−0.08	0.47	0.29	−0.14	−0.40	−0.78
CD40	−0.11	−0.33	−0.01	−0.24	0.41	−0.44
CD40LG	−0.06	0.25	0.21	−0.23	−0.87	−0.93
CD80	0.02	0.27	0.04	−0.51	0.15	−0.94
EDN1	0.37	−0.07	−0.07	−0.28	−0.01	−1.78
IKBKB	0.12	0.40	0.45	0.20	−0.13	−0.70
IL10	−0.04	−0.05	0.33	0.33	0.46	1
IL6	−0.47	0.04	−0.33	−0.33	−1.80	−1.72
IL6	−0.47	−0.18	−0.17	−0.06	−1.80	−1.72
NOS2	−0.42	−0.26	0.03	−0.25	−0.82	−1.13
SKI	0.06	0.03	−0.06	0.08	−0.42	−0.46

[a] Neonate group (age: 3 days to 38 days).
[b] Child group (age:1 year to 13 years).
[c] Neonate and child group.
NA = not available.

this study, we profiled the expression pattern of 92 genes in peripheral blood of two different groups, children with DS and controls, to identify differentially expressed genes that might be of pathogenetic importance for the development of the immunological alterations observed in individuals with DS. A set of 17 differentially expressed genes involved in immune and inflammatory pathways was identified including 13 genes (*BCL2, CCL3, CCR7, CD19, CD28, CD40, CD40LG, CD80, EDN1, IKBKB, IL6, NOS2* and *SKI*) significantly down-regulated and four genes (*BCL2L1, CCR2, CCR5* and *IL10*) significantly up-regulated in children with DS.

In our DS population we found a decreased number of typical lymphocytes and leukocytes and no alteration in the number of neutrophils, basophils, monocytes and eosinophils compared with controls. The reduced number of typical lymphocytes and leukocytes observed in our DS group is in agreement with prior literature data [21–23]. Changes in the lymphocyte number have been hypothesized to be due to thymus dysfunction and B and T cell apoptosis [24,25]. All these findings suggest that the alterations of such parameters are the core of the immune system problem observed in individuals with DS. On the other hand, as pointed out by Kusters and collegues [26], children with congenital heart disease that go through cardiac surgery with (partial) thymectomy end up with permanent changes in T lymphocyte numbers however, in contrast with individuals with DS, their frequency of infections and autoimmune diseases is not increased. Thus, the underlying mechanisms for the immune dysfunction in DS remain unclear and have been considered to be associated with the gene dosage imbalance caused by the presence of an additional chromosome 21 (HSA21). The different ratio of lymphocytes and leukocytes to myeloid cells in individuals with DS versus controls observed in our study may lead one to argue that the reduction in leukocytes and lymphocytes is the responsible for the differentially expressed genes observed in our study. Although we cannot completely rule out this assumption, when we look at genes expressed in leukocytes and lymphocytes, such as *CCR2* and *CCR5*, one would expect them to be down-regulated in our DS group according to the difference in the ratio of leukocytes and lymphocytes to other white blood cells, which is not true.

Gene expression profiling studies using hybridization-based methodologies, such as microarray and PCR-based assays, offer a promising approach to understanding the complex network of gene changes that are associated with complex traits such immune impairment. Previous genome-wide expression studies have successfully applied microarray technology to investigate the transcriptional consequences of trisomy 21 in several different types of biomaterials such as leukocytes [7], adult brain tissue [8], PBMCs [9], lymphoblastoid cell lines [10] and fetal fibroblasts [11]. We decided to use PBMCs, a reservoir to collect information from various physiologic processes once it permeates almost all tissues and cells, therefore it is a potentially the best biomaterial for sampling for overall immune function and health.

We identified 17 immune-related genes differentially expressed in our group of individuals with DS. The main functions of the differentially expressed genes are summarized in Table 2. Confirming data in the literature, the reduced expression of *BCL2* observed in our study was previously reported in DS leukocytes in comparison to normal controls [7]. This antiapoptotic gene is essential for the survival of mature lymphocytes and memory B cells [27,28]. Also, the overexpression of *IL10* in our DS group was also previously reported [29]. *IL10* overexpression can result in exacerbated inflammatory response leading to the development of hyper inflammatory disorders such as autoimmune diseases [30,31], a well known phenomena observed in individuals with DS.

In order to further investigate the findings in our study, we evaluated the degree of overlap between our data and that from three other gene expression studies [8,9,11] for the 17 differentially expressed genes observed in our study (Table 3). Gene expression values of the 17 genes of each study had little overlap. The genes *CD40LG*, *Il6* and *NOS2* where down-regulated in our study and in study by Letourneau et al. [11], and the gene *CD19* was found significant down-regulated in our study and in Li et al. [9] when neonate and child groups were combined, a finding that confirms previous studies of lymphocyte subpopulations in fetuses [32] and in children with DS [33]. Little overlap between the individual genes identified in our study and the literature is not surprising. There are several possible reasons for this discordance notably differences in cell types used for analysis at different developmental stages and small sample size. Moreover, there are many experimental factors such as array platform, tissue handling, RNA isolation method and hybridization procedure which are likely to contribute to the observed divergence.

A strength of this study that make it different from previous gene expression studies is that we attempted to identify a selected pathway associated to a specific DS feature, the immunological impairment. While others have applied microarray analysis to perform global gene expression and then chose one or more genes for further investigation, we decided to investigate a selected number of genes associated to the specific immunological alteration observed in DS. For that matter, some confounding factors including medication ingestion, personal history of chronic infection, and clinical manifestations suggestive of acute infection were controlled. Also, the majority of the previous transcriptome studies were performed using microarrays methods. Despite a high level of agreement between qPCR and microarrays, it has been demonstrated that microarrays tend to have a low dynamic range, which could lead to under-representation of changes in gene expression, whereas qPCR has a higher dynamic range [34]. Our observations are clearly limited by the small number of individuals analyzed; a larger study population would provide a higher statistical power. Nevertheless, our findings identify a number of genes with relevant functions in immune cells that are dysregulated in DS children; in any case it remains of interest to investigate the expression pattern of these genes at the protein. The expectation is that the identification of such dosage imbalance may provide insights to identify promising candidate genes underlying DS phenotype and thus bring more effective therapy that will lead to future advances for a safer and more targeted therapeutic approach in the treatment of individuals with DS for everyday clinical care. It is also important to mention that all the genes observed with altered expression in this study are located on chromosomes other than HSA21, what gives further evidence to the theory that secondary transcriptional changes throughout the genome occur as a result of trisomy 21.

Supporting Information

Table S1 Immune genes contained in the TaqMan Array Human Immune, Fast 96-Well Plate (Applied Biosystems, Carlsbad, California, USA).

Acknowledgments

The authors thank the collaboration of the day care center at Instituto de Biociências, Letras e Ciências Exatas - Universidade Estadual Paulista "Júlio de Mesquita Filho" (IBILCE-UNESP), the children and their families as well as the patients from the Genetics and Down syndrome Outpatient Pediatric Clinic and Outpatient Pediatric Clinic at Hospital de Base de São José do Rio Preto (HB) and their families.

Author Contributions

Conceived and designed the experiments: BLZ JMBP. Performed the experiments: BLZ JMBP. Analyzed the data: JESS MCB. Contributed reagents/materials/analysis tools: WASJ EMGB ECP. Wrote the paper: BLZ. Reviewed the manuscript for important intellectual content: JMBP WASJ EMGB ECP.

References

1. Chistiakov D (2007) Down syndrome and coexistent autoimmune diseases. J Appl Biomed 5: 71–76.
2. Xavier AC, Ge Y, Taub J (2010) Unique clinical and biological features of leukemia in Down syndrome children. Expert Rev Hematol 3: 175–186.
3. Ram G, Chinen J (2011) Infections and immunodeficiency in Down syndrome Clin Exp Immunol 164: 9–16.
4. Broers CJ, Gemke RJ, Weijerman ME, Kuik DJ, van Hoogstraten IM, et al. (2012) Frequency of lower respiratory tract infections in relation to adaptive immunity in children with Down syndrome compared to their healthy siblings. Acta Paediatr 101: 862–867.
5. Englund A, Jonsson B, Zander CS, Gustafsson J, Annerén G (2013) Changes in mortality and causes of death in the Swedish Down syndrome population. Am J Med Genet A 161: 642–649.
6. Fitzgerald P, Leonard H, Pikora TJ, Bourke J, Hammond G (2013) Hospital admissions in children with down syndrome: experience of a population-based cohort followed from birth. PLoS One 8: e70401.
7. Malagó W Jr, Sommer CA, Del Cistia Andrade C, Soares-Costa A, Abrao Possik P, et al. (2005) Gene expression profile of human Down syndrome leukocytes. Croat Med J 46: 647–656.
8. Lockstone HE1, Harris LW, Swatton JE, Wayland MT, Holland AJ, et al. (2007) Gene expression profiling in the adult Down syndrome brain. Genomics 90: 647–660.
9. Li C, Jin L, Bai Y, Chen Q, Fu L, et al. (2012) Genome-wide expression analysis in Down syndrome: insight into immunodeficiency. PLoS One 7: e49130.
10. Granese B, Scala I, Spatuzza C, Valentino A, Coletta M, et al. (2013) Validation of microarray data in human lymphoblasts shows a role of the ubiquitin-proteasome system and NF-kB in the pathogenesis of Down syndrome. BMC Med Genomics 6: 24.
11. Letourneau A, Santoni FA, Bonilla X, Sailani MR, Gonzalez D, et al. (2014) Domains of genome-wide gene expression dysregulation in Down's syndrome. Nature 508: 345–350.
12. Burczynski ME, Dorner AJ (2006) Transcriptional profiling of peripheral blood cells in clinical pharmacogenomic studies. Pharmacogenomics 7: 187–202.
13. Mohr S, Liew CC (2007) The peripheral-blood transcriptome: new insights into disease and risk assessment. Trends Mol Med 13: 422–432.
14. Livak KJ, Schmittgen TD (2001) Analysis of relative gene expression data using real-time quantitative PCR and the 2 (-Delta Delta C(T)) Method. Methods 25: 402–408.
15. Vandesompele J, De Preter K, Pattyn F, Poppe B, Van Roy N, et al. (2002) Accurate normalization of real-time quantitative RT-PCR data by geometric averaging of multiple internal control genes. Genome Biol 3: RESEARCH0034.
16. R Core Team (2013) R: A language and environment for statistical computing R Foundation for Statistical Computing, Vienna, Austria. Available from: http://wwwR-projectorg/
17. Gentleman RC, Carey VJ, Bates DM, Bolstad B, Dettling M, et al. (2004) Bioconductor: open software development for computational biology and bioinformatics. Genome Biol 5: R80.
18. Dvinge H, Bertone P (2009) HTqPCR: high-throughput analysis and visualization of quantitative real-time PCR data in R. Bioinformatics 25: 3325–3326.
19. Smyth GK (2004) Linear models and empirical bayes methods for assessing differential expression in microarray experiments. Stat Appl Genet Mol Biol 3: Article3.
20. Benjamini Y, Hochberg Y (1995) Controlling the false discovery rate: A practical and powerful approach to multiple testing. J R Stat Soc Series B Stat Methodol 57: 289–300.

21. Cossarizza A, Monti D, Montagnani G, Ortolani C, Masi M, et al. (1990) Precocious aging of the immune system in Down syndrome: alteration of B lymphocytes, T-lymphocyte subsets, and cells with natural killer markers. Am J Med Genet Suppl 7: 213–218.
22. de Hingh YC, van der Vossen PW, Gemen EF, Mulder AB, Hop WC, et al. (2005) Intrinsic abnormalities of lymphocyte counts in children with down syndrome. J Pediatr 147: 744–747.
23. Cocchi G, Mastrocola M, Capelli M, Bastelli A, Vitali F, et al. (2007) Immunological patterns in young children with Down syndrome: is there a temporal trend? Acta Paediatr 96: 1479–1482.
24. Elsayed SM, Elsayed GM (2009) Phenotype of apoptotic lymphocytes in children with Down syndrome. Immun Ageing 6: 2.
25. Kusters MA, Jol-van der Zijde CM, van Tol MJ, Bolz WE, Bok LA, et al. (2011) Impaired avidity maturation after tetanus toxoid booster in children with Down syndrome. Pediatr Infect Dis J 30: 357–359.
26. Kusters MA, Verstegen RH, Gemen EF, de Vries E (2009) Intrinsic defect of the immune system in children with Down syndrome: a review. Clin Exp Immunol 156: 189–193.
27. Nakayama K, Nakayama K, Negishi I, Kuida K, Sawa H, et al. (1994) Targeted disruption of Bcl-2 alpha beta in mice: occurrence of gray hair, polycystic kidney disease, and lymphocytopenia. Proc Natl Acad Sci U S A 91: 3700–3704.
28. Bhattacharya D, Cheah MT, Franco CB, Hosen N, Pin CL, et al. (2007) Transcriptional profiling of antigen-dependent murine B cell differentiation and memory formation. J Immunol 179: 6808–6819.
29. Guazzarotti L, Trabattoni D, Castelletti E, Boldrighini B, Piacentini L, et al. (2009) T lymphocyte maturation is impaired in healthy young individuals carrying trisomy 21 (Down syndrome). Am J Intellect Dev Disabil 114: 100–109.
30. O'Garra A, Barrat FJ, Castro AG, Vicari A, Hawrylowicz C (2008) Strategies for use of IL-10 or its antagonists in human disease. Immunol Rev 223: 114–131.
31. Dace DS, Khan AA, Stark JL, Kelly J, Cross AH, et al. (2009) Interleukin-10 overexpression promotes Fas-ligand-dependent chronic macrophage-mediated demyelinating polyneuropathy. PLoS One 4: e7121.
32. Zizka Z, Calda P, Fait T, Haakova L, Kvasnicka J, et al. (2006) Prenatally diagnosable differences in the cellular immunity of fetuses with Down's and Edwards' syndrome. Fetal Diagn Ther 21:510–514
33. Yilmaz C, Dogan M, Basarslan F, Yilmaz N, Yuca S, et al. (2013) Evaluation of Lymphocyte Subgroups in Children With Down Syndrome. Clin Appl Thromb Hemost. doi: 101177/1076029613511521
34. Mutch DM, Berger A, Mansourian R, Rytz A, Roberts MA (2002) The limit fold change model: a practical approach for selecting differentially expressed genes from microarray data. BMC Bioinformatics 3: 17.
35. Ma A, Pena JC, Chang B, Margosian E, Davidson L, et al. (1995) Bclx regulates the survival of double-positive thymocytes. Proc Natl Acad Sci U S A 92: 4763–4767.
36. Maurer M, von Stebut E (2004) Macrophage inflammatory protein-1. Int J Biochem Cell Biol 36: 1882–1886.
37. Charo IF, Peters W (2003) Charo IF, Peters W (2003) Chemokine receptor 2 (CCR2) in atherosclerosis, infectious diseases, and regulation of T-cell polarization. Microcirculation 10: 259–264.
38. Oppermann M (2004) Chemokine receptor CCR5: insights into structure, function, and regulation. Cell Signal 16: 1201–1210.
39. Forster R, Davalos-Misslitz AC, Rot A (2008) CCR7 and its ligands: balancing immunity and tolerance. Nat Rev Immunol 8: 362–871.
40. Tedder TF, Inaoki M, Sato S (1997) The CD19/21 complex regulates signal transduction thresholds governing humoral immunity and autoimmunity. Immunity 6: 107–118.
41. Salomon B, Lenschow DJ, Rhee L, Ashourian N, Singh B, et al. (2000) B7/CD28 costimulation is essential for the homeostasis of the CD4+CD25+ immunoregulatory T cells that control autoimmune diabetes. Immunity 12: 431–440.
42. Bour-Jordan H, Blueston JA (2002) CD28 function: a balance of costimulatory and regulatory signals. J Clin Immunol 22: 1–7.
43. Suttles J, Stout RD (2009) Macrophage CD40 signaling: a pivotal regulator of disease protection and pathogenesis. Semin Immunol 21: 257–264.
44. Gimmi CD, Freeman GJ, Gribben JG, Sugita K, Freedman AS, et al. (1991) B-cell surface antigen B7 provides a costimulatory signal that induces T cells to proliferate and secrete interleukin 2. Proc Natl Acad Sci U S A 88: 6575–6579.
45. Ruetten H, Thiemermann C (1997) Endothelin-1 stimulates the biosynthesis of tumour necrosis factor in macrophages: ET-receptors, signal transduction and inhibition by dexamethasone. J Physiol Pharmacol 48: 675–688.
46. Hofman FM, Chen P, Jeyaseelan R, Incardona F, Fisher M, et al. (1998) Endothelin-1 induces production of the neutrophil chemotactic factor interleukin-8 by human brain-derived endothelial cells. Blood 92: 3064–3072.
47. Browatzki M, Schmidt J, Kübler W, Kranzhöfer R (2000) Endothelin-1 induces interleukin-6 release via activation of the transcription factor NF-kappaB in human vascular smooth muscle cells. Basic Res Cardiol 95: 98–105.
48. Li Q, Verma IM (2002) NF-kappaB regulation in the immune system. Nat Rev Immunol 2: 725–734.
49. Mihara M, Hashizume M, Yoshida H, Suzuki M, Shiina M (2012) IL-6/IL-6 receptor system and its role in physiological and pathological conditions. Clin Sci (Lond) 122: 143–159.
50. Moore KW, de Waal Malefyt R, Coffman RL, O'Garra A (2001) Interleukin-10 and the interleukin-10 receptor. Annu Rev Immunol 19: 683–765.
51. Bogdan C (2001) Nitric oxide and the immune response. Nat Immunol 2: 907–916.
52. Li MO, Wan YY, Sanjabi S, Robertson AK, Flavell RA (2006) Transforming growth factor-beta regulation of immune responses. Annu Rev Immunol 24: 99–146.

Permissions

All chapters in this book were first published in PLOS ONE, by The Public Library of Science; hereby published with permission under the Creative Commons Attribution License or equivalent. Every chapter published in this book has been scrutinized by our experts. Their significance has been extensively debated. The topics covered herein carry significant findings which will fuel the growth of the discipline. They may even be implemented as practical applications or may be referred to as a beginning point for another development.

The contributors of this book come from diverse backgrounds, making this book a truly international effort. This book will bring forth new frontiers with its revolutionizing research information and detailed analysis of the nascent developments around the world.

We would like to thank all the contributing authors for lending their expertise to make the book truly unique. They have played a crucial role in the development of this book. Without their invaluable contributions this book wouldn't have been possible. They have made vital efforts to compile up to date information on the varied aspects of this subject to make this book a valuable addition to the collection of many professionals and students.

This book was conceptualized with the vision of imparting up-to-date information and advanced data in this field. To ensure the same, a matchless editorial board was set up. Every individual on the board went through rigorous rounds of assessment to prove their worth. After which they invested a large part of their time researching and compiling the most relevant data for our readers.

The editorial board has been involved in producing this book since its inception. They have spent rigorous hours researching and exploring the diverse topics which have resulted in the successful publishing of this book. They have passed on their knowledge of decades through this book. To expedite this challenging task, the publisher supported the team at every step. A small team of assistant editors was also appointed to further simplify the editing procedure and attain best results for the readers.

Apart from the editorial board, the designing team has also invested a significant amount of their time in understanding the subject and creating the most relevant covers. They scrutinized every image to scout for the most suitable representation of the subject and create an appropriate cover for the book.

The publishing team has been an ardent support to the editorial, designing and production team. Their endless efforts to recruit the best for this project, has resulted in the accomplishment of this book. They are a veteran in the field of academics and their pool of knowledge is as vast as their experience in printing. Their expertise and guidance has proved useful at every step. Their uncompromising quality standards have made this book an exceptional effort. Their encouragement from time to time has been an inspiration for everyone.

The publisher and the editorial board hope that this book will prove to be a valuable piece of knowledge for researchers, students, practitioners and scholars across the globe.

List of Contributors

Qiang Liu, Heng Liu, Pin Wang and Xiulian Sun
Key Lab of Otolaryngology, Qilu Hospital of Shandong University, Jinan, China

Na Liu, Shaolei Zang and Chunyan Ji
Department of Hematology, Qilu Hospital of Shandong University, Jinan, China

Mara Dierssen, Gloria Arqué, Jerome McDonald, Nuria Andreu and Cristina Fillat
Genes and Disease Program, Centre for Genomic Regulation (CRG), Barcelona Biomedical Research Park (PRBB), and CIBER de Enfermedades Raras (CIBERER), Barcelona, Catalonia, Spain

Carmen Martínez-Cué
Department of Physiology and Pharmacology, Faculty of Medicine, University of Cantabria, Santander, Spain

Jesús Flórez
Department of Physiology and Pharmacology, Faculty of Medicine, University of Cantabria, Santander, Spain
Fundación Síndrome de Down de Cantabria, Fundación Iberoamericana Down21, Santander, Spain

Isobel J. Whitehouse, Elizabeth B. C. Glennon, Katherine A. B. Kellett and Nigel M. Hooper
School of Molecular and Cellular Biology, Faculty of Biological Sciences, University of Leeds, Leeds, United Kingdom

J. Scott Miners, Patrick G. Kehoe and Seth Love
Dementia Research Group, School of Clinical Sciences, Institute of Clinical Neurosciences, University of Bristol, Bristol, United Kingdom

Elena Biagi, Marco Candela, Manuela Centanni, Simone Rampelli, Silvia Turroni and Patrizia Brigidi
Department of Pharmacy and Biotechnology, University of Bologna, Bologna, Italy

Clarissa Consolandi, Marco Severgnini and Clelia Peano
Institute of Biomedical Technologies - Italian National Research Council, Milan, Italy

Alessandro Ghezzo
Department of Experimental, Diagnostic and Specialty Medicine, University of Bologna, Bologna, Italy

Maria Scurti, Stefano Salvioli and Claudio Franceschi
Department of Experimental, Diagnostic and Specialty Medicine, University of Bologna, Bologna, Italy
Interdepartmental Centre "L. Galvani" (CIG), University of Bologna, Bologna, Italy

Yulin Zhou and Qiwei Guo
Molecular Diagnostics Laboratory, Department of Medical Genetics, Prenatal Diagnosis Center, Xiamen Maternal and Child Health Hospital, Xiamen, Fujian, China

Yihan Li and Jinchun Chen
Xiamen Hospital of Traditional Chinese Medicine, Fujian University of Traditional Chinese Medicine, Xiamen, Fujian, China

Shengmao Quan, Ahong Zhang, Hailing Zheng, Xingqiang Zhu, Jin Lin, Huan Xu and Hongliang Chen
Xiamen Vangenes BioTech, Xiamen, Fujian, China

Ayang Wu
Zhangzhou Affiliated Hospital of Fujian Medical University, Zhangzhou, Fujian, China

Young Joo Jeon, Sin-Gi Park and Hee Jae Joo
TheragenEtex Bio Institute, Suwon, Republic of Korea
Genome Care, Seoul, South Korea

Byung Chul Kim
Clinomics, Ulsan, Republic of Korea
Personal Genomics Institute, Genome Research Foundation, Suwon, Republic of Korea

Jong Bhak
TheragenEtex Bio Institute, Suwon, Republic of Korea
Genome Care, Seoul, South Korea
Personal Genomics Institute, Genome Research Foundation, Suwon, Republic of Korea
BioMedical Engineering, UNIST, Ulsan, Republic of Korea

Juliet A. Moncaster, Suqian Lu, Mark A. Burton, Joy G. Ghosh, Anca Mocofanescu and Lee E. Goldstein
Molecular Aging & Development Laboratory, Department of Surgery, Brigham and Women's Hospital, Harvard Medical School, Boston, Massachusetts, United States of America

Roberto Pineda
Department of Ophthalmology, Massachusetts Eye and Ear Infirmary, Harvard Medical School, Boston, Massachusetts, United States of America

Robert D. Moir, Stephanie J. Soscia and Rudolph E. Tanzi
Genetics and Aging Research Unit, Department of Neurology, Massachusetts General Hospital, Harvard Medical School, Charlestown, Massachusetts, United States of America

Maria Ericsson
Electron Microscopy Facility, Department of Cell Biology, Harvard Medical School, Boston, Massachusetts, United States of America

Rebecca D. Folkerth
Department of Pathology, Brigham and Women's Hospital, Harvard Medical School, Boston, Massachusetts, United States of America

Richard M. Robb and David G. Hunter
Department of Ophthalmology, Children's Hospital Boston, Harvard Medical School, Boston, Massachusetts, United States of America

Jer R. Kuszak
Departments of Ophthalmology and Pathology, Rush University Medical Center, Chicago, Illinois, United States of America

John I. Clark
Departments of Biological Structure and Ophthalmology, University of Washington, Seattle, Washington, United States of America

Jeroen L. A. Pennings, Wendy Rodenburg, Sandra Imholz, Conny T. M. van
Oostrom and Annemieke de Vries
Laboratory for Health Protection Research (GBO), National Institute for Public Health and the Environment (RIVM), Bilthoven, The Netherlands

Maria P. H. Koster and Peter C. J. I. Schielen
Laboratory for Infectious Diseases and Perinatal Screening (LIS), National Institute for Public Health and the Environment (RIVM), Bilthoven, The Netherlands

Timo M. Breit
MicroArray Department (MAD), University of Amsterdam (UvA), Amsterdam, The Netherlands

Sonya Girdler
School of Occupational Therapy and Social Work, Curtin University, Perth, Australia

Jenny Bourke, Peter Jacoby and Helen Leonard
Telethon Kids Institute, University of Western Australia, Perth, Australia

Gwynnyth Llewellyn
Faculty of Health Sciences, University of Sydney, Sydney, Australia

Bruce Tonge
Centre for Developmental Psychiatry and Psychology, Monash University, Melbourne, Australia

Trevor R. Parmenter
Sydney Medical School, University of Sydney, Sydney, Australia

Kitty-Rose Foley
Telethon Kids Institute, University of Western Australia, Perth, Australia
Department of Developmental Disability Neuropsychiatry, School of Psychiatry, The University of New South Wales, Sydney, Australia

Stewart Einfeld
Faculty of Health Sciences, University of Sydney, Sydney, Australia
Brain and Mind Research Institute, University of Sydney, Sydney, Australia

Tychele Turner, Vasyl Pihur and Aravinda Chakravarti
Center for Complex Disease Genomics, McKusick-Nathans Institute of Genetic Medicine, Johns Hopkins University School of Medicine, Baltimore, Maryland, United States of America

Huntington Potter
Department of Neurology and Linda Crnic Institute for Down Syndrome, University of Colorado School of Medicine, Aurora, Colorado, United States of America

Antoneta Granic
Department of Neurology and Linda Crnic Institute for Down Syndrome, University of Colorado School of Medicine, Aurora, Colorado, United States of America
Institute for Ageing and Health, Campus for Ageing and Vitality, Newcastle University, Newcastle upon Tyne, United Kingdom

Candace D. Middlebrooks, Stuart W. Tinker, Emily Graves Allen, Lora J. H. Bean and Stephanie L. Sherman
Department of Human Genetics, Emory University School of Medicine, Atlanta, Georgia, United States of America

Ferdouse Begum
Department of Biostatistics, Graduate School of Public Health, University of Pittsburgh, Pittsburgh, Pennsylvania, United States of America

Reshmi Chowdhury
Department of Human Genetics, Graduate School of Public Health University of Pittsburgh, Pittsburgh, Pennsylvania, United States of America

Tiffany Renee Oliver
Department of Human Genetics, Emory University School of Medicine, Atlanta, Georgia, United States of America
Department of Biology, Spelman College, Atlanta, Georgia, United States of America

Eleanor Feingold
Department of Biostatistics, Graduate School of Public Health, University of Pittsburgh, Pittsburgh, Pennsylvania, United States of America
Department of Human Genetics, Graduate School of Public Health University of Pittsburgh, Pittsburgh, Pennsylvania, United States of America

Vivian Cheung
Howard Hughes Medical Institute, University of Michigan, Ann Arbor, Michigan, United States of America
Department of Human Genetics, University of Michigan, Ann Arbor, Michigan, United States of America

Ji Hyae Lim, Shin Young Kim, So Yeon Park, Shin Yeong Lee and Mi Jin Kim
Laboratory of Medical Genetics, Medical Research Institute, Cheil General Hospital and Women's Healthcare Center, Seoul, Korea

You Jung Han, Si Won Lee, Jin Hoon Chung, Moon Young Kim and Jae Hyug Yang
Department of Obstetrics and Gynecology, Cheil General Hospital and Women's Healthcare Center, KwanDong University college of Medicine, Seoul, Korea

Hyun Mee Ryu
Laboratory of Medical Genetics, Medical Research Institute, Cheil General Hospital and Women's Healthcare Center, Seoul, Korea
Department of Obstetrics and Gynecology, Cheil General Hospital and Women's Healthcare Center, KwanDong University college of Medicine, Seoul, Korea

Damien L. Bruno
Victorian Clinical Genetics Services Cytogenetics Laboratory, Murdoch Childrens Research Institute, Melbourne, Australia

Yuval Benjamini
Department of Statistics, University of California, Berkeley, California, United States of America

Dineika Chandrananda and Natalie P. Thorne
Bioinformatics Division, The Walter and Eliza Hall Institute of Medical Research, Melbourne, Australia
Department of Medical Biology, University of Melbourne, Melbourne, Australia

Devika Ganesamoorthy and Howard R. Slater
Victorian Clinical Genetics Services Cytogenetics Laboratory, Murdoch Childrens Research Institute, Melbourne, Australia
Department of Paediatrics, University of Melbourne, Melbourne, Australia

Terence P. Speed
Bioinformatics Division, The Walter and Eliza Hall Institute of Medical Research, Melbourne, Australia
Department of Statistics, University of California, Berkeley, California, United States of America

Melanie Bahlo
Bioinformatics Division, The Walter and Eliza Hall Institute of Medical Research, Melbourne, Australia
Department of Mathematics and Statistics, University of Melbourne, Melbourne, Australia

Octavio Garcia, Maria Torres, Pablo Helguera, Pinar Coskun and Jorge Busciglio
Department of Neurobiology and Behavior, Institute for Memory Impairments and Neurological Disorders (iMIND), Center for the Neurobiology of Learning and Memory (CNLM), University of California Irvine, Irvine, California, United States of America

Hazem S. Abou-Youssef, Manal M. Kamal and Dina A. Mehaney
Clinical and Chemical Pathology Department, Faculty of Medicine, Cairo University, Cairo, Egypt

Nicholas J. Wald and Jonathan P. Bestwick
Wolfson Institute of Preventive Medicine, Barts and the London School of Medicine and Dentistry, London, United Kingdom

Jacobus P. van Wouwe, Helma B. M. van Gameren-Oosterom, Paul H. Verkerk and Minne Fekkes
Department of Child Health, Netherlands Organization for Applied Scientific Research TNO, Leiden, the Netherlands

Paula van Dommelen
Department of Life Style, Netherlands Organization for Applied Scientific Research TNO, Leiden, the Netherlands

Clémentine Ripoll, Emilie Ait Yahya-Graison, Evelyne Paly, Nicole Créau and Jean Maurice Delabar
Univ Paris Diderot, Sorbonne Paris Cité, Unitéde Biologie Fonctionnelle et Adaptative, EAC4413 CNRS, Paris, France,

Luce Dauphinot
CRICM, CNRS UMR7225, INSERM UMR975, UPMC Hôpital de la Pitié-Salpêtriére, Paris, France

Clothilde Mircher, Aimé Ravel, Yann Grattau and Henri Bléhaut
Institut Médical Jérôme Lejeune et Fondation Jérome Lejeune, Paris, France

Guy Dembour
Cardiologie pédiatrique, Cliniques Universitaires St Luc, Bruxelles, Belgique

Bénédicte de Fréminville and Renaud Touraine
Service de Génétique, Centre Hospitalier Universitaire de Saint-Etienne, Saint-Etienne, France

André Mégarbane
Institut Médical Jérôme Lejeune et Fondation Jérome Lejeune, Paris, France
Unité de Génétique Mé dicale, Faculté de Médecine, Université Saint-Joseph, Beirut, Lebanon

Terri J. Pikora, Jenny Bourke and Helen Leonard
Telethon Kids Institute, The University of Western Australia, Perth, Western Australia, Australia

Nicholas Lennox
Queeensland Centre for Intellectual and Developmental Disability, University of Queensland, South Brisbane, Queensland, Australia

Katherine Bathgate
Telethon Kids Institute, The University of Western Australia, Perth, Western Australia, Australia
School of Public Health, Curtin University, Bentley, Western Australia,
Australia

Kitty-Rose Foley
Telethon Kids Institute, The University of Western Australia, Perth, Western Australia, Australia
Queeensland Centre for Intellectual and Developmental Disability, University of Queensland, South Brisbane, Queensland, Australia

Kyung Ah Han, Hye Seon Kang, Jee Won Lee, Lang Yoo, Eunju Im, Ahyoung Hong, Yun Ju Lee, Woo Hyun Shin and Kwang Chul Chung
Department of Systems Biology, College of Life Science and Biotechnology, Yonsei University, Seoul, Korea

Isaac Kinde, Nickolas Papadopoulos, Kenneth W. Kinzler and Bert Vogelstein
The Ludwig Center for Cancer Genetics and Therapeutics and The Howard Hughes Medical Institute, Johns Hopkins Kimmel Cancer Center, Baltimore, Maryland, United States of America

Mylissa M. Slane
Developmental Neuropsychology Laboratory, Geisinger-Bucknell Autism and Developmental Medicine Institute, Lewisburg, Pennsylvania, United States of America

F. Lee Kleinpeter
Department of Psychology, River Parishes Community College, Sorrento, Louisiana, United States of America

K. B. Boomer
Department of Mathematics, Bucknell University, Lewisburg, Pennsylvania, United States of America

David W. Evans
Developmental Neuropsychology Laboratory, Geisinger-Bucknell Autism and Developmental Medicine Institute, Lewisburg, Pennsylvania, United States of America
Department of Mathematics, Bucknell University, Lewisburg, Pennsylvania, United States of America

Nicholas J. Wald, Jonathan P. Bestwick, Lynne M. George and Wayne J. Huttly
Wolfson Institute of Preventive Medicine, Barts and the London School of Medicine and Dentistry, Queen Mary University of London, London, United Kingdom

Jacobus P. Van Wouwe
Department of Child Health, Netherlands Organization for Applied Scientific Research (TNO), Leiden, The Netherlands

Paula Van Dommelen
Department of Life Style, Netherlands Organization for Applied Scientific Research (TNO), Leiden, The Netherlands

Anne Marie Oudesluys-Murphy
Department of Pediatrics, Leiden University Medical Centre, Leiden, The Netherlands

Simone E. Buitendijk
Leiden University Medical Centre, Leiden, The Netherlands

Helma B. M. Van Gameren-Oosterom
Department of Child Health, Netherlands Organization for Applied Scientific Research (TNO), Leiden, The Netherlands
Department of Life Style, Netherlands Organization for Applied Scientific Research (TNO), Leiden, The Netherlands

Stef Van Buuren
Department of Life Style, Netherlands Organization for Applied Scientific Research (TNO), Leiden, The Netherlands

Bruna Lancia Zampieri, Joice Matos Biselli-Périco, Eny Maria Goloni-Bertollo and Érika Cristina Pavarino
Unidade de Pesquisa em Genética e Biologia Molecular, Departamento de Biologia Molecular, Faculdade de Medicina de São Jose´ do Rio Preto (FAMERP), São José do Rio Preto, São Paulo, Brazil

Wilson Araújo Silva Júnior
Department of Genetics and, Ribeirão Preto Medical School University of São Paulo, São Paulo, Brazil
National Institute of Science and Technology in Stem Cell and Cell Therapy and Center For Cell Based Therapy, Ribeirao Preto, São Paulo, Brazil

Jorge Estefano Santana de Souza and Matheus Carvalho Bürger
Department of Genetics and, Ribeirão Preto Medical School University of São Paulo, São Paulo, Brazil
Institute of Bioinformatics and Biotechnology (2bio), São Paulo, Brazil
National Institute of Science and Technology in Stem Cell and Cell Therapy and Center For Cell Based Therapy, Ribeirao Preto, São Paulo, Brazil

Index